Delivery Systems in Gene Therapy

Delivery Systems in Gene Therapy

Edited by

Handan Kayhan

Cambridge Scholars Publishing

Delivery Systems in Gene Therapy

Edited by Handan Kayhan

This book first published 2026

Cambridge Scholars Publishing

Lady Stephenson Library, Newcastle upon Tyne, NE6 2PA, UK

British Library Cataloguing in Publication Data
A catalogue record for this book is available from the British Library

ISBN: 978-1-0364-7390-7
ISBN (Ebook): 978-1-0364-7391-4

TABLE OF CONTENTS

Preface viii

Part I: Viral Vectors

Chapter 1 2
Gene Therapy Evolution: Adenovirus Vectors and Novel Delivery Systems for Improved Efficacy
Praveenya Tirunagari, Kotthapalli Prashanth, Sumana Kumar

Chapter 2 48
A Safe, Favorable and Effective Viral Vector for Gene Therapy: Adeno-Associated Virus (AAV)
Asuman Özgöz

Chapter 3 76
Lentiviral Delivery System in Gene Therapy
Tatiana da Silva Authier, Bieke Bekaert, Vincent Timmerman

Chapter 4 113
Engineering Safety and Clinical Perspectives of Herpes Simplex Virus-Based Gene Delivery Systems
Cihan Taştan, Beyza Aydin

Chapter 5 151
Poxviruses
Cihan Inan

Chapter 6 175
Retrovıral Delıvery Systems in Gene Therapy
Berrak Kurt

Part II: Nonviral Delivery Systems

Chapter 7 210
Recent Developments in Extracellular Vesicle-Based Nanomedicines, Highlighting Technological Improvements and Clinical Prospects
Zoi Kardasi·, Efstathia Triantafyllopoulou, Natassa Pippa, Maria G. Roubelakis, Maria Gazouli

Chapter 8 259
Exosomes
Nihan Örüklü

Chapter 9 301
Peptide Delivery Systems
Durmus Ayan

Chapter 10 355
Liposomes
Sanem Gökçen

Chapter 11 386
Polymer-Based Delivery Systems for Nucleic Acid Therapeutics: Advances and Applications
Nurcan Gümüş, Umut Can Öz

Chapter 12 428
Synthetic Cationic Polymers for Gene Therapy
Ahmet Cesur, Umut Can Öz

Chapter 13 475
Inorganic Nanoparticles
Hüseyin Izgordü

Chapter 14 509
Transposon-Based Delivery Systems as a Strategic Pioneer in Gene Therapy: A Comprehensive Overview
Yasemin Kartal

Part III: Physical Methods for Gene Delivery

Chapter 15 574
Sonoporation
Simge Unay, Mehmet Dincer Bilgin, Mehmet Bilgen

Chapter 16 592
Photoporation for Membrane Transfer in Cells
Mehran Aksel, Mehmet Dinçer Bilgin, Mehmet Bilgen

Chapter 17 611
Electroporation Principles and Applications
Elçin Özgür Büyükatalay, Handan Kayhan

Chapter 18 629
Microinjection Precision Delivery at the Cellular Level
Muhammed Ali Nalbant

PREFACE

"Delivery Systems in Gene Therapy" is a comprehensive book that explores the various methods and technologies utilized for delivering therapeutic genes to cells. With an increasing focus on targeted and personalized treatments, gene therapy has emerged as a promising approach for combating cancer, and efficient delivery systems are essential for ensuring the successful delivery and expression of therapeutic genes.

The book begins by delving into viral vectors, which have long been utilized as efficient carriers of therapeutic genes. The chapters cover adenovirus, Adenovirus, Adeno-Associated Virus (AAV), Lentivirus, Herpes Virus, Poxvirus, and Retrovirus providing detailed insights into their characteristics, advantages, and limitations as delivery systems for gene therapy.

Furthermore, the book explores nonviral delivery systems, offering an alternative to viral vectors. It covers a wide range of approaches, including extracellular vesicles, peptide delivery systems, liposomes, polymeric delivery systems, synthetic cationic polymers, and inorganic nanoparticles (such as silicon, iron oxide, calcium phosphate, and carbon nanotubes), transposon-mediated delivery. Each chapter discusses the mechanisms, features, and potential applications of these nonviral delivery systems in gene therapy.

Additionally, the book highlights the significance of physical methods for gene delivery. It explores various techniques such as electroporation, sonoporation, photoporation, magnetofection, and microinjection, shedding light on their principles, advantages, and challenges in delivering therapeutic genes to the cells.

With contributions from leading experts in the field, "Delivery Systems in Gene Therapy" provides a comprehensive overview of the diverse delivery systems available for effectively delivering therapeutic genes to cells. It addresses the technical aspects, potential applications, and future directions in the field, making it an invaluable resource for researchers, clinicians, and students interested in gene therapy and targeted treatment approaches. This book serves as a valuable reference and guide for understanding the current landscape and advancing the field of gene therapy delivery systems.

PART I:

VIRAL VECTORS

CHAPTER 1

GENE THERAPY EVOLUTION: ADENOVIRUS VECTORS AND NOVEL DELIVERY SYSTEMS FOR IMPROVED EFFICACY

PRAVEENYA TIRUNAGARI[1], KOTTHAPALLI PRASHANTH[2], SUMANA KUMAR[2]

[1] Institute of Cardiovascular Physiology, Goethe University, Theodor-Stern-Kai 7, Frankfurt am Main 60590, Germany
[2] Department of Microbiology, JSS Academy of Higher Education and Research, Mysuru, Karnataka, 570015, India

Abstract

Gene therapy has transformed significantly since its inception, with adenovirus vectors playing a pivotal role. Adenoviral vectors are powerful tools in gene therapy, offering high transduction efficiency and broad tropism, making them ideal for various therapeutic applications. Adenovirus vectors have been instrumental in both in vivo and ex vivo gene therapies. Their versatility has made them a preferred choice in applications ranging from cancer treatment to vaccination and regenerative medicine. Recent advancements include codon optimization and incorporating tissue-specific regulatory elements to enhance transgene expression while minimizing immune response. Moreover, engineering efforts have focused on reducing vector immunogenicity and enabling precise control of gene expression through inducible systems, paving the way for personalized therapeutic approaches. The integration of adenovirus vectors with emerging delivery technologies, such as nanoparticle-based carriers and hybrid systems. These novel platforms aim to overcome limitations like DNA packaging constraints and improve targeted delivery to specific tissues or cells. Additionally, insights from clinical trials have informed the refinement of preparative condition protocols and vector safety profiles, addressing concerns about insertional mutagenesis and adverse immune reactions. Innovations have addressed these issues through developing advanced adenoviral vector generations, including helper-dependent adenoviral vectors that enhance safety and capacity. The integration of microRNA-targeted regulation and CRISPR/Cas9 technology for precise genome editing represents a new frontier in adenoviral vector design. Applications in cancer and monogenic disease have shown promising results, with adenoviral vectors being used in oncolytic therapy and gene replacement therapies. The combination of adenoviral vectors with other vector types and emerging technologies like nanotechnology and biomaterials is expected to enhance delivery efficiency. Recent clinical trials have demonstrated the potential of adenoviral vectors in treating complex disease, although regulatory frameworks and ethical considerations remain crucial in their development. This chapter provides in-depth exploration of the latest advancements in adenoviral vector technology, highlighting their potential to revolutionize therapeutic delivery and transform the landscape of gene therapy.

Keywords: Adenovirus, Viral vectors, Gene therapy, Personalized medicine, Vaccine development

1. Introduction to Adenoviral Vectors in Gene Therapy

Adenoviruses (Ad) are medium-sized, non-enveloped viruses with a linear double-stranded DNA (dsDNA) genome typically between 26-45 kilobases (kb). The genome is flanked by two inverted terminal repeats (ITRs) and contains multiple heavily spliced transcripts. Genes are categorized into early genes (E1-E4) involved in viral replication and host manipulation, and late genes (L1-L5) mainly coding for structural proteins necessary for assembling viral particles. Major capsid proteins include fiber, pentone base, and hexon, which plays a role sin virus attachment and entry into host cells. Adenoviral vectors are engineered viruses derived from adenoviruses, which are DNA viruses commonly associated with mild respiratory infections in humans (Hoeben & Uil, 2013). Adenoviruses have multiple serotypes, more than 50 distinct human adenovirus serotypes classified into seven species (A to G). These serotypes differ in their tissue tropism, clinical manifestations, and immune recognition, which makes them useful for various gene therapy and vaccine vector applications. Different serotypes are associated with different disease such as respiratory infections (mainly species B and C), conjunctivitis and gastroenteritis (species F). the backbone of the vector comes commonly from species C serotypes like Ad5 or Ad2, due to their well-characterized biology and high gene transfer efficiency. Different serotypes can be used as vector backbones to evade pre-existing immunity, alter tissue targeting, or improve safety profiles. Vectors based on Ad26 or Ad35 serotypes (species D or B) are used in vaccine platforms to avoid Ad5 immunity (Crenshaw et al., 2019; Lynch & Kajon, 2016; MacNeil et al., 2023).

Over the past few decades, these vectors have become a pivotal tool for delivering therapeutic genes in both research and clinical gene therapy applications, as well as in vaccine development. Adenoviral vectors efficiently transfer genetic material into diverse cell types, including both dividing and non-dividing cells. They have a large genome that accommodates substantial therapeutic genes, distinguishing them from other viral vectors. Unlike retroviruses, adenoviral DNA remains episomal and does not integrate into the host genome, reducing insertional mutagenesis risks and potential genetic disruptions (Araújo et al., 2022; Desfarges & Ciuffi, 2012; Salauddin et al., 2024). Adenoviral vectors can deliver large or multiple gene inserts typically up to 8-36kb, exceeding capacity of adeno-associated virus (AAV) vectors. They effectively infect dividing and non-dividing cells across various tissues. While their strong immune stimulation benefits vaccine development, it challenges gene therapy by reducing expression duration and causing adverse reactions. Unlike lentiviral vectors, adenovirus do not integrate into the host genome, resulting in transient gene expression. Adenoviral vectors can be easily produced at high titres, making them suitable for industrial-scale manufacturing and mass vaccination campaigns. They possess intrinsic adjuvant-like properties, often inducing potent humoral and cellular immune responses useful in vaccine development. These vectors can deliver genes to specialized tissues, such as muscle, heart, lung, and brain, which broadens their therapeutic application. Adenoviral vectors are characterized by transient gene expression due to their DNA's inability to integrate into the host genome, thereby limiting their application in contexts necessitating sustained therapeutic protein production. The administration of high doses of adenoviral vectors can elicit significant innate and adaptive immune responses, potentially leading to toxicity, acute inflammation, or severe adverse effects, particularly in individuals with pre-existing immunity to adenovirus. A substantial portion of the population possesses neutralizing antibodies from prior natural exposure to adenoviruses, which diminishes the efficacy of vector-mediated gene delivery and vaccines. Strategies to address this issue include utilizing rare human serotypes or vectors derived from non-human adenoviruses. The risk of generating replication-competent adenoviruses due to contamination during manufacturing poses concerns regarding tumorigenesis and other safety issues. Advances in packaging cell lines have reduced this risk, yet vigilant monitoring remains essential. To counteract vector clearance by the immune system, higher doses may be administered; however, this approach increases the likelihood of adverse events. Although efforts have been made to retarget adenoviral vectors to specific cell types, technical challenges persist, such as achieving efficient ligand incorporation and maintaining vector stability(Kajon et al., 2019; H. Zhang et al., 2023).

The milestone for recombinant, replication-defective adenovirus vectors occurred later, predominantly in the late 1980s and early 1990s. Researchers have excised the E1 gene, and the E3 gene, from the adenoviral genome. This excision serves a dual purpose: it inhibits undesired viral replication and enhances the capacity for the insertion of therapeutic genes (Hackett & Crystal, 2025; Roy-Chowdhury & Horwitz, 2002; Syyam et al., 2022). The construction of the vector involves the creation of two plasmids: a genomic plasmid containing the full-length adenoviral genome devoid of the E1/E3 regions, and a shuttle plasmid carrying the promoter, transgene, and polyadenylation sequences, which is designed to recombine with the genomic plasmid in E. coli through homologous recombination. The recombinant genome is subsequently purified and introduced into HEK293 cells, which provide E1 in trans for vector production(Bulcha et al., 2021; Wersto et al., 1998). The first successful use of replication-deficient adenovirus ($E1^-E3^-$) for gene transfer in vivo occurred around 1989-1990. Collaborations between two countries enabled the adaptation of adenoviral vectors (with the E1 and E3 deletions) and their propagation in *HEK293* cells, facilitating efficient gene delivery to target tissues(Crystal, 2014). Rosenfeld et al used $E1^-E3^-$ adenovirus to deliver genes for b-galactosidase in vivo, demonstrating robust, organ-specific expression. The technology rapidly entered clinical trials, in 1993, the first human received an $E1^-E3^-$ adenovirus vector carrying the normal CFTR gene for cystic fibrosis via nasal administration, marking an historic moment in gene therapy (Rosenfeld et al., 1991). A phase I clinical trial evaluated the safety and feasibility of direct intramyocardial delivery of an $E1^-E3^-$ adenovirus vector encoding human vascular endothelial growth factor (VEGF121) cDNA as a strategy to promote therapeutic angiogenesis in patients with severe, treatment-refractory coronary artery disease (CAD) who were unsuitable for conventional revascularization. Twenty-one patients received injections either as an adjunct during coronary artery bypass grafting or via minimally invasive thoracotomy alone., the therapy was well tolerated, with no significant cardiac or systemic adverse events reported during six months of follow up. Preliminary efficacy signals included improved myocardial perfusion, enhanced wall motion in treated cases, reduced angina class, and increased exercise tolerance, with benefits persisting at six months and encouraging long-term safety and survival trends over 10 years, without increased risks such as malignancy or retinopathy(Rosengart et al., 1999). Another landmark study explored the use of replication-deficient adenoviral vector (*Ad-CFTR*) to deliver a recombinant human a1-antitrypsin (a1AT) gene directly to the lung epithelium in vivo. This approach represented an early and important step toward somatic gene therapy for hereditary disorders such as a1-antitrypsin deficiency, which leads to emphysema, and cystic fibrosis. When freshly isolated tracheobronchial epithelia cells from cotton rats were infected with Ad-a1AT, the cells produced and secreted human a1AT, as confirmed by the presence of both messenger RNA and the protein itself. After intratracheal administration of Ad-a1AT into the respiratory tract of live cotton rats, human a1AT mRNA transcripts were detected in lung epithelial cells. Lung tissue synthesized and secreted genuine human a1AT protein, human a1AT was detectable in the epithelial lining fluid for at least 1-week post-administration. The study suggested that adenovirus vectors could directly target the respiratory epithelium, making gene transfer feasible for treatment of lung diseases resulting from genetic deficiencies. The expression of physiologically relevant levels of a1-AT in lung tissue highlights the possibility of local protein replacement therapy for inherited lung conditions (Rosenfeld et al., 1992).

a. Elements of Adenovirus genome

There are cis and trans elements of adenovirus vectors which are critical for their function in gene delivery and viral replication. Cis-acting elements are located within the adenovirus genome, essential for replication, packaging, and stability of the vector DNA. Inverted terminal repeats (ITRs) are found at both ends of the adenoviral genome (100-150 bp long), the ITRs serve as origins of replication and are necessary for viral DNA replication. They act as self-priming structures for primase-independent replication. Packaging signal (ψ) is located to the left ITR at the left end of the genome, this cis-acting element is essential for packaging the viral genome into the capsid. It consists of a series of redundant "A-repeats" within the packaging domain and must be near the genome ends to function. Terminal protein (pTP) are covalently linked to 5' ends of the viral genome, it plays a role in replication initiation and possibly assist with packaging. These cis elements are retained in even the most gutted (helper-dependent) adenoviral vectors to maintain replication and packaging capability of the vector genome (Gräble & Hearing, 1992; Hearing & Shenk, 1986). Trans-acting elements are typically viral proteins or gene products supplied in trans by the helper virus or packaging cell lines, which assist in viral replication, transcription, assembly, and host interaction but are not part of the vector genome itself. Early genes encode proteins that regulate viral gene expression, DNA replication, and modulation of host cell function. E1A is essential for activating transcription of other viral genes, and E1B helps counteract host apoptotic responses. Late genes encode structural proteins used for viral capsid assembly. In vector production systems, early and late viral functions are provided in trans by helper viruses or helper plasmids, supply all needed viral proteins for assembly and replication except for the viral DNA sequences removed from the recombinant vector (Ryu, 2017; J. H. Wang et al., 2024).

b. Entry and trafficking mechanisms

Adenoviral vectors enter host cells primarily via binding to specific receptors such as the Coxsackievirus and Adenovirus Receptor (CAR). However, viral capsid proteins, especially the fiber knob with and RGD motif, also interact with cellular integrins, promoting internalization through clathrin-mediated endocytosis and other secondary pathways like caveolin-mediated endocytosis and micropinocytosis. Human serotype 5 adenovirus (hAd5) utilizes CAR as the main receptor, the fiber knob proteins of several other serotypes of adenovirus, including hAd3, hAd11, hAd26, hAd35, hAd52, can bind to CD46, desmoglein 2 (DSG-2), polysialic acid (polySia), and/or GD1agylcan (GD1a) on the cell surface for cell entry. The virus then traffics through the cytosol utilizing the microtubule network and docks at the nuclear pore complex to deliver its genome into the nucleus for gene expression. This allows for engineered modifications in vector tropism and efficiency (Nicklin et al., 2005; Sharma et al., 2009; Thomas et al., 2002).

c. Generations of Adenoviral vectors

Adenoviruses were first identified in 1953 during studies of tonsil and adenoid tissues, which sought to find unknown viruses causing respiratory diseases. In 1977, the *HEK293* cell line was developed by stably integrating adenovirus type 5 (Ad5) E1 gene fragments into human embryonic kidney cells. This cell line became crucial for propagating recombinant adenoviruses whose E1 region had been deleted, making them incapable of replicating in normal cells. Adenoviral vectors are typically engineered from human adenovirus serotype 5 (Ad5), with deletions in certain genome regions to make them replication-deficient. Adenoviral vectors have evolved through several generations to improve their utility for gene therapy, primarily by increasing safety, reducing immunogenicity, and boosting their capacity for foreign gene delivery (Ghebremedhin, 2014; Kovesdi & Hedley, 2010).

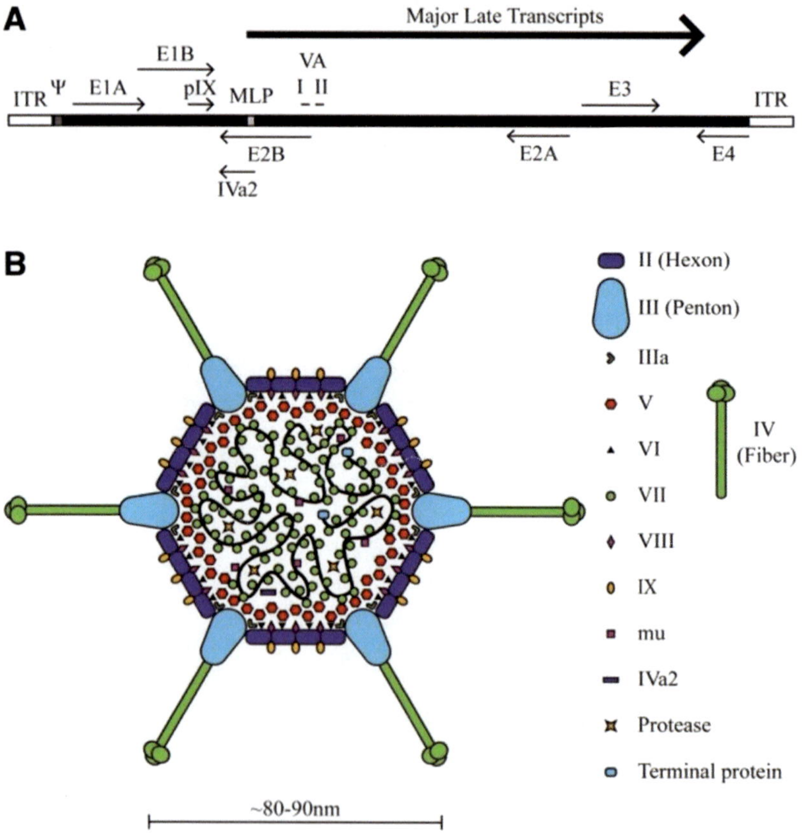

Figure 1: Structural Framework of Adenoviruses. (A) Schematic representation of adenovirus genome organization; (B) Structural composition of adenovirus virion with labeled proteins.

Table No. 1: Generational Advances in Adenoviral Vectors

Generation	Viral gene deletions	Transgene capacity	Immunogenicity	Production complexity	Key advantages	limitations
First-generation	E1 & E3	~6.5kb	High	Moderate	High transgene expression, high titer	Risk of RCA formation, immunogenicity
Second-generation	E1, E3+E2 and/or E4	~10.5-14kb	Reduced vs. 1st gen	More complex	Reduced immune response (partial), larger transgene capacity	Lower viral yields, unstable expression
Third-generation	All viral genes except ITRs and packaging signal	~36kb	Lowest	Most complex, requires helper virus	Large capacity, minimal immune response, prolonged expression	Complex production, potential helper virus contamination

i. First-Generation Adenovirus Vectors:

First-generation vectors are engineered by excising the E1 region (comprising E1A and E1B) and the E3 region from the wild-type adenoviral genome. These deletions both disable viral replication and create space for the insertion of therapeutic or research gene cassettes. The removal of E1 renders the vectors replication-incompetent and allows for the insertion of therapeutic genes up to 6.5 kb in size. Although the deletion of E3 further augments the available cargo space, it is not imperative for vector production. The production process necessitates a packaging cell line, typically *HEK293*, which provides E1 proteins in trans. First-generation vectors have relatively high immunogenicity, which can limit their use in certain therapeutic contexts. These vectors allow high transgene expression but have a risk of generating replication-competent adenoviruses (RCAs) through recombination with the packaging cell genome(Bernt et al., 2002; Leikas et al., 2023).

ii. Second-Generation Adenovirus Vectors:

Second-generation vectors incorporate additional deletions in the E2 and/or E4 regions, in conjunction with E1 and E3 deletions found in first-generation vectors. This further reduces the leaky expression of viral genes, with the objective of decreasing immunogenicity and the formation of replication-competent adenoviruses (RCA). These vectors have an increased capacity for genetic cargo, accommodating up to 10.5 kb. The E2 and E4 functions are complemented in trans by specialized packaging cell lines during production. However, they necessitate more advanced packaging cell lines that provide all deleted regions in trans. However, these vectors often face challenges such as reduced viral yields and less stable or weaker long-term transgene expression compared to first-generation vectors. Advances include inducible expression systems controlling E2/E4 gene expression to enhance vector production without harming host cells. Thus, while they represent an advancement in reducing immune responses and expanding transgene capacity, the practical and production difficulties have limited their widespread adoption. Common cell lines include modified HEK293, 911, and A549 derivatives optimized for these purposes (Kreppel & Hagedorn, 2021).

iii. Third-Generation Helper-Dependent Adenoviral (HDAd) Vectors:

Third-generation adenoviral vectors, also referred to as helper-dependent or gutless vectors, are characterized by the deletion of all viral coding sequences, retaining only the inverted terminal repeats (ITRs) and the packaging signal (ψ). These vectors can accommodate up to 36-37 kilobases of genetic material, making them suitable for the delivery of large or multiple transgenes. Their immunogenicity is significantly reduced due to the absence of viral genes. The production of these vectors necessitates the use of a helper virus or plasmid, which supplies the deleted adenoviral proteins in trans. They require co-infection with a helper virus supplying necessary viral proteins in trans. Innovations such as Cre-loxP recombination systems prevent packaging of helper virus DNA, ensuring safety and purity of vector preparations (Józkowicz & Dulak, 2005; Rosewell et al., 2011).

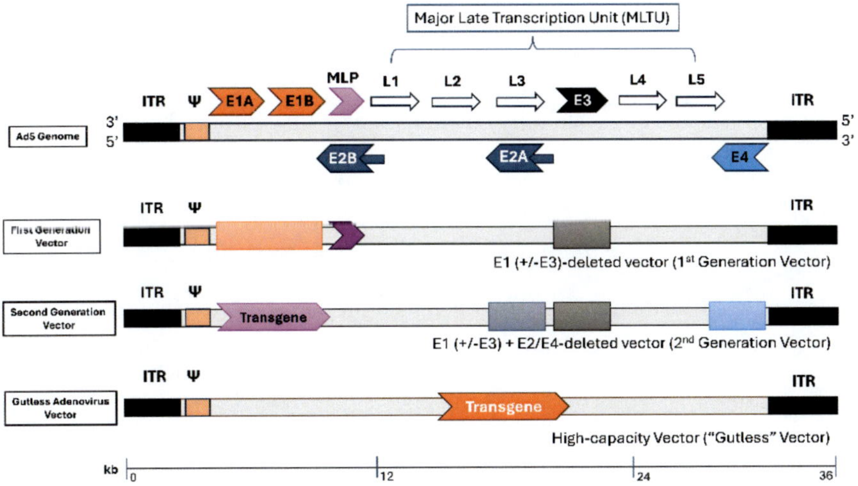

Figure 2: Genome Map of Adenoviruses and Derived Vectors

2. Engineering Innovations for Enhanced Delivery

a. Codon Optimization for Improved Transgene Expression

Codon optimization is a powerful strategy to enhance transgene expression in adenovirus vectors, but its application requires a careful balance between boosting expression and preserving viral fitness. By adjusting codon usage to better match, the preference of host, initial transgene expression can be increased. However, fully optimized codons may negatively affect viral replication, resulting in reduced long-term expression. In contrast, the use of partially suboptimal codons, while lowering initial expression levels, can better sustain viral replication and maintain transgene expression overtime. This balance is particularly important in oncolytic adenovirus therapies, where both viral replication and gene expression contribute to therapeutic efficacy. Adenoviral genes themselves display varied codon usage, with many late structural proteins using optimal human codons, while others, such as fiber protein, rely on suboptimal codons crucial for replication (Núñez-Manchón et al., 2021; Paremskaia et al., 2024). In gene therapy, especially in vaccine development, codon optimization may be employed to boost antigen production while intentionally attenuating viral growth. More advanced approaches like localized codon optimization (LCO) aim to enhance expression without disrupting essential viral functions, experimental studies show that while codon optimization can significantly increase protein levels, it may impair replication unless finely tuned. Combining codon usage adjustments with promoter selection, regulatory element tuning, and gene-protective strategies can help achieve both high expression and vector stability, demonstrating that in adenoviral vector design, partial codon optimization often offers better therapeutic outcomes than full optimization (Giménez-Roig et al., 2021).

b. Capsid engineering for tissue targeting

Genetic modifications to adenoviral capsid proteins such as fiber, pentone base, enable retargeting to specific cell types by modifying receptor usage and allows modification of viral tropism. However, early interactions of adenovirus vectors with host components, such as blood factors and immune cells, pose significant challenges. These interactions occur immediately upon systemic delivery, influencing distribution of vector, clearance, and immune recognition before it reaches target cells. The vector surface properties, including size, shape, and capsid proteins composition, trigger these early host responses. This tunable tropism is key to improving therapeutic specificity and reducing off-target effects. Capsid engineering aims to modify the surface of adenovirus vectors at the genetic or chemical level to avoid recognition and neutralization by the immune system and blood components and retarget the vector away from natural tropism and enhance delivery to specific tissues or cell types of therapeutic interest (Weklak et al., 2021). Techniques such as capsid pseudo-typing, replacing adenoviral capsid proteins with those from other viruses, serotype switching, and fiber protein alterations have been employed to redirect vectors towards specific tumor cell receptors, increasing specificity and reducing off-target effects. The fiber protein on the adenovirus capsid is a primary determinant of tropism. Approaches include fiber pseudo-typing, where fiber or knob domain from the different adenovirus serotypes with alternative receptor specificities are used to redirect vector tropism, ligand incorporation into fiber knob to target non-CAR receptors and fiber "deknobbing" with added targeting ligands. The integration of ligands, or motifs that specifically target integrins or other tumor-associated antigens facilitates the selective infection of cancer cells, thereby enhancing the efficacy of oncolytic and gene therapy applications. The incorporation of peptides or ligands into the hexon protein, which is the most abundant capsid protein with exposed hypervariable regions, or into minor capsid proteins such as polypeptide IX, allows for increased ligand valency and unique targeting opportunities while preserving particle stability (Muravyeva & Smirnikhina, 2024). High-capacity or "gutless" adenoviral vectors can be engineered as empty capsid shells with minimal viral gene expression, reducing immunogenicity and toxicity. These particles can incorporate targeting, imaging (e.g., positron emission tomography (PET) reporter enzymes), and therapeutic functions simultaneously, enabling precise delivery and monitoring of therapy. Imaging with PET receptor enzymes in adenovirus vectors involves incorporating specific genes encoding enzymes that can be detected noninvasively using PET. These reporter gene produce enzymes that phosphorylate or metabolize PET reporter proves, radioactive molecules administered to the subject, that can then be imaged with PET scanning to visualize and quantify the location and level of gene expression in living organism. A classic use of herpes simplex virus type 1 thymidine kinase (HSV1-tk) gene or its mutant versions, HSV1-sr39TK, as a PET reporter gene, when expressed by an adenovirus vector in tissues such as liver or tumors, these enzymes phosphorylate specific PET probe substrates like 18F-FHBG or 18F-FEAU, leading to intracellular trapping of the radioactive probe. This accumulation results in PET signal that correlate with the level of transgene expression (Glasgow et al., 2006; Sakhuja et al., 2003). Studies have demonstrated the ability to repeatedly and quantitively image HSV1-tk gene expression mice, including non-invasive visualization of adenovirus-mediated gene delivery to the liver or tumors (Gambhir et al., 2000; Yaghoubi & Gambhir, 2007).

Besides genetic engineering, chemical approaches modify the capsid surfaces to alter receptor binding or evade neutralizing antibodies without altering the viral genome. One widely used chemical modification is the covalent attachment of hydrophilic polymers such as polyethylene glycol (PEG) or poly-N-(2-hydroxypropyl) methacrylamide (HPMA) to surface-exposed amino acids on capsid proteins. This "PEGylation" or polymer coating masks viral epitopes recognized by the immune system, reducing neutralization and clearance by antibodies and immune cells. It can also extend the vector's circulation time in the bloodstream and decrease undesired liver uptake and inflammation. Some polymers can be further functionalized with targeting ligands to facilitate receptor-specific uptake by desired cells. Chemical modifications typically target exposed lysine or cysteine residues on capsid proteins using reactive groups that form stable or reversible bonds under mild conditions. This preserves capsid structural integrity and avoids the potential vector production and stability issues sometimes seen with genetic modifications. The chemical methods are relatively quick and can generate heterogenous capsid modifications, offering flexibility in designing vectors. More advanced chemical strategies include site-specific modification through incorporation of special chemical tags or unnatural amino acids, enabling precise conjugation of targeting molecules or fluorophores to defined capsid locations. This can increase targeting precision or enable in vivo tracking of vectors (C. Chen et al., 2020; Kreppel & Kochanek, 2008; Lam et al., 2021).

c. Tissue-Specific Promoters and Regulatory Elements

Adenoviruses can be engineered to incorporate tissue-specific promoters, enabling selective gene expression in desired cell types for applications such as targeted gene therapy or cancer treatment. These promoters are chosen based on their activity profiles and ability to minimize off-target toxicity. Some of the promoters used in adenoviruses are surfactant protein B (SPB), Alpha-fetoprotein (AFP), Myosin Light Chain-2v (MLC-2V), Alpha-Myosin Heavy Chain (a-MHC), and CXCR4. SPB/SPC is active in type II alveolar and bronchial epithelial cells and used to restrict adenoviral replication and gene expression specifically to lung tissues, maximizing safety in non-lung tissues. Alpha-fetoprotein (AFP) is an oncofetal protein highly expressed during fetal liver development, but its expression is minimal in healthy adult tissue sand strong in liver tissues and certain cancer cells as cancer/tissue-specific control element. Reactivation of AFP expression is commonly observed in hepatocellular carcinoma (HCC) and certain other malignancies making the AFP promoter a valuable regulatory element for tissue- or cancer-specific gene expression. The activity of the AFP promoter alone is relatively weak. Linked enhancer regions can substantially boost expression, resulting in stronger and more selective activity in HCC or AFP-positive cells. Hepatocyte nuclear factor 1 (HNF-1) is critical for the tissue-specific transcription of AFP, binding to its promoter region and facilitating liver-specific expression. The combined use of enhancer and promoter sequences enables highly selective expression in cancer gene therapy applications(Barnett et al., 2002; Głowska-Ciemny et al., 2023; Ucdal et al., 2025). In a clinical study by Butterfield et al, a vaccine strategy aimed to stimulate an immune response targeting AFP-expressing tumor by using a “DNA Prime”, a plasmid encoding AFP, followed by an “adenovirus boost”, adenovirus encoding AFP. Patients received three plasmid DNA injections encoding AFP and GM-CSF, followed by a single replication-deficient adenovirus injection encoding AFP. The treatment was well tolerated with no significant toxicities. One exhibited a weak AFP-positive tumor recurrence but strong adenovirus-specific immunity and experienced AFP-positive tumor recurrence. Other mounted robust AFP-specific CD8+ and CD+ T cell responses, along with adenovirus-neutralizing antibodies, and relapsed with an AFP-negative tumor and no rise in serum AFP. Baseline anti-adenovirus appeared associated with longer progression-free survival. These findings suggest that the AFP DNA prime-adenovirus boost approach is safe, immunogenic, and may delay recurrence in patients achieving strong antigen-specific immunity, warranting further evaluation in larger clinical trials(Butterfield et al., 2014).

Promoters that are active primarily in cancer cells, such as prostate-specific antigen (PSA) promoter for prostate cancer, and the hTERT promoter for telomerase-positive cancers, drive the replication-essential genes, restricting viral propagation. These promoters are mainly active in cancer cells, not in normal cells, and drive the expression of therapeutic genes (e.g., suicide genes, replication-essential viral genes) only within tumors, thus restricting off-target effects and viral propagation to cancerous tissues. The PSA promoter is specifically active in prostate epithelial cells and most prostate cancer cells, including androgen-independent clones. This promoter enables the selective expression of therapeutic or replication-essential genes within prostate tumors while sparing normal tissues and other cell types. PSA-driven gene therapy constructs have been used to direct prodrug-activating enzymes and oncolytic virus replication specifically to prostate cancer cells. The hTERT promoter is active in most human cancers because telomerase is reactivated in these cells but is silenced in most normal somatic cells. This promoter can drive the expression of viral replication genes or cytotoxic genes selectively in telomerase-positive cancer cells. Oncolytic viruses, like Telomelysin/OBP-301, use the hTERT promoter to replicate and cause cell death only in cancerous tissues, minimizing normal tissue toxicity. Other promoters with cancer-specificity include those from COX-2, CXCR4,

BIRC5 (Survivin), EGFR, HER2/NEU, and others, each enriched in various cancer types(Kyo et al., 2008; Yang et al., 2022).

Recombinant adenoviruses containing cardiac-specific promoters are a powerful approach for gene delivery targeting heart tissue, aiming to minimize off-target effects and increase safety for therapeutic applications in cardiomyopathies. Both MLC-2V and a-MHC are utilized for myocardial-specific gene expression, ideal in heart muscle gene delivery. Particularly, MLC-2V shows high selectivity for the ventricular myocardium. MLC-2V promoter is known for its high selectivity towards the ventricular myocardium, making it particularly suitable for targeting ventricular cells in gene therapy approaches. Its activity is developmentally regulated and strongest at specific heart development stages and in adult ventricular myocardium. However, recent research suggests that MLC-2V, which mainly ventricular, can occasionally be detected in atrial tissue, especially under stress or certain physiological conditions, though its primary function and utility remain ventricular focused. a-MHC promoter is generally used for broader cardiac-specific gene expression but does not provide the same level of chamber (ventricular versus atrium) selectivity as MLC-2V. MLC-2V is thus preferred when high specificity for ventricular heart muscle is required, whereas a-MHC is chosen for general cardiac targeting (Griscelli et al., 1998; Suzuki et al., 1998). In a study by Franz et al, recombinant adenoviral vectors were engineered to express a reporter gene, luciferase, under the regulation of cardiac-specific promoters. These vectors, designated as Ad-MHCLuc and Ad-MLCLuc, were administered into neonatal rat hearts and quadriceps femoris muscles, followed by the assessment of luciferase activity across nine different tissues. Injection into the cardiac cavity resulted in markedly elevated expression in cardiac tissue, particularly with the MLC-2V promoter, which exhibited the highest selectivity and potency for ventricular myocardium. The virus driven by the MLC-2V promoter demonstrated only baseline reporter activity in non-cardiac tissues, confirming its tissue specificity (Franz et al., 1997). Conversely, the α-MHC promoter exhibited minor, yet detectable, off-target activity in the liver and lung. Although adenoviral genomes were detectable in various tissues, transgene expression was confined to the target tissue due to the specificity of the cardiac promoters. Studies show the MLC-2 promoter drives selective expression in ventricular myocardium, a key advantage for cardiac gene therapy by preventing unintended transgene activity. A 250-bp fragment of the MLC-2V gene enables robust cardiomyocyte expression while reducing non-cardiac tissue expression compared to standard viral promoters such as cytomegalovirus (CMV) promoter. In comparisons with promoters like MLC-2V or a-MHC, the

CMV promoter typically yields higher transgene expression, but much less specificity. Therefore, it is often used as "gold standard" for benchmarking expression levels, but not for targeted cardiac expression. Cardiac-restricted expression occurs through cis-regulatory elements activated by cardiac-specific transcription factors like MEF-2 and SRF. The cardiac-specific sequence (CSS) within the promoter represses activity in skeletal muscle and other tissues, with its removal causing loss of tissue specificity. Many tissue-specific promoters do not achieve the high activity levels characteristic of viral or robust constitutive promoters such as CMV, CAG, and EF1a, which can limit their efficacy. Specificity and leakiness are significant concerns, as promoters may express genes outside the intended tissue, leading to undesirable effects(Hunter et al., 1995; Schröder et al., 2023). Consequently, the recombinant adenovirus system employs tissue-specific promoters to direct gene delivery and expression specifically to cardiac, pulmonary, or cancer cells. This approach is crucial in the development of safer gene therapies. The use of tumor- or tissue-specific promoters reduces toxicity and enhances the therapeutic index by confining adenovirus replication and cytotoxicity to cancer cells or targeted tissues. Strategies such as double-unit vectors, which combine a tissue-specific promoter with a strong inducible promoter, or the incorporation of insulator sequences, enhance both specificity and gene expression levels in adenoviral constructs (Boecker et al., 2004; Chai et al., 2023; Norrman et al., 2010; Suarez-Amaran et al., 2025).

Adenoviral gene expression and replication are controlled by regulatory elements. Adenoviral early genes E1, E2, E3, and E4 are regulated by promoter regions responsive to viral and cellular transcription factors. E1A protein serves as the master regulator for adenovirus early gene expression, stimulating transcription from viral early promoters for efficient replication. E1A modulates cellular genes by acting as a transcriptional activator or repressor by binding to cellular regulatory proteins. The E1A-289R protein contains conserved regions critical for transactivation, with CR3 domain required for strong activation. E1A interacts with cellular factors like DREF nuclear factor to modulate chromatin structure and early viral gene expression. E1A drives G0-arrested cells into S phase for viral replication through activation of cellular and viral promoters. E1A ensures downstream regions are activated by remodelling the cellular transcriptional environment and supporting immune evasion and cell cycle activation (Fessler & Young, 1998).

Among adenoviral genes, the virus-associated (VA) RNA genes are notable for not encoding proteins but instead producing small non-coding RNAs that fulfil regulatory functions, particularly in modulating host antiviral responses and enhancing viral gene expression. One such gene is VARNA1, which is transcribed by RNA polymerase III. Due to its well-defined promoter structure and compact regulatory regions, the VARNA1 gene has been instrumental in elucidating the functional organization of transcriptional control elements in eukaryotes. The control region of the VARNA1 gene, specific to adenovirus type 2, contains positive regulatory elements that facilitate transcription and virus-restricted expression. Investigations employing linker-scanning mutations from positions -33 to +77 have identified five critical regulatory elements. The B block is vital for transcription and the stable formation of transcription factor complexes, while the A block, though necessary, is less critical. The A and B blocks constitute core promoter elements for the assembly of basal transcription machinery. An additional element is present in the interblock region, and two regulatory elements in the 5' flanking region contribute to transcription and moderate complex formation (Punga et al., 2020; Schwartz et al., 2023; Zhao et al., 2013).

A persistent challenge in adenoviral vector systems is the unintended influence of viral enhancer elements and chromatin position effects, leading to leaky basal transcription or inappropriate transgene activation. To address this, the HS-4 insulator from chicken b-globin locus has been integrated into vector designs. HS-4 is a chromatin insulator that regulates gene expression by shielding tissue-specific promoters from viral enhancers, blocking enhancer activity and lowering background transcription in non-induced states. It maintains tight regulation of transgene expression while limiting off-target expression, though its effectiveness varies by integration site. Studies show that placing an insulator between viral genome and hepatoma-specific promoter shields from unwanted regulation. Recombinant adenoviruses with HS-4 showed higher reporter gene (e.g., alkaline phosphatase) expression in hepatocellular carcinoma cells such as HepG2, Hep3B, HuH7, with minimal expression in AFP-negative tumor lines and normal cells. In vivo, reporter expression localized exclusively to transplanted hepatoma cells, showing higher expression compared to non-insulated vectors (Burcin et al., 1999; Railey & Wu, 1988; Wong et al., 2013; Yahata et al., 2007).

3. Applications in Cancer and Monogenic Diseases

a. Adenoviral Vectors in Oncolytic Therapy

Adenoviral vectors are among the earliest and most widely utilized tools in both gene delivery and oncolytic virotherapy for cancer. Their effectiveness stems from several unique strengths. Oncolytic adenoviruses selectively infect and replicate within tumor cells, causing cell lysis and the release of viral progeny that can infect neighbouring tumor cells, promoting further tumor destruction. Lysis of tumor cells results in the release of tumor antigens and viral antigens, which are presented to T cells by dendritic cells, thereby stimulating local and systemic antitumor immune responses. Dendritic cells, which are specialized antigen-presenting cells, engulf the release tumor and viral antigens. They process these antigens and present them on their surface to T cells using major histocompatibility complex (MHC) molecules. The presented antigens stimulate both local and systemic immune responses. The combined effect of direct tumor lysis and immune activation leads to immunogenic cell death, amplifying the antitumor effect(Alberts et al., 2002; Cerullo et al., 2012). This dual mechanism, viral oncolysis and immune stimulation, can potentially induce long-lasting immune memory against tumor antigens, providing durable responses and protection against recurrence. Oncolytic adenoviruses can be engineered to express molecules that modify the tumor microenvironment to enhance viral spread and immune activation, like vectors expressing hyaluronidase or cytokines such as granulocyte macrophage colony-stimulating factor (GM-CSF). Clinical trials are ongoing for such armed vectors, showing promising efficacy with minimal side effects(Kaufman et al., 2015; Marelli et al., 2018). Oncolytic adenoviruses engineered to express positron emission tomography (PET) reporter genes have been utilized to monitor their presence in tumors and other tissues. This approach offers dynamic insights into viral replication, dissemination, and therapeutic efficacy in both preclinical cancer models and clinical trials. These models encompass a range of solid tumors, including breast cancer, prostate carcinoma, and myeloma, as well as hematologic malignancies. This imaging approach enhances safety and efficacy assessment by revealing vector biodistribution and therapeutic gene activity without invasive biopsies(Matsunaga & Gotoh, 2023; Trivedi et al., 2023).

Conditionally replicating adenovirus (CRAD) are engineered viral antigens to replicate only in tumor cells, using tumor-specific promoter, such as those regulating midkine or telomerase expression, minimizing off-target effects and increasing safety. CRAD typically replace the promoter of essential viral replication genes like E1A or E1B, with a tumor-specific promoter, such as midkine and human telomerase reverse transcriptase (hTERT). These promoters are highly active in many tumor cells due to their elevated expression or activity, while remaining largely inactive in normal tissue, which sharply limits off-target effects. In cancer cells, high-activity of these promoters drives expression of adenoviral replication genes, allowing the virus to replicate and destroy the tumor cells. In non-cancerous cells, low promoter activity prevents significant expression of these genes, blocking viral replication. Midkine promoter-based conditionally replicate adenovirus (CRAD) therapy is an innovative approach for treating midkine-expressing human pancreatic cancer. The strategy leverages the fact that midkine, a heparin-binding growth factor, is overexpressed in numerous cancers, including human pancreatic cancer cell lines, while its expression in healthy adult tissues is typically low (Jounaidi et al., 2007; Shim et al., 2009; H. Zhang et al., 2009). A recombinant adenovirus (Ad5MK) was engineered whereby viral replication is controlled by the midkine promoter. This specificity allows the virus to preferentially replicate in cancer cells expressing midkine, sparing normal tissue. In preclinical studies, Ad5MK was tested on seven human pancreatic cancer cell lines. Most of these lines exhibited moderate to strong midkine expression, the promoter activity was significantly higher in midkine-positive cells, enhancing virus replication and cytotoxicity against these cancer cells. In vivo experiments involved intratumoral injection of Ad5MK into nude mice with Suit-2 pancreatic cancer xenografts. Ad5MK-treated mice showed higher expression of viral-replication-related genes in tumor tissue, significant inhibition of tumor growth, and extended survival compared to controls(Toyoda et al., 2008). In another study, a midkine promoter-based CRA (Ad-MK-E1a) is a gene therapy strategy designed to target human bladder cancer cells, that overexpress midkine mRNA. The approach utilizes the tumor-specific activity of the MK promoter and Ad-MK-E1a demonstrated significant antitumor efficacy in bladder cancer models. In human bladder cancer cell lines overexpressing MK mRNA, especially KK47 and 5637, Ad-MK-E1a replicated selectively and inhibited cancer cell growth. In animal studies, direct injection of Ad-MK-E1a into tumors suppressed tumor growth in nude mice with bladder cancer xenografts(Terao et al., 2007).

Nonreplicating adenoviral vectors are a prominent platform in cancer gene therapy due to their efficient gene delivery capabilities to both dividing and nondividing cells. They have distinct advantages such as in vivo stability, ease of manufacturing, and capacity to carry therapeutic genes that stimulate antitumor immune responses. However, challenges arise from their broad native tropism, nonspecific transduction of normal cells, liver sequestration, neutralization by antibodies during systemic administration, and host antiviral immune responses that can limit therapeutic efficacy (Tessarollo et al., 2021). Combining a conditionally replicating adenovirus with an E1-deleted adenovirus carrying the therapeutic gene TRAIL (tumor necrosis factor-related apoptosis inducing ligand), markedly enhances gene replication efficiency and the anticancer effect in head and neck squamous cell carcinoma (HNSCC). Experiments showed that co-administering CRAD with E1-deleted adenovirus dramatically increases expression of therapeutic and reporter genes (luciferase, LacZ, GFP) by 10-to-50-fold compared to the adenovirus alone. Triple-regulated conditionally replicating adenovirus (CRA) is an advanced form of oncolytic viral therapy developed to improve both the effectiveness and safety of treating peritoneal carcinomatosis (PC), especially from gastric and colorectal cancers. These CRAs are engineered to selectively replicate in and destroy cancer cells by being regulated through three cancer-specific factors like surviving promoter, carcinoembryonic antigen (CEA) promoter, and cytomegalovirus immediate early gene enhancer/promoter. This ensures high specificity, minimizing the risk to normal cells. By exploiting high expression levels of surviving and CEA in cancer cells and their absence in normal cells. The virus can selectively target and kill malignant cells while sparing healthy tissues(Shim et al., 2010). The carcinoembryonic antigen (CEA)-producing cell-specific oncolytic adenovirus, known as OV798, has been developed as a targeted therapy for colorectal cancer due to the high expression of CEA in most colorectal cancers. OV798 uses transcriptional regulatory elements from the CEA gene to control adenoviral gene expression and replication, making the virus replicate preferentially in CEA-producing colon cancer cells. This design enables OV798 to selectively target and kill CEA-positive colorectal cancer cells (e.g., LoVo and SW1463 cell lines), with a 1000-fold lower replication rate in CEA-negative cell lines, this minimizes collateral damage to normal or CEA-negative tissues(Shen et al., 2002; Yuanhao Li et al., 2003). In a mouse xenograft model bearing human colon tumors, a single intratumoral injection of OV798 resulted in marked tumor growth inhibition. Six weeks after treatment, tumor volume stabilized, while untreated tumors grew significantly. Preclinical studies in mice showed that triple-regulated Conditionally replicating adenoviruses could dramatically improve survival and body weight compared to no treatment(E. C. Chen et al., 2015; Ning et al., 1996). Notably, cancers expressing CEA responded better, with minimal toxicity to normal cells. This multi-factor regulation enhances the safety profile substantially. Tumor specificity is improved, decreasing side effects commonly seen in earlier generations of oncolytic adenoviruses. A study developed a therapy for colorectal cancer by incorporating ST13 tumor suppressor gene into a double-regulated oncolytic adenovirus, controlled by the CEA promoter and E1A region deletion. The therapy, Ad. (ST13). CEA.E1A (24) or CTGVT-CRC (cancer targeting gene-viro-therapy for colorectal cancer), targets CEA-expressing cells, which comprise 90% of colorectal cancers. E1A deletion restricts viral replication to retinoblastoma-deficient cancer cells. ST13 gene inclusion enhances tumor inhibition in xenograft models, inducing apoptosis via p38 MAPK pathway through CHOP and ATF-2 upregulation, and activates mitochondrial-mediated apoptosis through caspase-9 and caspase-3 expression (D. Bin Yu et al., 2009; Zhou et al., 2012).

Several adenoviral therapies have been approved for cancer treatment. Notably, Gendicine, a replication-defective human p53 adenoviral vector, has been approved in China for the treatment of squamous cell carcinoma. It is specifically designed to reintroduce the wild-type p53 gene into cancer cells. This strategy exploits the fact that over 50% of human cancers harbour mutations or inactivation in the TP53 gene, leading to uncontrolled cellular proliferation, resistance to cell death, and tumor progression. Gendicine uses a modified adenovirus, typically serotype 5 (Ad5), with its replication genes (early region 1) excised, thereby preventing it from multiplying in human cells and reducing risks of unwanted viral replication. The adenoviral vector carries and expresses the wild-type human p53 gene, under control of a robust promoter, in cancer cells. The "restored" p53 protein functions as a checkpoint to induce cell-cycle arrest, promote DNA repair, and trigger apoptosis or senescence in response to cellular stress or DNA damage (G. X. Chen et al., 2014; W. W. Zhang et al., 2018). Introducing functional p53 disrupts tumor growth and can drive cancer cells, especially those unable to repair DNA, into cell death, thus shrinking tumors and potentially sensitizing them to conventional therapies like chemotherapy and radiotherapy. Gendicine is usually administered via direct intratumoral injection, intracavity, or intravascular infusion, to maximize local effects while minimizing systemic exposure. Additionally, oncolytic adenoviruses such as ONYX-015 (dl1520) and Oncorine (H101), which selectively replicate in p53-deficient tumor cells, have been approved and are utilized for head and neck cancers (Khuri et al., 2000; Mulvihill et al., 2001). ONYX-015 is a genetically engineered adenovirus carries deletions in the E1B-55kDa gene, which normally encodes a protein that helps the virus inactivate the p53 tumor suppressor. In normal cell cycle arrest or apoptosis, thus preventing productive viral replication. However, in tumor cells that lack functional p53 due to mutation or deletion, the virus can replicate efficiently, causing cell lysis and selective destruction of cancer cells. While ONYX-015 demonstrated a favorable safety profile and modest efficacy in clinical trials for recurrent head and neck cancer, as a single agent its benefit was limited. Its use is mostly in clinical trials settings, often combined with chemotherapeutic agents like cisplatin or 5-FU, or radiotherapy, where additive anti-tumor effects have been observed (Dix et al., 2001; Larson et al., 2015). Oncorine, on the other hand, developed in China, is closely related to ONYX-015 and similarly lacks the ability to counteract p53. This allows it to replicate preferentially in p53-deficent cells. The virus destroys cancer cells either by direct oncolysis or by stimulating anti-tumor immune responses through release of tumor antigens. Oncorine was the first oncolytic virus to the commercially available for the treatment of head and neck cancers specifically nasopharyngeal carcinoma. Clinical trials showed that combining Oncorine with chemotherapy nearly doubled the short-term response rate compared to chemotherapy alone. It is especially effective when injected directly into tumors (Liang, 2018; Russell & Peng, 2018).

Table 2: Oncolytic Adenovirus Vectors in Clinical Cancer Therapy

Oncolytic Adenovirus Vector	Target	Cancer Type	Transgene expression	References
ONYX-015	p53-deficient cells	Head & Neck, Colorectal	Native vector (E1B-55K deleted)	(McCormick, 2000)
Oncorine (H101)	p53 pathway	Head & Neck	P53 gene	(Castellanos & Pan, 2016; Geoerger et al., 2004; W. Yu & Fang, 2007; W. Zhang et al., 2025)
ZD55-TRAIL	hTERT promoter, TRAIL-active	Hepatocellular Carcinoma	TRAIL (apoptosis-induing ligand)	(Y. G. Wang et al., 2016)
Ad5-CD/TKrep	Prostate-specific antigens	Prostate Cancer	CD-TK fusion suicide gene	(Ahn et al., 2008)
TILT-123	Multiple tumor markers	Several solid tumors	TNF-alpha and IL-2 immunostimulatory genes	(Jirovec et al., 2024)

Ad5-yCD/utTK~SR~rep-hNIS	Prostate tissue	Prostate Cancer	CD and TK suicide genes, hNIS	(Nyati et al., 2023)
ZD55-Smac	hTERT promoter	Hepatocellular Carcinoma	SMAC pro-apoptotic gene	(Pei et al., 2004)
CG7870	PSA promoter E1A/E1B modifications	Prostate cancer	PSA promoter drives tumor-selective replication	(Small et al., 2006)
DNX-2401 (Ad-delta24)	Altered RB1 pathway	Glioblastoma melanoma	Selective replication in RB-mutated cells	(Lang et al., 2018)
ICOVIR (Ad-delta24-RGD)	Integrin avb receptor (RGD motif)	Glioblastoma melanoma	Enhanced cell entry via RGD motif; combined with immunotherapy	(Van Putten et al., 2022)
coloAd1 (enadenotucirev)	Multiple-immune modulators	Colorectal and solid tumors	Potent oncolytic activity; armed with co-stim factors	(Garcia-Carbonero et al., 2017)

4. Gene Replacement Therapies by adenoviruses for Monogenic Disorders

Gene replacement therapies using adenoviral vectors represent a significant avenue in treating monogenic disorders. Adenoviral gene replacement therapies have been tested across several monogenic diseases, especially in pre-clinical and some clinical trials. For monogenic disorders, gene replacement involves inserting an exogenous, functional gene to compensate for the protein loss of malfunctioning due to the mutation (Lee et al., 2017).

a. Hemophilia A and B (deficient Factor VIII and IX, respectively)

Adenoviral vectors carrying the relevant gene have shown transient correction in animal models (dogs and mice), with improved long-term results using newer generations, helper-dependent, "gutted" adenoviruses, or integration-promoting systems like transposases (e.g., Sleeping beauty transposase). These integration-promoting systems have been combined with adenoviral vectors to enable somatic integration of therapeutic genes into the host genome. This approach helps stabilize transgene expression and extends the therapeutic effect, especially in dividing cells. Hyperactive versions of transposases such as SB100X & HSB5, delivered by high-capacity adenoviral vectors can lead to persistent gene expression and long-term phenotypic correction in animal models, such as mice and dogs, as demonstrated for diseases requiring continual expression of correction factors such as hemophilia (Hausl et al., 2010; Ricobaraza et al., 2020). In research by Zhang et al, adenovirus/transposase hybrid vectors utilizing hyperactive sleeping beauty transposases (HSB5) for somatic integration has addressed both integration profile and safety aspects, mostly in murine models and in dogs for hemophilia B. Genome-wide analysis using LM-PCR and LAM-PCR in mice revealed a close-to-random integration profile. SB-HSB5 mediated integration events were spread across gene and non-gene areas without significant bias, reducing concerns about insertional mutagenesis commonly seen with some other integrating vectors. A minority of integration events occurred in the delivered adenoviral genome, attributed to transposon excision and reinsertion(W. Zhang et al., 2013). Stabilized transgene expression was observed and correlated with vector dose. However, at the highest vector dose tested (2×10^{11} TU/kg), fatalities occurred in mice, indicating dose-dependent toxicity, lower doses were well tolerated. Gutless adenoviral vectors, which lacks all coding regions, offer less cytotoxicity, reduced immunogenicity, and a much greater coding capacity than earlier generation adenoviral vectors such as Av3H8101 (E1/E2a/E3-deficient adenoviral vector) (Bilbao et al., 2005). Research has demonstrated that systemic delivery of gutless adenoviral vectors (AGV14-HFVIII & AGV15-HFVIII) encoding human Factor VIII (HFVIII) in hemophilia A mice leads to sustained and effective clotting factor expression, with important safety and therapeutic implications. In hemophilia A mice, systemic (intravenous) delivery of a gutless adenoviral vector resulted in FVIII expression levels up to 10-fold higher than conventional adenoviral vectors. The sustained expression was maintained for at least 9 months, with gutless vector-mediated plasma HFVIII levels declining only gradually overtime but remaining robust and detectable. These vectors were less likely to trigger immune responses, like anti-FVIII antibodies or inhibitors, than recombinant protein administration or conventional vectors. Administration of gutless FVIII vectors, especially via neonatal injection, can induce tolerance to HFVIII, further reducing the risk of inhibitor formation in treated subjects(Andrews et al., 2001; Reddy et al., 2002).

b. Alpha-1 Antitrypsin deficiency

Gene therapy for alpha-1 antitrypsin deficiency (AATD) lung disease is rapidly advancing, offering hope for more effective and lasting treatments compared to standard augmentation therapy. AATD is a genetic disorder leading to low levels of AAT protein, crucial for protecting the lungs from damage by neutrophil elastase. This deficiency results in lung diseases like emphysema and COPD and can also cause liver disease due to protein buildup. The primary therapy involves regular intravenous infusions of purified human AAT protein to maintain protective plasma levels. This is known as augmentation therapy but is costly, requires frequent dosing, and carries risks of viral contamination and allergic reactions(Pires Ferreira et al., 2023; Wozniak et al., 2015). Early clinical trials and preclinical studies in a-1 antitrypsin (AAT) deficiency have demonstrated that gene therapy approaches can successfully express the replacements AAT gene in both liver and lung cells. One promising advancement is the development of a myeloid cell-binding adenovirus (Ad.MBP), which specifically targets myeloid lineage leukocytes to enhance lung-directed gene delivery. This vector incorporates a myeloid cell-binding peptide (MBP) into the fiber protein of an adenovirus, that shifts viral tropism towards myeloid cells, enabling efficient transduction of target immune cells primarily residing in the lung microvasculature. This approach is especially relevant for disease where inflammatory myeloid cell infiltrates are central, as is the case with AATD-related lung destruction (Buggio et al., 2014). For AATD, a combinatorial gene therapy approach includes the use of microRNA targeting of the mutant AAT protein alongside a miR-resistance wild-type transgene, as strategy which has been efficacious in mouse models. The use of Ad.MBP with such bicistronic transgenes could optimize both lung and liver targeting, offering a platform for durable expression and disease modification. Interestingly, beyond its role in inherited deficiency disorders, changes in AAT levels have also been observed in acute inflammatory conditions(Lorincz & Curiel, 2020; Mueller et al., 2012). Gupta et al demonstrated AAT and serum albumin levels in tear fluids increase significantly during acute adenovirus conjunctivitis, as measured by electro immunodiffusion comparing 63 patients with the condition to 76 healthy subjects. The protein elevation correlated with disease severity, with no significant difference between virus-isolated and non-isolated cases, indicating these proteins mainly reflect conjunctival inflammation rather than direct infection. The protein levels normalized as symptoms improved, suggesting AAT and serum albumin serve as reversible indicators of conjunctival inflammation severity in acute adenovirus conjunctivitis (Gupta et al., 1988).

c. Ornithine transcarbamylase deficiency (OTCD)

Pre-clinical models have demonstrated the correction of metabolic defects in Ornithine Transcarbamylase Deficiency (OTCD); however, clinical trials have encountered challenges such as low efficiency and significant immune-related side effects. Research on the phenotypic correction of ornithine transcarbamylase deficiency (OTCD) using low-dose helper-dependent adenoviral (HDAd) vectors (HDAd-hOTC-W & HDAd-hOTC-WL) indicates promising advancements in gene therapy for this urea cycle disorder. HDAd vectors are engineered viral particles designed to deliver a healthy OTC gene to the liver without expressing viral proteins that trigger immune responses, thereby facilitating long-term gene expression. While high doses of HDAd vectors can correct the metabolic phenotype in mouse models of OTCD, such doses may induce systemic inflammatory responses and acute toxicity in humans, necessitating dose reduction for clinical translation. In SPF-ASH mice, a model of OTCD, vectors with optimized expression cassettes have achieved correction of orotic acid overproduction, the primary biochemical marker of OTCD, at lower doses (1×10^{12}), whereas other vectors required doses as high as 1×10^{13} to show similar correction. Lower doses also correlated with longer-lasting phenotypic correction (Brunetti-Pierri et al., 2008). Genetic and mRNA-based therapies in mice, including the spf and spf-J mutant strains, resulted in the restoration or enhancement of OTC enzyme activity, improved metabolic profiles, and protection against lethal hyperammonemia. This was particularly evident with the use of LNP-encapsulated OTC-mRNA (LUNAR-OTC) and ARCUS nuclease methodologies (Prieve et al., 2018; Tarasenko et al., 2015). These results confirm the feasibility of gene and mRNA therapies in preclinical models. Gene therapy approaches, especially those using adenoviral vectors, have led to significant immune reactions in humans. Serious incidents, including systemic inflammatory response syndrome, cytokine storm, and multi-organ failure, have been documented. Notable adverse events, including systemic inflammatory response syndrome, cytokine storm, and multi-organ failure, have been reported. A particularly significant case involved the death of an 18-year-old with partial ornithine transcarbamylase deficiency (OTCD), an X-linked urea cycle disorder, following participation in an adenoviral vector-based gene therapy trial. This incident was attributed to elevated levels of inflammatory cytokines, specifically interleukin-6 and interleukin-10, indicating an acute innate immune response to the vector. This case represented a pivotal moment in the consideration of safety in gene therapy (Lowenstein et al., 2007; Sibbald, 2001).

d. Vaccinal Approaches Using Adenoviral Vectors

Adenoviral vector-based vaccinal strategies utilize modified adenoviruses as vectors to deliver genetic material encoding antigens from pathogens, thereby stimulating the host immune system to elicit a protective response without inducing disease. Adenoviral-vectored vaccines have been clinically developed for pathogens such as SARS-CoV-2 (e.g., Ad5-nCOV vaccine), HIV (e.g., MRKAd5/HIV-1), and respiratory syncytial virus (RSV) (e.g., Ad5.RSV-F) (Barouch, 2010; Chavda et al., 2023; Jang et al., 2025; Michael, 2012). These vectors can be administered intranasally, to target respiratory or other mucosal surfaces, thereby inducing robust IgA responses and tissue-resident memory T cells, which offer superior protection against mucosal infections compared to systemic immunity alone(Afkhami et al., 2016; Vemula & Mittal, 2010). An adenoviral vector vaccine encoding the RSV fusion protein, when combined with an immune modulator, demonstrated enhanced mucosal immune responses and superior protection compared to natural infection (Sampson et al., 2025). In animal studies, intranasal administration of Ad5-nCOV provided complete protection in the respiratory tracts, although intramuscular delivery was selected for clinical trials due to safety concerns in certain populations. Adenovirus vectors are produced by inserting influenza antigen gene into replication-defective adenovirus genomes, which are then propagated in complementing cell lines like HEK293 in bioreactors for large-scale vaccine production. These vectors are purified through multiple steps to achieve high titres and safety(Freitag et al., 2023; Wu et al., 2021). Used as delivery systems for influenza vaccines, adenovirus vectors offer rapid vaccine generation, strong humoral and cellular immune responses, and flexibility in antigen design without requiring liver virus, making them suitable for pandemic preparedness (Hoelscher et al., 2006).

5. Future Directions and Emerging Technologies

Adenoviruses have traditionally been employed as vectors due to their substantial capacity for foreign DNA, their ability to infect both dividing and non-dividing cells, and their pronounced immunogenicity, which is advantageous in certain therapeutic contexts. Strategies to mitigate immune responses against adenoviral vectors include immunosuppression, immunomodulation, serotype switching, and the utilization of nonhuman or rare human adenovirus serotypes to circumvent pre-existing immunity (Shirley et al., 2020; Thacker et al., 2009). Additionally, capsid modifications and microencapsulation techniques are being investigated to alleviate acute inflammatory responses and enhance vector safety. Scalable bioreactor systems with suspension cell lines enhance production yield and batch consistency of adenoviral vectors, facilitating broader clinical application. Engineering adenoviral fiber proteins or capsid motifs, such as RGD insertion, facilitates the selective targeting of specific cell types, including cancer cells that downregulate natural adenovirus receptors, thereby enhancing transduction efficiency and therapeutic efficacy, which is crucial for oncolytic adenovirus therapies(Ballard et al., 2012; Swift et al., 2022). The integration of CRISPR-Cas9 for precise genome editing in adenoviruses involves using adenoviral vectors to efficiently deliver the CRISPR-Cas9 system into target cells. Hybrid vectors, combining adenoviruses with other viruses such as adeno-associated viruses or Epstein-Barr virus, are being developed for stable gene transfer and integration. High-capacity, replication-deficient adenoviral vectors, devoid of all viral genes, are employed to safely carry the Cas9 gene and guide RNA (gRNA) components for precise genome editing. Adenoviruses can deliver CRISPR-Cas9 components for targeted knockout or transcriptional regulation of genes, such as oncogenes in cancer therapy, using either active Cas9 for DNA cleavage or dead Cas9 fused to activator or repressor domains to modulate gene expression without inducing double-strand breaks. The combination of adenoviral vectors carrying CRISPR-Cas9 nucleases with adeno-associated vectors (AAVs) that deliver donor DNA templates significantly enhances precise editing outcomes by promoting homology-directed repair (HDR) (Boucher et al., 2020; Khoshandam et al., 2024; Li et al., 2020). Recent strategies employ advanced third-generation adenoviral vectors with optimized, high-specificity Cas9 variants to reduce off-target effects and cytotoxicity, thereby enabling more efficient and safe gene editing. These integrated systems have been explored for cancer gene therapy, allowing for the selective knockout or repression of mutated oncogenes, with ongoing clinical research focused on improving safety, efficacy, and delivery (Azeez et al., 2024; Xu et al., 2025).

6. Conclusion

Adenovirus vectors are advantageous due to their ability to be produced in high titers, their broad host range, and their suitability for in vivo delivery. However, several significant challenges must be addressed to facilitate their broader and systemic application. One of the primary challenges is the transient nature of gene expression, which limits their use to applications that do not require sustained expression. At present, adenoviral vectors show promise for localized gene delivery where prolonged expression is not necessary, such as in synovial ablation for arthritis and as gene delivery vehicles in cancer therapy trials. Additionally, the immunogenicity of adenoviral vectors poses a critical issue, as it triggers strong immune responses that can hinder repeat dosing and lead to the elimination of transduced cells (Chuang et al., 2022). Strategies to mitigate this include using rare human serotypes such as Ad26, Ad35, or non-human adenoviruses (chimpanzee-derive), as well as capsid engineering to evade neutralizing antibodies. The potential to genetically modify adenoviral proteins to achieve targeted tissue tropism offers valuable flexibility for specific therapeutic applications, such as oncolytic therapies (Tang et al., 2025). While adenoviral vectors remain a powerful and versatile tool in gene therapy, their future success hinges on continued vector engineering, including de-immunization strategies, use of helper-dependent “gutless” adenoviruses for long-term expression with reduced toxicity and combinatorial approaches with immune suppression, to address challenges related to immune responses and expression longevity, thereby broadening their safe applicability in diverse therapeutic contexts. With ongoing advancements and careful clinical application, adenoviral vectors are poised to remain a powerful and versatile component of gene therapy, oncolytic virotherapy and vaccine development, balancing their inherent strength with minimized safety concerns.

References

Afkhami, S., Yao, Y., & Xing, Z. (2016). Methods and clinical development of adenovirus-vectored vaccines against mucosal pathogens. *Molecular Therapy Methods and Clinical Development*, *3*, 16030. https://doi.org/10.1038/MTM.2016.30/ASSET/30D159D6-6A28-4625-A38E-572DCDDF4383/MAIN.ASSETS/GR3.JPG

Ahn, M., Lee, S. J., Li, X., Jiménez, J. A., Zhang, Y. P., Bae, K. H., Mohammadi, Y., Kao, C., & Gardner, T. A. (2008). Enhanced combined tumor-specific oncolysis and suicide gene therapy for prostate cancer using M6 promoter. *Cancer Gene Therapy*, *16*(1), 73. https://doi.org/10.1038/CGT.2008.59

Alberts, B., Johnson, A., Lewis, J., Raff, M., Roberts, K., & Walter, P. (2002). *T Cells and MHC Proteins*. https://www.ncbi.nlm.nih.gov/books/NBK26926/

Andrews, J. L., Kadan, M. J., Gorziglia, M. I., Kaleko, M., & Connelly, S. (2001). Generation and characterization of E1/E2a/E3/E4-deficient adenoviral vectors encoding human factor VIII. *Molecular Therapy*, *3*(3), 329–336. https://doi.org/10.1006/mthe.2001.0264

Araújo, N. M., Rubio, I. G. S., Toneto, N. P. A., Morale, M. G., & Tamura, R. E. (2022). The use of adenoviral vectors in gene therapy and vaccine approaches. *Genetics and Molecular Biology*, *45*(3 Suppl 1), e20220079. https://doi.org/10.1590/1678-4685-GMB-2022-0079

Azeez, S. S., Hamad, R. S., Hamad, B. K., Shekha, M. S., & Bergsten, P. (2024). Advances in CRISPR-Cas technology and its applications: revolutionising precision medicine. *Frontiers in Genome Editing*, *6*, 1509924. https://doi.org/10.3389/FGEED.2024.1509924/FULL

Ballard, E. N., Trinh, V. T., Hogg, R. T., & Gerard, R. D. (2012). Peptide Targeting of Adenoviral Vectors to Augment Tumor Gene Transfer. *Cancer Gene Therapy*, *19*(7), 476. https://doi.org/10.1038/CGT.2012.23

Barnett, B. G., Tillman, B. W., Curiel, D. T., & Douglas, J. T. (2002). Dual Targeting of Adenoviral Vectors at the Levels of Transduction and Transcription Enhances the Specificity of Gene Expression in Cancer Cells. *Molecular Therapy*, *6*(3), 377–385. https://doi.org/10.1006/MTHE.2002.0670

Barouch, D. H. (2010). Novel Adenovirus Vector-Based Vaccines for HIV-1. *Current Opinion in HIV and AIDS*, *5*(5), 386. https://doi.org/10.1097/COH.0B013E32833CFE4C

Bernt, K., Liang, M., Ye, X., Ni, S., Li, Z.-Y., Ye, S. L., Hu, F., & Lieber, A. (2002). A New Type of Adenovirus Vector That Utilizes Homologous Recombination To Achieve Tumor-Specific Replication. *Journal of Virology*, *76*(21), 10994. https://doi.org/10.1128/JVI.76.21.10994-11002.2002

Bilbao, R., Reay, D. P., Wu, E., Zheng, H., Biermann, V., Kochanek, S., & Clemens, P. R. (2005). Comparison of high-capacity and first-generation adenoviral vector gene delivery to murine muscle in utero. *Gene Therapy*, *12*(1), 39–47. https://doi.org/10.1038/sj.gt.3302392

Boecker, W., Bernecker, O. Y., Wu, J. C., Zhu, X., Sawa, T., Grazette, L., Rosenzweig, A., del Monte, F., Schmidt, U., & Hajjar, R. J. (2004). Cardiac-Specific Gene Expression Facilitated by an Enhanced Myosin Light Chain Promoter. *Molecular Imaging*, *3*(2). https://doi.org/10.1162/15353500200404103

Boucher, P., Cui, X., & Curiel, D. T. (2020). Adenoviral Vectors for In Vivo Delivery of CRISPR-Cas Gene Editors. *Journal of Controlled Release: Official Journal of the Controlled Release Society*, *327*, 788. https://doi.org/10.1016/J.JCONREL.2020.09.003

Brunetti-Pierri, N., Clarke, C., Mane, V., Palmer, D. J., Lanpher, B., Sun, Q., O'Brien, W., & Lee, B. (2008). Phenotypic Correction of Ornithine Transcarbamylase Deficiency Using Low Dose Helper Dependent Adenoviral Vectors. *The Journal of Gene Medicine*, *10*(8), 890. https://doi.org/10.1002/JGM.1218

Buggio, M., Towe, C., & Curiel, D. T. (2014). Development of a myeloid cell-binding adenovirus for the potential gene therapy of alpha-1 anti-trypsin deficiency. *European Respiratory Journal*, *44*(Suppl 58). https://doi.org/10.1183/13993003/ERJ.44.SUPPL_58.P852

Bulcha, J. T., Wang, Y., Ma, H., Tai, P. W. L., & Gao, G. (2021). Viral vector platforms within the gene therapy landscape. *Signal Transduction and Targeted Therapy 2021 6:1*, *6*(1), 1–24. https://doi.org/10.1038/s41392-021-00487-6

Burcin, M. M., Schiedner, G., Kochanek, S., Tsai, S. Y., & O'Malley, B. W. (1999). Adenovirus-mediated regulable target gene expression in vivo. *Proceedings of the National Academy of Sciences of the United States of America*, *96*(2), 355. https://doi.org/10.1073/PNAS.96.2.355

Butterfield, L. H., Economou, J. S., Gamblin, T. C., & Geller, D. A. (2014). Alpha fetoprotein DNA prime and adenovirus boost immunization of two hepatocellular cancer patients. *Journal of Translational Medicine*, *12*(1). https://doi.org/10.1186/1479-5876-12-86,

Castellanos, M. R., & Pan, Q. (2016). Novel p53 therapies for head and neck cancer. *World Journal of Otorhinolaryngology - Head and Neck Surgery*, *2*(2), 68. https://doi.org/10.1016/J.WJORL.2016.05.005

Cerullo, V., Koski, A., Vähä-Koskela, M., & Hemminki, A. (2012). Oncolytic Adenoviruses for Cancer Immunotherapy: Data from Mice, Hamsters, and Humans. *Advances in Cancer Research*, *115*, 265–318. https://doi.org/10.1016/B978-0-12-398342-8.00008-2

Chai, S., Wakefield, L., Norgard, M., Li, B., Enicks, D., Marks, D. L., & Grompe, M. (2023). Strong ubiquitous micro-promoters for recombinant adeno-associated viral vectors. *Molecular Therapy. Methods & Clinical Development*, *29*, 504. https://doi.org/10.1016/J.OMTM.2023.05.013

Chavda, V. P., Bezbaruah, R., Valu, D., Patel, B., Kumar, A., Prasad, S., Kakoti, B. B., Kaushik, A., & Jesawadawala, M. (2023). Adenoviral Vector-Based Vaccine Platform for COVID-19: Current Status. *Vaccines*, *11*(2), 432. https://doi.org/10.3390/VACCINES11020432

Chen, C., Ng, D. Y. W., & Weil, T. (2020). Polymer bioconjugates: Modern design concepts toward precision hybrid materials. *Progress in Polymer Science*, *105*, 101241. https://doi.org/10.1016/J.PROGPOLYMSCI.2020.101241

Chen, E. C., Karl, T. A., Kalisky, T., Gupta, S. K., O'Brien, C. A., Longacre, T. A., Van De Rijn, M., Quake, S. R., Clarke, M. F., & Rothenberg, M. E. (2015). KIT Signaling Promotes Growth of Colon Xenograft Tumors in Mice and is Upregulated in a Subset of Human Colon Cancers. *Gastroenterology*, *149*(3), 705. https://doi.org/10.1053/J.GASTRO.2015.05.042

Chen, G. X., Zhang, S., He, X. hua, Liu, S. Y., Ma, C., & Zou, X. P. (2014). Clinical utility of recombinant adenoviral human p53 gene therapy: current perspectives. *OncoTargets and Therapy*, *7*, 1901. https://doi.org/10.2147/OTT.S50483

Chuang, S. T., Conklin, B., Stein, J. B., Pan, G., & Lee, K. B. (2022). Nanotechnology-enabled immunoengineering approaches to advance therapeutic applications. *Nano Convergence 2022 9:1*, *9*(1), 1–31. https://doi.org/10.1186/S40580-022-00310-0

Crenshaw, B. J., Jones, L. B., Bell, C. R., Kumar, S., & Matthews, Q. L. (2019). Perspective on Adenoviruses: Epidemiology, Pathogenicity, and Gene Therapy. *Biomedicines*, *7*(3), 61. https://doi.org/10.3390/BIOMEDICINES7030061

Crystal, R. G. (2014). Adenovirus: The First Effective In Vivo Gene Delivery Vector. *Human Gene Therapy*, *25*(1), 3. https://doi.org/10.1089/HUM.2013.2527

Desfarges, S., & Ciuffi, A. (2012). Viral Integration and Consequences on Host Gene Expression. *Viruses: Essential Agents of Life*, *9789400748996*, 147. https://doi.org/10.1007/978-94-007-4899-6_7

Dix, B. R., Edwards, S. J., & Braithwaite, A. W. (2001). Does the Antitumor Adenovirus ONYX-015/dl1520 Selectively Target Cells Defective in the p53 Pathway? *Journal of Virology*, *75*(12), 5443. https://doi.org/10.1128/JVI.75.12.5443-5447.2001

Fessler, S. P., & Young, C. S. H. (1998). Control of Adenovirus Early Gene Expression during the Late Phase of Infection. *Journal of Virology*, *72*(5), 4049. https://doi.org/10.1128/JVI.72.5.4049-4056.1998

Franz, W. M., Rothmann, T., Frey, N., & Katus, H. A. (1997). Analysis of tissue-specific gene delivery by recombinant adenoviruses containing cardiac-specific promoters. *Cardiovascular Research*, *35*(3), 560–566. https://doi.org/10.1016/S0008-6363(97)00154-5

Freitag, T. L., Fagerlund, R., Karam, N. L., Leppänen, V. M., Ugurlu, H., Kant, R., Mäkinen, P., Tawfek, A., Jha, S. K., Strandin, T., Leskinen, K., Hepojoki, J., Kesti, T., Kareinen, L., Kuivanen, S., Koivulehto, E., Sormunen, A., Laidinen, S., Khattab, A., … Saksela, K. (2023). Intranasal administration of adenoviral vaccines expressing SARS-CoV-2 spike protein improves vaccine immunity in mouse models. *Vaccine*, *41*(20), 3233. https://doi.org/10.1016/J.VACCINE.2023.04.020

Gambhir, S. S., Bauer, E., Black, M. E., Liang, Q., Kokoris, M. S., Barrio, J. R., Iyer, M., Namavari, M., Phelps, M. E., & Herschman, H. R. (2000). A mutant herpes simplex virus type 1 thymidine kinase reporter gene shows improved sensitivity for imaging reporter gene expression with positron emission tomography. *Proceedings of the National Academy of Sciences of the United States of America*, *97*(6), 2785. https://doi.org/10.1073/PNAS.97.6.2785

Garcia-Carbonero, R., Salazar, R., Duran, I., Osman-Garcia, I., Paz-Ares, L., Bozada, J. M., Boni, V., Blanc, C., Seymour, L., Beadle, J., Alvis, S., Champion, B., Calvo, E., & Fisher, K. (2017). Phase 1 study of intravenous administration of the chimeric adenovirus enadenotucirev in patients undergoing primary tumor resection. *Journal for Immunotherapy of Cancer*, *5*(1), 71. https://doi.org/10.1186/S40425-017-0277-7

Geoerger, B., Vassal, G., Opolon, P., Dirven, C. M. F., Morizet, J., Laudani, L., Grill, J., Giaccone, G., Vandertop, W. P., Gerritsen, W. R., & Van Beusechem, V. W. (2004). Oncolytic activity of p53-expressing conditionally replicative adenovirus AdΔ24-p53 against human malignant glioma. *Cancer Research*, *64*(16), 5753–5759. https://doi.org/10.1158/0008-5472.CAN-04-0499

Ghebremedhin, B. (2014). Human adenovirus: Viral pathogen with increasing importance. *European Journal of Microbiology & Immunology*, *4*(1), 26. https://doi.org/10.1556/EUJMI.4.2014.1.2

Giménez-Roig, J., Núñez-Manchón, E., Alemany, R., Villanueva, E., & Fillat, C. (2021). Codon Usage and Adenovirus Fitness: Implications for Vaccine Development. *Frontiers in Microbiology*, *12*, 633946. https://doi.org/10.3389/FMICB.2021.633946/BIBTEX

Glasgow, J. N., Everts, M., & Curiel, D. T. (2006). Transductional targeting of adenovirus vectors for gene therapy. *Cancer Gene Therapy*, *13*(9), 830. https://doi.org/10.1038/SJ.CGT.7700928

Głowska-Ciemny, J., Szymański, M., Kuszerska, A., Malewski, Z., von Kaisenberg, C., & Kocyłowski, R. (2023). The Role of Alpha-Fetoprotein (AFP) in Contemporary Oncology: The Path from a Diagnostic Biomarker to an Anticancer Drug. *International Journal of Molecular Sciences*, *24*(3), 2539. https://doi.org/10.3390/IJMS24032539

Gräble, M., & Hearing, P. (1992). cis and trans requirements for the selective packaging of adenovirus type 5 DNA. *Journal of Virology*, *66*(2), 723. https://doi.org/10.1128/JVI.66.2.723-731.1992

Griscelli, F., Gilardi-Hebenstreit, P., Hanania, N., Franz, W. M., Opolon, P., Perricaudet, M., & Ragot, T. (1998). Heart-specific targeting of β-galactosidase by the ventricle-specific cardiac myosin light chain 2 promoter using adenovirus vectors. *Human Gene Therapy*, *9*(13), 1919–1928. https://doi.org/10.1089/hum.1998.9.13-1919

Gupta, A. K., Sarin, G. S., Mathur, M. D., & Ghosh, B. (1988). α1-Antitrypsin and serum albumin in tear fluids in acute adenovirus conjunctivitis. *British Journal of Ophthalmology*, *72*(5), 390–393. https://doi.org/10.1136/BJO.72.5.390,

Hackett, N. R., & Crystal, R. G. (2025). Four decades of adenovirus gene transfer vectors: History and current use. *Molecular Therapy*, *33*(5), 2192–2204. https://doi.org/10.1016/J.YMTHE.2025.03.062

Hausl, M. A., Zhang, W., Müther, N., Rauschhuber, C., Franck, H. G., Merricks, E. P., Nichols, T. C., Kay, M. A., & Ehrhardt, A. (2010). Hyperactive Sleeping Beauty Transposase Enables Persistent Phenotypic Correction in Mice and a Canine Model for Hemophilia B. *Molecular Therapy*, *18*(11), 1896. https://doi.org/10.1038/MT.2010.169

Hearing, P., & Shenk, T. (1986). The adenovirus type 5 E1A enhancer contains two functionally distinct domains: One is specific for E1A and the other modulates all early units in cis. *Cell*, *45*(2), 229–236. https://doi.org/10.1016/0092-8674(86)90387-9

Hoeben, R. C., & Uil, T. G. (2013). Adenovirus DNA Replication. *Cold Spring Harbor Perspectives in Biology*, *5*(3), a013003. https://doi.org/10.1101/CSHPERSPECT.A013003

Hoelscher, M. A., Garg, S., Bangari, D. S., Belser, J. A., Lu, X., Stephenson, I., Bright, R. A., Katz, J. M., Mittal, S. K., & Sambhara, S. (2006). Development of adenoviral-vector-based pandemic influenza vaccine against antigenically distinct human H5N1 strains in mice. *Lancet*, *367*(9509), 475. https://doi.org/10.1016/S0140-6736(06)68076-8

Hunter, J. J., Tanaka, N., Rockman, H. A., Ross, J., & Chien, K. R. (1995). Ventricular expression of a mlc-2v-ras fusion gene induces cardiac hypertrophy selective diastolic dysfunction in transgenic mice. *Journal of Biological Chemistry*, *270*(39), 23173–23178. https://doi.org/10.1074/jbc.270.39.23173

Jang, E., Lee, S., Han, J., & Chang, J. (2025). Single-dose intranasal adenovirus-based RSV vaccines targeting G and M2. *Npj Vaccines*, *10*(1), 1–6. https://doi.org/10.1038/S41541-025-01186-X;SUBJMETA=250,254,590,631;KWRD=INFECTION,VACCINES

Jirovec, E., Quixabeira, D. C. A., Clubb, J. H. A., Pakola, S. A., Kudling, T., Arias, V., Haybout, L., Jalkanen, K., Alanko, T., Monberg, T., Khammari, A., Dreno, B., Svane, I. M., Block, M. S., Adamo, D. A., Mäenpää, J., Kistler, C., Sorsa, S., Hemminki, O., … Hemminki, A. (2024). Single intravenous administration of oncolytic adenovirus TILT-123 results in systemic tumor transduction and immune response in patients with advanced solid tumors. *Journal of Experimental & Clinical Cancer Research: CR*, *43*(1), 297. https://doi.org/10.1186/S13046-024-03219-0

Jounaidi, Y., Doloff, J. C., & Waxman, D. J. (2007). Conditionally Replicating Adenoviruses for Cancer Treatment. *Current Cancer Drug Targets*, *7*(3), 285. https://doi.org/10.2174/156800907780618301

Józkowicz, A., & Dulak, J. (2005). Helper-dependent adenoviral vectors in experimental gene therapy. *Acta Biochimica Polonica*, *52*(3), 589. https://doi.org/10.18388/abp.2005_3419

Kajon, A. E., Weinberg, J. B., & Spindler, K. R. (2019). Adenoviruses. *Reference Module in Biomedical Sciences*. https://doi.org/10.1016/B978-0-12-801238-3.00086-6

Kaufman, H. L., Kohlhapp, F. J., & Zloza, A. (2015). Oncolytic viruses: a new class of immunotherapy drugs. *Nature Reviews. Drug Discovery*, *14*(9), 642. https://doi.org/10.1038/NRD4663

Khoshandam, M., Soltaninejad, H., Mousazadeh, M., Hamidieh, A. A., & Hosseinkhani, S. (2024). Clinical applications of the CRISPR/Cas9 genome-editing system: Delivery options and challenges in precision medicine. *Genes & Diseases*, *11*(1), 268–282. https://doi.org/10.1016/J.GENDIS.2023.02.027

Khuri, F. R., Nemunaitis, J., Ganly, I., Arseneau, J., Tannock, I. F., Romel, L., Gore, M., Ironside, J., MacDougall, R. H., Heise, C., Randlev, B., Gillenwater, A. M., Bruso, P., Kaye, S. B., Hong, W. K., & Kirn, D. H. (2000). A controlled trial of intratumoral ONYX-015, a selectively-replicating adenovirus, in combination with cisplatin and 5-fluorouracil in patients with recurrent head and neck cancer. *Nature Medicine*, *6*(8), 879–885. https://doi.org/10.1038/78638

Kovesdi, I., & Hedley, S. J. (2010). Adenoviral Producer Cells. *Viruses*, *2*(8), 1681. https://doi.org/10.3390/V2081681

Kreppel, F., & Hagedorn, C. (2021). Capsid and Genome Modification Strategies to Reduce the Immunogenicity of Adenoviral Vectors. *International Journal of Molecular Sciences*, *22*(5), 2417.

https://doi.org/10.3390/IJMS22052417

Kreppel, F., & Kochanek, S. (2008). Modification of Adenovirus Gene Transfer Vectors With Synthetic Polymers: A Scientific Review and Technical Guide. *Molecular Therapy*, *16*(1), 16–29. https://doi.org/10.1038/SJ.MT.6300321

Kyo, S., Takakura, M., Fujiwara, T., & Inoue, M. (2008). Understanding and exploiting hTERT promoter regulation for diagnosis and treatment of human cancers. *Cancer Science*, *99*(8), 1528. https://doi.org/10.1111/J.1349-7006.2008.00878.X

Lam, A. K., Frabutt, D., Li, L., & Xiao, W. (2021). Chemical Modifications of the Capsid for Redirecting and Improving the Efficacy of Adeno-Associated Virus Vectors. *Human Gene Therapy*, *32*(23–24), 1433. https://doi.org/10.1089/HUM.2021.124

Lang, F. F., Conrad, C., Gomez-Manzano, C., Alfred Yung, W. K., Sawaya, R., Weinberg, J. S., Prabhu, S. S., Rao, G., Fuller, G. N., Aldape, K. D., Gumin, J., Vence, L. M., Wistuba, I., Rodriguez-Canales, J., Villalobos, P. A., Dirven, C. M. F., Tejada, S., Valle, R. D., Alonso, M. M., … Fueyo, J. (2018). Phase I Study of DNX-2401 (Delta-24-RGD) Oncolytic Adenovirus: Replication and Immunotherapeutic Effects in Recurrent Malignant Glioma. *Journal of Clinical Oncology*, *36*(14), 1419. https://doi.org/10.1200/JCO.2017.75.8219

Larson, C., Oronsky, B., Scicinski, J., Fanger, G. R., Stirn, M., Oronsky, A., & Reid, T. R. (2015). Going viral: a review of replication-selective oncolytic adenoviruses. *Oncotarget*, *6*(24), 19976. https://doi.org/10.18632/ONCOTARGET.5116

Lee, C. S., Bishop, E. S., Zhang, R., Yu, X., Farina, E. M., Yan, S., Zhao, C., Zeng, Z., Shu, Y., Wu, X., Lei, J., Li, Y., Zhang, W., Yang, C., Wu, K., Wu, Y., Ho, S., Athiviraham, A., Lee, M. J., … He, T. C. (2017). Adenovirus-mediated gene delivery: Potential applications for gene and cell-based therapies in the new era of personalized medicine. *Genes & Diseases*, *4*(2), 43–63. https://doi.org/10.1016/J.GENDIS.2017.04.001

Leikas, A. J., Ylä-Herttuala, S., & Hartikainen, J. E. K. (2023). Adenoviral Gene Therapy Vectors in Clinical Use—Basic Aspects with a Special Reference to Replication-Competent Adenovirus Formation and Its Impact on Clinical Safety. *International Journal of Molecular Sciences 2023, Vol. 24, Page 16519*, *24*(22), 16519. https://doi.org/10.3390/IJMS242216519

Li, Q., Wang, H., Gong, C. yu, Chen, Z., Yang, J. xing, Shao, H. wei, & Zhang, W. feng. (2020). Efficient Editing of an Adenoviral Vector Genome with CRISPR/Cas9. *Indian Journal of Microbiology*, *61*(1), 91. https://doi.org/10.1007/S12088-020-00905-3

Liang, M. (2018). Oncorine, the World First Oncolytic Virus Medicine and its Update in China. *Current Cancer Drug Targets*, *18*(2), 171–176. https://doi.org/10.2174/1568009618666171129221503,

Lorincz, R., & Curiel, D. T. (2020). Advances in alpha-1 antitrypsin gene therapy. *American Journal of Respiratory Cell and Molecular Biology*, *63*(5), 560–570. https://doi.org/10.1165/RCMB.2020-0159PS/SUPPL_FILE/DISCLOSURES.PDF

Lowenstein, P. R., Mandel, R. J., Xiong, W., Kroeger, K., & Castro, M. G. (2007). Immune Responses to Adenovirus and Adeno-Associated Vectors Used for Gene Therapy of Brain Diseases: The Role of Immunological Synapses in Understanding the Cell Biology of Neuroimmune Interactions. *Current Gene Therapy*, *7*(5), 347. https://doi.org/10.2174/156652307782151498

Lynch, J. P., & Kajon, A. E. (2016). Adenovirus: Epidemiology, Global Spread of Novel Serotypes, and Advances in Treatment and Prevention. *Seminars in Respiratory and Critical Care Medicine*, *37*(4), 586. https://doi.org/10.1055/S-0036-1584923

MacNeil, K. M., Dodge, M. J., Evans, A. M., Tessier, T. M., Weinberg, J. B., & Mymryk, J. S. (2023). Adenoviruses in medicine: innocuous pathogen, predator, or partner. *Trends in Molecular Medicine*, *29*(1), 4–19. https://doi.org/10.1016/J.MOLMED.2022.10.001

Marelli, G., Howells, A., Lemoine, N. R., & Wang, Y. (2018). Oncolytic Viral Therapy and the Immune System: A Double-Edged Sword Against Cancer. *Frontiers in Immunology*, *9*(APR), 866. https://doi.org/10.3389/FIMMU.2018.00866

Matsunaga, W., & Gotoh, A. (2023). Adenovirus as a Vector and Oncolytic Virus. *Current Issues in Molecular Biology*, *45*(6), 4826. https://doi.org/10.3390/CIMB45060307

McCormick, F. (2000). Interactions between adenovirus proteins and the p53 pathway: The development of ONYX-015. *Seminars in Cancer Biology*, *10*(6), 453–459. https://doi.org/10.1006/scbi.2000.0336

Michael, N. L. (2012). Rare serotype adenoviral vectors for HIV vaccine development. *The Journal of Clinical Investigation*, *122*(1), 25–27. https://doi.org/10.1172/JCI60988

Mueller, C., Tang, Q., Gruntman, A., Blomenkamp, K., Teckman, J., Song, L., Zamore, P. D., & Flotte, T. R. (2012). Sustained miRNA-mediated Knockdown of Mutant AAT With Simultaneous Augmentation of Wild-type AAT Has Minimal Effect on Global Liver miRNA Profiles. *Molecular Therapy*, *20*(3), 590. https://doi.org/10.1038/MT.2011.292

Mulvihill, S., Warren, R., Venook, A., Adler, A., Randlev, B., Heise, C., & Kirn, D. (2001). Safety and feasibility of injection with an E1B-55 kDa gene-deleted, replication-selective adenovirus (ONYX-015) into primary carcinomas of the pancreas: A phase I trial. *Gene Therapy*, *8*(4), 308–315. https://doi.org/10.1038/sj.gt.3301398

Muravyeva, A., & Smirnikhina, S. (2024). Strategies for Modifying Adenoviral Vectors for Gene Therapy. *International Journal of Molecular Sciences*, *25*(22), 12461. https://doi.org/10.3390/IJMS252212461

Nicklin, S. A., Wu, E., Nemerow, G. R., & Baker, A. H. (2005). The influence of adenovirus fiber structure and function on vector development for gene therapy. *Molecular Therapy*, *12*(3), 384–393. https://doi.org/10.1016/J.YMTHE.2005.05.008/ASSET/C8DC2401-8391-4BD2-9463-05F6E93BAC15/MAIN.ASSETS/GR1.JPG

Ning, S., Trisler, K., Brown, D. M., Yu, N. Y., Kanekal, S., Lundsten, M. J., & Knox, S. J. (1996). Intratumoral radioimmunotherapy of a human colon cancer xenograft using a sustained-release gel. *Radiotherapy and Oncology*, *39*(2), 179–189. https://doi.org/10.1016/0167-8140(96)01718-5

Norrman, K., Fischer, Y., Bonnamy, B., Sand, F. W., Ravassard, P., & Semb, H. (2010). Quantitative Comparison of Constitutive Promoters in Human ES cells. *PLOS ONE*, *5*(8), e12413–e12413. https://doi.org/10.1371/JOURNAL.PONE.0012413

Núñez-Manchón, E., Farrera-Sal, M., Otero-Mateo, M., Castellano, G., Moreno, R., Medel, D., Alemany, R., Villanueva, E., & Fillat, C. (2021). Transgene codon usage drives viral fitness and therapeutic efficacy in oncolytic adenoviruses. *NAR Cancer*, *3*(2), zcab015. https://doi.org/10.1093/NARCAN/ZCAB015

Nyati, S., Stricker, H., Barton, K. N., Li, P., Elshaikh, M., Ali, H., Brown, S. L., Hwang, C., Peabody, J., Freytag, S. O., Movsas, B., & Siddiqui, F. (2023). A phase I clinical trial of oncolytic adenovirus mediated suicide and interleukin-12 gene therapy in patients with recurrent localized prostate adenocarcinoma. *PLOS ONE*, *18*(9), e0291315. https://doi.org/10.1371/JOURNAL.PONE.0291315

Paremskaia, A. I., Kogan, A. A., Murashkina, A., Naumova, D. A., Satish, A., Abramov, I. S., Feoktistova, S. G., Mityaeva, O. N., Deviatkin, A. A., & Volchkov, P. Y. (2024). Codon-optimization in gene therapy: promises, prospects and challenges. *Frontiers in Bioengineering and Biotechnology*, *12*, 1371596. https://doi.org/10.3389/FBIOE.2024.1371596

Pei, Z., Chu, L., Zou, W., Zhang, Z., Qiu, S., Qi, R., Gu, J., Qian, C., & Liu, X. (2004). An Oncolytic Adenoviral Vector of Smac Increases Antitumor Activity of TRAIL Against HCC in Human Cells and in Mice. *Hepatology*, *39*(5), 1371–1381. https://doi.org/10.1002/HEP.20203,

Pires Ferreira, D., Gruntman, A. M., & Flotte, T. R. (2023). Gene therapy for alpha-1 antitrypsin deficiency: an update. *Expert Opinion on Biological Therapy*, *23*(3), 283–291. https://doi.org/10.1080/14712598.2023.2183771,

Prieve, M. G., Harvie, P., Monahan, S. D., Roy, D., Li, A. G., Blevins, T. L., Paschal, A. E., Waldheim, M., Bell, E. C., Galperin, A., Ella-Menye, J. R., & Houston, M. E. (2018). Targeted mRNA Therapy for Ornithine Transcarbamylase Deficiency. *Molecular Therapy*, *26*(3), 801. https://doi.org/10.1016/J.YMTHE.2017.12.024

Punga, T., Darweesh, M., & Akusjärvi, G. (2020). Synthesis, Structure, and Function of Human Adenovirus Small Non-Coding RNAs. *Viruses*, *12*(10), 1182. https://doi.org/10.3390/V12101182

Railey, J. F., & Wu, G.-J. (1988). Organization of multiple regulatory elements in the control region of the adenovirus type 2-specific VARNA1 gene: fine mapping with linker-scanning mutants. *Molecular and Cellular Biology*, *8*(3), 1147–1159. https://doi.org/10.1128/MCB.8.3.1147-1159.1988

Reddy, P. S., Sakhuja, K., Ganesh, S., Yang, L., Kayda, D., Brann, T., Pattison, S., Golightly, D., Idamakanti, N., Pinkstaff, A., Kaloss, M., Barjot, C., Chamberlain, J. S., Kaleko, M., & Connelly, S. (2002). Sustained human factor VIII expression in hemophilia A mice following systemic delivery of a gutless adenoviral vector. *Molecular Therapy*, *5*(1), 63–73. https://doi.org/10.1006/mthe.2001.0510

Ricobaraza, A., Gonzalez-Aparicio, M., Mora-Jimenez, L., Lumbreras, S., & Hernandez-Alcoceba, R. (2020). High-Capacity Adenoviral Vectors: Expanding the Scope of Gene Therapy. *International Journal of Molecular Sciences*, *21*(10), 3643. https://doi.org/10.3390/IJMS21103643

Rosenfeld, M. A., Siegfried, W., Yoshimura, K., Yoneyama, K., Fukayama, M., Stier, L. E., Pääkkö, P. K., Gilardi, P., Stratford-Perricaudet, L. D., Perricaudet, M., Jallat, S., Pavirani, A., Lecocq, J.-P., & Crystal, R. G. (1991). Adenovirus-Mediated Transfer of a Recombinant α1-Antitrypsin Gene to the Lung Epithelium in Vivo. *Science*, *252*(5004), 431–434. https://doi.org/10.1126/SCIENCE.2017680,

Rosenfeld, M. A., Yoshimura, K., Trapnell, B. C., Yoneyama, K., Rosenthal, E. R., Dalemans, W., Fukayama, M., Bargon, J., Stier, L. E., Stratford-Perricaudet, L., Perricaudet, M., Guggino, W. B., Pavirani, A., Lecocq, J. P., & Crystal, R. G. (1992). In vivo transfer of the human cystic fibrosis transmembrane conductance regulator gene to the airway epithelium. *Cell*, *68*(1), 143–155. https://doi.org/10.1016/0092-8674(92)90213-V,

Rosengart, T. K., Lee, L. Y., Patel, S. R., Sanborn, T. A., Parikh, M., Bergman, G. W., Hachamovitch, R., Szulc, M., Kligfield, P. D., Okin, P. M., Hahn, R. T., Devereux, R. B., Post, M. R., Hackett, N. R., Foster, T., Grasso, T.

M., Lesser, M. L., Isom, O. W., & Crystal, R. G. (1999). Angiogenesis gene therapy: Phase I assessment of direct intramyocardial administration of an adenovirus vector expressing VEGF121 cDNA to individuals with clinically significant severe coronary artery disease. *Circulation*, *100*(5), 468–474. https://doi.org/10.1161/01.CIR.100.5.468,

Rosewell, A., Vetrini, F., & Ng, P. (2011). Helper-Dependent Adenoviral Vectors. *Journal of Genetic Syndrome & Gene Therapy*, *Suppl 5*(2), 001. https://doi.org/10.4172/2157-7412.S5-001

Roy-Chowdhury, J., & Horwitz, M. S. (2002). Evolution of adenoviruses as gene therapy vectors. *Molecular Therapy*, *5*(4), 340–344. https://doi.org/10.1006/mthe.2001.0575

Russell, L., & Peng, K. W. (2018). The emerging role of oncolytic virus therapy against cancer. *Chinese Clinical Oncology*, *7*(2), 16. https://doi.org/10.21037/CCO.2018.04.04

Ryu, W.-S. (2017). Virus Vectors. *Molecular Virology of Human Pathogenic Viruses*, 263–275. https://doi.org/10.1016/B978-0-12-800838-6.00019-9

Sakhuja, K., Connelly, S., Reddy, P. S., Ganesh, S., Cantaniag, F., Pattison, S., Limbach, P., Kayda, D. B., Kadan, M. J., & Kaleko, M. (2003). Optimization of the generation and propagation of gutless adenoviral vectors. *Human Gene Therapy*, *14*(3), 243–254. https://doi.org/10.1089/10430340360535797;WGROUP:STRING:PUBLICATION

Salauddin, M., Saha, S., Hossain, M. G., Okuda, K., & Shimada, M. (2024). Clinical Application of Adenovirus (AdV): A Comprehensive Review. *Viruses*, *16*(7), 1094. https://doi.org/10.3390/V16071094

Sampson, A. T., Hlaváč, M., Gillman, A. C. T., Douradinha, B., & Gilbert, S. C. (2025). Developing the next-generation of adenoviral vector vaccines. *Human Vaccines & Immunotherapeutics*, *21*(1), 2514356. https://doi.org/10.1080/21645515.2025.2514356

Schröder, L. C., Frank, D., & Müller, O. J. (2023). Transcriptional Targeting Approaches in Cardiac Gene Transfer Using AAV Vectors. *Pathogens*, *12*(11), 1301. https://doi.org/10.3390/PATHOGENS12111301

Schwartz, U., Komatsu, T., Huber, C., Lagadec, F., Baumgartl, C., Silberhorn, E., Nuetzel, M., Rayne, F., Basyuk, E., Bertrand, E., Rehli, M., Wodrich, H., & Laengst, G. (2023). Changes in adenoviral chromatin organization precede early gene activation upon infection. *The EMBO Journal*, *42*(19), e114162–e114162. https://doi.org/10.15252/EMBJ.2023114162

Sharma, A., Li, X., Bangari, D. S., & Mittal, S. K. (2009). Adenovirus receptors and their implications in gene delivery. *Virus Research*, *143*(2), 184. https://doi.org/10.1016/J.VIRUSRES.2009.02.010

Shen, L. Z., Wu, W. X., Xu, D. H., Zheng, Z. C., Liu, X. Y., Ding, Q., Hua, Y. B., & Yao, K. (2002). Specific CEA-producing colorectal carcinoma cell killing with recombinant adenoviral containing cytosine deaminase gene. *World Journal of Gastroenterology*, *8*(2), 270–275. https://doi.org/10.3748/wjg.v8.i2.270

Shim, S. H., Lee, C. T., Hun Hah, J., Lee, J. J., Park, S. W., Heo, D. S., & Sung, M. W. (2009). Conditionally replicating adenovirus improves gene replication efficiency and anticancer effect of E1-deleted adenovirus carrying TRAIL in head and neck squamous cell carcinoma. *Cancer Science*, *101*(2), 482. https://doi.org/10.1111/J.1349-7006.2009.01409.X

Shim, S. H., Lee, C. T., Hun Hah, J., Lee, J. J., Park, S. W., Heo, D. S., & Sung, M. W. (2010). Conditionally replicating adenovirus improves gene replication efficiency and anticancer effect of E1-deleted adenovirus carrying TRAIL in head and neck squamous cell carcinoma. *Cancer Science*, *101*(2), 482–487. https://doi.org/10.1111/J.1349-7006.2009.01409.X,

Shirley, J. L., de Jong, Y. P., Terhorst, C., & Herzog, R. W. (2020). Immune Responses to Viral Gene Therapy Vectors. *Molecular Therapy*, *28*(3), 709. https://doi.org/10.1016/J.YMTHE.2020.01.001

Sibbald, B. (2001). Death but one unintended consequence of gene-therapy trial. *CMAJ: Canadian Medical Association Journal*, *164*(11), 1612. https://pmc.ncbi.nlm.nih.gov/articles/PMC81135/

Small, E. J., Carducci, M. A., Burke, J. M., Rodriguez, R., Fong, L., van Ummersen, L., Yu, D. C., Aimi, J., Ando, D., Working, P., Kirn, D., & Wilding, G. (2006). A Phase I Trial of Intravenous CG7870, a Replication-Selective, Prostate-Specific Antigen–Targeted Oncolytic Adenovirus, for the Treatment of Hormone-Refractory, Metastatic Prostate Cancer. *Molecular Therapy*, *14*(1), 107–117. https://doi.org/10.1016/J.YMTHE.2006.02.011

Suarez-Amaran, L., Song, L., Tretiakova, A. P., Mikhail, S. A., & Samulski, R. J. (2025). AAV vector development, back to the future. *Molecular Therapy*, *33*(5), 1903–1936. https://doi.org/10.1016/J.YMTHE.2025.03.064

Suzuki, M., Singh, R. N., & Crystal, R. G. (1998). Pharmacological expression in rat hepatocytes of a gene transferred by an adenovirus vector enabled by a chimeric promoter containing multiple cyclic adenosine monophosphate response elements. *Hepatology*, *27*(1), 160–165. https://doi.org/10.1002/hep.510270125

Swift, E. A., Pollard, S. M., & Parker, A. L. (2022). Engineering Cancer Selective Virotherapies: Are the Pieces of the Puzzle Falling into Place? *Human Gene Therapy*, *33*(21–22), 1109. https://doi.org/10.1089/HUM.2022.178

Syyam, A., Nawaz, A., Ijaz, A., Sajjad, U., Fazil, A., Irfan, S., Muzaffar, A., Shahid, M., Idrees, M., Malik, K., & Afzal, S. (2022). Adenovirus vector system: construction, history and therapeutic applications. *BioTechniques*, *73*(6), 297–305. https://doi.org/10.2144/BTN-2022-0051;WEBSITE:WEBSITE:TFOPB;REQUESTEDJOURNAL:JOURNAL:IBTN20;PAGEGROUP:STRING:PUBLICATION

Tang, J., Amin, M. Al, & Campian, J. L. (2025). Past, Present, and Future of Viral Vector Vaccine Platforms: A Comprehensive Review. *Vaccines*, *13*(5), 524. https://doi.org/10.3390/VACCINES13050524

Tarasenko, T. N., Rosas, O. R., Singh, L. N., Kristaponis, K., Vernon, H., & McGuire, P. J. (2015). A New Mouse Model of Mild Ornithine Transcarbamylase Deficiency (spf-j) Displays Cerebral Amino Acid Perturbations at Baseline and upon Systemic Immune Activation. *PLoS ONE*, *10*(2), e0116594–e0116594. https://doi.org/10.1371/JOURNAL.PONE.0116594

Terao, S., Shirakawa, T., Kubo, S., Bishunu, A., Lee, S. J., Goda, K., Tsukuda, M., Hamada, K., Tagawa, M., Takenaka, A., Fujisawa, M., & Gotoh, A. (2007). Midkine Promoter-Based Conditionally Replicative Adenovirus for Targeting Midkine-Expressing Human Bladder Cancer Model. *Urology*, *70*(5), 1009–1013. https://doi.org/10.1016/j.urology.2007.07.003

Tessarollo, N. G., Domingues, A. C. M., Antunes, F., da Luz, J. C. D. S., Rodrigues, O. A., Cerqueira, O. L. D., & Strauss, B. E. (2021). Nonreplicating Adenoviral Vectors: Improving Tropism and Delivery of Cancer Gene Therapy. *Cancers*, *13*(8), 1863. https://doi.org/10.3390/CANCERS13081863

Thacker, E. E., Timares, L., & Matthews, Q. L. (2009). Strategies to overcome host immunity to adenovirus vectors in vaccine development. *Expert Review of Vaccines*, *8*(6), 761. https://doi.org/10.1586/ERV.09.29

Thomas, C. E., Edwards, P., Wickham, T. J., Castro, M. G., & Lowenstein, P. R. (2002). Adenovirus Binding to the Coxsackievirus and Adenovirus Receptor or Integrins Is Not Required To Elicit Brain Inflammation but Is Necessary To Transduce Specific Neural Cell Types. *Journal of Virology*, *76*(7), 3452. https://doi.org/10.1128/JVI.76.7.3452-3460.2002

Toyoda, E., Doi, R., Kami, K., Mori, T., Ito, D., Koizumi, M., Kida, A., Nagai, K., Ito, T., Masui, T., Wada, M., Tagawa, M., & Uemoto, S. (2008). Midkine promoter-based conditionally replicative adenovirus therapy for midkine-expressing human pancreatic cancer. *Journal of Experimental and Clinical Cancer Research*, *27*(1), 1–13. https://doi.org/10.1186/1756-9966-27-30/FIGURES/6

Trivedi, P. D., Byrne, B. J., & Corti, M. (2023). Evolving Horizons: Adenovirus Vectors' Timeless Influence on Cancer, Gene Therapy and Vaccines. *Viruses*, *15*(12), 2378. https://doi.org/10.3390/V15122378

Ucdal, M., Yazarkan, Y., Sonmez, G., Celtikci, B., & Balaban, Y. (2025). Alpha-fetoprotein: A Multifaceted Player in Cancer Biology. *Euroasian Journal of Hepato-Gastroenterology*, *15*(1), 72. https://doi.org/10.5005/JP-JOURNALS-10018-1458

Van Putten, E. H. P., Kleijn, A., Van Beusechem, V. W., Noske, D., Lamers, C. H. J., De Goede, A. L., Idema, S., Hoefnagel, D., Kloezeman, J. J., Fueyo, J., Lang, F. F., Teunissen, C. E., Vernhout, R. M., Bakker, C., Gerritsen, W., Curiel, D. T., Vulto, A., Lamfers, M. L. M., & Dirven, C. M. F. (2022). Convection Enhanced Delivery of the Oncolytic Adenovirus Delta24-RGD in Patients with Recurrent GBM: A Phase I Clinical Trial Including Correlative Studies. *Clinical Cancer Research*, *28*(8), 1572. https://doi.org/10.1158/1078-0432.CCR-21-3324

Vemula, S. V, & Mittal, S. K. (2010). Production of adenovirus vectors and their use as a delivery system for influenza vaccines. *Expert Opinion on Biological Therapy*, *10*(10), 1469–1487. https://doi.org/10.1517/14712598.2010.519332

Wang, J. H., Gessler, D. J., Zhan, W., Gallagher, T. L., & Gao, G. (2024). Adeno-associated virus as a delivery vector for gene therapy of human diseases. *Signal Transduction and Targeted Therapy 2024 9:1*, *9*(1), 1–33. https://doi.org/10.1038/s41392-024-01780-w

Wang, Y. G., Huang, P. P., Zhang, R., Ma, B. Y., Zhou, X. M., & Sun, Y. F. (2016). Targeting adeno-associated virus and adenoviral gene therapy for hepatocellular carcinoma. *Http://Www.Wjgnet.Com/*, *22*(1), 326–337. https://doi.org/10.3748/WJG.V22.I1.326

Weklak, D., Pembaur, D., Koukou, G., Jönsson, F., Hagedorn, C., & Kreppel, F. (2021). Genetic and Chemical Capsid Modifications of Adenovirus Vectors to Modulate Vector–Host Interactions. *Viruses*, *13*(7), 1300. https://doi.org/10.3390/V13071300

Wersto, R. P., Rosenthal, E. R., Seth, P. K., Eissa, N. T., & Donahue, R. E. (1998). Recombinant, Replication-Defective Adenovirus Gene Transfer Vectors Induce Cell Cycle Dysregulation and Inappropriate Expression of Cyclin Proteins. *Journal of Virology*, *72*(12), 9491–9502. https://doi.org/10.1128/JVI.72.12.9491-9502.1998,

Wong, C. M., McFall, E. R., Burns, J. K., & Parks, R. J. (2013). The role of chromatin in adenoviral vector function. *Viruses*, *5*(6), 1500–1515. https://doi.org/10.3390/v5061500

Wozniak, J., Wandtke, T., Kopinski, P., & Chorostowska-Wynimko, J. (2015). Challenges and Prospects for Alpha-1 Antitrypsin Deficiency Gene Therapy. *Human Gene Therapy*, *26*(11), 709. https://doi.org/10.1089/HUM.2015.044

Wu, S., Huang, J., Zhang, Z., Wu, J., Zhang, J., Hu, H., Zhu, T., Zhang, J., Luo, L., Fan, P., Wang, B., Chen, C., Chen, Y., Song, X., Wang, Y., Si, W., Sun, T., Wang, X., Hou, L., & Chen, W. (2021). Safety, tolerability, and immunogenicity of an aerosolised adenovirus type-5 vector-based COVID-19 vaccine (Ad5-nCoV) in adults: preliminary report of an open-label and randomised phase 1 clinical trial. *The Lancet. Infectious Diseases*, *21*(12), 1654. https://doi.org/10.1016/S1473-3099(21)00396-0

Xu, Y., Le, H., Wu, Q., Wang, N., & Gong, C. (2025). Advancements in CRISPR/Cas systems for disease treatment. *Acta Pharmaceutica Sinica B*, *15*(6), 2818–2844. https://doi.org/10.1016/J.APSB.2025.05.007

Yaghoubi, S. S., & Gambhir, S. S. (2007). PET imaging of herpes simplex virus type 1 thymidine kinase (HSV1-tk) or mutant HSV1-sr39tk reporter gene expression in mice and humans using [18F]FHBG. *Nature Protocols*, *1*(6), 3069–3075. https://doi.org/10.1038/NPROT.2006.459,

Yahata, K., Maeshima, K., Sone, T., Ando, T., Okabe, M., Imamoto, N., & Imamoto, F. (2007). cHS4 Insulator-mediated Alleviation of Promoter Interference during Cell-based Expression of Tandemly Associated Transgenes. *Journal of Molecular Biology*, *374*(3), 580–590. https://doi.org/10.1016/J.JMB.2007.09.054

Yang, Z., Bai, H., Hu, L., Kong, D., Li, G., Zhao, C., Feng, L., Cheng, S., Shou, J., Zhang, W., & Zhang, K. (2022). Improving the diagnosis of prostate cancer by telomerase-positive circulating tumor cells: A prospective pilot study. *EClinicalMedicine*, *43*, 101161. https://doi.org/10.1016/J.ECLINM.2021.101161

Yu, D. Bin, Zhong, S. Y., Yang, M., Wang, Y. G., Qian, Q. J., Zheng, S., & Liu, X. Y. (2009). Potent antitumor activity of double-regulated oncolytic adenovirus-mediated ST13 for colorectal cancer. *Cancer Science*, *100*(4), 678. https://doi.org/10.1111/J.1349-7006.2009.01110.X

Yu, W., & Fang, H. (2007). Clinical Trials with Oncolytic Adenovirus in China. *Current Cancer Drug Targets*, *7*(2), 141–148. https://doi.org/10.2174/156800907780058817

Yuanhao Li, Yu Chen, Jeanette Dilley, Trini Arroyo, Derek Ko, Peter Working, & De-Chao Yu. (2003). Carcinoembryonic antigen-producing cell-specific

oncolytic adenovirus, OV798, for colorectal cancer therapy. *Mol Cancer Ther*, *2*(10), 1003–1009.
Zhang, H., Takayama, K., Zhang, L., Uchino, J., Harada, A., Harada, T., Hisasue, J., Nakagaki, N., Zhou, C., & Nakanishi, Y. (2009). Tetracycline-inducible promoter-based conditionally replicative adenoviruses for the control of viral replication. *Cancer Gene Therapy*, *16*(5), 415–422. https://doi.org/10.1038/CGT.2008.101;KWRD=BIOMEDICINE
Zhang, H., Wang, H., An, Y., & Chen, Z. (2023). Construction and application of adenoviral vectors. *Molecular Therapy. Nucleic Acids*, *34*, 102027. https://doi.org/10.1016/J.OMTN.2023.09.004
Zhang, W., Marte, I., Seuthe, C., Gadepalli, R., Pareek, P., Gupta, A., & Chavan, S. R. (2025). Oncolytic viruses in head and neck cancers: clinical applications and therapeutic potential. *Frontiers in Microbiology*, *16*, 1641267. https://doi.org/10.3389/FMICB.2025.1641267
Zhang, W., Muck-Hausl, M., Wang, J., Sun, C., Gebbing, M., Miskey, C., Ivics, Z., Izsvak, Z., & Ehrhardt, A. (2013). Integration Profile and Safety of an Adenovirus Hybrid-Vector Utilizing Hyperactive Sleeping Beauty Transposase for Somatic Integration. *PLOS ONE*, *8*(10), e75344. https://doi.org/10.1371/JOURNAL.PONE.0075344
Zhang, W. W., Li, L., Li, D., Liu, J., Li, X., Li, W., Xu, X., Zhang, M. J., Chandler, L. A., Lin, H., Hu, A., Xu, W., & Lam, D. M. K. (2018). The First Approved Gene Therapy Product for Cancer Ad-p53 (Gendicine): 12 Years in the Clinic. *Human Gene Therapy*, *29*(2), 160–179. https://doi.org/10.1089/HUM.2017.218,
Zhao, H., Chen, M., & Pettersson, U. (2013). Identification of adenovirus-encoded small RNAs by deep RNA sequencing. *Virology*, *442*(2), 148–155. https://doi.org/10.1016/J.VIROL.2013.04.006
Zhou, X., Xie, G., Wang, S., Wang, Y., Zhang, K., Zheng, S., Chu, L., Xiao, L., Yu, Y., Zhang, Y., & Liu, X. (2012). Potent and Specific Antitumor Effect for Colorectal Cancer by CEA and Rb Double Regulated Oncolytic Adenovirus Harboring ST13 Gene. *PLOS ONE*, *7*(10), e47566. https://doi.org/10.1371/JOURNAL.PONE.0047566

Author Biographies

Praveenya Tirunagari is a multidisciplinary life-science researcher whose work bridges genomics, bioinformatics, and molecular biomedical research. She has contributed to scholarly work on the application of genomics for identifying novel microbial species. She is currently pursuing her Ph. D at the Institute for Cardiovascular Physiology, Goethe University, Frankfurt, underscoring her involvement in advanced translational research at the interface of computational biology and human disease mechanisms

Kotthapalli Prashanth is a biologist whose research primarily focuses on infectious disease biology, with a particular emphasis on virology. He also possesses a strong interest in food science, nanotechnology, microbiome, and cancer studies, having contributed to related projects. He has authored several book chapters and research articles published in peer-reviewed journals.

Dr. Sumana Kumar is an Associate Professor in the Department of Microbiology, holds Ph.D. in Microbiology specializing in Mycology, Plant Pathology, Microbial Biotechnology, and Disease Diagnostics. She has over two decades of teaching and research experience and published over 60 articles in national and international journals.

CHAPTER 2

A SAFE, FAVORABLE AND EFFECTIVE VIRAL VECTOR FOR GENE THERAPY: ADENO-ASSOCIATED VIRUS (AAV)

ASUMAN ÖZGÖZ, PHD

Department of Medical Genetics, Kastamonu University, Kastamonu, Türkiye.

Abstract

Gene therapy is a revolutionary therapeutic approach that aims to treat genetic disorders by modifying gene expression within target cells through viral, non-viral, or physical delivery approaches. Among these approaches, gene replacement therapy, involving delivery of a functional version of a defective gene into living cells, is one of the most widely applied strategies. FDA approval of Luxturna for Leber congenital amaurosis type 2 (LCA2) in 2017 represented a major milestone for gene replacement therapy. Adeno-associated viruses (AAVs) are among the most commonly used vectors in gene therapy applications. AAVs are non-enveloped viral vectors carrying a single-stranded DNA genome enclosed within a capsid, and different serotypes of AAVs differ in their capsid structures and genomic characteristics. Because of their relatively low pathogenicity and their ability to support sustained transgene expression across multiple tissues, AAV vectors have become important delivery systems in clinical gene therapy. In addition, AAV vectors possess broad tissue tropism, adaptable manufacturing strategies, and generally favorable safety profiles. Importantly, AAV rarely integrates into the host genome. Certain AAV serotypes can efficiently enter target cells and achieve effective transgene expression, thereby enhancing transduction efficiency. Recombinant AAV (rAAV) vectors have been developed and modified to improve specificity for treatment of various disorders, including ophthalmologic, neurological, metabolic, hematologic, neuromuscular, cardiovascular diseases, and cancers. Several AAV-mediated gene therapies have progressed to Phase III clinical trials, and FDA-approved AAV-based therapeutics are currently available for disorders including spinal muscular atrophy (SMA), Leber congenital amaurosis type 2 (LCA2), hemophilia A, and hemophilia B.

Keywords: Gene therapy, Adeno-Associated Virus (AAV), viral vector, EMA-FDA approvals, low pathogenicity.

1. Introduction

Gene therapy represents an important therapeutic strategy for treatment of genetic disorders through transfer of specific genetic material into cells in order to modify cellular function. The main objective of gene therapy is to restore or compensate for defective or missing genes associated with development of genetic diseases. Successful application of gene therapy largely depends on efficient delivery of therapeutic genetic material into appropriate target cells and tissues within the body (Bulcha et al., 2021; Mendell et al., 2021).

The systems used to transport therapeutic genes are known as vectors or gene delivery vehicles and are generally classified as viral or non-viral vectors. Current viral vector-based gene therapy mainly employs in vivo and ex vivo delivery approaches. In in vivo applications, viral vectors are administered directly into the patient to transfer therapeutic transgenes into target tissues. In current gene therapy applications, retroviruses, adenoviruses (Ads), and adeno-associated viruses (AAVs) are among the most preferred viral vectors. In contrast, ex vivo gene therapy involves obtaining cells from the patient, modifying these cells outside the body through viral vector-mediated transgene delivery, and subsequently reintroducing the genetically modified cells into the patient (Bulcha et al., 2021; Mendell et al., 2021). Retrovirus-derived vectors are suitable for hematopoietic and different stem cell types in ex vivo gene therapies, whereas AAVs and Ads are primarily utilized in in vivo gene therapy applications involving postmitotic cells (Wu et al., 2022).

Gene therapy can repair pathogenic mutations through three principal approaches: (1) enhancing expression of a therapeutic gene or gene product; (2) silencing the mutant gene; and (3) substituting the defective gene with a functional counterpart. Gene silencing approaches may be achieved using methods such as short hairpin RNA (shRNA)-mediated approaches or zinc finger silencing techniques. These approaches may be performed either permanently through genome modification technologies such as zinc finger nucleases (ZFNs) or transiently through episomal vector-mediated delivery systems. AAV vectors can support both transient and permanent therapeutic approaches (Garriga-Canut et al., 2012; Agustín-Pavón et al., 2016; Pereira et al., 2017; Chandrasegaran, 2017; Bulcha et al., 2021; Mendell et al., 2021).

Because of their low immunogenicity, acceptable safety profile, and capacity to maintain continuous transgene expression across multiple tissues, AAV vectors are widely preferred for gene therapy applications. The low frequency of integration into the host genome decreases the risk of insertional mutagenesis. AAVs also demonstrate broad tissue tropism and efficient transduction. Their usefulness as gene delivery vehicles is further supported by FDA-approved therapies using AAV vectors, such as Luxturna and Zolgensma, which have shown successful outcomes in genetic disorders. Furthermore, recent developments in vector design and capsid engineering continue to improve transduction efficiency and immune evasion properties, making AAVs a flexible platform for various therapeutic targets (Zwi-Dantsis et al., 2025). Besides capsid engineering, different immune evasion approaches have also demonstrated promising results. In a study conducted by Mehta et al., engineered CpG-depleted vectors (pNC182) were generated by reducing the total CpG content by 38% together with alteration of CpG-S motifs within the vector. CpG reduction did not negatively affect transgene expression or therapeutic efficacy in mouse models of familial lipoprotein lipase deficiency (LPLD), and CpG-depleted vectors achieved comparable therapeutic outcomes, including normalization of lipid levels, with a reduced immunogenic profile (Mehta et al., 2025).

Gene-coding DNA regions must be accompanied by regulatory sequences required for expression, including promoters, poly(A) signals, and AAV inverted terminal repeat sequences (ITRs), in order to facilitate gene transfer and sustained transgene expression in AAV vectors. However, inclusion of these elements reduces the available transgene capacity of AAV-based gene therapies. The packaging limit of an efficiently assembled AAV genome is approximately 4.8 kb. It is generally accepted that recombinant AAV (rAAV) vectors most efficiently accommodate transgenes up to approximately 3.5 kb in size. Numerous minigenes, which are minimally functional forms of larger transgenes compatible with AAV packaging capacity, have been rationally designed and functionally evaluated. The recent approval of Elevidys for Duchenne muscular dystrophy (DMD), utilizing a micro-dystrophin construct to compensate for the native dystrophin gene larger than 2200 kb, demonstrates the practical importance of the minigene strategy.

In addition to directly influencing vector capacity, transduction efficiency, and transgene expression patterns, optimization of AAV expression cassettes may also improve AAV packaging capacity. These expression cassettes include ITRs, enhancers, promoters, introns, post-transcriptional regulatory elements (PREs), and poly(A) signals, all of which may influence transgene expression patterns. Another strategy, known as dual or triple AAV vector delivery, increases vector capacity by separating large cDNA fragments into multiple components and packaging each fragment into separate AAV vectors (Kolesnik et al., 2024).

2. The Structure and Genome of the AAVs

In 1965, adeno-associated virus (AAV) was identified by Atchison and his colleagues as a contaminant during studies involving simian adenovirus type 1 (SV15) in rhesus monkey kidney cells (RMK). Since the virus was initially detected in adenovirus preparations, it was subsequently named adeno-associated virus (Atchison et al., 1965; Carter, 2004).

Because AAV is replication-deficient, it depends on helper viruses for productive replication in mammalian cells. Adenoviruses and herpesviruses are generally recognized as the primary helper viruses that support completion of the AAV life cycle. Although AAV can coexist in humans together with its helper viruses, early investigations indicated that it is not linked to any clearly defined human disease (Carter, 2004).

AAVs are small, non-enveloped viruses belonging to the Parvoviridae family and Dependoparvovirus genus. Their nomenclature and taxonomic classification are based on the requirement for helper viruses during replication. AAVs are capable of infecting multiple vertebrate species, including humans and non-human primates. AAV contains a hexagonal capsid approximately 26 nm in diameter and carries a single-stranded DNA (ssDNA) genome of nearly 4.7 kb. The viral genome contains T-shaped ITRs positioned at both ends and can exist in either sense (plus) or antisense (minus) orientations. Three principal coding regions are present within the AAV genome: AAP, which encodes an assembly-activating protein required for capsid formation; Cap, which encodes the structural capsid proteins responsible for cell attachment and genome protection; and Rep, which participates in viral replication and genome packaging (Naso et al., 2017; Au et al., 2022).

VP1, VP2, and VP3 are the three structural proteins forming the viral capsid and are present at an approximate ratio of 1:1:10 (VP1:VP2:VP3), together generating sixty capsid subunits. The ITR regions located at both ends of the genome mainly function as replication origins and packaging signals. The Rep gene produces four proteins—Rep40, Rep52, Rep68, and Rep78—which are named according to their molecular weights and play essential roles during viral replication. The cap gene encodes the three capsid proteins through alternative splicing and utilization of different translation start codons. In addition, AAP is translated from an alternative reading frame located within the cap coding sequence and contributes to efficient viral assembly (Sonntag et al., 2010; Sonntag et al., 2011; Wang et al., 2019).

3. AAV Serotypes

AAV serotypes are classified based on variations in their capsid proteins, which influence their ability to infect distinct cells and tissues. Different serotypes exhibit distinct tissue tropisms and immunogenic profiles, making them relevant for targeted gene therapy applications. The six historically well-characterized AAV serotypes include AAV1–6, each with unique properties and target tissue specificities. For instance, AAV2 is the most extensively studied serotype and has wide tissue tropism in the central nervous system and liver, while AAV4 is notable for its distinct antigenic profile and preference for sialic acid residues. The choice of serotype is crucial for optimizing gene delivery efficiency and minimizing immune responses in therapeutic applications (Issa et al., 2023).

Although more than one hundred divergent AAV serotypes or unique AAV variants have been identified in monkeys, bats, sea lions, goats, snakes, and other animals, it is generally accepted that 13 AAV serotypes (AAV1–13) have been identified to date. Each serotype displays distinct tissue and organ tropisms with different transduction efficiencies depending on the target site. Gene therapy applications strategically utilize the variability among AAV serotypes in order to target different cell and tissue types for therapeutic purposes (Zwi-Dantsis et al., 2025).

Two serotypes, AAV4 and AAV5, differ more from the others in terms of capsid amino acid sequences. AAV5 is the most phylogenetically distinct serotype, sharing approximately 58% capsid similarity with AAV2 and AAV8, as well as 57% similarity with AAV10. However, the other serotypes frequently used in gene transfer applications exhibit nearly 80% capsid similarity. Sequence variations are primarily associated with conformationally distinct loops within the VP architecture, which are linked to receptor interaction, transduction efficiency, and antigenic properties. These loops are important when considering variations in tissue tropism, antigenic properties, and the probability of cross-reactive immune responses among serotypes (Pupo et al., 2022).

Tissue tropism is associated with interactions between cell glycans, cell receptors, and serotype-specific features of the rAAV capsid. Many AAV serotypes initially bind to primary receptors, including glycans and proteoglycans such as terminal galactose (Gal), heparan sulfate, and different sialic acid (SA) linkage variations (Pipe et al., 2019).

AAV serotypes can be divided into three groups according to their glycan receptor usage: AAV1, AAV4, AAV5, and AAV6 utilize sialic acid (SA); AAV9 utilizes Gal; and AAV2 utilizes Heparan Sulfate Proteoglycan (HSPG). For AAV7, AAV8, AAVrh10, AAV11, and AAV12–15, it remains unclear whether they possess major glycan receptors. Classification based on glycan receptor utilization is likely oversimplified; however, the actual profile of glycan recognition is more complex (Pupo et al., 2022).

AAV1 gained clinical importance because Glybera, the first approved AAV-based gene therapy in Europe, used an AAV1 vector for the treatment of lipoprotein lipase deficiency (Pupo et al., 2022). AAV1 is characterized by sialic acid-mediated cell entry and lack of heparin binding (Huang et al., 2016). Its ability to transduce several tissues, including skeletal and cardiac muscle (Palomeque et al., 2007; Su et al., 2008), retina (Auricchio et al., 2001), and endothelial and vascular smooth muscle cells (Chen et al., 2005), supports its relevance for gene therapy applications.

AAV2, which was first identified in 1965, is the most extensively studied serotype and is widely utilized in both research and clinical studies because of its affinity for heparan sulfate. The tissue tropism of AAV2 includes skeletal muscle (Lisowski et al., 2015), the central nervous system (CNS) (Griffey et al., 2006), retina (Wassmer et al., 2017), hepatocytes (Logan et al., 2017), and renal tissue (Haddad et al., 2021).

AAV3 was initially disregarded because of its poor in vitro transduction efficiency in murine cell lines; however, it subsequently showed strong potential for targeting hepatocytes and human liver cancer cells (Hadi et al., 2024; Vercauteren et al., 2016). AAV4 and AAV5 exhibit unique transduction capacities because of their different antigenic profiles and receptor usage patterns, particularly in retinal cells (Weber et al., 2003) and the central nervous system (Davidson et al., 2000). AAV6 demonstrates high transduction efficiency in multiple tissues, including skeletal muscle (Qiao et al., 2010) and airway epithelia (Duncan et al., 2018). AAV7, AAV8, and AAV9, which are derived from humans and non-human primates, exhibit strong tropism for hepatic, skeletal, and cardiac muscle tissues (Issa et al., 2023). AAV9 is particularly important for neurological therapy because it is able to cross the blood–brain barrier (BBB) (Duque et al., 2009). The field of AAV research continues to expand through identification of AAV10, AAV11, AAV12, and AAV13, which exhibit broad tissue tropisms and distinct cellular targets and contribute to current understanding of AAV cell entry pathways and therapeutic applications (Issa et al., 2023) **(Table 1-1).**

Table 1-1. Reported tissue tropism, receptor/glycan usage, and selected capsid-associated post-translational modifications of natural AAV serotypes (Pupo et al., 2022; Issa et al., 2023; Matsuzaka & Yashiro, 2024)

AAV Serotype	Organ/Tissue Tropism	Post-Translational Modifications (PTMs)	Glycan Ligand Specificity	Additional Information
AAV1	Skeletal muscle, heart, glial and ependymal cells	Limited evidence available	Sialic acid	Efficient transduction of muscle and heart tissues
AAV2	Retina, liver, kidney, CNS, skeletal muscle	Limited evidence available	Heparan sulfate proteoglycan (HSPG)	Well-studied; broad tissue tropism
AAV3	Liver hepatocytes, cochlear inner hair cells	Acetylation, phosphorylation, glycosylation	HSPG, FGFR1, LR, hHGFR	High transduction efficiency, especially in liver

AAV Serotype	Organ/Tissue Tropism	Post-Translational Modifications (PTMs)	Glycan Ligand Specificity	Additional Information
AAV4	Limited data; possibly nerve and muscle tissues	Limited evidence available	Sialic acid	Limited information available
AAV5	Retinal cells, airway epithelia, liver, CNS	Ubiquitination, phosphorylation, SUMOylation, glycosylation	Sialic acid	Transduces neural and airway tissues effectively
AAV6	Muscles, liver	Limited evidence available, likely HSPG related	Heparin, possibly HSPG	Similar to AAV2; efficient in muscle and liver transduction
AAV7	Murine skeletal muscle, liver, neurons	Glycosylation, phosphorylation, SUMOylation, acetylation	Does not bind heparin; interacts with other glycans	Low human seroprevalence, potential for clinical applications
AAV8	Liver, muscle, pancreas, cardiac tissue	Phosphorylation, glycosylation, acetylation	Not binding heparin; likely galactose	Very high hepatotropism and transduction efficiency
AAV9	Liver, muscle, CNS (crosses blood-brain barrier)	Glycosylation, ubiquitination, phosphorylation, SUMOylation, acetylation	Terminal N-linked galactose	Broad tissue transduction, especially CNS
AAV10	NHP intestine, hepatocytes, lymph nodes, CNS	Limited evidence available	Limited evidence available	Limited data available

AAV Serotype	Organ/Tissue Tropism	Post-Translational Modifications (PTMs)	Glycan Ligand Specificity	Additional Information
AAV11	NHP CNS neurons, astrocytes	Limited evidence available	Limited evidence available	Emerging serotype, limited data
AAV13	Likely HSPG binding	Limited evidence available	HSPG (unknown primary receptor)	Shares structural similarity with AAV2/3

4. How AAVs Act as Vectors

Viruses are biological agents that enter host cells and replicate their genomes within these cells. As a virus, AAV also has the ability to deliver its genome into host cells (Naso et al., 2017; Matsuzaka & Yashiro, 2024).

AAV enters human cells through clathrin-coated vesicles, a process triggered by interactions between the viral capsid and cell surface receptors. The steps involved in this process are as follows: (1) attachment to the cell membrane; (2) endocytosis (plasma membrane penetration); (3) endosomal transport; (4) escape from late endosomes and lysosomes; (5) transport to the nucleus; (6) formation of the replicative form of the AAV genome (double-stranded DNA); (7) Rep gene expression; (8) genome replication; (9) Cap gene expression and production of the next-generation single-stranded DNA genomes; (10) assembly of complete viral particles; and (11) release from infected cells (Ryu, 2017).

AAV primarily utilizes cell surface proteoglycans as receptors to attach to the cell surface and enter cells. After cellular entry, AAV is transported through the endocytic pathway. During this process, the virus avoids degradation by escaping from endosomes through disruption of the endosomal lipid bilayer, a mechanism known as endosomal escape. The VP1 protein located within the AAV capsid contains a phospholipase A2 (PLA2) domain, which plays an important role in endosomal and lysosomal escape as well as viral infectivity. Experimental studies demonstrated that the PLA2 region of the murine minute virus contributes to endosomal escape through formation of lipolytic pores (Matsuzaka & Yashiro, 2024).

5. rAAV Manufacturing Methods

Mammalian cells, mainly human embryonic kidney 293 (HEK293) cells and their derivatives, as well as less frequently HeLa, baby hamster kidney (BHK), and Chinese hamster ovary (CHO) cells, are used in AAV production platforms. These systems employ viral transduction or plasmid transfection to provide the genetic material required for recombinant AAV (rAAV) production. In addition, baculovirus-based systems using Spodoptera frugiperda (Sf9) insect cells are also utilized as non-mammalian production platforms. Producer cell lines and stable packaging systems have likewise been applied for rAAV production following induction by chemicals or helper viruses. Currently, two commercially approved AAV products are produced using the Sf9-baculovirus system, whereas five are produced using HEK293-based systems (Reid et al., 2024).

The production of rAAV drug products is commonly divided into two stages: upstream and downstream processing. The upstream stage determines important vector properties, including yield, integrity, infectivity, and potency. Parameters such as post-translational capsid modifications, residual plasmid and host-cell DNA packaging, full-to-empty capsid ratios, and other product-related contaminants are assessed during this stage. The downstream process generally includes cell lysis, nuclease treatment, capture and purification by chromatography, concentration and buffer exchange, ion-exchange chromatography, ultracentrifugation, enrichment of full capsids, formulation, and final filling procedures (Smith et al., 2018; Srivastava et al., 2021).

Over the past two decades, many novel AAV vectors have been developed in addition to naturally occurring AAV serotypes. Different engineering approaches have been used to generate hybrid vectors with improved transduction efficiency, altered immunogenicity, or restricted tissue tropism toward specific cell types. These engineered vectors include combinatorial, chimeric, and mosaic vector systems. Mosaic capsids contain subunits derived from different serotypes selected according to receptor interaction and intracellular trafficking characteristics. In contrast, chimeric vectors generally contain modified capsid proteins generated through DNA shuffling and domain-swapping techniques intended to alter specific amino acid residues (Issa et al., 2023).

Capsid engineering methods: Intermolecular joining strategies have been shown to help overcome limitations associated with rAAV packaging capacity, enabling delivery of transgenes larger than the conventional carrying capacity of standard AAV vectors, including human coagulation factor VIII cDNA. Capsid engineering is considered one of the more practical approaches for improving the therapeutic potential of AAV vectors because of the close association between capsid structure and vector function. Early studies investigating AAV capsid modification were based on observations that capsid proteins derived from different AAV serotypes share substantial structural similarity and are capable of assembling into functional chimeric particles. Chimeric AAVs have been reported to combine characteristics of individual parental serotypes while also displaying properties not observed in the original vectors (Lisowski et al., 2015).

The structural and functional diversity of viral proteins is influenced by post-translational modifications (PTMs), which may affect viral infectivity and transduction efficiency. PTMs include acetylation, glycosylation, SUMOylation, phosphorylation, and ubiquitination. Previous studies have shown that certain PTMs can enhance AAV transduction efficiency under both in vitro and in vivo conditions. These modifications enable viruses to adapt to host cellular barriers and increase infectivity. The type and abundance of PTMs acquired by capsid proteins during AAV packaging may vary depending on serotype. Such modifications in recombinant AAV vectors, including AAV1-rh10, likely contribute to infectivity within host cells. Restrictive effects associated with capsid-specific PTMs have also been reported, and in silico analyses have contributed to identification of these regions. For example, AAV transduction efficiency has been enhanced both in vitro and in vivo through capsid mutations targeting phosphorylation sites involving serine, tyrosine, and threonine residues, as well as ubiquitination sites involving lysine residues (Mary et al., 2019).

Epidermal growth factor receptor protein tyrosine kinase (EGFR-PTK) phosphorylates tyrosine residues on AAV2 capsids, resulting in ubiquitination and reduced intracellular transport toward the nucleus. Improved transduction efficiency at lower vector doses may be achieved using surface-exposed tyrosine residues such as Y444F and Y730F carrying point mutations. Compared with wild-type AAV2, vectors containing the triple mutation Y444F/Y500F/Y730F demonstrated approximately 130-

fold greater transgene expression in murine fibroblasts and 30–80-fold higher levels of in vivo gene transfer to murine hepatocytes (Pupo et al., 2022).

The mutant AAV2 vector K258Q demonstrated minimal transduction together with reduced levels of SUMO-1/2/3 proteins. PTMs identified in AAV5 include glycosylation at N292, ubiquitination at K122, K451, and K639, and HexNAcylation at residues N308, T376, and N428. In AAV5 mutant vectors carrying phosphorylation-neutralizing mutations at threonine (T107A) and serine residues (S268A, S652A, and S658A), gene transfer efficiency was increased both in vitro and in vivo (Mary et al., 2019).

Different capsid engineering approaches have also been developed to modify AAV tropism, transduction efficiency, and immunogenicity. Among these approaches, peptide/protein insertions and capsid DNA shuffling are commonly used methods for generating modified AAV capsids (Issa et al., 2023).

1. Insertions of proteins and peptides: AAV chimeric capsids can be generated by inserting peptides or proteins into specific VP regions as an alternative to transferring motifs between different serotypes. The primary objective of these insertions is to alter the tropism of the native AAV serotype. In one study, a chimeric AAV2 capsid containing a fusion protein (anti-CD34 scAb-VP2) instead of VP2 was generated to selectively target CD34-positive hematopoietic stem cells. The chimeric vector demonstrated significantly increased infectivity toward the ordinarily refractory $CD34^+$ KG-1 human acute myeloid leukemia cell line (Yang et al., 1998).

To introduce a selective and specifically targeted tumor cell, an anti-Her2/neu DARPin was inserted into the N-terminal region of AAV2 VP2. DARPins are 14–17 kDa high-affinity binding proteins considered alternatives to antibodies. DARPin-modified AAV vectors significantly inhibited Her2/neu-positive tumor growth without inducing lethal liver toxicity (Münch et al., 2013).

2. Capsid DNA shuffling: DNA shuffling is a recombination-based technique that generates diversity through integration of beneficial mutations derived from multiple genes. This approach enables rapid evolution of both single-gene and multigene traits requiring multiple sequence variations for improved phenotypes. As an example of this method, a highly infectious strain termed Chimeric-1829 was selected from a chimeric capsid library composed of randomly fragmented and reassembled capsid DNA sequences derived from AAV serotypes 1–9. This clone contains genomic segments originating from AAV1, AAV2, AAV8, and AAV9. Although Chimeric-1829 utilizes heparan sulfate as its primary receptor similarly to AAV2, it demonstrates distinct immunological characteristics, enhanced transduction efficiency in melanoma cells, and altered tropism toward liver, skeletal muscle, and brain tissues (Li et al., 2008).

6. Preclinical and Clinical Study Examples Using AAV Vectors

More than three hundred clinical trials have so far evaluated AAV-based products for the treatment of 55 different disorders, reflecting the rapid development of AAV-mediated gene therapy. These extensive investigations have resulted in multiple approvals in both the United States and Europe. In the early 2000s, a Phase I clinical study investigated the safety and efficacy of an AAV2 vector in patients with cystic fibrosis. Analysis of transgene expression revealed several limitations of this Phase I AAV-based therapy, including poor transduction of target cells and restricted transgene expression caused by immune responses. Nevertheless, the trial confirmed the safety of the therapy and supported further development of AAV vectors as safer and more adaptable alternatives to adenovirus-based treatments. Lessons learned from cystic fibrosis studies contributed to development of Glybera, the first approved AAV gene therapy in Europe for lipoprotein lipase deficiency. Administration of Glybera as a single dose resulted in long-term reductions in both the frequency and severity of acute pancreatic inflammation and hospitalization, together with sustained therapeutic protein expression. However, despite its favorable safety profile, the manufacturing company (UniQure) did not renew the marketing authorization application, and the product was withdrawn because of its high cost (Zwi-Dantsis et al., 2025).

Ophthalmologic Disorders: Gene therapy studies targeting the retina account for approximately thirty-four percent of all clinical studies, with 30 of these trials employing AAV vectors for targeted delivery. A considerable proportion of these studies has progressed to advanced clinical phases, including Phase III and Phase II/III trials. Although AAV2, AAV4, AAV5, and AAV8 have been investigated in most studies, serotypes such as AAV7m8 and AAV2tYF have also been evaluated, and no severe AAV-associated adverse effects have been reported. Improvements observed in some patients suggest potential therapeutic benefits; however, despite numerous clinical studies, no new retinal gene therapy product has been approved since Luxturna in 2017 (Zwi-Dantsis et al., 2025).

Neurodegenerative Disorders (NDDs): Huntington's disease is an autosomal dominant neurodegenerative disorder associated with expanded CAG repeats. Although clinical studies investigating AAV-mediated gene therapy for Huntington's disease have been conducted, no definitive therapeutic outcomes have yet been achieved. Current approaches mainly focus on reducing levels of mutated huntingtin (mHTT) and its pathogenic effects. In one Phase I/II clinical study, twenty-six patients received bilateral caudate injections of AAV5-miHTT with magnetic resonance imaging (MRI) guidance in order to promote cleavage and degradation of mutated huntingtin mRNA. Although several animal studies demonstrated transgene expression in both injected and distant regions, the clinical study was limited by restricted tissue distribution and uncertainties related to the delivery approach (Kang et al., 2023).

Alzheimer's disease (AD) is a neurodegenerative disorder associated with age-related dementia and characterized by extracellular neuritic plaques and amyloid-β accumulation. These pathological changes contribute to degeneration of cholinergic neurons in the basal forebrain. More than one hundred clinical trials have investigated therapeutic approaches for AD. Apart from immunotherapy, there is currently no effective treatment capable of slowing disease progression in patients with cognitive impairment. AAV-mediated gene therapy approaches for AD remain limited. In one Phase I clinical study, ten patients with mild or moderate AD received bilateral administration of AAV2-nerve growth factor into the nucleus basalis. No serious adverse effects were observed, and the treatment was well tolerated. However, despite administration of a higher dose in a subsequent Phase II trial, no significant differences in cognitive or cerebral metabolic function were observed between treatment and placebo groups. Autopsy findings from three patients demonstrated that limited AAV2 diffusion prevented efficient entry into the nucleus basalis, making interpretation of therapeutic efficacy difficult. Therefore, restricted AAV distribution caused by tau, amyloid, and heparan sulfate proteoglycans may represent a major limitation for AD gene therapy (Kang et al., 2023).

In the nervous system, apoE is a multifunctional lipid transport protein that plays important roles in lipid metabolism and maintenance of neural homeostasis. The major apoE isoforms, E2, E3, and E4, exert distinct effects on neuronal recovery following injury. Increased expression of apoE4 has been associated with development of AD, whereas apoE2 appears to exert protective effects on neurons. Genome editing approaches using CRISPR/Cas9 may help convert apoE4 to apoE3 in induced pluripotent stem cells (iPSCs) associated with AD-related disorders. In addition, delivery of apoE2 cDNA (AAV-E2) through AAV vectors may increase apoE2 expression in order to protect neurons and reduce amyloid-β accumulation. Because the pathophysiology of AD remains incompletely understood, further clarification of these mechanisms will be important for development of future gene therapy approaches (Wang et al., 2025).

Lysosomal Storage Disorders: During the last decades, preclinical studies investigating gene therapy approaches for mucopolysaccharidosis type I (MPS I) have shown that restoration of α-L-iduronidase (IDUA) activity may provide therapeutic benefit. However, these studies have encountered difficulties in maintaining long-term IDUA expression, both systemically and within the central nervous system (CNS), in addition to limitations related to safety concerns associated with certain vector-based strategies.

Glycosaminoglycans accumulate within lysosomes as a consequence of IDUA enzyme dysfunction in MPS I, an inherited metabolic disorder. Most gene therapy studies investigating MPS I have utilized AAV vectors designed to deliver therapeutic DNA while lacking most viral coding sequences. Numerous investigations have successfully transduced MPS I cells through both in vitro and in vivo approaches. However, these methods have also raised concerns regarding insertional mutagenesis and transduction efficiency. Combined with gene-editing approaches such as CRISPR/Cas9, recent advances in AAV vector systems may provide a feasible therapeutic alternative for MPS I by improving vascular endothelial targeting while reducing hepatotoxicity (Hurt et al., 2021).

Using AAV8-mediated delivery of IDUA cDNA into the CNS of an MPS I murine model, studies demonstrated reduced lysosomal storage and increased IDUA activity mainly within the CNS without substantial effects on other organ systems. Multiple investigations using canine, feline, and rhesus macaque models have also evaluated AAV-mediated IDUA gene transfer into the CNS. Following treatment, cerebrospinal fluid analysis demonstrated persistent but limited IDUA activity in canine and feline models despite the absence of reduction in the number of transduced cells. These findings suggested that limited therapeutic efficacy might result from immune responses directed specifically against the IDUA enzyme. Consequently, it was proposed that immune responses against human IDUA may have limited therapeutic efficacy in these models (Wolf et al., 2011; Hurt et al., 2021).

Targeting Aging and Age-related Disorders with Gene Therapy: AAV vectors are being investigated for several aging-related therapeutic targets, including klotho for improving cognitive function and TERT for promoting longevity. In murine models of sarcopenia, AAV-mediated delivery of PGC-1α and Zfx3 has been shown to restore muscle function. In several age-associated disease models, AAV-based therapies targeting longevity-associated genes such as FGF21, α-klotho, and TGFβR2 improved both health status and lifespan. New approaches involving AAV-mediated delivery of Yamanaka factors (Oct4, Sox2, Klf4, and c-Myc; OSKM), including partial cellular reprogramming, aim to rejuvenate cells and tissues with the potential to extend lifespan and alleviate age-related disorders (Zwi-Dantsis et al., 2025).

Cardiovascular Disorders: Percutaneous delivery of AAV2/1-hSERCA2a enhanced SERCA2a expression and duration of expression in large animal models, significantly improving left ventricular function in a sheep model of heart failure and showing no adverse effects on myocardial fibrosis or necrosis (Mariani et al., 2011). A Phase I/2a clinical trial further demonstrated the safety of AAV1/SERCA2a therapy in patients with severe heart failure (Zhang et al., 2022). The calcineurin-NFAT signaling pathway regulates myocardial hypertrophic remodeling, which may eventually contribute to heart failure (HF) development. In murine models of severe HF, Remes et al. utilized AAV9-mediated delivery of decoy oligodeoxynucleotides (dODNs) targeting NFATc1-c4 in cardiomyocytes, thereby reducing NFAT activity and preserving cardiac function under conditions of excessive stress (Remes et al., 2021).

Normal cardiolipin production depends on the mitochondrial protein tafazzin (TAZ), and mutations in the TAZ gene are associated with Barth syndrome, a disorder linked to mitochondrial inner membrane dysfunction. AAV9-hTAZ gene therapy effectively improved cardiac function in a Taz-knockout animal model. Research investigating major contributors to cardiovascular disease (CVD), including hereditary and metabolic disorders such as atherosclerosis, hyperglycemia, and hypercholesterolemia, has produced promising findings. In controlled experimental studies, overexpression of proprotein convertase subtilisin/kexin type 9 (PCSK9) induced atherosclerosis in murine models. Liver-directed degradation of the low-density lipoprotein receptor (LDLR) using AAV-CRISPR vectors has also been proposed as a practical experimental strategy for investigating atherosclerosis. In two separate clinical trials, AAV-mediated LDLR gene therapy reduced plasma cholesterol levels in a limited number of patients (Zhang et al., 2022).

Another preclinical study investigated the role of SIRT6 using a mouse model of carotid plaque through AAV-SIRT6-mediated overexpression of SIRT6. By preventing degradation of HIF-1α and stimulating angiogenesis-related signaling pathways, SIRT6 was associated with increased cardiovascular risk. These findings suggested that suppression of SIRT6 may represent a potential strategy for limiting progression of atherosclerosis (Yang et al., 2021).

7. AAV-Based Approved Clinical Therapeutics

The number of approved AAV-based gene therapy products remains limited. Despite considerable progress in AAV-mediated gene therapy, many preclinical and clinical studies have been discontinued or terminated without resulting in approved therapeutics. Consequently, effective treatment options are still unavailable for many disorders, particularly rare diseases. One contributing factor may be the incomplete understanding of gene therapy mechanisms, especially those associated with AAV vectors. Further studies aimed at optimizing vector design are therefore needed to improve the efficacy of AAV-mediated therapies (Issa et al., 2023).

The European Medicines Agency (EMA) authorized **Glybera, the first AAV1-based therapy**, in 2012 for treatment of LPLD, a rare monogenic disorder characterized by accumulation of triglycerides in plasma due to mutations in the lipoprotein lipase gene. Nevertheless, despite showing therapeutic promise, Glybera was ultimately unsuccessful commercially because of its high cost and limited clinical demand. The therapy was later withdrawn from the market, highlighting the continuing challenges associated with financing and reimbursement strategies for rare disease treatments within healthcare systems (Pupo et al., 2022).

Luxturna (Roche) is another AAV-based gene therapy that received approval from the United States Food and Drug Administration (FDA) in 2017 and from the EMA in 2019 for treatment of inherited retinal disorders. This therapy is used for retinal dystrophy caused by biallelic mutations in the RPE65 gene, which encodes an enzyme required for regeneration of light-sensitive pigments in retinal cells. Therapeutic delivery of RPE65 aims to restore retinal function through recovery of RPE65 protein expression (Issa et al., 2023; Reid et al., 2024).

Zolgensma (Novartis), which was approved by the FDA in 2019 and by the EMA in 2020 for treatment of spinal muscular atrophy (SMA), represents another important development in AAV-mediated gene therapy. SMA is a genetic disorder characterized by degeneration of spinal motor neurons, resulting in progressive loss of motor function. Zolgensma delivers cDNA encoding survival motor neuron 1 (SMN1) through adeno-associated virus serotype 9 (AAV9) vectors. Following intravenous administration, AAV9 can cross the BBB and deliver the SMN1 gene to motor neurons. Clinical studies have demonstrated that this treatment can improve motor function and reduce disease severity in patients with SMA (Issa et al., 2023; Reid et al., 2024).

Hemgenix (CSL Behring), a gene therapy approved by the FDA in 2022 and by the EMA in 2023, is used for treatment of hemophilia B caused by inherited factor IX deficiency. Hemgenix utilizes an adeno-associated virus serotype 5 (AAV5) vector to deliver the factor IX gene. Similarly, **Roctavian** (BioMarin), which received EMA approval in 2022 and FDA approval in 2023 for treatment of hemophilia A, uses an AAV5 vector to deliver the factor VIII gene under control of a liver-specific promoter (Ozelo et al., 2022; Reid et al., 2024).

Pathogenic variants in the dopa decarboxylase (DDC) gene cause aromatic L-amino acid decarboxylase (AADC) deficiency, an extremely rare autosomal recessive neurotransmitter metabolic disorder. The AADC enzyme is required for the final step in biosynthesis of monoamine neurotransmitters. Deficiency of this enzyme reduces production of dopamine, epinephrine, and norepinephrine, leading to severe neurological and developmental impairments together with increased risk of premature mortality. Clinical manifestations include motor delay, dystonia, hypotonia, oculogyric crises, behavioral abnormalities, and autonomic symptoms (Abukhaled et al., 2023). **Upstaza** (PTC Therapeutics), which utilizes an AAV2 vector for treatment of AADC deficiency, received EMA approval in 2022 (Reid et al., 2024).

Duchenne muscular dystrophy (DMD) results from deficiency of dystrophin, a structural protein required for maintenance of muscle cell integrity. Dystrophin deficiency causes progressive muscle weakness and degeneration, which represent the major clinical features of DMD. FDA approval of **Elevidys** (Sarepta Therapeutics) in 2023 represented an important advancement in therapeutic options for pediatric patients with DMD beyond conventional symptomatic management. Elevidys utilizes an AAVrh74 vector to deliver micro-dystrophin, a modified version of the dystrophin gene designed to compensate for dystrophin deficiency in patients with DMD. Administered as a single intravenous dose, Elevidys has been shown to increase micro-dystrophin expression and support preservation of muscle cell structure and function (Zwi-Dantsis et al., 2025; Reid et al., 2024).

Since the preparation of this chapter, additional AAV-based therapeutics have received regulatory approval, including Beqvez for hemophilia B, Kebilidi for AADC deficiency, and Itvisma for SMA, while the regulatory status of Elevidys has also been updated (U.S. Food and Drug Administration, 2026).

8. Novel Strategies with AAVs

Approximately 10% of GNAO1-related disorders are associated with the GNAO1 c.607G>A (p.G203R) variant, which causes a severe phenotype characterized by involuntary movements and early-onset epilepsy. Gene therapy targeting the genetic basis of the disease may provide a personalized therapeutic approach for encephalopathy associated with GNAO1 c.607G>A. Suppression of pathogenic variants may offer therapeutic benefit in both dominant-negative and gain-of-function conditions. In this strategy, AAV vectors carrying RNA interference components (AAV-RNAi) are used to deliver RNA interference (RNAi) effectors, including short hairpin RNA (shRNA) or artificial miRNA, to target tissues. Following transcription, hairpin RNAs are processed by the enzymes Drosha and/or Dicer into double-stranded RNA composed of passenger and guide strands. The guide strand subsequently mediates sequence-specific silencing of the disease-causing transcript through the RNAi machinery. In the next-generation vector system, an artificially designed miRNA (miR1500) was used to reduce passenger strand activity, while the hSyn promoter restricted expression to neurons. Systemic administration of miR1500-expressing AAV9 in Gnao1-GGA mice successfully promoted guide strand production and targeted Gαo-positive neurons. No adverse effects were observed in mice within six weeks following AAV administration. However, potential risks associated with human application cannot yet be completely excluded (Lunev et al., 2025).

Introduction of CRISPR-based genome editing technologies has facilitated development of more comprehensive therapeutic strategies for a wide range of genetic disorders. Numerous preclinical and clinical studies have reported promising findings. Recombinant AAV vectors combined with CRISPR-based approaches have considerable potential for development of therapies aimed at permanently correcting disease-causing genetic abnormalities. Targeted replacement of wild-type nucleotides to restore gene function represents an attractive therapeutic strategy regardless of mutation type. In addition, use of AAV vectors for CRISPR delivery may reduce pathogenicity and provide tissue selectivity despite the limited packaging capacity of these vectors (Hadi et al., 2024).

The CRISPR/Cas system may represent a promising strategy against oncogenic viruses. Development of hepatocellular carcinoma (HCC) has been associated with hepatic fibrosis and chronic hepatitis C virus (HCV) infection (Hadi et al., 2024). RNA interference approaches combined with genome editing strategies have shown potential for reducing HCC risk in patients with HCV infection. In one approach, an anti-HCV shmiRNA, a short hairpin RNA incorporated into a miRNA structure, was introduced using an AAV-delivered CRISPR/Cas9 system targeting the miR-122 region. Combined treatment involving CRISPR/Cas and RNA interference demonstrated marked suppression of HCV proliferation in vitro (Senís et al., 2017).

Originally developed for viral RNA detection, Cas13a has also been investigated as a gene interference tool for cancer therapy. In this approach, DCUg, a vector expressing Cas13a, was designed to regulate expression of Cas13a and its guide RNA (gRNA) through different promoters. DCUg effectively suppressed oncogenes together with TERT, EZH2, and RelA reporter genes in HepG2 human hepatoma cells, leading to apoptosis and inhibition of cell proliferation while preserving normal liver cells. In addition, packaging of this system into an AAV vector suppressed tumor growth in animal models and inhibited proliferation of cancer cells in culture. By enabling selective Cas13a expression in tumor tissues, this study demonstrated the potential tumor-specific efficacy of an AAV-delivered CRISPR-Cas13a system (Gao et al., 2020).

9. Conclusion

The first worldwide approval of an AAV-based gene therapy, Glybera (2012) for LPLD, followed by Luxturna (2017) for LCA2 and Zolgensma (2019) for SMA, has highlighted the translational potential of AAV vectors despite their long-standing history in gene therapy research. AAV vectors possess several genetic and antigenic characteristics that support their widespread use in gene delivery applications. These include relatively low immunogenicity of the viral capsid, availability of large-scale manufacturing platforms, favorable safety profiles of both wild-type and recombinant AAV vectors, adaptable genetic structures that allow development of molecular AAV variant libraries, and the ability to provide long-term transgene expression in both dividing and non-dividing cells (Kolesnik et al., 2024).

According to a meta-analysis, 136 clinical trials investigating 134 AAV-based therapeutic compounds for treatment of 55 disorders have been reported. Approximately 64% of these studies consisted of Phase I/II or Phase II/III clinical trials, and most targeted rare diseases (Au et al., 2022). Considering the ongoing technological developments, favorable properties of AAV vectors, increasing number of clinical studies, and currently approved AAV-based therapies, AAV vectors are expected to maintain an important role in both current and future gene therapy applications.

References

Abukhaled, M., Al Muqbil, M., Alghamdi, M. A., Hundallah, K., Suleiman, J., Ben-Omran, T., Alfadhel, M., Almannai, M., Alsaleh, R., & Tabarki, B. (2023). Aromatic L-amino acid decarboxylase deficiency in countries in the Middle East: a case series and literature review. *Eur J Pediatr, 182(6),* 2535–2545. https://doi.org/10.1007/s00431-023-04886-5

Agustín-Pavón, C., Mielcarek, M., Garriga-Canut, M., & Isalan, M. (2016). Deimmunization for gene therapy: host matching of synthetic zinc finger constructs enables long-term mutant Huntingtin repression in mice. *Mol Neurodegener, 11(1),* 64. https://doi.org/10.1186/s13024-016-0128-x

Atchison, R. W., Casto, B. C., & Hammon, W. M. (1965). Adenovirus-Associated Defective Virus Particles. *Science (New York, N.Y.), 149(3685),* 754–756. https://doi.org/10.1126/science.149.3685.754

Au, H. K. E., Isalan, M., & Mielcarek, M. (2022). Gene Therapy Advances: A Meta-Analysis of AAV Usage in Clinical Settings. *Front Med (Lausanne), 8,* 809118. https://doi.org/10.3389/fmed.2021.809118

Auricchio, A., Kobinger, G., Anand, V., Hildinger, M., O'Connor, E., Maguire, A. M., Wilson, J. M. & Bennett, J. (2001). Exchange of surface proteins impacts on viral vector cellular specificity and transduction characteristics: the retina as a model. *Hum Mol Genet, 10(26),* 3075–3081. https://doi.org/10.1093/hmg/10.26.3075

Bulcha, J. T., Wang, Y., Ma, H., Tai, P. W. L., & Gao, G. (2021). Viral vector platforms within the gene therapy landscape. *Signal Transduct Target Ther, 6(1),* 53. https://doi.org/10.1038/s41392-021-00487-6

Carter, B. J. (2004). Adeno-associated virus and the development of adeno-associated virus vectors: a historical perspective. *Mol Ther, 10(6),* 981–989. https://doi.org/10.1016/j.ymthe.2004.09.011

Chandrasegaran, S. (2017). Recent advances in the use of ZFN-mediated gene editing for human gene therapy. *Cell Gene Ther Insights, 3(1),* 33–41. https://doi.org/10.18609/cgti.2017.005

Chen, S., Kapturczak, M., Loiler, S. A., Zolotukhin, S., Glushakova, O. Y., Madsen, K. M., Samulski, R. J., Hauswirth, W. W., Campbell-Thompson, M., Berns, K. I., Flotte, T. R., Atkinson, M. A., Tisher, C. C., & Agarwal, A. (2005). Efficient transduction of vascular endothelial cells with recombinant adeno-associated virus serotype 1 and 5 vectors. *Hum Gene Ther, 16(2),* 235–247. https://doi.org/10.1089/hum.2005.16.235

Davidson, B. L., Stein, C. S., Heth, J. A., Martins, I., Kotin, R. M., Derksen, T. A., Zabner, J., Ghodsi, A., & Chiorini, J. A. (2000). Recombinant adeno-associated virus type 2, 4, and 5 vectors: transduction of variant cell types and regions in the mammalian central nervous system. *Proc Natl Acad Sci U S A, 97(7),* 3428–3432. https://doi.org/10.1073/pnas.97.7.3428

Duncan, G. A., Kim, N., Colon-Cortes, Y., Rodriguez, J., Mazur, M., Birket, S. E., Rowe, S. M., West, N. E., Livraghi-Butrico, A., Boucher, R. C., Hanes, J., Aslanidi, G., & Suk, J. S. (2018). An Adeno-Associated Viral Vector Capable of Penetrating the Mucus Barrier to Inhaled Gene Therapy. *Mol Ther Methods Clin Dev, 9,* 296–304. https://doi.org/10.1016/j.omtm.2018.03.006

Duque, S., Joussemet, B., Riviere, C., Marais, T., Dubreil, L., Douar, A. M., Fyfe, J., Moullier, P., Colle, M. A., & Barkats, M. (2009). Intravenous administration of self-complementary AAV9 enables transgene delivery to adult motor neurons. *Mol Ther, 17(7),* 1187–1196. https://doi.org/10.1038/mt.2009.71

Gao, J., Luo, T., Lin, N., Zhang, S., & Wang, J. (2020). A New Tool for CRISPR-Cas13a-Based Cancer Gene Therapy. *Mol Ther Oncolytics, 19,* 79–92. https://doi.org/10.1016/j.omto.2020.09.004

Garriga-Canut, M., Agustín-Pavón, C., Herrmann, F., Sánchez, A., Dierssen, M., Fillat, C., & Isalan, M. (2012). Synthetic zinc finger repressors reduce mutant huntingtin expression in the brain of R6/2 mice. *Proc Natl Acad Sci U S A, 109(45),* E3136–E3145. https://doi.org/10.1073/pnas.1206506109

Griffey, M. A., Wozniak, D., Wong, M., Bible, E., Johnson, K., Rothman, S. M., Wentz, A. E., Cooper, J. D., & Sands, M. S. (2006). CNS-directed AAV2-mediated gene therapy ameliorates functional deficits in a murine model of infantile neuronal ceroid lipofuscinosis. *Mol Ther, 13(3),* 538–547. https://doi.org/10.1016/j.ymthe.2005.11.008

Haddad, G., Kölling, M., Wegmann, U. A., Dettling, A., Seeger, H., Schmitt, R., Soerensen-Zender, I., Haller, H., Kistler, A. D., Dueck, A., Engelhardt, S., Thum, T., Mueller, T. F., Wüthrich, R. P., & Lorenzen, J. M. (2021). Renal AAV2-Mediated Overexpression of Long Non-Coding RNA H19 Attenuates Ischemic Acute Kidney Injury Through Sponging of microRNA-30a-5p. *J Am Soc Nephrol, 32(2),* 323–341. https://doi.org/10.1681/ASN.2020060775

Hadi, M., Qutaiba B Allela, O., Jabari, M., Jasoor, A. M., Naderloo, O., Yasamineh, S., Gholizadeh, O., & Kalantari, L. (2024). Recent advances in various adeno-associated viruses (AAVs) as gene therapy agents in hepatocellular carcinoma. *Virol J, 21(1),* 17. https://doi.org/10.1186/s12985-024-02286-1

Huang, L. Y., Patel, A., Ng, R., Miller, E. B., Halder, S., McKenna, R., Asokan, A., & Agbandje-McKenna, M. (2016). Characterization of the Adeno-Associated Virus 1 and 6 Sialic Acid Binding Site. *J Virol. 90(11),* 5219–5230. https://doi.org/10.1128/JVI.00161-16

Hurt, S. C., Dickson, P. I., & Curiel, D. T. (2021). Mucopolysaccharidoses type I gene therapy. *J Inherit Metab Dis, 44*(5), 1088–1098. https://doi.org/10.1002/jimd.12414

Issa, S. S., Shaimardanova, A. A., Solovyeva, V. V., & Rizvanov, A. A. (2023). Various AAV Serotypes and Their Applications in Gene Therapy: An Overview. *Cells, 12(5),* 785. https://doi.org/10.3390/cells12050785

Kang, L., Jin, S., Wang, J., Lv, Z., Xin, C., Tan, C., Zhao, M., Wang, L., & Liu, J. (2023). AAV vectors applied to the treatment of CNS disorders: Clinical status and challenges. *J Control Release, 355,* 458–473. https://doi.org/10.1016/j.jconrel.2023.01.067

Kolesnik, V. V., Nurtdinov, R. F., Oloruntimehin, E. S., Karabelsky, A. V., & Malogolovkin, A. S. (2024). Optimization strategies and advances in the research and development of AAV-based gene therapy to deliver large transgenes. *Clin Transl Med, 14(3),* e1607. https://doi.org/10.1002/ctm2.1607

Li, W., Asokan, A., Wu, Z., Van Dyke, T., DiPrimio, N., Johnson, J. S., Govindaswamy, L., Agbandje-McKenna, M., Leichtle, S., Eugene Redmond, D., Jr, McCown, T. J., Petermann, K. B., Sharpless, N. E., & Samulski, R. J. (2008). Engineering and Selection of Shuffled AAV Genomes: A New Strategy for Producing Targeted Biological Nanoparticles. *Mol Ther, 16(7),* 1252–1260. https://doi.org/10.1038/mt.2008.100

Lisowski, L., Tay, S. S., & Alexander, I. E. (2015). Adeno-associated virus serotypes for gene therapeutics. *Curr Opin Pharmacol, 24,* 59–67. https://doi.org/10.1016/j.coph.2015.07.006

Logan, G. J., Dane, A. P., Hallwirth, C. V., Smyth, C. M., Wilkie, E. E., Amaya, A. K., Zhu, E., Khandekar, N., Ginn, S. L., Liao, S. H. Y., Cunningham, S. C., Sasaki, N., Cabanes-Creus, M., Tam, P. P. L., Russell, D. W., Lisowski, L., & Alexander, I. E. (2017). Identification of liver-specific enhancer-promoter activity in the 3' untranslated region of the wild-type AAV2 genome. *Nat Genet, 49(8),* 1267–1273. https://doi.org/10.1038/ng.3893

Lunev, E. A., Klementieva, N. V., Vassilieva, S. G., Volovikov, E. A., Jappy, D., Savchenko, I. M., Svetlova, E. A., Polikarpova, A. V., Shubina, M. Y., Spirin, D. M., Anufrieva, K. S., Lebedev, P. R., Pokrovsky, V. M., Utkina, M. V., Krut', V. G., Sintsov, M., Popov, S., Deykin, A. V., Rozov, A., Egorova, T. V., & Bardina, M. V. (2025). Development of an AAV-RNAi strategy to silence the dominant variant GNAO1 c.607G>A linked to encephalopathy. *Gene Ther,* 10.1038/s41434-025-00532-x. Advance online publication. https://doi.org/10.1038/s41434-025-00532-x

Mariani, J. A., Smolic, A., Preovolos, A., Byrne, M. J., Power, J. M., & Kaye, D. M. (2011). Augmentation of left ventricular mechanics by recirculation-mediated AAV2/1-SERCA2a gene delivery in experimental heart failure. *Eur J Heart Fail, 13(3),* 247–253. https://doi.org/10.1093/eurjhf/hfq234

Mary, B., Maurya, S., Arumugam, S., Kumar, V., & Jayandharan, G. R. (2019). Post-translational modifications in capsid proteins of recombinant adeno-associated virus (AAV) 1-rh10 serotypes. *FEBS J, 286(24),* 4964–4981. https://doi.org/10.1111/febs.15013

Matsuzaka, Y., & Yashiro, R. (2024). Therapeutic Application and Structural Features of Adeno-Associated Virus Vector. *Curr Issues Mol Biol, 46(8),* 8464–8498. https://doi.org/10.3390/cimb46080499

Mehta, N., Gilbert, R., Chahal, P. S., Moreno, M. J., Nassoury, N., Coulombe, N., Gingras, R., Mullick, A., Drouin, S., Sasseville, M., Latawa, J., Tiwari, K., Lin, W., Harvey, E. M., Miao, F., Ross, C. J. D., & Hayden, M. R. (2025). Optimization of adeno-associated viral (AAV) gene therapies vectors for balancing efficacy, longevity and safety for clinical application. *Gene Ther,* 10.1038/s41434-025-00524-x. Advance online publication. https://doi.org/10.1038/s41434-025-00524-x

Mendell, J. R., Al-Zaidy, S. A., Rodino-Klapac, L. R., Goodspeed, K., Gray, S. J., Kay, C. N., Boye, S. L., Boye, S. E., George, L. A., Salabarria, S., Corti, M., Byrne, B. J., & Tremblay, J. P. (2021). Current Clinical

Applications of In Vivo Gene Therapy with AAVs. *Mol Ther, 29(2),* 464–488. https://doi.org/10.1016/j.ymthe.2020.12.007

Münch, R. C., Janicki, H., Völker, I., Rasbach, A., Hallek, M., Büning, H., Buchholz, C. J. (2013). Displaying high-affinity ligands on adeno-associated viral vectors enables tumor cell-specific and safe gene transfer. *Mol Ther, 21(1),* 109–118. https://doi.org/10.1038/mt.2012.186

Naso, M. F., Tomkowicz, B., Perry, W. L., 3rd, Strohl, W. R. (2017). Adeno-Associated Virus (AAV) as a Vector for Gene Therapy. *BioDrugs, 31(4),* 317–334. https://doi.org/10.1007/s40259-017-0234-5

Ozelo, M. C., Mahlangu, J., Pasi, K. J., Giermasz, A., Leavitt, A. D., Laffan, M., Symington, E., Quon, D. V., Wang, J. D., Peerlinck, K., Pipe, S. W., Madan, B., Key, N. S., Pierce, G. F., O'Mahony, B., Kaczmarek, R., Henshaw, J., Lawal, A., Jayaram, K., Huang, M., & GENEr8-1 Trial Group, (2022). Valoctocogene Roxaparvovec Gene Therapy for Hemophilia A. *N Engl J Med, 386(11),* 1013–1025. https://doi.org/10.1056/NEJMoa2113708

Palomeque, J., Chemaly, E. R., Colosi, P., Wellman, J. A., Zhou, S., Del Monte, F., & Hajjar, R. J. (2007). Efficiency of eight different AAV serotypes in transducing rat myocardium in vivo. *Gene Ther, 14(13),* 989–997. https://doi.org/10.1038/sj.gt.3302895

Pereira, P., Queiroz, J. A., Figueiras, A., & Sousa, F. (2017). Current progress on microRNAs-based therapeutics in neurodegenerative diseases. *Wiley Interdiscip Rev RNA, 8(3*), 10.1002/wrna.1409. https://doi.org/10.1002/wrna.1409

Pipe, S., Leebeek, F. W. G., Ferreira, V., Sawyer, E. K., & Pasi, J. (2019). Clinical Considerations for Capsid Choice in the Development of Liver-Targeted AAV-Based Gene Transfer. Molecular therapy. *Mol Ther Methods Clin Dev, 15,* 170–178. https://doi.org/10.1016/j.omtm.2019.08.015

Pupo, A., Fernández, A., Low, S. H., François, A., Suárez-Amarán, L., & Samulski, R. J. (2022). AAV vectors: The Rubik's cube of human gene therapy. *Mol Ther, 30(12),* 3515–3541. https://doi.org/10.1016/j.ymthe.2022.09.015

Qiao, C., Zhang, W., Yuan, Z., Shin, J. H., Li, J., Jayandharan, G. R., Zhong, L., Srivastava, A., Xiao, X., & Duan, D. (2010). Adeno-associated virus serotype 6 capsid tyrosine-to-phenylalanine mutations improve gene transfer to skeletal muscle. *Hum Gene Ther, 21(10),* 1343–1348. https://doi.org/10.1089/hum.2010.003

Reid, C. A., Hörer, M., & Mandegar, M.A. (2024). Advancing AAV production with high-throughput screening and transcriptomics. *Cell Gene Ther Insights, 10(6),* 821–840. DOI: 10.18609/CGTI.2024.095

Remes, A., Wagner, A. H., Schmiedel, N., Heckmann, M., Ruf, T., Ding, L., Jungmann, A., Senger, F., Katus, H. A., Ullrich, N. D., Frey, N., Hecker, M., & Müller, O. J. (2021). AAV-mediated expression of NFAT decoy oligonucleotides protects from cardiac hypertrophy and heart failure. *Basic Res Cardiol, 116(1),* 38. https://doi.org/10.1007/s00395-021-00880-w

Ryu W-S, Chapter 3-Virus Life Cycle, Editor: Ryu W-S, In: Molecular Virology of Human Pathogenic Viruses, *Academic Press,* (2017), Pages 31-45, ISBN 9780128008386, https://doi.org/10.1016/B978-0-12-800838-6.00003-5. (https://www.sciencedirect.com/science/article/pii/B9780128008386000035)

Senís, E., Mockenhaupt, S., Rupp, D., Bauer, T., Paramasivam, N., Knapp, B., Gronych, J., Grosse, S., Windisch, M. P., Schmidt, F., Theis, F. J., Eils, R., Lichter, P., Schlesner, M., Bartenschlager, R., & Grimm, D. (2017). TALEN/CRISPR-mediated engineering of a promoterless anti-viral RNAi hairpin into an endogenous miRNA locus. *Nucleic Acids Res, 45(1),* e3. https://doi.org/10.1093/nar/gkw805

Smith J, Grieger J, & Samulski RJ. (2018). Overcoming bottlenecks in AAV manufacturing for gene therapy. *Cell Gene Ther Insights, 4(8),* 815–825.

Sonntag, F., Köther, K., Schmidt, K., Weghofer, M., Raupp, C., Nieto, K., Kuck, A., Gerlach, B., Böttcher, B., Müller, O. J., Lux, K., Hörer, M., & Kleinschmidt, J. A. (2011). The assembly-activating protein promotes capsid assembly of different adeno-associated virus serotypes. *J Virol, 85(23),* 12686–12697. https://doi.org/10.1128/JVI.05359-11

Sonntag, F., Schmidt, K., & Kleinschmidt, J. A. (2010). A viral assembly factor promotes AAV2 capsid formation in the nucleolus. *Proc Natl Acad Sci U S A, 107(22),* 10220–10225. https://doi.org/10.1073/pnas.1001673107

Srivastava, A., Mallela, K. M. G., Deorkar, N., & Brophy, G. (2021). Manufacturing Challenges and Rational Formulation Development for AAV Viral Vectors. *J Pharm Sci, 110(7),* 2609–2624. https://doi.org/10.1016/j.xphs.2021.03.024

Su, H., Yeghiazarians, Y., Lee, A., Huang, Y., Arakawa-Hoyt, J., Ye, J., Orcino, G., Grossman, W., & Kan, Y. W. (2008). AAV serotype 1 mediates more efficient gene transfer to pig myocardium than AAV serotype 2 and plasmid. *J Gene Med, 10(1),* 33–41.

https://doi.org/10.1002/jgm.1129
U.S. Food and Drug Administration. (2026). *Approved Cellular and Gene Therapy Products*, Retrieved May 16, 2026, from: https://www.fda.gov/vaccines-blood-biologics/cellular-gene-therapy-products/approved-cellular-and-gene-therapy-products
Vercauteren, K., Hoffman, B. E., Zolotukhin, I., Keeler, G. D., Xiao, J. W., Basner-Tschakarjan, E., High, K. A., Ertl, H. C., Rice, C. M., Srivastava, A., de Jong, Y. P., & Herzog, R. W. (2016). Superior In vivo Transduction of Human Hepatocytes Using Engineered AAV3 Capsid. *Mol Ther, 24(6),* 1042–1049. https://doi.org/10.1038/mt.2016.61
Wang, L., Ma, L., Gao, Z., Wang, Y., & Qiu, J. (2025). Significance of gene therapy in neurodegenerative diseases. *Front Neurosci,* 19:1515255. https://doi.org/10.3389/fnins.2025.1515255
Wang, D., Tai, P. W. L., & Gao, G. (2019). Adeno-associated virus vector as a platform for gene therapy delivery. Nature reviews. *Nat Rev Drug Discov, 18(5),* 358–378. https://doi.org/10.1038/s41573-019-0012-9
Wassmer, S. J., Carvalho, L. S., György, B., Vandenberghe, L. H., & Maguire, C. A. (2017). Exosome-associated AAV2 vector mediates robust gene delivery into the murine retina upon intravitreal injection. *Sci Rep, 7,* 45329. https://doi.org/10.1038/srep45329
Weber, M., Rabinowitz, J., Provost, N., Conrath, H., Folliot, S., Briot, D., Chérel, Y., Chenuaud, P., Samulski, J., Moullier, P., & Rolling, F. (2003). Recombinant adeno-associated virus serotype 4 mediates unique and exclusive long-term transduction of retinal pigmented epithelium in rat, dog, and nonhuman primate after subretinal delivery. *Mol Ther, 7(6),* 774–781. https://doi.org/10.1016/s1525-0016(03)00098-4
Wolf, D. A., Lenander, A. W., Nan, Z., Belur, L. R., Whitley, C. B., Gupta, P., Low, W. C., & McIvor, R. S. (2011). Direct gene transfer to the CNS prevents emergence of neurologic disease in a murine model of mucopolysaccharidosis type I. *Neurobiol Dis, 43(1),* 123–133. https://doi.org/10.1016/j.nbd.2011.02.015
Wu, X., He, X., Liu, F., Jiang, X., Wang, P., Zhang, J., & Jiang, J. (2022). Development and clinical translation of ex vivo gene therapy. *Comput Struct Biotechnol J, 20,* 2986–3003. https://doi.org/10.1016/j.csbj.2022.06.015
Yang, Q., Mamounas, M., Yu, G., Kennedy, S., Leaker, B., Merson, J., Wong-Staal, F., Yu, M., & Barber, J. R. (1998). Development of novel cell surface CD34-targeted recombinant adenoassociated virus vectors for gene therapy. *Hum Gene Ther, 9(13),* 1929–1937. https://doi.org/10.1089/hum.1998.9.13-1929

Yang, Z., Huang, Y., Zhu, L., Yang, K., Liang, K., Tan, J., & Yu, B. (2021). SIRT6 promotes angiogenesis and hemorrhage of carotid plaque via regulating HIF-1α and reactive oxygen species. *Cell Death Dis, 12(1),* 77. https://doi.org/10.1038/s41419-020-03372-2

Zhang, H., Zhan, Q., Huang, B., Wang, Y., & Wang, X. (2022). AAV-mediated gene therapy: Advancing cardiovascular disease treatment. *Front Cardiovasc Med, 9,* 952755. https://doi.org/10.3389/fcvm.2022.952755

Zwi-Dantsis, L., Mohamed, S., Massaro, G., & Moeendarbary, E. (2025). Adeno-Associated Virus Vectors: Principles, Practices, and Prospects in Gene Therapy. *Viruses, 17(2),* 239. https://doi.org/10.3390/v17020239

Author Biography

Dr. Asuman ÖZGÖZ has been a PhD in Medical Genetics since 2010. She worked as an assistant in Afyon Kocatepe University, School of Medicine, Department of Medical Genetics between 2005-2012 and as a lecturer in Kastamonu University, Faculty of Health Sciences, Department of Nutrition and Dietetics between 2012-2017 where she was a Vice Dean of the faculty during this period. She is a lecturer and Head of Department in Kastamonu University, School of Medicine, Department of Medical Genetics since 2017. She received Associate Professor degree in Medical Genetics in 2022. Her studies mostly focus on molecular mechanisms of human genetic disorders and malignancies.

CHAPTER 3

LENTIVIRAL DELIVERY SYSTEM IN GENE THERAPY

TATIANA DA SILVA AUTHIER, BIEKE BEKAERT, VINCENT TIMMERMAN

Peripheral Neuropathy Research Group, Department of Biomedical Sciences, University of Antwerp, Belgium

Abstract

Lentivirus vectors (LVs) have emerged as a promising tool for gene therapy due to their ability to efficiently deliver and integrate genetic material into both dividing and non-dividing cells, allowing stable and long-term gene expression. Additionally, their ability to accommodate large cargos further broaden their therapeutic applications, rendering them useful for a large range of genetic disorders and cancers. While most lentiviral gene therapy make use of vectors derived from the human immunodeficiency virus, non-human lentiviruses also appear as an attractive platform due to their lack of pathogenicity in humans. Nevertheless, over the past decades, continuous efforts were made to modify and engineer LVs structures to improve their safety, efficiency, and specificity. For instance, advances in self-inactivating (SIN) vectors and integration site targeting have further enhanced precise insertion and reduced risks of insertional mutagenesis and oncogenesis. Moreover, their tropism was improved through tissue-specific promoters and versatile envelope pseudotyping. To date, LVs continue to be involved in many clinical trials, most of them performed in an *ex-vivo* modality allowing for safer transduction, and more controlled and efficient gene modification. Furthermore, the regulatory approval of several lentiviral gene therapies has played a crucial role in advancing gene therapy for rare genetic diseases and cancer, but also demonstrated the safety and efficacy of lentiviral delivery systems in clinical applications. Despite promising ongoing research being focused on optimizing vector design, expanding therapeutic applications, and enhancing cell targeting and safety, the challenges of large-scale manufacturing and cost production remain important obstacles that still need to be overcome to allow widespread clinical adoption. Novel manufacturing techniques, including producer cell lines and continuous bioprocessing are being investigated to improve lentiviral stability, purity and titre, and meet clinical-grade standards. This book chapter provides an overview of the lentivirus biology and development, highlighting recent advancements in gene therapy, clinical successes, and ongoing efforts to overcome key limitations.

Keywords: Lentiviral vectors, gene therapy, vector manufacturing, quality control, lentivirus biology, immune response.

1. Introduction

Lentiviral vectors (LVs) are gaining popularity as a delivery tool in modern gene therapy due to the many attractive features they possess (Ginn et al. 2024). Derived from the lentivirus, a member of the *Retroviridae* family, these carriers stand out from their counterparts for their capacity to infect both dividing and non-dividing cells. This property broadens their targeting range, allowing efficient delivery towards hematopoietic stem cells and neurons, among others (Wang et al. 2021). Furthermore, LVs offer the unique advantage for long-term and stable expression of the delivered therapeutic material due to their property to integrate into the host genome. Their cargo capacity of ~9 kb allows them to deliver large or multiple transgenes, but can also accommodate other materials, such as the CRISPR/Cas editing tool (Askou et al., 2015; Dong et al., 2021). These features significantly broaden the therapeutic potential of LVs, especially in comparison to adeno-associated viruses (AAVs), which often require dual-vector systems to deliver similarly sized payloads (Riedmayr et al., 2023). LVs have also demonstrated a favourable safety profile in clinical applications, due in part to their lower immunogenicity and reduced risk of triggering host immune responses. This confers an additional advantage over the widely used AAV and adenovirus vectors, which have been associated with strong immune response and dose-limiting adverse events. However, despite their favourable safety profile, LVs still carry a risk of insertional oncogenesis that must be carefully considered in clinical applications. In recent decades, ongoing efforts have been made to modify and engineer the structures of LVs to enhance their safety, efficiency, and specificity. To date, LVs may not be the leading platform in viral-based gene therapy, but they have been successfully used in preclinical and clinical studies to treat a large spectrum of disease, including cancers, hematologic and neurodegenerative disorders, among others. While the choice of the delivery vehicle in gene therapy depends on the desired application and outcome, LVs appear as the predominant platform for long-term gene expression in the *ex vivo* setting (Baranyi et al., 2014). Despite their promising use in gene therapy, the complexity of production process and the challenges of scaling up remain one the main limitation of lentiviral vectors (Macchiarulo et al., 2018). Indeed, these multistep processes must comply to stringent regulatory requirements to ensure high titres and quality (Shi et al., 2022). In addition, LVs manufacturing implicates considerable costs, which in turn, also limits the accessibility of certain therapies and hinder their clinical development. Hence, ongoing technological developments are trying to address these challenges.

2. Biology of Lentivirus

2.1. Structure and Genome

Lentiviruses are spherical, enveloped viruses with a diameter of approximately 125 nm and share characteristic virion morphology with most retroviruses (Briggs et al., 2006). The outer viral envelope of the virion consists of a lipid bilayer and proteins acquired from the host cell during the budding process, and viral spike-like projections proteins formed by glycoprotein complexes (Fig. 3-1A). This lipid bilayer is essential for maintaining viral structural integrity, while the embedded glycoproteins are critical for receptor-mediated entry into host cells during the infection process. The lentivirus envelope, arranged in a circular manner, surrounds the matrix and encloses the viral capsid that contains essential proteins and two identical copies of positive-sense single-stranded RNA (ssRNA). The core genome of lentiviruses comprises three structural genes, namely *gag*, *pol* and *env*, that are required for the survival and function of the virus, along with a combination of regulatory and accessory genes (Fig. 3-1B) (Poletti et al., 2021). The *gag* region encodes structural proteins that assemble into the viral core. In contrast, the *pol* region encodes critical enzymes, such as reverse transcriptase and integrase. These enzymes are essential for reverse transcription and integration into the host cell genome. The *env* region encodes the viral envelope glycoproteins which recognize and bind to host cell surface receptors. While the type and number of accessory and regulatory genes may differ among primate and non-primate lentiviruses, they all share similar functions that are essential for the viral life cycle, including replication, transcription, exportation and infection process (Munis, 2020). The human immunodeficiency virus type 1 (HIV-1), the most studied lentivirus, possesses four accessory genes, including *vif*, *vpr*, *vpu*, *nef*, and two regulatory genes *rev* and *tat* (Gurumoorthy et al., 2022). The proviral genome is flanked by long terminal repeats (LTRs), which are essential for regulating its expression and facilitating its integration into the host cell's genome (Fig. 3-1B). Each LTRs possesses identical regions that are comprised by promoter and enhancer sequences (U3), a conserved repeated sequence (R), and a polyadenylation signal (U5). Finally, the packaging signal Ψ, encompassing part of the U5 region, the primer-binding site (PBS) and a part of the gag region, plays an important role in the packaging of the viral RNA into the virion.

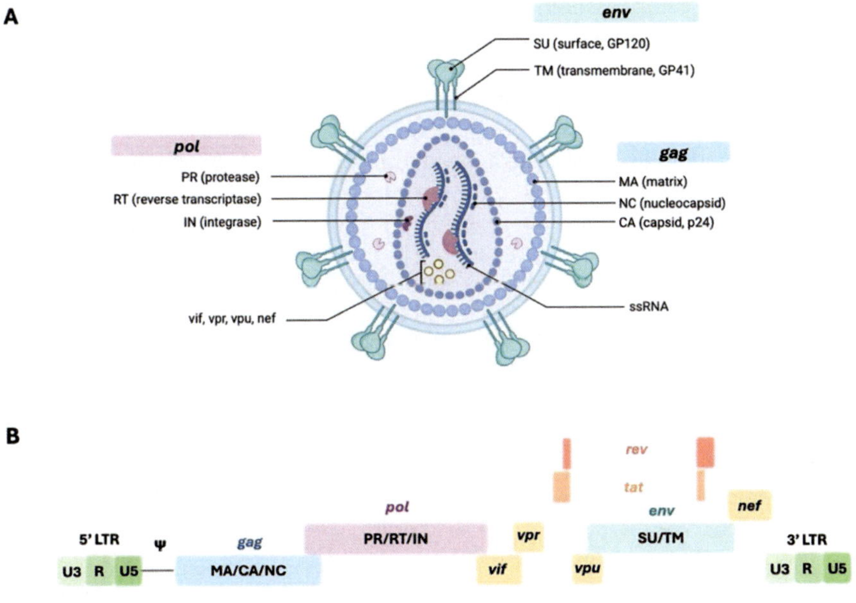

Figure 3-1. Structure and Genome of HIV-1. A. HIV virion morphology. **B.** Proviral genome of HIV-1. The LTRs of proviral DNA differ from the RNA LTRs. During reverse transcription, the U3 region is copied to the 5'LTR. The proviral DNA is a full copy of the viral RNA, with extra sequences added at both the 5' and 3'ends, ensuring that the viral DNA features have identical U3RU5 sequences at both LTRs. LTR, long terminal repeat. (Created in BioRender. Da Silva Authier, T. (2026) https://BioRender.com/80psoky)

2.2. Life Cycle

The life cycle begins with the binding of the mature virus to the host cell surface, where viral glycoproteins gp120 recognize their primary CD4 receptors as well as their co-receptors CCR5 (present on monocytes) or CXCR4 (present on T-lymphocytes) (Fig. 3-2) (Kwong et al., 1998). This binding facilitates the fusion between the viral and cellular membranes, mediated by conformational changes in gp41, allowing the viral capsid to enter the cell (Chan et al., 1997). Once inside the cytoplasm, progressive shedding of capsid protein units begins together with reverse transcription. The viral genome and proteins form, together with host cell factors, the reverse transcription complex (RTC) that is critical for the replication of lentiviruses. As the RTC is transported towards the nucleus, the ssRNA undergoes a complex multistep reverse transcription process to generate a double-stranded DNA (dsDNA) molecule, also known as proviral DNA (Milone et al., 2018). This process starts with the binding of a specific cellular transfer RNA (tRNA-lys3) to the PBS, located downstream the U5 region of the viral RNA (Fig. 3-3). The viral reverse transcriptase binds to the tRNA complex and begins to synthesize a short negative-strand DNA, using the 5'end of the viral RNA as a template. At this stage, an RNA/DNA duplex is created, and the copied R-U5 region is degraded by the ribonuclease H (RNase H) activity of the reverse transcriptase, liberating the small newly synthesized DNA fragment. The latter is then relocated to the 3'end of the viral RNA to function as a primer for the synthesis of the rest of the negative strand DNA. Although most of the RNA strand is degraded during reverse transcription, two polypurine tracts (PPTs), one located at the centre of the RNA and the other upstream of the U3 region, are resistant to RNase H and serve as primers toward the positive strand DNA synthesis. At the end of the reverse transcription process, the partial dismantled core containing the proviral dsDNA is subsequently imported to the nucleus via the preintegration complex (PIC) that comprises several viral and cellular proteins (Demeulemeester et al., 2015; Yamashita et al., 2004). The PIC of lentiviruses differs from other retroviruses and has gain the ability to exploit the nuclear transport machinery. Hence, the interaction of the PIC with the components of the nuclear pore complex facilitates the importation of the provirus into the nucleus and its subsequent integration. The integration of the provirus is catalysed by the integrase, a key component of the lentiviral PIC, which is preferentially recruited to actively transcribed chromatin regions through interactions with host proteins such as Lens Epithelium-Derived Growth Factor/p75 (LEDGF/p75) (Demeulemeester et al., 2015). Once integrated, the provirus relies on the host machinery to be transcribed into a canonical full-length mRNA, which can undergo multiple

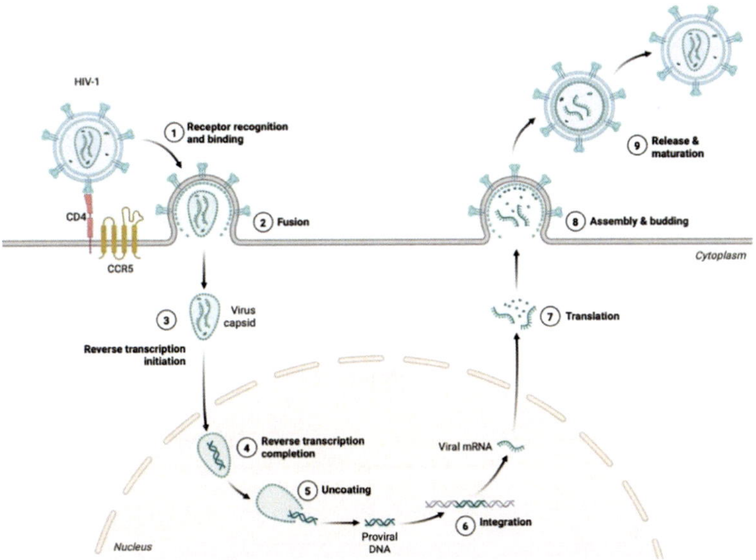

Figure 3-2. Life Cycle of HIV-1. 1, The HIV life cycle begins with the virus recognizing and binding to its specific receptor, CD4, along with a co-receptor (either CCR5 or CXCR4) on the host cell surface. **2**, This interaction facilitates fusion of the viral envelope with the host cell membrane, allowing the entry of the viral core into the cytoplasm. **3**, Once inside, the reverse transcriptase, present inside the viral capsid along with the viral RNA and other enzymes, initiates the reverse transcription process, converting the viral RNA into dsDNA. This process occurs while the viral capsid is translocated toward the nucleus. **4**, Upon importation into the nucleus, reverse transcription is completed, **5**, and complete uncoating occurs, releasing the viral DNA into the nucleus. **6**, Here, integrase, an essential enzyme encoded by the HIV genome, facilitates the integration of the proviral DNA into the host genome, establishing a dormant viral reservoir for future transcription and replication. The integrated viral DNA is then transcribed into viral mRNA by the host's RNA polymerase. **7**, This mRNA is spliced to create various forms of viral transcripts, which are transported to the cytoplasm for translation. **8**, The accumulation of viral structural proteins and enzymes in the cytoplasm signals the commencement of the assembly process, where these components gather in the inner membrane space of the host cell. The newly formed viral particle buds off from the host cell, acquiring a portion of the host membrane as its own envelope. **9**, After budding, the viral particle is released into the extracellular environment. Following release, maturation occurs, where proteases cleave polyproteins into functional proteins, ultimately producing a fully infectious viral particle, ready to initiate a new cycle of infection. dsDNA, double-stranded DNA. (Created in BioRender. Da Silva Authier, T. (2026) https://BioRender.com/9u6z6ai)

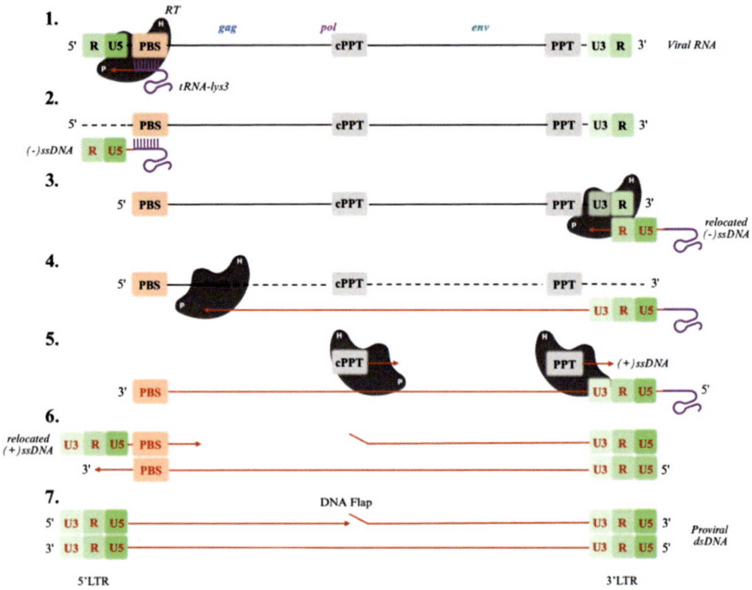

Figure 3-3. Reverse Transcription Process of HIV-1 ssRNA. 1, The reverse transcription process begins when a specific cellular transfer RNA (tRNA-lys3) binds to the PBS downstream of the viral RNA's U5 region, enabling the viral reverse transcriptase to engage the RNA-tRNA complex and initiates the synthesis of a small portion of the (-)ssDNA. **2**, Concurrently, the RNA segment that had just been copied is degraded (indicated by the dotted line) by the ribonuclease H activity of the reverse transcriptase. **3**, The newly synthesized (-)ssDNA fragment is then transferred towards the 3'end of the viral RNA and binds to the R region through complementary base pairing, establishing a stable interaction. **4**, As the reverse transcription proceeds, the (-)ssDNA continues to be synthesized, while the RNA strand is further degraded. However, the PPTs on the RNA strand, which are resistant to ribonuclease H activity, serve as new primer sites for the synthesis of the future (+)ssDNA molecule. **5**, The synthesis of the (+)ssDNA (using the (-)ssDNA as a template) begins, resulting in two fragments: one originating from the cPPT and the other from the 3'end PPT. **6**, The latter is then translocated near the 3'end of the (-)ssDNA, and binds through complementary to its PBS. This allows for the synthesis of the remaining portions of both the (-)DNA and the (+)DNA strands. **7**, As the synthesis of the (+)DNA reaches its conclusion, a structure known as the DNA flap emerges. This flap is formed from the excess sequence at the 5'end of one of the synthesized (+)DNA fragment, which remains unpaired with the (-)DNA strand. The presence of this flap is crucial for the subsequent activities of integrase, as it provides a structure necessary for the integration of the viral DNA into the host genome. PBS, primer binding site; U5, unique region 5; RT, reverse transcriptase; (-)ssDNA, negative single-stranded DNA; R, repeat; PPT, polypurine tract; (+)ssDNA, positive single-stranded DNA; cPPT, central polypurine tract; U3, unique region 3; dsDNS, double-stranded DNA. (Created in BioRender. Da Silva Authier, T. (2026) https://BioRender.com/4wi7uik)

alternative splicing, generating mRNAs that encode structural and regulatory proteins. Only the fully spliced mRNA encoding the proteins Rev, Tat, and Nef can exit the nucleus for translation (Cullen, 2003). The partially spliced and unspliced mRNA require the binding of the Rev protein to the Rev responsive element (RRE), found in the intronic region within the *env*, to further be exported from the nucleus. As the viral proteins are translated and accumulate at the inner surface of the host cell membrane, the Gag polyprotein mediates the essential events of virion assembly (Sundquist et al., 2012). These events include packaging of the genomic RNA through direct interaction with the Ψ, protein-protein interactions essential for the formation of spherical particles, incorporation of viral Env protein, and binding to the plasma membrane. The membrane wraps around the viral core and releases the newly formed virion through a budding process involving the cellular endosomal sorting complexes required for transport (ESCRT) machinery, which facilitates membrane deformation and scission. Although initially non-infectious, the virion matures through proteolytic processing of Gag proteins, mediated by viral proteases, and can finally start a new infection cycle.

Understanding the life cycle of lentiviruses is crucial for designing and engineering more efficient and specific delivery methods in gene therapy. For instance, the integration site of the provirus can disrupt normal cellular genes or regulatory elements, potentially leading to oncogenesis or other cellular dysfunctions. As such, latent infection is a double-edged sword, allowing for stable expression of a therapeutic gene while also carrying the risk of insertional mutagenesis and its significant consequences. Therefore, thorough investigation of the integration mechanisms and their effects on host cell biology is essential for minimizing adverse outcomes. Additionally, it is vital to consider the roles of other key players in the viral life cycle, such as viral proteins like Gag, Pol, and Env, as well as host cell factors that influence viral entry, replication, and integration. By understanding these interactions, researchers can optimize the design of lentiviral vectors to enhance transduction efficiency and specificity while reducing toxic effects. Ultimately, a comprehensive understanding of the lentiviral life cycle not only informs safer vector designs but also contributes to the overall efficacy and reliability of gene therapy as a treatment modality.

3. Lentiviral Vector

3.1. The Evolution of Lentiviral Vectors

Lentiviral vectors, derived from HIV-1, have evolved through several generations, each with distinct features, advantages, and limitations. The development of these vectors has significantly advanced gene therapy and molecular biology. The first-generation of LVs emerged in the 1990s and was characterized by the initial attempts to harness the lentiviral system for therapeutic use. This system has retained most of the viral genome and is divided in three expression plasmids (Fig. 3-4). The packaging vector contains the structural and enzymatic genes *gag* and *pol,* along with the accessory and regulatory genes, driven by a minimal cytomegalovirus (CMV) promoter. The HIV-1 Env proteins were removed and replaced by the spike glycoprotein G of the vesicular stomatitis virus (VSV-G), forming the envelope plasmid. The presence of VSV-G increases the tropism of the lentiviral vector, as it recognizes the low-density lipoprotein (LDL) receptor present in many cell types, including hepatocytes, muscle cells, T-lymphocytes and neurons, among others. The third plasmid, known as the transfer plasmid, comprises the transgene expression cassette. This cassette is driven by a heterologous promoter and is flanked by the parental HIV-1 *cis*-acting sequences, such as LTRs, Ψ, and RRE. First-generation vectors can efficiently transduce both dividing and non-dividing cells; however, their design retained many HIV-1 genes, raising safety concerns due to the potential generation of replication-competent lentiviruses (RCLs). For instance, the accessory genes are known to contribute further to the virus's adaptability and pathogenicity. Indeed, during HIV-1 infection cycle, Vpu enhances viral release from infected cells by promoting the degradation of host protein BST-2/tetherin, which normally restricts the release of newly formed virions (McNatt et al., 2013). Furthermore, Vif can bind and degrade cellular antiviral proteins, such as the apolipoprotein B editing complex (APOBEC3G), which can induce mutations in the viral genome to inhibit replication (Li et al., 2023). While Vpr facilitates the nuclear import of the viral genome, it also regulates host cellular functions, including cell cycle arrest and apoptosis (Andersen et al., 2008). HIV-1 LTRs are particularly active during the G2 phase of the cell cycle; therefore, by inducing G2 arrest, Vpr enhances transcription of the LTRs, which subsequently leads to increased viral production. Additionally, Nef enhances viral replication, infectivity, and transmission by modulating the host immune response. This is achieved through down-regulation of surface proteins such as CD4 and major histocompatibility complex class I (MHC I) and II (MHC II), among others (Landi et al., 2011). Since the removal of these virulent genes did not

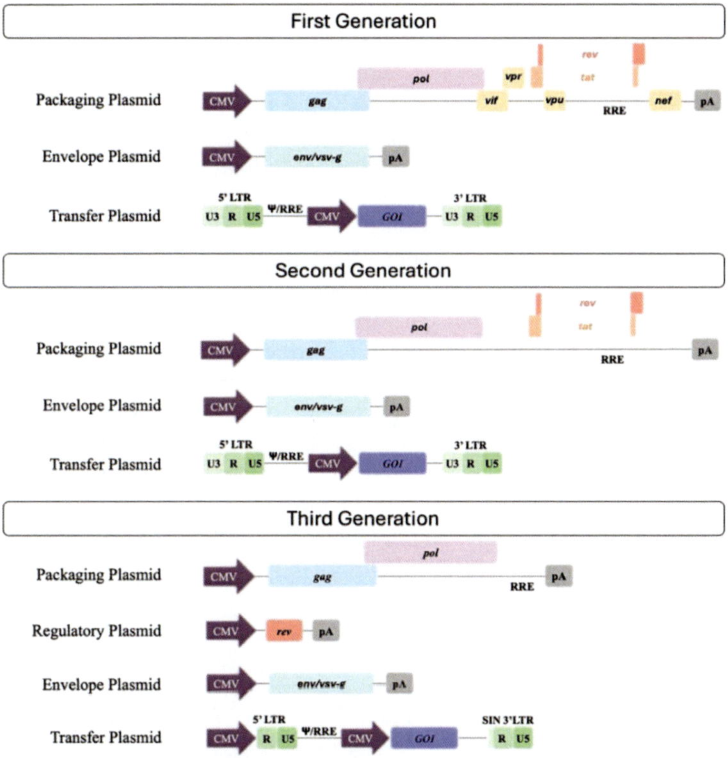

Figure 3-4. Evolution of Lentiviral Vectors. The **first generation** retains most of the HIV-1 genome and is divided into three plasmids: the packaging plasmids is composed of the regulatory and accessory genes, together with the structural proteins, except *env*, which is transferred into a separate plasmid, namely the envelope plasmid. The third plasmid contains the GOI driven by a promoter and flanked by the viral LTRs. In the **second generation**, the design is further streamlined for enhanced safety: the accessory genes are removed from the packaging plasmids, while the envelope and transfer plasmids remain unchanged. To further enhance safety and efficiency, a **third generation** of lentiviral vector is developed. The regulatory gene *rev* is relocated to a newly created regulatory plasmid, while *tat* is permanently eliminated. Additionally, the transfer plasmid undergoes further optimization, which includes replacing the U3 region of the LTR with a heterologous promoter to enhance expression control, together with the introduction of a self-inactivating (SIN) deletion of a large portion of the U3 region in the 3'end. This alteration ensures that the integrated lentiviral genome does not have the ability to produce infectious viral particles, thereby increasing the overall biosafety of the vector. GOI, gene of interest; LTRs, long terminal repeats; CMV, cytomegalovirus; vsv-g, vesicular stomatitis virus G; pA, polyadenylation; RRE, Rev Responsive element.

compromise the *in vivo* production of lentiviral particles, second-generation LVs were developed from the first-generation and designed to exclude these accessory genes to enhance safety (Zufferey et al., 1997). The design of a third generation set a new standard for enhancing biosafety and efficiency by introducing a more refined system. Tat, that is normally required for activation of the transcription through transactivation of the HIV-1 LTR, becomes dispensable once a constitutive heterologous promoter is inserted upstream the LTR of the transfer plasmid (Dull et al., 1998). As such, *tat* is removed from the packaging vector and the remaining viral genes are divided into two separate plasmids: one harbouring the structural and enzymatic genes *gag* and *pol,* plus the *cis*-acting RRE sequence, and the other containing the regulatory gene *rev*. Further optimization was achieved through a significant deletion of the U3 region, creating self-inactivating (SIN) LVs that prevent the transcription of any potential replication-competent RNA (Zufferey et al., 1998). This 400-nucleotide deletion encompasses essential elements that regulate HIV-1 LTR promoter activity, leading to a nearly complete loss of its functionality. Moreover, the insertion of cis-acting post-transcriptional regulatory elements (PREs) into the 3'UTR of the transfer gene can significantly improve its expression (Zufferey et al., 1999). Other new features were incorporated, such as the displacement of the parental HIV-1 elements including PBS, Ψ, and RRE, downstream the SIN 3'LTR of the transfer plasmid (Vink et al., 2017). This new configuration prevents their integration into the host genome and reduces the viral genome to just 4.8% of the full-length parental genome. Within the third generation of LVs, a variety of transfer plasmids have been developed, showcasing significant differences among numerous commercially available vectors as well as those under investigation in clinical trials (Johnson et al., 2021). This highlights the diverse iterations of transfer plasmids designed to address specific requirements and improve their effectiveness in gene delivery applications.

3.2. Lentiviral Vector Design for Selective Cell Targeting

Pseudotyping LVs with viral glycoproteins has significantly broadened their tropism and increased their utility as therapeutic tools (Joglekar et al., 2017). Some of these proteins demonstrate a broad tropism, allowing them to interact with a wide variety of receptors found on various cell types. For instance, VSV-G is notorious for its adaptability, enabling efficient transduction across many cell types, which contributes to its status as one of the most used viral glycoproteins (Deng et al., 2023). VSV-G recognizes and binds to LDL receptors, facilitating entry into target cells through endocytosis.

However, T and B cells exhibit low permissiveness to VSV-G pseudotyping, partly due to their reduced levels of LDL receptors expression (Gutierrez-Guerrero et al., 2020). As a result, cells with higher expression levels of specific receptors are more readily infected than those with lower levels, leading to differential infection efficiency. A recent study demonstrated that a dual-pseudotyped LV incorporating envelope proteins from VSV-G and Sendai virus hemagglutinin-neuraminidase (HN) could significantly improve transduction efficiency across various cell types, including human hematopoietic stem cells (HSCs). This may provide an alternative approach for improving gene therapy targeting in cells with low VSV-G permissiveness (Jargalsaikhan et al., 2024). Furthermore, N-acetylneuraminic acid serves as a critical binding component for the Sendai virus HN protein in the dual system, facilitating the viral entry process. The synergistic effect of the two envelope proteins not only broadens the range of target cells but also enhances overall cellular entry efficiency, ultimately leading to improved gene expression in those cells. In contrast, certain glycoproteins exhibit more selective tropism, favouring specific cell populations over others. For instance, the rabies virus naturally infects both the peripheral nervous system and the central nervous system through retrograde axonal transport (Davis et al., 2015). The rabies viral envelope glycoprotein G (RabG) recognizes several neuronal receptors such as the neurotrophic receptor (p75NTR), the neuronal cell adhesion molecule (NCAM), the nicotinic acetylcholine receptor (nAChR), and the metabotropic glutamate receptor 2 (mGluR2) (Lafon, 2005; Wang et al., 2018). Viral entry of RabG pseudotyping is mediated through endocytosis following recognition of these neuronal receptors (Mazarakis et al., 2001). While tropism of rabies virus is primarily towards neuronal tissues, NCAM receptors are also found in immune cells leading to possible off-targets (Van Acker et al., 2017). Similarly, glycoproteins from the measles virus preferentially infect immune cells, demonstrating a tropism for hematopoietic lineages (de Swart et al., 2007). The measles virus has two glycoproteins: H (hemagglutinin), found on the surface of the viral envelope, and F (fusion), which facilitate viral entry in a similar manner to HIV-1. The glycoprotein H primarily recognizes the signalling lymphocytic activation molecule (SLAM), which is expressed on hematopoietic cells, while CD46, a type I transmembrane protein found on all cells except erythrocytes, is less favoured as a receptor (Yanagi et al., 2006).

Lack of specificity can present significant challenges as some therapies require targeted delivery to minimize unintended off-target effects and associated complications. To achieve selective cell targeting, modifications can be made to the envelope glycoproteins of lentiviral vectors, along with the incorporation of specific ligands or antibodies. These modifications entail mutations that inhibit the envelope proteins from binding to their natural receptors while maintaining the ability to enter target cells through a retargeting moiety. This system offers notable targeting versatility. Indeed, once established, it can facilitate the targeting of multiple cell types by simply changing the ligands or antibodies used. This flexibility significantly refines the potential applications of lentiviral vectors in gene therapy, allowing researchers to tailor the delivery system for specific therapeutic contexts and improve treatment outcomes. These systems have already been developed and tested *in vitro* and *in vivo*. For instance, a study focused on the development of a bispecific antibody (bsAb) capable of binding directly to both the viral envelope and specific antigens present on target cells (Parker et al., 2020). The system utilized a non-integrated LV pseudotyped with a modified alphavirus Sindbis envelope. The E2 glycoprotein, responsible for binding to its cognate receptor was mutated to abolish tropism, while E1 that mediates cell fusion, was retained. Subsequently, the chimeric bsAb was engineered by combining human IgG1 backbones of the HER2-negative (a transmembrane receptor of breast cells) and the E2 field domain of Sindbis. The results indicated that the bsAb-LV system significantly improved the cell specificity of gene delivery, achieving high transduction efficiency across various cell types. In another study, a versatile targeting system for LVs, utilizing biotinylated targeting antibody, was designed to enhance specificity and efficiency of gene delivery (Situ et al., 2018). The system involved a LV that was pseudotyped with a multi-mutated E2 domain alphavirus Sindbis together with a membrane-anchored biotin-binding protein. The latter mediate the non-covalently binding of a biotinylated antibody to the pseudotyped LV to redirect tropism. The system was successfully tested *in vitro* in different cell types. Another recent interesting approach involved an innovative and versatile modular platform, DIRECTED (Delivery to Intend REcipient Cells Through Envelope Design), that allows for the customization of several of its components to achieve efficient cell type-specific delivery of therapeutic agents. Three modular systems, namely pAG-DIRECT, scFv-DIRECT, and SNAP-DIRECT were engineered for the recruitment or immobilization of the targeting moiety (Strebinger et al., 2023). The first strategy consisted in the internalization of protein A/G (i.e., bacterial proteins that recognize IgG from various species) coding sequence between the secretion signal and the transmembrane domain of the VSV-G viral envelope. After viral assembly, the protein A/G, displayed on the surface of the viral particle, interacts with targeting antibodies. The second system employed the single-chain variable fragment (scFv), an engineered molecule formed by the variable regions of heavy (V_H) and light (V_L) immunoglobulin chains, linked together by a flexible peptide connector. This molecule preserves the antigen-binding capacities of the corresponding IgG antibody. The coding sequence of scFv is incorporated within the secretion signal and the transmembrane domain of the VSV-G, allowing it to be covalently anchored on the virion surface. Finally, SNAP-DIRECT uses a self-labelling protein, SNAP-tag, that is inserted in LV's envelope, similarly to its counterpart. The SNAP-tagged LVs reacts covalently with benzylguanine derivates, hence requiring a prior modification of targeting antibodies. In all three systems, attenuation of natural tropism was achieved by mutating the receptor binding domain of VSV-G. Subsequently, successful results were obtained when testing these systems with different antibodies in different cell lines, achieving significant enhancement of their transducibility, with residual off-targets. Moreover, the authors tested several fusogenic envelope proteins from different viruses and demonstrated their compatibility with DIRECTED systems (Strebinger et al., 2023). The versatility of this system with various viral envelopes is particularly appealing, as VSV-G, while popular *in vitro*, faces limitations *in vivo* due to its susceptibility to inactivation by human serum proteins and its immunogenicity. The study's findings suggest that these alternative fusogenic proteins could effectively address the limitations of VSV-G *in vivo*, resulting in improved transduction efficiency and outcomes.

3.3. Non-Integrating Lentiviral Vectors

Despite significant advancements in vector design, safety, and efficiency of conventional integrating lentiviral vectors, the risk of insertional mutagenesis remains. The elaboration of non-integrating lentiviral vectors (NILVs) aims to address these concerns by providing a safer alternative for gene delivery. The therapeutic material is expressed transiently and adopt an episomal form (Vargas et al., 2004; Yáñez-Muñoz et al., 2006). The integration process can be impaired or reduced in several ways: by mutating the key enzymatic player, integrase; by modifying the attachment sites in the LTRs recognized by the integrase; or by deleting the PPT site (Apolonia et al., 2007; Kantor et al., 2011; Shaw et al., 2017). NILVs express higher efficiency and loading capacity than other non-integrated methods, such as AAVs (Gurumoorthy et al., 2022). However, they have been associated with lower expression levels when compared to conventional integrating LVs. Various approaches have been developed to enhance the expression of therapeutic materials. One promising strategy involves the optimization of vector design, such as the SIN vectors, which have demonstrated a notable improvement in gene expression (Bayer et al., 2008). However, this alteration still falls short compared to the expression level achieved with their integrated counterparts. Conversely, the addition of a minimal scaffold-matrix attachment regions (S/MAR), derived from the human β-interferon gene downstream of the transgene, has been shown to lead to sustained expression levels in dividing cells (Xu et al., 2016). Furthermore, the administration of specific drugs to transduced cells can enhance the expression levels of NILVs (Apolonia, 2020). While the limitations of the NILVs make them less suitable for certain applications, it is essential to weigh these disadvantages against the benefits when determining the most appropriate delivery method for specific research or therapeutic purposes. For instance, the use of NILVs in conjunction with CRISPR technology offers several advantages, making them an attractive option for various genetic and therapeutic applications (Hu et al., 2018; Ortinski et al., 2017; Uchida et al., 2021). Indeed, their genetic cargo is sufficient to accommodate the CRISPR components such as the Cas9 protein and guide RNA, while the transient nature of these vectors allows for limited-duration expression. This can be beneficial in reducing potential off-target effects and unwanted changes to the genome over an extended period.

3.4. Non-Human Lentiviral Vectors

Non-human lentiviral vectors (NHLVs) are derived from the lentivirus genomes of non-human species, such as simian immunodeficiency virus (SIV), feline immunodeficiency virus (FIV), and equine infectious anaemia virus (EIAV), among others (Munis, 2020). They are an interesting alternative to human-derived lentiviral vectors, particularly in gene therapy and research applications. Not only do they offer a safer alternative because of their clear inability to replicate in human cells, but they also provide a more reassuring solution to the psychological impact and reticence that patients experience regarding the use of HIV-1 derived lentiviral vectors. As mentioned previously, non-human lentiviruses exhibit similar morphology, genomic structure and life cycle to their human counterparts, but they differ in the number, type and organization of the accessory and regulatory genes (Munis, 2020). As such, the development of non-human lentiviral vector systems was easily adapted from the design principles and cutting-edge advancements of HIV-1 lentiviral vector technology. The underlying principle remains the same: removal of accessory and regulatory genes except *rev*, splitting of remaining viral genome, generation of SIN in the 3' LTR, inclusion of cis-acting elements, and the use of heterologous promoters, and polyadenylation to enhance transgene expression (Barraza et al., 2008; Nègre et al., 2002; Rholl et al., 2002). NHLVs can transduce a wide variety of cells across different species through appropriate pseudotyping. Indeed, several envelope genes of other viruses were used to achieve broader tropism, and successful transduction efficiency, both *in vitro* and *in vivo* (Duisit et al., 2002; Munis, 2020; Poeschla et al., 1998). Despite their promising characteristics, NHLVs encounter significant immunogenicity challenges when introduced into human cells. However, some NHLVs are more susceptible to host immune responses than others. This variability arises from their evolutionary adaptations to the unique immune landscapes of their respective species. HIV and SIV share a common lineage, as SIV evolved in primates, and the similarity in immune responses among primates enhances SIV's ability to better evade the human immune system (Meyerson et al., 2011). In contrast, FIV is adapted to felines and has not faced the same evolutionary pressures intrinsic to interacting with humans, allowing it to remain less adapted to evade the human immune system. Part of the immunogenicity in humans is due to the presence of various intrinsic restriction factors, such as APOBEC3, tripartite motif-containing protein 5α (TRIM5α), sterile alpha motif and histidine-aspartate domain-containing protein 1 (SAMHD1), and tetherin, among others (Sakuma et al., 2012; Zielonka et al., 2011). While some of these antiviral factors can be mitigated by viral accessory genes found in SIV, such as *vif*, which inhibits APOBEC3; *vpu*, which protects the virus from tetherin; and *vpx*, a potent inhibitor of SAMHD1, not all non-human lentiviruses are equipped with the same arsenal (Ahn et al., 2012; Binning et al, 2019; Brandariz-Nuñez et al., 2012; Meyerson et al., 2011). For instance, feline immunodeficiency virus (FIV) possesses only a single accessory gene, *vif*. Additionally, third-generation vectors lack these viral protective genes, further complicating NHLVs' effectiveness in overcoming the immune barriers presented by human cells and affecting their utility in gene therapy applications.

4. Manufacturing and Quality Control

4.1. Large-Scale Production

4.1.1. Upstream Processing

Lentivirus production is a critical component in various biotechnological applications, particularly in gene therapy. The choice of the cell culture system plays a significant role in determining the efficiency and yield of the viral vectors. Cells can be cultured either in adherent, suspension or perfusion cultures, each possessing distinct advantages and limitations

(Ferreira et al., 2021; Macchiarulo et al., 2018; Perry et al., 2021). Adherent cells, which require a solid surface for growth, are typically suited for small to moderate scales, going from petri dishes to bioreactors. However, operational control of cell culture can be labour-intensive, and the reliance on foetal bovine serum (FBS), as a common supplement in culture media, increases the risk of contamination and variability. In contrast, suspension cells grow freely in stirred tanks or rocking platforms, generally in serum free culture medium, and are better monitored and controlled to ensure optimal conditions. They are more suited for large-scale production and can go from small volumes of a few litres to larger tank of thousands of litres. Perfusion systems take cell culturing a step further by continuously supplying fresh media and removing waste, allowing for very high cell densities and viabilities. The human embryonic kidney 293T (HEK293T) cells exhibit several characteristics that make them the preferred choice for lentivirus production (Ferreira et al., 2020). The predominant method for producing lentiviruses involves the transient transfection of cells with the necessary plasmid DNA (Ferreira et al., 2021; Perry et al., 2021). This process is typically carried out using cationic agents, resulting in viral production within 48 to 72 hours, with titres of approximately 10^7 TU.ml^{-1}. While this method is rapid and efficient for generating lentiviral particles, it has several limitations, including toxicity and variability between batches. Furthermore, it is not well-suited for large-scale production, as it requires significant amounts of purified DNA for transfection, as well as subsequent media changes to remove toxic transfection agents, making the process costly. Alternatively, stable production through packaging cells offers a more reproducible and scalable approach in a cost-effective manner, but with lower titres. This drawback is principally due to the cytotoxic or cytostatic effect of viral gene products, such as VSV-G and viral proteases, due to long term expression (Nie et al., 2007). Inducible producer cell, such as the Tet-On and Tet-Off systems, may provide valuable strategies for mitigating this toxicity. Under the presence of tetracycline or doxycycline, the Tet-on system allows for activation of gene expression, while the Tet-off system shuts down the gene expression. Several strategies have been developed for such systems, which are thoroughly examined in the review paper by Ferreira *et al.* (Ferreira et al., 2021).

4.1.2. Downstream Processing

The downstream bioprocessing of LVs focuses on the clearance of undesirable cellular components that could adversely affect the efficacy or the safety of the final product. This process is critical for ensuring that LVs maintain their therapeutic potential and are suitable for clinical applications, while for small-scale purposes, high purity is typically not essential. Equally important is the economic viability of these processes, as they must balance high recovery rates and purity standards with cost-effectiveness. Achieving this balance is essential for scaling up production in a manner that meets both regulatory requirements and market demands, ultimately contributing to the successful development and commercialization of LV-based therapies. The downstream processing involves several key steps including clarification, purification, polishing, formulation and sterilization.

After harvesting LVs-medium content, cell, cell debris and any other large impurity are removed by clarification. The process initiates with a pre-filtration through low-speed centrifugation, preventing possible clogging in the next step. Filtration is then applied to the suspension, noting that the choice of filter can significantly impact the efficiency of clarification if not selected appropriately (Perry et al., 2021). Next, the LV-containing media undergoes a purification process that is achieved through ultracentrifugation and/or chromatography. While this part of the downstream process is crucial for isolating high-quality viral particles from remaining cellular components and contaminants, its extent is dependent on the final usage of LVs (Moleirinho et al., 2020). At this point, a nucleic cleavage reaction can be performed on the concentrated LVs, to eliminate any residual plasmid or host cell DNA, ensuring biosafety compliance (Moreira et al., 2021). This action is generally performed before clarification but performing it on concentrate is more cost-effective than in large volumes. Afterwards, one or multiple chromatography techniques, such as ion-exchange, affinity or mixed-mode chromatography can be employed to further purify the lentiviral particles (Moleirinho et al., 2020; Perry et al., 2021; Shi et al., 2022). Prior to exchanging the LV-containing media into the final formulation, LVs undergo a polishing process to ensure high potency and quality at the final stage. As such, an additional purification step is added to the process, which is achieved by ultracentrifugation or chromatography. In either approach, the lentiviral particles are separated through size from the remaining low molecular weight impurities, and are further concentrated (Moreira et al., 2021; Perry et al., 2021). At the end of the downstream process, the lentiviral particles need to be adequately formulated and sterilized to ensure proper isolation for storage, distribution, and clinical or research applications (Moleirinho et al., 2020).

4.2. Quality Control

To minimize production variability, it is essential to adhere to guidelines that establish a robust framework for the entire manufacturing process. Such guidelines have been provided by the European Medicines Agency (EMA/CAT/80183/2014) and the American Food and Drug Administration (Current Good Manufacturing Practice). However, it is challenging to establish uniform and consensus quality requirements for all LV products due to the significant variations in their vector designs. Nevertheless, certain quality attributes, such as identity, purity, potency, and safety, have been established and must be applied to each lentiviral vector batch intended for clinical applications. This quality control involves the utilization of validated analytical assays that ensure compliance with these attributes to maintain the integrity and efficacy of the products. Example of these assays can be found in Table 3-1. The genetic identity of the LV product must be verified and confirmed, and its potency and efficiency should be assessed (Moreira et al., 2021; Shi et al., 2022). All impurities, whether product-related (such as plasmid DNA, viral proteins, etc) or process-related (including serum, host cell DNA, cell debris, and raw materials, among others), should be identified, specified, and quantified. Acceptance limits for these impurities must be established and justified to prevent or minimize immunogenic responses or other adverse outcomes in future patients. The safety profile is set to rule out any potential extraneous agents and detect any potential RCL.

5. Clinical Landscape

Lentiviral vectors (LVs) have emerged as a versatile tool in gene therapy and are employed across various modalities, addressing a wide range of diseases (Wang et al., 2021). Their long-lasting gene expression combined with their reasonable payload capacity make them suitable for several therapeutic approaches. In gene transfer, LVs facilitate the introduction of therapeutic genes into target cells, potentially improving or restoring normal function. For instance, positive results of *in vivo* LV-mediated delivery of mini-dystrophin provided new insights into potential treatment strategies for Duchenne muscular dystrophy (Wang et al., 2024). Additionally, gene addition therapies leverage LVs to either introduce functional copies of a defective gene or add a different gene that can improve the phenotype, thereby providing a therapeutic benefit in various genetic disorders, such as Huntington's disease. Indeed, a recent study explored the potential protective effects of the *erythropoietin* gene in a transgenic mouse model of Huntington's disease, which harbours a CAG repeat expansion in the human *huntingtin* gene (Rolfes et al., 2020). Results showed that a single injection of an LV encoding *erythropoietin* was sufficient to improve cognitive impairments associated with the disease. Furthermore, an innovative study

Table 3-1. Technical Assays for the Quality Control Assessment of LV Products

	Sample Attribute	Assays	Ref
Identity	Viral genome	qPCR, sequencing	Paugh et al., 2021
	Viral capsid	WB, RP-HPLC, LC, MS	
Potency	Functional titre	FC, qPCR, ddPCR	Leinonen et al., 2019; Soldi et al., 2020; Wu et al., 2024
	Physical titre	p24 ELISA, qPCR	
Purity	Host cell DNA	qPCR, fluorimetry	Merten et al., 2011; Soldi et al., 2020
	Host cell protein	ELISA	
	Plasmid	qPCR, SB, ddPCR	
	Total DNA	Fluorimetry	
	Total protein	Bradford, BCA protein assay	
	DNA size distribution	Electrophoresis	
	Residual BSA	ELISA	
	Endonuclease	Restriction digestion	
Safety	Sterility	Bacterial and fungal sterility	Corre et al., 2016; Soldi et al., 2020
	Endotoxins	LAL	
	Mycoplasma	Culture-based method, PCR	
	Adventitious agents	PCR	
	RCL	Amplification in suitable line followed by PCR, p24 ELISA	

ddPCR, digital droplet polymerase chain reaction; ELISA, enzyme-linked immunosorbent assay; FC, flow cytometry; LAL, *limulus amoebocyte* lysate; LC, liquid chromatography; MS, mass spectrometry; qPCR, quantitative polymerase chain reaction; RCL, Replication-competent lentivirus; RP-HPLC, reversed-phase high-performance liquid chromatography; SB, Southern blotting; WB, western blotting.

has illustrated the dual action of an LV engineered to deliver a therapeutic version of a modified anti-sickling β-globin (βAS3) transgene while also incorporating an artificial microRNA (miR7m) that silences the mutated allele responsible for sickle cell disease (Brusson et al., 2023). As a result, the βAS3m/miR7m LV was efficient in transducing hematopoietic stem and progenitor cells derived from patients and successfully depicted its therapeutic effect. In our study, LVs containing a short hairpin RNA targeting the small heat shock protein B8 (HSPB8) were successfully transduced into motor neurons derived from induced pluripotent stem cells (iPSCs) (Vendredy et al., 2025). Results showed an improvement in mitochondrial morphology, which is typically impaired in axonal Charcot-Marie-Tooth disease. In parallel, CRISPR/Cas9 technology, in conjunction with LVs, has been explored as a promising strategy for treating a wide range of diseases associated with genetic disorders, as well as infectious diseases. This approach enables precise gene editing and targeted delivery of therapeutic agents (Khamaikawin et al., 2024; Raikwar et al., 2019; Yao et al., 2024). A recent study demonstrated the use of the synergistic activation mediator (SAM) CRISPR system to activate the endogenous *tyrosine hydroxylase* gene in rat astrocytes, leading to the production of dopamine (Narváez-Péres et al., 2024). Subsequently, the genetically modified astrocytes were implanted into the brains of a rat model of Parkinson's disease. The resulting generation of dopamine was found to rescue the behavioural motor phenotype associated with the disease.

While many preclinical studies are exploring the potential of lentiviral therapies, it is important to note that a number of these approaches have advanced into clinical trials as well. These trials aim to assess the safety and efficacy of lentiviral vectors in treating a range of diseases, highlighting the promising role that lentiviral therapies may play in future clinical applications. A recent groundbreaking advancement in the field of gene medicine showcased a first-in-class inhaled gene therapy designed to treat cystic fibrosis (Davies et al., 2024). This therapy utilizes LVs pseudotyped with the Sendai virus F and HN envelope proteins, which specifically target receptors on the apical surface of airway epithelial cells to deliver the *cystic fibrosis transmembrane conductance regulator* transgene. Following promising results in preclinical studies, this innovative strategy has advanced to Phase 1/2 clinical trials (NCT06515002).

As of now, several lentiviral vectors have received regulatory approval for clinical use, reflecting their significant potential in gene therapy (Table 3-2). Notably, these approved vectors include those used in treatments for various genetic disorders, such as beta-thalassemia. The efficacy and safety profiles of these therapies have been rigorously evaluated in clinical trials, demonstrating not only the ability of lentiviral vectors to deliver therapeutic genes effectively but also their capacity for stable, long-term expression within target cells. These advancements have paved the way for the ongoing exploration of lentiviral vectors in the treatment of a broader range of diseases, reinforcing their role as a cornerstone of modern gene therapy.

Table 3-2. List of Approved Lentiviral-Based Gene Therapies

Gene Therapy	Indication	Date of Approval	
		EMA	FDA
Kymriah	B-cell acute lymphoblastic leukaemia, adult large B-cell lymphoma	2022	2017
Libmeldy	Metachromatic leukodystrophy	2020	2024
Elivaldogene	Cerebral adrenoleukodystrophy	2021	2022
Breyanzi	Large B-cell lymphoma	2022	2021
Zynteglo	β-thalassemia	2019	2022
Lyfgenia	Sickle Cell disease	-	2023
Abecma	Multiple myeloma	2021	2021
Waskyra	Wiskott-Aldrich syndrome	2026	2025
Kresladi	Leukocyte Adhesion Deficiency Type I	-	2026

EMA, European Medicines Agency; FDA, U.S Food and Drug Agency

6. Immune Response Modulation

Despite being engineered to enhance safety, lentiviral vectors still encounter immune responses when introduced into their hosts. LVs tend to induce a less robust immune response compared to adeno-associated viruses (AAVs), primarily because a significant portion of the human population has not been exposed to the parental virus, HIV-1. However, the activation of both the innate and adaptive immune systems can be influenced by specific components of the lentiviral particles, including the envelope, the capsid, and its nucleic acids, which may compromise the effectiveness of the intended therapy (Annoni et al., 2019). The innate immune system plays a critical role as it employs pattern recognition receptors, such as Toll-like receptor, that triggers the release of pro-inflammatory cytokines and interferons (Breckpot et al., 2010; Rossetti et al., 2011). In parallel, the adaptive immune response can be activated, resulting in the production of antibodies and the activation of cytotoxic T cells that specifically target and destroy transduced cells harbouring the lentiviral vectors (Annoni et al., 2019). Understanding the interplay between the immune system and LVs is crucial for developing strategies to evade or mitigate the immune response in treated patients. This knowledge allows researchers to design LVs that minimize immunogenicity and enhance therapeutic outcomes. For instance, approaches such as transient immunosuppression, where the immune system is temporarily suppressed during the administration of LVs, can help reduce the likelihood of an immune reaction. This was the case when HSCs were treated with cyclosporine H, which effectively mitigated the innate immune response and improved lentiviral transduction efficiency (Petrillo et al., 2018). The study demonstrated that cyclosporine treatment led to decreased expression of interferon-stimulated genes in HSCs, facilitating enhanced transgene integration and sustained expression. On the other hand, engineering LVs with modified envelope proteins may help circumvent the anti-envelope antibodies, thereby enhancing the vectors' ability to deliver therapeutic genes while minimizing immune-mediated neutralization. For instance, two heterologous VSV-G derived from Cocal virus (COCV.G) and Pity virus (PIRYV.G) were pseudotyped in LV and were able to evade the neutralizing response, thereby enhancing the efficacy of gene delivery *in vivo* (Munis et al., 2019). The use of PIRYV.G demonstrated significant effectiveness in improving transduction efficiency, while COCV.G was also efficient but to a lesser extent. Interestingly, PIRYV.G shares only 40% amino acid homology with VSV-G, which is probably what prevented the antibodies from recognizing and neutralizing the modified vector. In a recent study, an LV engineered with mammalian fusogenic proteins derived from myogenic cells was efficiently transduced to target skeletal muscle cells without eliciting a neutralizing immune response (Hindi et al., 2023). Alternatively, incorporating immune-modulatory agents can also help evade the immune response. A study has demonstrated that biotinylated LV capped with a chimeric CD47 protein could significantly reduce their uptake by phagocytic cells *in vitro*, enhancing the efficiency of transduction (Alyami et al., 2022). Another interesting example involves the genetic modification of producer cell lines to disrupt *beta-2-microglobulin*, which prevents the expression of major histocompatibility complex class I (MHC-I) molecules (Milani et al., 2017). Normally, LVs incorporate MHC-I proteins into their envelope as they bud from the host cell, where these proteins are naturally present on the cellular membrane. MHC-I molecules are crucial for presenting antigenic peptides to CD8+ T cells, playing a vital role in the immune response. As a result, the LVs produced by these modified cells lack the MHC-I complex and demonstrate enhanced resistance to antibody-mediated inactivation. In tests conducted with human serum, the MHC-I-free LVs exhibited greater resilience compared to LVs pseudotyped with GP64, which are known to be resistant to immune responses.

7. Conclusion and Future Perspectives

Over the years, LVs have been utilized in numerous preclinical and clinical studies, demonstrating their utility across a wide range of therapeutic applications, from genetic disorders to cancer treatment. While some studies have shown remarkable therapeutic success, others have underscored the complexities and challenges associated with their use. It is precisely these challenges that have spurred extensive research and innovation, driving the evolution of LVs and inspiring scientists to pursue continuous improvements.

Current advancements in LV engineering aim to refine their integration mechanisms to minimize the risk of insertional mutagenesis and enhance control over gene expression levels. Researchers are exploring various strategies, including pseudotyping, which alters viral envelope proteins to improve stability, host range, and cellular tropism, thus enabling more targeted delivery to specific cell types. These ongoing efforts are essential for optimizing lentiviral vector design and expanding their therapeutic potential for a diverse array of genetic disorders and diseases. Furthermore, as highlighted by the complexities of immune responses to LVs, it is crucial to consider immunogenicity in the design process. Researchers can significantly enhance the efficacy of lentiviral therapies by integrating strategies to mitigate immune activation. These strategies may employ immune-modulatory techniques, such as engineered envelope proteins that evade neutralizing antibodies. This dual focus on both vector optimization and immune evasion is vital for maximizing therapeutic outcomes and ensuring sustained efficacy in clinical applications.

Moreover, addressing the limitations in the production of LVs is crucial for their broader applicability, especially given that several LV products have already received clinical approval. To enhance the efficiency and scalability of LV production, it is essential to improve the development of packaging and producer cell lines, thereby increasing vector yield and reducing associated costs. Although purification steps have shown progress, recovery yields remain suboptimal, which in turn affects viral titres. Future advancements in these areas, including the exploration of novel technologies and optimization strategies, will be vital for maximizing the therapeutic potential of LVs and expanding their use in gene therapy.

Moving forward, the design of LVs must be meticulously tailored to align with intended therapeutic outcomes, ensuring optimal efficacy and safety. By continuing to address the challenges associated with production, integration, and delivery, the future of lentiviral vectors holds great promise for revolutionizing gene therapy and providing effective treatments for a broad spectrum of diseases.

List of Abbreviations

AAVs – Adeno-associated viruses
cPPT – central polypurine tract
CRISPR - Clustered Regularly Interspaced Short Palindromic Repeats
HIV-1 – Human immunodeficiency virus 1
HSCs – Hematopoietic Stem Cells
LTR – Long terminal repeat
LVs – Lentiviral vectors
NILVs – Non-integrating lentiviral vectors
PBS – Primer binding site
PPT – Polypurine tract
RCL – Replication-competent lentivirus
RRE – Rev responsive element
SIN – Self-inactivating
VSV-G – Vesicular stomatitis virus protein G

Acknowledgement

T.D.S.A. is supported by the University of Antwerp (TOP-BOF research grant N°38694 to V.T.). B.B. is supported by a postdoc fellowship of the Flanders Research Foundation (FWO-Flanders, fellowship N°1241725N).

References

Ahn, J., Hao, C., Yan, J., DeLucia, M., Mehrens, J., Wang, C., Gronenborn, A. M., & Skowronski, J. (2012). HIV/Simian immunodeficiency virus (SIV) accessory virulence factor Vpx loads the host cell restriction factor SAMHD1 onto the E3 ubiquitin ligase complex CRL4DCAF1. *Journal of Biological Chemistry, 287*(15), 12550–12558. https://doi.org/10.1074/jbc.M112.340711

Alyami, E. M., Tarar A., & Peng, C.-A. (2022). Less phagocytosis of viral vectors by tethering with CD47 ectodomain. *Journal of Materials Chemistry B, 1*, 64-77. https://doi.org/10.1039/D1TB01815A

Andersen, J. L., Le Rouzic, E., & Planelles, V. (2008). HIV-1 Vpr: Mechanisms of G2 arrest and apoptosis. *Experimental and Molecular Pathology, 85*(1), 2–10. https://doi.org/10.1016/j.yexmp.2008.03.015

Annoni, A., Gregori, S., Naldini, L., & Cantore, A. (2019). Modulation of immune responses in lentiviral vector-mediated gene transfer. *Cellular Immunology, 342*, 1-8. https://doi.org/10.1016/j.cellimm.2018.04.012

Apolonia, L., Waddington, S. N., Fernandes, C., Ward, N. J., Bouma, G., Blundell, M. P., Thrasher, A. J., Collins, M. K., & Philpott, N. J. (2007). Stable gene transfer to muscle using non-integrating lentiviral vectors. *Molecular Therapy, 15*(11), 1947–1954. https://doi.org/10.1038/sj.mt.6300281

Apolonia, L. (2020). The old and the new: Prospects for non-integrating lentiviral vector technology. *Viruses, 12*(10), 1-14. https://doi.org/10.3390/v12101103

Askou, A. L., Aagaard, L., Kostic, C., Arsenijevic, Y., Hollensen, A. K., Bek, T., Jensen, T. G., Mikkelsen, J. G., & Corydon, T. J. (2015). Multigenic lentiviral vectors for combined and tissue-specific expression of miRNA- and protein-based antiangiogenic factors. *Molecular Therapy - Methods & Clinical Development, 2*, 1-11. https://doi.org/10.1038/mtm.2014.64

Baranyi, L., Slepushkin, V., & Dropulic, B. (2014). Ex vivo gene therapy: Utilization of genetic vectors for the generation of genetically modified cell products for therapy. In C. E. C. Lattime & S. L. Gerson (Eds.) *Gene Therapy of Cancer: Translational Approaches from Preclinical Studies to Clinical Implementation*, (3rd ed., pp. 3–18). Elsevier.

Barraza, R. A., & Poeschla, E. M. (2008). Human gene therapy vectors derived from feline lentiviruses. *Veterinary Immunology and Immunopathology, 123*(1), 23–31. https://doi.org/10.1016/j.vetimm.2008.01.009

Bayer, M, Kantor, B., Cockrell, A., Ma, H., Zeithaml, B., Li, X., McCown, T., & Kafri, T. (2008). A large U3 deletion causes increased in vivo expression from a nonintegrating lentiviral vector. *Molecular Therapy, 16*(12), 1968–1976. https://doi.org/10.1038/mt.2008.199

Binning, J. M., Chesarino, N. M., Emerman, M., & Gross, J. D. (2019). Structural basis for a species-specific determinant of an SIV Vif protein toward hominid APOBEC3G antagonism. *Cell Host & Microbe, 26*(6), 739-747. https://doi.org/10.1016/j.chom.2019.10.014

Brandariz-Nuñez, A., Valle-Casuso, J. C., White, T. E., Laguette, N., Benkirane, M., Brojatsch, J., & Diaz-Griffero, F. (2012). Role of SAMHD1 nuclear localization in restriction of HIV-1 and SIVmac. *Retrovirology, 9*(49), 1-12. https://doi.org/10.1186/1742-4690-9-49

Breckpot, K., Escors, D., Arce, F., Lopes, L., Karwacz, K., Van Lint, S., Keyaerts, M., & Collins, M. (2010). HIV-1 lentiviral vector immunogenicity is mediated by toll-like receptor 3 (TLR3) and TLR7. *Journal of Virology, 84*(11), 5627–5636. https://doi.org/10.1128/JVI.00014-10

Briggs, J. A. G., Grünewald, K., Glass, B., Förster, F., Kräusslich, H.-G., & Fuller, S. D. (2006). The mechanism of HIV-1 core assembly: Insights from three-dimensional reconstructions of authentic virions. *Structure, 14*(1), 15–20. https://doi.org/10.1016/j.str.2005.09.010

Brusson, M., Chalumeau, A., Martinucci, P., Romano, O., Felix, T., Poletti, V., Scaramuzza, S., Ramadier, S., Masson, C., Ferrari, G., Mavilio, F., Cavazzana, M., Amendola, M., & Miccio, A. (2023). Novel lentiviral vectors for gene therapy of sickle cell disease combining gene addition and gene silencing strategies. *Molecular Therapy - Nucleic Acids, 32*, 229–246. https://doi.org/10.1016/j.omtn.2023.03.012

Chan, D. C., Fass, D., Berger, J. M., & Kim, P. S. (1997). Core structure of gp41 from the HIV envelope glycoprotein. *Cell, 89*(2), 263–273. https://doi.org/10.1016/S0092-8674(00)80205-6

Corre, G., Dessainte, M., Marteau, J.-B., Dalle, B., Fenard, D., & Galy, A. (2016). RCL-pooling assay: A simplified method for the detection of replication-competent lentiviruses in vector batches using sequential pooling. *Human Gene Therapy, 27*(2), 202–210. https://doi.org/10.1089/hum.2015.166

Cullen, B. R. (2003). Nuclear mRNA export: Insights from virology. *Trends in Biochemical Sciences, 28*(8), 419–424. https://doi.org/10.1016/S0968-0004(03)00142-7

Davis, B. M., Rall, G. F., & Schnell, M. J. (2015). Everything you always wanted to know about rabies virus (but were afraid to ask). *Annual Review of Virology, 2*(1), 451–471. https://doi.org/10.1146/annurev-virology-100114-055157

Davies, J. C., Polineni, D., Boyd, A. C., Donaldson, S., Gill, D. R., Griesenbach, U., Hyde, S. C., Jain, R., McLachlan, G., Mall, M. A, & Alton, E. W. F. W. (2024). Lentiviral gene therapy for cystic fibrosis: A promising approach and first-in-human trial. *American Journal of Respiratory and Critical Care Medicine, 210*(12), 1398–1408. https://doi.org/10.1164/rccm.202402-0389CI

de Swart, R. L., Ludlow, M., de Witte, L., Yanagi, Y., van Amerongen, G., McQuaid, S., Yüksel, S., Geijtenbeek, T. B. H., Duprex, W. P., & Osterhaus, A. D. M. E. (2007). Predominant infection of CD150+ lymphocytes and dendritic cells during measles virus infection of macaques. *PLoS Pathogens, 3*(11), 1771–1781. https://doi.org/10.1371/journal.ppat.0030178

Demeulemeester, J., De Rijck, J., Gijsbers, R., & Debyser, Z. (2015). Retroviral integration: Site matters. Mechanisms and consequences of retroviral integration site selection. *BioEssays, 37*(11), 1202–1214. https://doi.org/10.1002/bies.201500051

Deng, L., Liang, P., & Cui, H. (2023). Pseudotyped lentiviral vectors: Ready for translation into targeted cancer gene therapy? *Genes & Diseases, 10*(5), 1937–1955. https://doi.org/10.1016/j.gendis.2022.03.007

Dong, W, & Kantor, B. (2021). Lentiviral vectors for delivery of gene-editing systems based on CRISPR/Cas: Current state and perspectives. *Viruses, 13*(7), 1-17. https://doi.org/10.3390/v13071288

Dull, T., Zufferey, R., Kelly, M., Mandel, R. J., Nguyen, M., Trono, D., & Naldini, L. (1998). A third-generation lentivirus vector with a conditional packaging system. *Journal of Virology, 72*(11), 8463-8471. https://journals.asm.org/journal/jvi

Duisit, G., Conrath, H., Saleun, S., Folliot, S., Provost, N., Cosset, F. L., Sandrin, V., Moullier, P., & Rolling, F. (2002). Five recombinant simian immunodeficiency virus pseudotypes lead to exclusive transduction of retinal pigmented epithelium in rat. *Molecular Therapy, 6*(4), 446–454. https://doi.org/10.1006/mthe.2002.0690

Ferreira, C. B., Sumner, R. P., Rodriguez-Plata, M. T., Rasaiyaah, J., Milne, R. S., Thrasher, A. J., Qasim, W., & Towers, G. J. (2020). Lentiviral vector production titer is not limited in HEK293T by induced intracellular innate immunity. *Molecular Therapy - Methods & Clinical Development, 17*, 209-219. https://doi.org/10.1016/j.omtm.2019.11.021

Ferreira, M. V., Cabral, E. T., & Coroadinha, A. S. (2021). Progress and perspectives in the development of lentiviral vector producer cells. *Biotechnology Journal, 16*(1), 1-12. https://doi.org/10.1002/biot.202000017

Ginn, S. L., Mandwie, M., Alexander, I. E., Edelstein, M., & Abedi, M. R. (2024). Gene therapy clinical trials worldwide to 2023-an update. *The Journal of Gene Medicine, 26*(8), 1-25. https://doi.org/10.1002/jgm.3721

Gurumoorthy, N., Nordin, F., Tye, G. J., Wan Kamarul Zaman, W. S., & Ng, M. H. (2022). Non-integrating lentiviral vectors in clinical applications: A glance through. *Biomedicines, 10*(1), 1-19.

https://doi.org/10.3390/biomedicines10010107
Gutierrez-Guerrero, A., Cosset, F.-L., & Verhoeyen, E. (2020). Lentiviral vector pseudotypes: Precious tools to improve gene modification of hematopoietic cells for research and gene therapy. *Viruses, 12*(9), 1-20. https://doi.org/10.3390/v12091016
Hindi, S. M., Petrany, M. J., Greenfeld, E., Focke, L. C., Cramer, A. A. W., Whitt, M. A., Khairallah, R. J., Ward, C. W., Chamberlain, J. S., Prasad, V., Podbilewizc, B., & Millay, D. P. (2023). Enveloped viruses pseudotyped with mammalian myogenic cell fusogens target skeletal muscle for gene delivery. *Cell, 186*(10), 2062-2077. https://doi.org/10.1016/j.cell.2023.03.033
Hu, J., Schokrpur, S., Archang, M., Hermann, K., Sharrow, A. C., Khanna, P., Novak, J., Signoretti, S., Bhatt, R. S., Knudsen, B. S., Xu, H., & Wu, L. (2018). A non-integrating lentiviral approach overcomes Cas9-induced immune rejection to establish an immunocompetent metastatic renal cancer model. *Molecular Therapy - Methods & Clinical Development, 9*, 203–210. https://doi.org/10.1016/j.omtm.2018.02.009
Jargalsaikhan, B.-E., Muto, M., Been, Y., Matsumoto, S., Okamura, E., Takahashi, T., Narimichi, Y., Kurebayashi, Y., Takeuchi, H., Shinohara, T., Yamamoto, R., & Ema, M. (2024). The dual-pseudotyped lentiviral vector with VSV-G and sendai virus HN enhances infection efficiency through the synergistic effect of the envelope proteins. *Viruses, 16*(6), 1-20. https://doi.org/10.3390/v16060827
Joglekar, A. V., & Sandoval, S. (2017). Pseudotyped lentiviral vectors: One vector, many guises. *Human Gene Therapy Methods, 28*(6), 291-301. https://doi.org/10.1089/hgtb.2017.084
Johnson, N. M., Alvarado, A. F., Moffatt, T. N., Edavettal, J. M., Swaminathan, T. A., & Braun, S. E. (2021). HIV-based lentiviral vectors: Origin and sequence differences. *Molecular Therapy - Methods & Clinical Development, 21*, 451–465. https://doi.org/10.1016/j.omtm.2021.03.018
Kantor, B., Bayer, M., Ma, H., Samulski, J., Li, C., McCown, T., & Kafri, T. (2011). Notable reduction in illegitimate integration mediated by a PPT-deleted, nonintegrating lentiviral vector. *Molecular Therapy, 19*(3), 547–556. https://doi.org/10.1038/mt.2010.277
Khamaikawin, W., Saisawang, C., Tassaneetrithep, B., Bhukhai, K., Phanthong, P., Borwornpinyo, S., Phuphuakrat, A., Pasomsub, E., Chaisavaneeyakorn, S., Anurathapan, U., Apiwattanakul, N., & Hongeng, S. (2024). CRISPR/Cas9 genome editing of CCR5 combined with C46 HIV-1 fusion inhibitor for cellular resistant to R5 and X4 tropic HIV-1. *Scientific Reports, 14*(10852), 1-3.

https://doi.org/10.1038/s41598-024-61626-x

Kwong, P. D., Wyatt, R., Robinson, J., Sweet, R. W., Sodroski, J., & Hendrickson, W. A. (1998). Structure of an HIV gp120 envelope glycoprotein in complex with the CD4 receptor and a neutralizing human antibody. *Nature, 393*, 648–659. https://doi.org/10.1038/31405

Lafon, M. (2005). Rabies virus receptors. *Journal of NeuroVirology*, 11(1): 82–87. https://doi.org/10.1080/13550280590900427

Landi, A., Iannucci, V., Van Nuffel, A., Meuwissen, P., & Verhasselt, B. (2011). One protein to rule them all: Modulation of cell surface receptors and molecules by HIV Nef. *Current HIV Research, 9*(7), 496–504. https://doi.org/10.2174/157016211798842116

Leinonen, H. M., Lipponen, E. M., Valkama, A. J., Hynynen, H., Oruetxebarria, I., Turkki, V., Olsson, V., Kurkipuro, J., Samaranayake, H., Määttä, A.-M., Parker, N. R., Ylä-Herttuala, S., & Lesch, H. P. (2019). Preclinical proof-of-concept, analytical development, and commercial scale production of lentiviral vector in adherent cells. *Molecular Therapy - Methods & Clinical Development, 15*, 63–71. https://doi.org/10.1016/j.omtm.2019.08.006

Li, Y-L., Langley, C. A., Azumaya, C. M., Echeverria, I., Chesarino, N. M., Emerman, M., Cheng, Y., & Gross, J. D. (2023). The structural basis for HIV-1 Vif antagonism of human APOBEC3G. *Nature, 615*, 728–733. https://doi.org/10.1038/s41586-023-05779-1

Macchiarulo, E., Bassett, P., & Dudley, M. (2018). Challenges and progress in lentiviral vector bioprocessing. *Cell and Gene Therapy Insights, 4*(10), 915–923. https://doi.org/10.18609/cgti.2018.091

Mazarakis, N. D., Azzouz, M., Rohll, J. B., Ellard, F. M., Wilkes, F. J., Olsen, A. L., Carter, E. E., Barber, R. D., Baban, D. F., Kingsman, S. M., Kingsman, A. J., O'Malley, K., & Mitrophanous, K. A. (2001). Rabies virus glycoprotein pseudotyping of lentiviral vectors enables retrograde axonal transport and access to the nervous system after peripheral delivery. *Human Molecular Genetics, 10*(19), 2109–2121. https://doi.org/10.1093/hmg/10.19.2109

McNatt, M. W., Zang, T., & Bieniasz, P. D. (2013). Vpu binds directly to tetherin and displaces it from nascent virions. *PLOS Pathogens, 9*(4), 1-22. https://doi.org/10.1371/journal.ppat.1003299

Merten, O.-W., Charrier, S., Laroudie, N., Fauchille, S., Dugué, C., Jenny, C., Audit, M., Zanta-Boussif, M.-A., Chautard, H., Radrizzani, M., Vallanti, G., Naldini, L., Noguiez-Hellin, P., & Galy, A. (2011). Large-scale manufacture and characterization of a lentiviral vector produced for clinical ex vivo gene therapy application. *Human Gene Therapy, 22*(3), 343–356. https://doi.org/10.1089/hum.2010.060

Meyerson, N. R., & Sawyer, S. L. (2011). Two-stepping through time: mammals and viruses. *Trends in Microbiology, 19*(6), 286–294. https://doi.org/10.1016/j.tim.2011.03.006

Milani, M., Annoni, A., Bartolaccini, S., Biffi, M., Russo, F., Di Tomaso, T., Raimondi, A., Lengler, J., Holmes, M. C., Scheiflinger, F., Lombardo, A., Cantore, A., & Naldini, L. (2017). Genome editing for scalable production of alloantigen-free lentiviral vectors for in vivo gene therapy. *EMBO Molecular Medicine, 9*(11), 1558–1573. https://doi.org/10.15252/emmm.201708148

Milone, M. C., & O'Doherty, U. (2018). Clinical use of lentiviral vectors. *Leukemia, 32*(7), 1529–1541. https://doi.org/10.1038/s41375-018-0106-0

Moleirinho, M. G., Silva, R. J. S., Alves, P. M., Carrondo, M. J. T., & Peixoto, C. (2020). Current challenges in biotherapeutic particles manufacturing. *Expert Opinion on Biological Therapy, 20*(5), 451–465. https://doi.org/10.1080/14712598.2020.1693541

Moreira, A. S., Guia Cavaco, D., Faria, T. Q., Alves, P. M., Carrondo, M. J. T., & Peixoto, C. (2021). Advances in lentivirus purification. *Biotechnology Journal, 16*(1), 1-11. https://doi.org/10.1002/biot.202000019

Munis, A. M. (2020). Gene therapy applications of non-human lentiviral vectors. *Viruses, 12*, 1-21. https://doi.org/10.3390/v12101106

Munis, A. M., Mattiuzzo, G., Bentley, E. M., Collins, M. K., Eyles, J. E., & Takeuchi, Y. (2019). Use of heterologous vesiculovirus g proteins circumvents the humoral anti-envelope immunity in lentivector-based in vivo gene delivery. *Molecular Therapy - Nucleic Acids, 17*, 126–137. https://doi.org/10.1016/j.omtn.2019.05.010

Narváez-Pérez, L. F., Paz-Bermúdez, F., Avalos-Fuentes, J. A., Campos-Romo, A., Florán-Garduño, B., & Segovia, J. (2024). CRISPR/sgRNA-directed synergistic activation mediator (SAM) as a therapeutic tool for Parkinson´s disease. *Gene Therapy, 31*, 31–44. https://doi.org/10.1038/s41434-023-00414-0

Nègre, D., & Cosset, F.-L. (2002). Vectors derived from simian immunodeficiency virus (SIV). *Biochimie, 84*(11), 1161–1171. https://doi.org/10.1016/S0300-9084(02)00036-6

Nie, Z., Bren, G. D., Vlahakis, S. T., Algeciras Schimnich, A., Brenchley, J. M., Trushin, S. A., Warren, S., Schnepple, D. J., Kovacs, C. M., Loutfy, M. R., Douek, D. C., & Bradley, A. D. (2007). Human immunodeficiency virus type 1 protease cleaves procaspase 8 in vivo. *Journal of Virology, 81*(13), 6947–6956. https://doi.org/10.1128/JVI.02798-06

Ortinski, P. I., O'Donovan, B., Dong, X., & Kantor, B. (2017). Integrase-deficient lentiviral vector as an all-in-one platform for highly efficient CRISPR/Cas9-mediated gene editing. *Molecular Therapy - Methods & Clinical Development, 5*, 153–164. https://doi.org/10.1016/j.omtm.2017.04.002

Parker, C. L., Jacobs, T. M., Huckaby, J. T., Harit, D., & Lai, S. K. (2020). Efficient and highly specific gene transfer using mutated lentiviral vectors redirected with bispecific antibodies. *mBio, 11*(1), 1-12. https://doi.org/10.1128/mBio.02990-19

Paugh, B. S., Baranyi, L., Roy, A., He, H-J., Harris, L., Cole, K. D., Artlip, M., Raimund, C., Langan, P. S., Jana, S., Orentas, R. J., Lin-Gibson, S., Krueger, W., & Dropulić, B. (2021). Reference standards for accurate validation and optimization of assays that determine integrated lentiviral vector copy number in transduced cells. *Scientific Reports, 11*(389), 1-9. https://doi.org/10.1038/s41598-020-79698-w

Perry, C, & Rayat, A. C. M. E. (2021). Lentiviral vector bioprocessing. *Viruses, 13*(268), 1-46. https://doi.org/10.3390/v13020268

Petrillo, C., Thorne, L. G., Unali, G., Schiroli, G., Giordano, A. M. S., Piras, F., Cuccovillo, I., Petit, S. J., Ahsan, F., Noursadeghi, M., Clare, S., Genovese, P., Gentner, B., Naldini, L., Towers, G. J., & Kajaste-Rudnitski, A. (2018). Cyclosporine H overcomes innate immune restrictions to improve lentiviral transduction and gene editing in human hematopoietic stem cells. *Cell Stem Cell, 23*(6), 820-832. https://doi.org/10.1016/j.stem.2018.10.008

Poletti, V., & Mavilio, F. (2021). Designing lentiviral vectors for gene therapy of genetic diseases. *Viruses, 13*, 1-14. https://doi.org/10.3390/v13081526

Poeschla, E. M., Wong-Staal, F., & Looney, D. J. (1998). Efficient transduction of nondividing human cells by feline immunodeficiency virus lentiviral vectors. *Nature Medicine, 4*(3), 354–357. https://doi.org/10.1038/nm0398-354

Raikwar, S. P., Kikkeri, N. S., Sakuru, R., Saeed, D., Zahoor, H., Premkumar, K., Mentor, S., Thangavel, R., Dubova, I., Ahmed, M. E., Selvakumar, G. P., Kempuraj, D., Zaheer, S., Iyer, S. S., & Zaheer, A. (2019). Next generation precision medicine: CRISPR-mediated genome editing for the treatment of neurodegenerative disorders. *Journal of Neuroimmune Pharmacology, 14*(4), 608–641. https://doi.org/10.1007/s11481-019-09849-y

Riedmayr, L. M., Hinrichsmeyer, K. S., Thalhammer, S. B., Mittas, D. M., Karguth, N., Otify, D. Y., Böhm, S., Weber, V. J., Bartoschek, M. D., Splith, V., Brümmer, M., Ferreira, R., Boon, N., Wögenstein, G. M.,

Grimm, C., Wijnholds, J., Mehfeld, V., Fenske, S. M. S., Biel, M., & Becirovic, E. (2023). mrna trans-splicing dual AAV vectors for (epi)genome editing and gene therapy. *Nature Communications, 14*, 1-14. https://doi.org/10.1038/s41467-023-42386-0

Rohll, J. B., Mitrophanous, K. A., Martin-Rendon, E., Ellard, F. M., Radcliffe, P. A., Mazarakis, N. D., & Kingsman, S. M. (2002). Design, production, safety, evaluation, and clinical applications of nonprimate lentiviral vectors. *Methods in Enzymology, 346*, 466–500. https://doi.org/10.1016/S0076-6879(02)46072-7

Rolfes, S., Munro, D. A. D., Lyras, E.-M., Matute, E., Ouk, K., Harms, C., Böttcher, C., & Priller, J. (2020). Lentiviral delivery of human erythropoietin attenuates hippocampal atrophy and improves cognition in the R6/2 mouse model of Huntington's disease. *Neurobiology of Disease, 144*, 1-12. https://doi.org/10.1016/j.nbd.2020.105024

Rossetti, M., Gregori, S., Hauben, E., Brown, B. D., Sergi, L. S., Naldini, L., & Roncarolo, M.-G. (2011). HIV-1-derived lentiviral vectors directly activate plasmacytoid dendritic cells, which in turn induce the maturation of myeloid dendritic cells. *Human Gene Therapy, 22*(2), 177–188. https://doi.org/10.1089/hum.2010.085

Sakuma, R., & Takeuchi, H. (2012). SIV replication in human cells. *Frontiers in Microbiology*, 3(162), 1-8. https://doi.org/10.3389/fmicb.2012.00162

Shaw, A. M., Joseph, G. L., Jasti, A. C., Sastry-Dent, L., Witting, S., & Cornetta, K. (2017). Differences in vector-genome processing and illegitimate integration of non-integrating lentiviral vectors. *Gene Therapy, 24*(1), 12–20. https://doi.org/10.1038/gt.2016.69

Shi, R., Jia, S., Liu, H., & Nie, H. (2022). Clinical grade lentiviral vector purification and quality control requirements. *Journal of Separation Science, 45*(12), 2093–2101. https://doi.org/10.1002/jssc.202100937

Situ, K., Chua, B. A., Bae, S. Y., Meyer, A. S., & Morizono, K. (2018). Versatile targeting system for lentiviral vectors involving biotinylated targeting molecules. *Virology, 525*, 170–181. https://doi.org/10.1016/j.virol.2018.09.017

Soldi, M., Sergi, L. S., Unali, G., Kerzel, T., Cuccovillo, I., Capasso, P., Annoni, A., Biffi, M., Rancoita, P. M. V., Cantore, A., Lombardo, A., Naldini, L., Squadrito, M. L., & Kajaste-Rudnitski, A. (2020). Laboratory-scale lentiviral vector production and purification for enhanced ex vivo and in vivo genetic engineering. *Molecular Therapy - Methods & Clinical Development, 19*, 411–425. https://doi.org/10.1016/j.omtm.2020.10.009

Strebinger, D., Frangieh, C. J., Friedrich, M. J, Faure, G., Macrae, R. K., & Zhang, F. (2023). Cell type-specific delivery by modular envelope design. *Nature Communications, 14*, 1-18. https://doi.org/10.1038/s41467-023-40788-8

Sundquist, W. I., & Krausslich, H.-G. (2012). HIV-1 assembly, budding, and maturation. *Cold Spring Harbor Perspectives in Medicine, 2*(7), 1-24. https://doi.org/10.1101/cshperspect.a006924

Uchida, N., Drysdale, C. M., Nassehi, T., Gamer, J., Yapundich, M., DiNicola, J., Shibata, Y., Hinds, M., Gudmundsdottir, B., Haro-Mora, J. J., Demirci, S., & Tisdale, J. F. (2021). Cas9 protein delivery non-integrating lentiviral vectors for gene correction in sickle cell disease. *Molecular Therapy - Methods & Clinical Development, 21*, 121–132. https://doi.org/10.1016/j.omtm.2021.02.022

Van Acker, H. H., Capsomidis, A., Smits, E. L., & Van Tendeloo, V. F. (2017). CD56 in the immune system: More than a marker for cytotoxicity? *Frontiers in Immunology, 8*, 1-9. https://doi.org/10.3389/fimmu.2017.00892

Vargas, J., Gusella, G. L., Najfeld, V., Klotman, M. E., & Cara, A. (2004). Novel Integrase-Defective Lentiviral Episomal Vectors for Gene Transfer. *Human Gene Therapy, 15*(4), 361–372. https://doi.org/10.1089/104303404322959515

Vendredy, L., De Winter, V., Van Lent, J., Orije, J., Da Silva Authier, T., Katona, I., Asselbergh, B., Adriaenssens, E., Weis, J., Verhoye, M., & Timmerman, V. (2025). RNA interference targeting small heat shock protein b8 failed to improve distal hereditary motor neuropathy in the mouse model. *The Journal of Gene Medicine, 27*(2): 1-18. https://doi.org/10.1002/jgm.70013

Vink, C. A., Counsell, J. R., Perocheau, D. P., Karda, R., Buckley, S. M. K., Brugman, M. H., Galla, M., Schambach, A., McKay, T. R., Waddington, S. N., & Howe, S. J. (2017). Eliminating HIV-1 packaging sequences from lentiviral vector proviruses enhances safety and expedites gene transfer for gene therapy. *Molecular Therapy, 25*(8), 1790–1804. https://doi.org/10.1016/j.ymthe.2017.04.028

Wang, J., Wang, Z., Liu, R., Shuai, L., Wang, X., Luo, J., Wang, C., Chen, W., Wang, X., Ge, J., He, X., Wen, Z., & Bu, Z. (2018). Metabotropic glutamate receptor subtype 2 is a cellular receptor for rabies virus. *PLOS Pathogens, 14* (7), 1-21. https://doi.org/10.1371/journal.ppat.1007189

Wang, X., Ma, C., Rodríguez Labrada, R., Qin, Z., Xu, T., He, Z., & Wei, Y. (2021). Recent Advances in Lentiviral Vectors for Gene Therapy. *Science China Life Sciences, 64*(11), 1842–1857. https://doi.org/10.1007/s11427-021-1952-5

Wang, X., Zhu, Y., Liu, T., Zhou, L., Fu, Y., Zhao, J., Li, Y., Zheng, Y., Yang, X., Di, X., Yang, Y., & He, Z. (2024). Duchenne muscular dystrophy treatment with lentiviral vector containing mini-dystrophin gene in vivo. *MedComm, 5*(1), 1-13. https://doi.org/10.1002/mco2.423

Wu, X., Zhou, X., Wang, Y., Wu, J., Liang, Q., Yang, X., Zhan, K., & Meng, S. (2024). Development and validation of a droplet digital PCR method for quantifying lentiviral vector infectious titer. *Heliyon, 10*, 1-12. https://doi.org/10.1016/j.heliyon.2024.e38512

Xu, Z., Chen, F., Zhang, L., Lu, J., Xu, P., Liu, G., Xie, X., Mu, W., Wang, Y., & Liu, D. (2016). Non-integrating lentiviral vectors based on the minimal S/MAR sequence retain transgene expression in dividing cells. *Science China Life Sciences, 59*(10), 1024–1033. https://doi.org/10.1007/s11427-016-0067-0

Yamashita, M., & Emerman, M. (2004). Capsid is a dominant determinant of retrovirus infectivity in nondividing cells. *Journal of Virology, 78*(11), 5670–5678. https://doi.org/10.1128/JVI.78.11.5670-5678.2004

Yanagi, Y, Takeda, M., & Ohno, S. (2006). Measles virus: Cellular receptors, tropism and pathogenesis. *Journal of General Virology, 87*(10), 2767–2779. https://doi.org/10.1099/vir.0.82221-0

Yáñez-Muñoz, R J., Balaggan, K. S., MacNeil, A., Howe, S. J., Schmidt, M., Smith, A. J., Buch, P., MacLaren, R. E., Anderson, P. N., Barker, S. E., Duran, Y., Bartholomae, C., von Kalle, C., Heckenlively, J. R., Kinnon, C., Ali, R. R., & Trasher, A. J. (2006). effective gene therapy with nonintegrating lentiviral vectors. *Nature Medicine, 12*(3), 348–353. https://doi.org/10.1038/nm1365

Yao, Z. Q., Schank, M. B., Zhao, J., El Gazzar, M., Wang, L., Zhang, Y., Hill, A. D., Banik, P., Pyburn, J., & Moorman, J. P. (2024). The potential of HBV cure: an overview of CRISPR-mediated HBV gene disruption. *Frontiers in Genome Editing, 6*, 1-23. https://doi.org/10.3389/fgeed.2024.1467449

Zielonka, J., & Münk, C. (2011). Cellular restriction factors of feline immunodeficiency virus. *Viruses, 3*(10), 1986–2005. https://doi.org/10.3390/v3101986

Zufferey, R, Donello, J. E., Trono, D., & Hope, T. J. (1999). Woodchuck hepatitis virus posttranscriptional regulatory element enhances expression of transgenes delivered by retroviral vectors. *Journal of Virology, 73*(4), 2886–2892. https://doi.org/10.1128/JVI.73.4.2886-2892.1999

Zufferey, R., Dull, T., Mandel, R. J., Bukovsky, A., Quiroz, D., Naldini, L., & Trono, D. (1998). Self-inactivating lentivirus vector for safe and efficient in vivo gene delivery. *Journal of Virology, 72*(12), 9873–9880.

https://doi.org/10.1128/JVI.72.12.9873-9880.1998
Zufferey, R., Nagy, D., Mandel, R. J., Naldini, L., & Trono, D. (1997). Multiply attenuated lentiviral vector achieves efficient gene delivery in vivo. *Nature Biotechnology, 15*(9), 871–875. https://doi.org/10.1038/nbt0997-871

Author Biographies

Tatiana da Silva Authier is a senior PhD student at the Peripheral Neuropathy Research Group, University of Antwerp, Belgium, led by Prof. Vincent Timmerman. She graduated from the University of Algarve, Portugal, where she acquired a bachelor's degree in *Biochemistry* and a Master's degree in *Molecular and Microbial Biology*. She gave an oral platform presentation at the Peripheral Nerve Society Annual Meeting 2024, highlighting the potential of CRISPR Cas9 system in ameliorating the axonal Charcot-Marie Tooth type 2L (CMT2L) phenotype. She has collaborated with colleagues within the Peripheral Neuropathy Research Group which resulted in two co-author papers (Van Lent et al., 2022; Vendredy et al., 2025). Currently, her research focuses on genome engineering with CRISPR/Cas9 as a precision medicine for CMT2L, using iPSCs-derived motor neurons and myoprogenitors as models.

Bieke Bekaert began her PhD research project as a FWO (Flemish fund for scientific research) aspirant at Ghent University. Her research focused on CRISPR/Cas9 gene editing in the mouse/human germline and human pluripotent disease stem cell models targeting genes related to infertility. This research resulted in one first-author review (Bekaert et al., 2022), one co-author paper (Stamatiadis et al., 2021), and two first-author articles (Bekaert et al., 2023, 2024) on gene editing. Currently, she is working as a post-doctoral researcher in the Peripheral Neuropathy Research Group in UAntwerp led by Prof. Vincent Timmerman. Her main focus is investigating Charcot-Marie-Tooth (CMT) disease using various 3D human stem cell models, supported by a junior postdoctoral fellowship from the FWO. She is also the Social Media Ambassador for the Peripheral Nerve Society.

Vincent Timmerman is a full professor at the University of Antwerp (Belgium). His peripheral neuropathy research team has identified several gene mutations associated with CMT disease. They are studying the effect of mutations in neuronal and non-neuronal cells, including neurons differentiated from human induced pluripotent stem cells. The molecular biology of mutations, compared with clinical, physiological and pathological data from CMT patients, contributes to genotype-phenotype correlations.

They have gained knowledge using various gene-cloning technologies and have generated mouse and Drosophila models of peripheral neuropathies. The recent development of human-derived organoids and assembloids complements the animal, cellular and molecular models and allows the study of disease mechanisms relevant to inherited sensory and/or motor neuropathies.
ORCID: https://orcid.org/0000-0002-2162-0933

CHAPTER 4

ENGINEERING SAFETY AND CLINICAL PERSPECTIVES OF HERPES SIMPLEX VIRUS-BASED GENE DELIVERY SYSTEMS

CIHAN TAŞTAN[1,2,3,4], BEYZA AYDIN[1,3,4,5]

[1] Transgenic Cell Technologies and Epigenetic Application and Research Center (TRGENMER), Üsküdar University, Istanbul, Turkiye
[2] Molecular Biology and Genetics Department, Faculty of Engineering and Natural Science, Üsküdar University, Istanbul, Türkiye
[3] Hidna Biotechnology Inc., Istanbul, Türkiye
[4] Synastra Biotechnology Inc., Istanbul, Türkiye
[5] Molecular Biology, Institute of Science and Technology, Üsküdar University, Istanbul, Türkiye

Abstract

Herpes simplex virus (HSV)-based vectors have emerged as one of the most versatile and clinically advanced gene delivery platforms due to their exceptional payload capacity (up to ~150 kb), natural neurotropism, and ability to establish stable, episomal persistence in both the central and peripheral nervous systems (**Graphical Abstract**). These features make HSV uniquely suitable for complex therapeutic strategies requiring long-term, high-level gene expression in neuronal populations, as well as for oncolytic applications targeting solid tumors. Over the last five years (2020–2025), HSV vector engineering has evolved substantially. Next-generation replication-defective (rdHSV) vectors have been developed with optimized promoter–insulator architectures that minimize cytotoxicity and adaptive immune responses while enabling durable transgene expression in neurons. Helper virus-free amplicon systems now allow safe, large-capacity delivery of multiplexed gene circuits, CRISPR/Cas9 payloads, and combinatorial therapeutic cassettes, opening new avenues for precision genome editing and multi-gene regulation. In parallel, oncolytic HSV (oHSV) platforms have advanced to clinical success, with talimogene laherparepvec (T-VEC) approved for melanoma, teserpaturev (G47Δ) approved in Japan for malignant glioma, and beremagene geperpavec (Vyjuvek) — a topical redosable HSV-1 vector — approved by the FDA in 2023 for treating dystrophic epidermolysis bullosa (DEB). These milestones underscore HSV's flexibility across diverse indications, including oncology, neurodegeneration, dermatology, and regenerative medicine. This chapter synthesizes recent advances in HSV molecular biology, vector engineering, delivery strategies, and translational manufacturing, integrating updated clinical trial data, immune modulation approaches, and synthetic biology-inspired payload control systems. We highlight cutting-edge innovations in capsid engineering, tissue-specific promoter design, and microRNA-guided detargeting, alongside strategies for overcoming challenges such as pre-existing immunity, vector re-administration, and large-scale GMP manufacturing. Special emphasis is placed on HSV-based therapies for central nervous system (CNS) disorders, where payload size and episomal stability provide unique advantages over AAV and lentiviral platforms. Together, these updates provide a comprehensive resource for researchers and clinicians developing HSV-based vectors, advancing the next generation of gene and oncolytic therapies.

Keywords: Herpes simplex virus, HSV, Gene delivery systems, Oncolytic virotherapy.

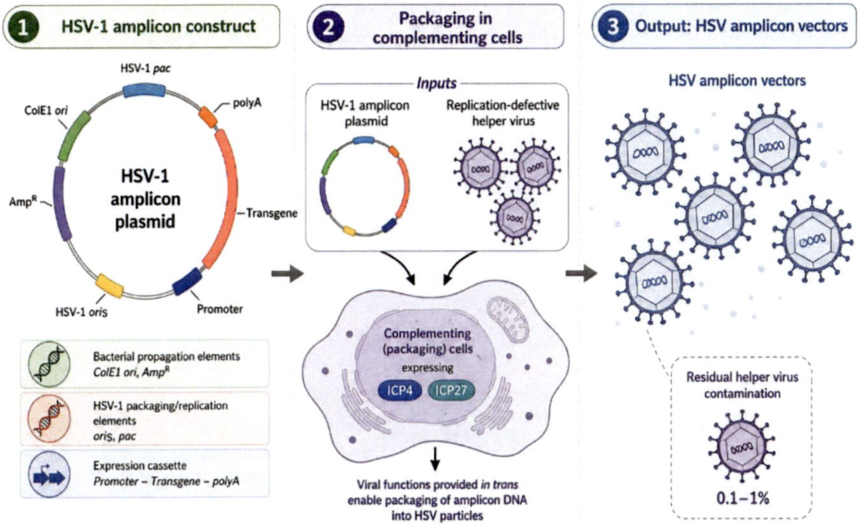

Graphical Abstract. Schematic overview of HSV-1 amplicon vector production. An amplicon plasmid carrying the transgene cassette and HSV-1 packaging/replication elements (oriS and pac), together with bacterial propagation elements (ColE1 ori and AmpR), is introduced into complementing cells in the presence of a replication-defective helper virus. Complementing cells expressing ICP4 and ICP27 provide essential viral functions in trans, enabling packaging of the amplicon DNA into HSV particles. The resulting preparation contains HSV amplicon vectors together with a low level of helper virus contamination, approximately 0.1–1%.

Table 1. Major clinical delivery routes for HSV vectors to the CNS: intraparenchymal, intrathecal/intraventricular, and systemic.

Delivery Route	Administration Method	Advantages	Limitations / Challenges	Representative Clinical Applications
Intraparenchymal	Direct stereotactic injection into specific brain regions	• High local vector concentration • Precise targeting • Ideal for focal lesions	•Invasive procedure •Limited distribution beyond injection site • Surgical risks	Glioblastoma (oHSV G207, G47Δ), Parkinson's disease
Intrathecal/ Intraventricular	Injection into cerebrospinal fluid (CSF) via lumbar puncture or ventricular catheter	• Broader CNS coverage • Less invasive than stereotactic delivery • Suitable for diffuse CNS involvement	• Dilution in CSF reduces local concentration • Potential immune activation • Variable biodistribution	Spinal muscular atrophy (SMA), ALS, lysosomal storage disorders
Systemic (Intravenous)	IV infusion of HSV vector into peripheral circulation	• Potential to reach widespread CNS targets • Non-invasive • Can be combined with BBB modulation techniques	• Limited BBB penetration •Requires capsid engineering or receptor-targeting • High risk of systemic immune responses	Experimental trials for Alzheimer's disease, metastatic CNS cancers

Table 2. Representative clinical applications: melanoma (T-VEC), glioma (G47Δ/G207), and DEB (Vyjuvek).

Therapy / Vector	Indication	Mechanism of Action	Administration Route	Key Trial(s)
Talimogene laherparepvec (T-VEC)	Metastatic melanoma	Oncolytic HSV-1 engineered with **ICP34.5** deletion and **GM-CSF** expression → selectively replicates in tumor cells, induces oncolysis, and promotes anti-tumor immunity.	Intralesional injection	NCT00769704
Teserpaturev (G47Δ)	Malignant glioma (GBM)	Third-generation oncolytic HSV with deletions in **ICP34.5**, **ICP47**, and **UL39**, enhancing tumor selectivity and immune activation.	Intratumoral injection (stereotactic)	NCT03152318
G207	Pediatric high-grade glioma	Second-generation oncolytic HSV engineered for tumor-selective replication, combined with low-dose radiation to enhance viral spread.	Intratumoral injection	NCT02457845
Beremagene geperpavec (Vyjuvek)	Dystrophic epidermolysis bullosa (DEB)	Non-replicating HSV-1 vector delivering **COL7A1** cDNA to restore type VII collagen expression and improve wound healing.	Topical application	GEM-1 / GEM-2 (NCT04491604)

Introduction

Herpes simplex virus type 1 (HSV-1) is a large, enveloped, double-stranded DNA virus known for its unique ability to undergo both productive lytic infection and long-term latency within sensory and autonomic neurons (**Fig. 1**). These characteristics have been harnessed to develop versatile gene delivery platforms, encompassing replication-defective (rdHSV) vectors—which eliminate viral gene expression to enable prolonged neuronal transduction—alongside helper-free amplicon systems capable of delivering large heterologous sequences (up to ~150 kb), and replication-selective oncolytic HSV (oHSV) designed to lyse tumor cells while activating anti-tumor immunity selectively (Epstein 2024). The clinical translation of HSV vectors has reached significant milestones. Talimogene laherparepvec (T-VEC; Imlygic®) became the first oncolytic viral therapy approved by the FDA in 2015 for unresectable melanoma, marking a pivotal step for oncolytic virotherapy in oncology (Bommareddy 2017; Kaufman et al. 2022). Japan approved teserpaturev (G47Δ; Delytact), an oHSV tailored for malignant glioma, demonstrating the potential of virotherapy in neuro-oncology (Wu & Alvarez-Breckenridge 2023). More recently, the FDA approved beremagene geperpavec (Vyjuvek), the first topical HSV-1–based gene therapy for dystrophic epidermolysis bullosa (DEB), showcasing HSV's versatility in delivering corrective gene therapy beyond oncologic applications (FDA 2023).

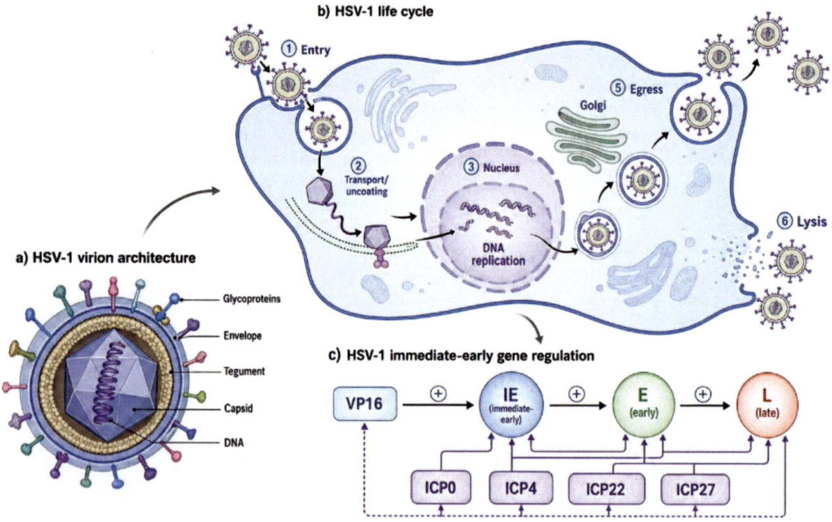

Fig. 1. Overview of herpes simplex virus type 1 (HSV-1) structure, life cycle, and transcriptional regulation. (a) HSV-1 virion architecture showing surface glycoproteins, the envelope, tegument, icosahedral capsid, and genomic DNA. (b) HSV-1 life cycle in a host cell: entry at the plasma membrane, transport and uncoating to the nucleus, viral DNA replication in the nucleus, assembly and trafficking through the Golgi, egress at the plasma membrane, and release of progeny by lysis. (c) Immediate-early gene regulation: VP16 initiates expression of immediate-early (IE) genes; IE gene products ICP0, ICP4, ICP22, and ICP27 coordinate and activate the transcriptional cascade from IE to early (E) and late (L) viral gene expression.

These approvals demonstrate that distinct HSV architectures can be finely tuned to achieve different therapeutic goals—ranging from immune-oncology and neuro-oncology to gene replacement in dermatological conditions—while leveraging the same foundational viral biology (**Fig. 2**). Recent reviews highlight that next-generation rdHSV vectors, which eliminate viral gene expression, exhibit minimal cytotoxicity and maintain robust transgene expression from episomal genomes in neurons. This success is often attributed to the incorporation of insulators, highly optimized promoters, and enhancer-blocking elements that prevent epigenetic silencing (Ingusci et al. 2025a; Ingusci et al. 2025b). Concurrently, amplicon vector systems have advanced with helper virus–free production methods, refined packaging cell lines, and insulator-flanked expression cassettes that reduce immune activation and transgene variability (Le Hars et al. 2025).

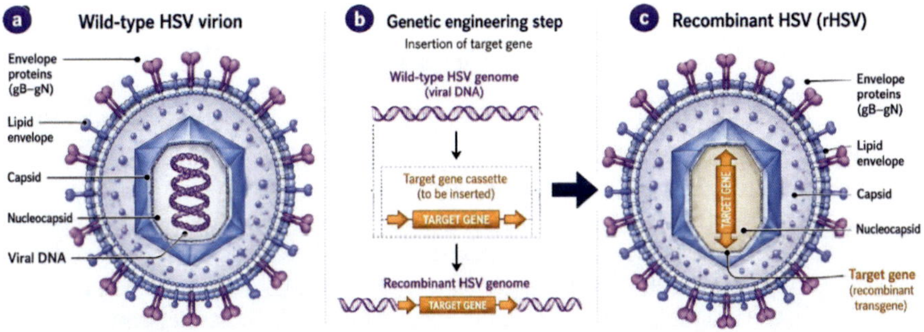

Fig. 2. Schematic comparison of wild-type herpes simplex virus (WT-HSV) and recombinant HSV (rHSV). (a) The wild-type HSV virion consists of envelope proteins (gB–gN) embedded in a lipid envelope surrounding the capsid and nucleocapsid, which contain the viral DNA genome. (b) Recombinant engineering of HSV introduces a target gene into the viral genome while preserving the overall virion architecture. (c) The resulting recombinant HSV (rHSV) retains the structural components of HSV but carries the inserted target gene as the key engineered genetic element.

For oncolytic platforms, safety and immunogenicity are enhanced through targeted deletions of neurovirulence genes (e.g., ΔICP34.5, ΔUL39) and the inclusion of immune-stimulatory payloads such as GM-CSF, cytokines, chemokines, or bispecific T-cell engagers (BiTEs), designed to promote immunogenic cell death, antigen presentation, and epitope spreading (Frampton 2022; Sethumadhavan et al. 2022). Therapeutically, delivery strategies vary depending on the disease context. Intralesional or intratumoral injection remains dominant for oncolytic and peripheral applications. In contrast, central nervous system (CNS) applications often require stereotactic intraparenchymal or intrathecal delivery to bypass the blood–brain barrier and achieve efficient transduction in neuronal tissues. Moreover, the field is merging synthetic biology tools—such as logic-gated payload expression, microRNA-mediated detargeting, and receptor-specific retargeting—with combination regimens integrating checkpoint blockade, radiotherapy, and chemotherapeutics to enhance efficacy across multiple disease models (Wu & Alvarez-Breckenridge 2023). Furthermore, the regulatory landscape for viral vectors has matured significantly. Current guidelines—and expectations around shedding, environmental risk assessments, long-term follow-up, and Good Manufacturing Practice (GMP) for Advanced Therapy Medicinal Products (ATMPs)—provide a well-structured pathway for bench-to-bedside translation of HSV vectors (European Commission 2018-2025; FDA 2023; Furlan et al. 2007).

Genome Organization

The herpes simplex virus type 1 (HSV-1) genome is approximately 152 kilobases (kb) in length and is composed of two unique segments, UL (unique long) and US (unique short), which are bounded by inverted repeat regions (TRL/IRL and IRS/TRS) (**Fig. 3**). This genomic arrangement enables the formation of four isomeric conformations within virions (McGeoch et al. 2006). HSV-1 genes are classified into immediate-early (IE), early (E), and late (L) kinetic expression classes, orchestrating the sequential cascade of gene expression during lytic replication (Roizman & Whitley, 2013). This genomic architecture provides multiple engineering entry points for vector development. For instance, disruption of essential IE genes such as ICP4/RS1, ICP27/UL54, ICP22/US1, and ICP0/RL2 yields replication-defective HSV (rdHSV) vectors that cannot express viral proteins, thereby improving biosafety (Wong et al. 2023). Similarly, ablation or mutation of the neurovirulence determinant ICP34.5/RL1 attenuates replication in normal tissues and enhances tumor tropism, forming the basis of oncolytic HSV (oHSV) platforms (Cassady & Parker, 2010). Moreover, amplicon vectors, in which the viral genome is replaced with plasmid DNA containing only the HSV origin of replication (oriS) and the packaging signal (pac), accommodate exceptionally large genetic payloads (Wade-Martins et al. 2001).

Advances in long-read sequencing technologies and synthetic genome reconstruction have refined our understanding of HSV repeat architecture, genomic termini, and recombination hotspots—features critical for the rational design of genetically stable vector genomes (Dolan et al. 1998; Nicoll et al. 2012). In parallel, structural and functional studies of tegument and capsid proteins (e.g., VP16, UL36, UL37) have highlighted their pivotal role in early nuclear delivery and IE gene transactivation. Engineered tegument modifications have been leveraged to enhance nuclear import of transgenes and regulatory payloads (Heldwein & Krummenacher, 2008). The UL/US inverted repeats further contribute versatile redundant insertion loci and bidirectional promoters, which can be repurposed to drive expression of synthetic cassettes under cell–type–specific transcriptional control (Karpoff et al. 2000). Collectively, these properties enable HSV-based vectors to stably accommodate multigene circuits, which is particularly advantageous for delivering large cDNAs (e.g., dystrophin microgenes that exceed the capacity of AAV vectors) or combinatorial payloads such as cytokine-expression modules coupled with immune checkpoint traps (Miyagawa et al. 2015).

State-of-the-art high-capacity rdHSV vectors are typically devoid of viral coding sequences. This design markedly reduces vector-associated antigenicity while preserving episomal persistence in post-mitotic neurons. This unique combination of features renders HSV-1 vectors exceptionally well suited for long-term gene delivery in the central nervous system (CNS) and related therapeutic contexts (Goins et al. 2020).

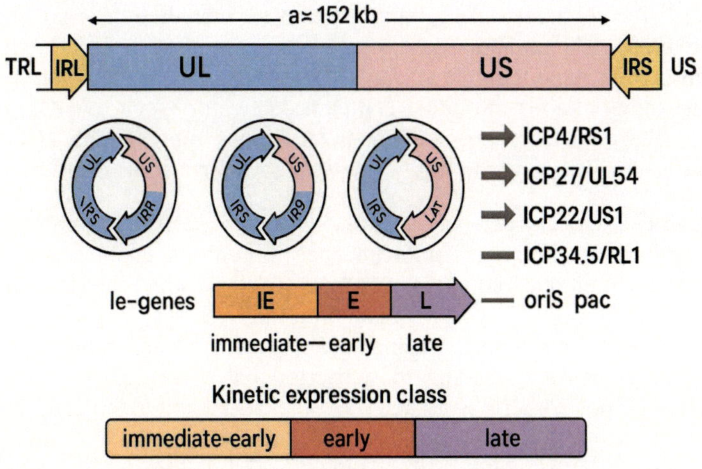

Fig. 3. Genome Organization of the herpes simplex virus type 1 (HSV-1).

Latency and Neurotropism

Herpes simplex virus type 1 (HSV-1) exhibits a hallmark capacity to establish lifelong latency in peripheral sensory and autonomic neurons, where the viral genome persists in an episomal state within the neuronal nucleus (**Fig. 4**). During latency, lytic gene expression is globally repressed through epigenetic silencing, and the viral DNA is incorporated into host chromatin enriched with repressive histone modifications, notably H3K27me3 and H3K9me3 (Canova et al. 2024; Bloom 2016). In this transcriptionally quiescent state, expression is largely restricted to the latency-associated transcript (LAT) locus and a subset of viral microRNAs, which act collectively to stabilize latency.

LAT has been shown to promote the establishment and maintenance of latency by exerting anti-apoptotic effects in infected neurons and by reinforcing heterochromatinization of lytic gene promoters, thereby preventing premature reactivation (Nicoll et al. 2016; Arbuckle et al. 2023; Pierce et al. 2023; Deng et al. 2024). In addition to viral determinants, neuronal microRNAs (miRNAs), such as miR-9, miR-138, and miR-155, interact with viral and host chromatin-modifying pathways to sustain epigenetic silencing of HSV genomes (Pan et al. 2014; da Silva & Jones 2013). These findings highlight how cell-intrinsic chromatin environments and neuronal transcriptional programs cooperate with viral non-coding RNAs to enforce a durable latent state. Reactivation from latency can be induced by a range of cellular stressors, including axonal injury, hyperthermia, UV irradiation, and psychological stress, all of which converge on chromatin-remodeling pathways. These signals disrupt repressive histone modifications, mobilize cellular coactivators such as HCF-1 and LSD1, and re-enable expression of viral IE genes, most notably ICP0 and ICP4, thereby initiating the full lytic cascade (Canova et al. 2024).

From a gene-delivery perspective, HSV-1 latency offers both opportunities and limitations. Episomal maintenance in neurons enables long-term persistence of engineered vector genomes while avoiding the risks of host genome integration. However, innate antiviral defenses, including cGAS-STING sensing, interferon signaling, and epigenetic silencing, may suppress transgene expression, leading to transcriptional extinction if expression cassettes are not properly insulated (Nicoll et al. 2016; Orzalli et al. 2015).

To address these challenges, modern replication-deficient HSV (rdHSV) vectors employ synthetic promoter–insulator architectures, neuron-specific enhancers, and viral ORF-free scaffolds, which collectively minimize immune stimulation and reduce susceptibility to heterochromatin-mediated shutdown (Packard et al. 2021; Soukupová et al. 2021; Su et al. 2024). Such approaches increase the likelihood of stable, cell-type–specific expression in vivo, particularly in postmitotic neuronal populations. Parallel therapeutic strategies, particularly in the context of herpetic keratitis and recurrent ocular disease, increasingly aim to permanently silence or excise latent viral genomes. Recent work has leveraged CRISPR-Cas9 nucleases, meganucleases, and other genome-editing platforms delivered via AAV or lentiviral vectors to target conserved HSV genes essential for reactivation or latency maintenance, such as ICP0, ICP4, and LAT. Preclinical studies demonstrate that such interventions can significantly reduce viral reactivation and associated pathology, underscoring the translational potential of genome-targeted anti-HSV therapies (Aubert et al. 2020; van Diemen et al. 2016; Yin et al. 2021).

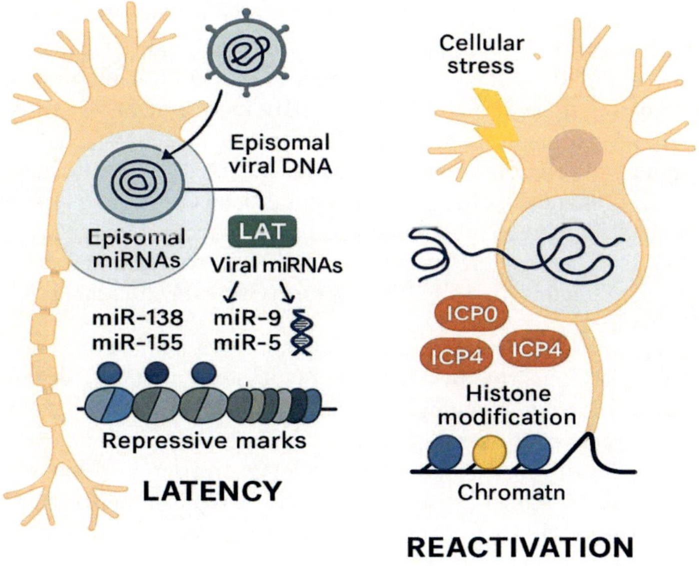

Fig. 4. Latency and Neurotropism of HSV-1.

Immune Evasion Mechanisms

Herpes simplex virus type 1 (HSV-1) has evolved an extensive repertoire of immune evasion strategies that enable viral persistence in the host by attenuating both innate and adaptive immune responses (**Fig. 5**). Among the most well-characterized is ICP47, an immediate-early protein that binds to the transporter associated with antigen processing (TAP), thereby blocking the translocation of viral peptides into the endoplasmic reticulum. This prevents peptide loading onto major histocompatibility complex class I (MHC-I) molecules, reducing $CD8^+$ T cell recognition of infected cells. Notably, ICP47 exhibits strong species specificity-potently inhibiting human TAP but showing weaker activity against murine TAP-thereby complicating the translational relevance of preclinical mouse models (Praest et al. 2018; Nagy et al. 2024). Recent studies further suggest that ICP47 differentially impacts HLA allotypes, particularly suppressing HLA-A and HLA-C antigen presentation while sparing HLA-B, with potential implications for the design of oncolytic HSV (oHSV) vectors combined with immune checkpoint blockade (Sethumadhavan et al. 2022). Beyond antigen presentation, HSV-1 manipulates innate immune signaling pathways. Viral proteins such as ICP0, UL36, UL37, and UL41 (vhs) interfere with cGAS–STING–TBK1–IRF3 signaling, thereby suppressing type I interferon induction and antiviral gene expression (Tabtieng 2022; Zhang et al. 2018). In parallel, HSV antagonizes the PKR–eIF2α pathway, a key antiviral stress response that normally halts protein synthesis. The viral γ134.5 protein recruits host protein phosphatase 1α (PP1α) to dephosphorylate eIF2α, restoring translation and facilitating continued viral replication (Takai et al. 2018). Additional mechanisms include modulation of non-classical antigen presentation pathways, such as downregulation of MHC class II and interference with NK cell recognition via altered expression of ligands for NKG2D receptors (Gao et al. 2025).

From a vector design perspective, these immune-evasion functions represent both risks and opportunities. For oncolytic HSV (oHSV), deletion or inactivation of genes encoding immune evasins (e.g., ICP47, γ134.5) is a well-established safety strategy that enhances tumor immunogenicity by restoring antigen presentation and boosting interferon responsiveness (Workenhe & Mossman 2014). Conversely, in replication-deficient HSV (rdHSV) vectors, viral gene expression is largely absent, preventing de novo synthesis of immune modulators while maintaining the viral capsid's inherent neurotropism.

This reduces antigenic load and diminishes the risk of chronic inflammation in the central nervous system (CNS) (Su et al. 2024). Emerging findings also reveal host genetic variability in immune defense against HSV. For example, certain TAP polymorphisms confer reduced susceptibility to ICP47 binding, potentially enhancing antigen presentation despite infection (Praest et al. 2018). These discoveries are informing novel approaches in both preclinical modeling and vector engineering. One promising avenue involves incorporating immunostimulatory payloads—such as secreted interferons, chemokines, or STING agonists—into oHSV backbones to overcome viral subversion and promote productive anti-tumor immunity (Kaur et al. 2012). Together, these insights underscore the importance of balancing safety, immunogenicity, and persistence in HSV vector platforms. Rational oHSV design increasingly favors attenuated genomes that both expose tumor antigens and stimulate innate immunity. At the same time, rdHSV approaches focus on minimizing innate activation to support durable, inflammation-free transgene expression in the CNS.

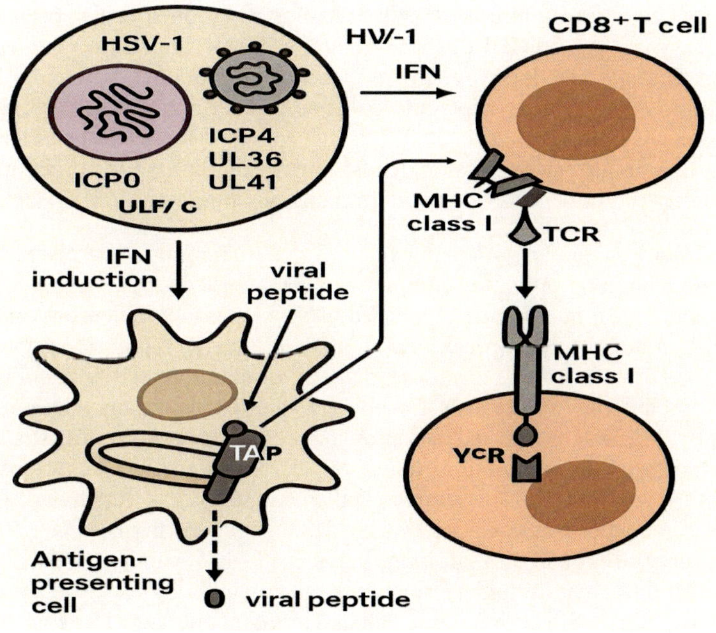

Fig. 5. Repertoire of immune evasion strategies of HSV-1.

Replication-Defective Vectors

Replication-defective HSV (rdHSV) vectors represent a mature and versatile platform for central nervous system (CNS) gene delivery, distinguished by their ability to accommodate payloads far exceeding the size constraints of adeno-associated virus (AAV) and lentiviral systems (**Fig. 6**). These vectors are typically engineered by deleting one or more essential immediate-early (IE) genes-most commonly ICP4 (RS1) and ICP27 (UL54), with additional deletions of ICP22 (US1) and ICP0 (RL2)-to abolish viral gene expression in transduced cells (Su et al. 2024; Canova et al. 2024). As a result, no de novo synthesis of viral proteins occurs, minimizing cytotoxicity and immune recognition while preserving the virus's inherent neurotropism. The vector genome remains episomal within the nucleus. It can support very large genetic payloads (>30–50 kb), enabling delivery of therapeutic cDNAs too large for AAV (e.g., full-length dystrophin), multicistronic operons, and synthetic gene regulatory circuits (Ingusci et al. 2025a; Ingusci et al. 2025b; Goins et al. 2020). Recent design iterations incorporate chromatin insulators (e.g., cHS4 derivatives) to reduce heterochromatin-mediated silencing, neuron-specific promoters (e.g., synapsin, CaMKIIα) to achieve cell-type precision, and post-transcriptional regulatory elements such as WPRE and optimized 5′/3′ UTRs to stabilize transcripts and enhance protein output (Su et al. 2024; Ingusci et al. 2025a; Ingusci et al. 2025b). Together, these strategies sustain long-term transgene expression in post-mitotic neurons while mitigating the promoter shutdown that often undermines non-optimized HSV systems.

Importantly, complete silencing of viral gene expression sharply reduces adaptive immune activation compared to oHSV or wild-type infection. This immunological quiescence supports durable expression in neurons and has demonstrated utility in preclinical models of enzyme replacement therapy (e.g., lysosomal storage diseases), delivery of neuroprotective factors, and neuromodulation approaches for epilepsy and chronic pain (Goins et al. 2020). Manufacturing technologies have also advanced significantly. Modern rdHSV production relies on bacterial artificial chromosome (BAC)-based genome assembly and recombineering methods, which streamline precise engineering of large HSV genomes (Ingusci et al. 2025a; Ingusci et al. 2025b). In addition, helper cell lines expressing deleted IE gene products in trans under stringent regulation have improved vector yield and scalability while minimizing helper-virus contamination (Su et al. 2024; Goins et al. 2020). These innovations facilitate Good Manufacturing Practice (GMP)-compliant production, a prerequisite for translation.

Early-phase clinical neurotherapeutic programs employing rdHSV vectors increasingly adopt stereotactic intraparenchymal or intrathecal administration, coupled with dose-escalation protocols and long-term monitoring for vector biodistribution, viral shedding, and immunogenicity. Collectively, these refinements position rdHSV as a robust gene-transfer system for CNS disorders in which AAV-based approaches are limited by payload size or restricted tropism (Ingusci et al. 2025a; Ingusci et al. 2025b; Goins et al. 2020).

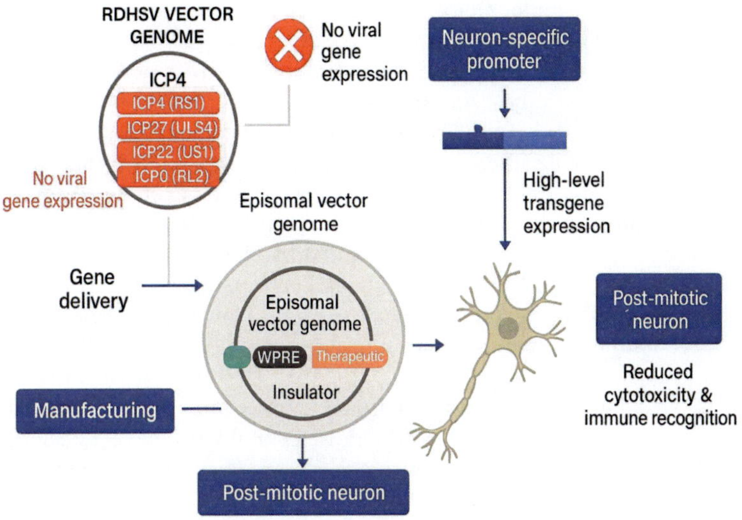

Fig. 6. Replication-defective HSV (rdHSV) vectors.

Amplicon Vectors

Herpes simplex virus (HSV) amplicon vectors represent one of the most flexible gene delivery platforms available, owing to their extraordinary cargo capacity and minimal viral coding sequence content (**Fig. 7**). Amplicons are non-replicating, helper-dependent constructs in which exogenous DNA-often up to ~150 kilobases (kb)-is flanked by the HSV origin of replication (oriS/oriL) and packaging signal (pac), enabling efficient encapsidation into HSV virions (Moralli et al. 2020; Ingusci et al. 2025a; Ingusci et al. 2025b).

Because amplicons lack all viral coding sequences, they are considered genetically safer than oncolytic or replication-defective HSV vectors, avoiding cytotoxic viral gene expression while preserving HSV's natural neurotropism and episomal maintenance in non-dividing neurons (Bailer et al. 2017). The defining strength of amplicon systems lies in their cargo capacity, which exceeds that of all other viral vector platforms. This enables delivery of large disease genes (e.g., full-length *dystrophin* or *CFTR*), multi-cistronic operons, regulatory networks, or CRISPR-based multiplexed payloads (including multiple gRNA arrays, nucleases, and accessory proteins) within a single vector (Cuchet et al. 2007; Ingusci et al. 2025a; Ingusci et al. 2025b). These features make amplicons particularly attractive for neurogenetic disorders, gene replacement therapies requiring multi-kilobase cDNAs, and immuno-oncology applications involving combinatorial payloads (e.g., cytokine + checkpoint inhibitor traps) (Toda et al. 1999). Despite these advantages, early amplicon systems were hindered by transgene silencing and variegated expression due to heterochromatinization of episomal DNA. To overcome these limitations, recent designs incorporate chromatin regulatory elements such as insulators (cHS4 variants), scaffold/matrix attachment regions (S/MARs), and ubiquitous chromatin-opening elements (UCOEs) to insulate payloads from repressive chromatin and maintain transcriptional activity (Su et al. 2024; Ingusci et al. 2025a; Ingusci et al. 2025b). These improvements have enabled sustained and uniform neuronal expression, even in long-term studies. Parallel advances in production technologies have accelerated translational potential. Traditional amplicon production relied on helper viruses, which complicated vector purification and raised regulatory hurdles.

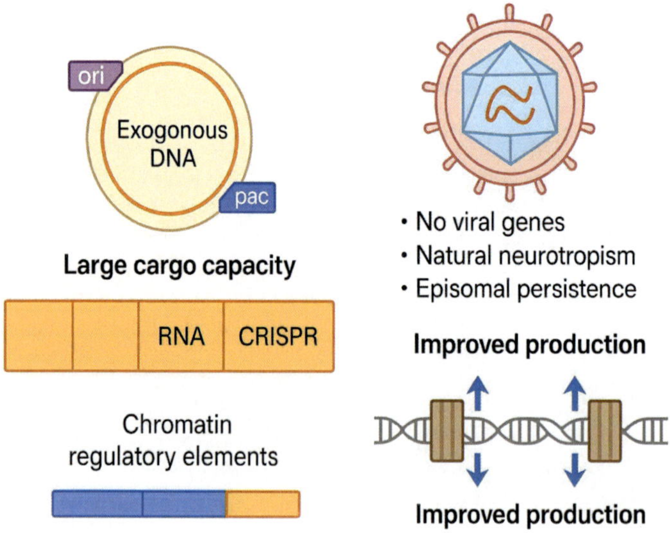

Fig. 7. Herpes simplex virus (HSV) amplicon vectors.

Modern systems employ helper virus–free production strategies, including split-helper plasmid approaches and refined producer cell lines, thereby eliminating helper-virus contamination while improving scalability (De Silva et al. 2009). Furthermore, optimized capsid and tegument compositions have been shown to enhance nuclear delivery and episomal stability, improving functional transduction efficiency (Toda et al. 1999; Ingusci et al. 2025a; Ingusci et al. 2025b). As Good Manufacturing Practice (GMP)-compliant production platforms continue to mature, HSV amplicon vectors are increasingly viewed as a next-generation option for CNS and ex vivo applications, particularly when payload size or genetic complexity exceeds the limits of AAV or lentiviral vectors. Collectively, these innovations position amplicons as a unique, scalable, and clinically relevant tool for large-gene delivery, multiplexed genome editing, and advanced cell and gene therapy paradigms.

Helper Virus-Free Production

The development of helper virus–free production systems has been pivotal for advancing HSV vectors toward clinical application (**Fig. 8**). Historically, HSV amplicon vectors required helper HSV genomes to supply viral proteins necessary for encapsidation and maturation. However, this approach carried substantial risks of contamination with replication-competent HSV (rcHSV), creating both biosafety and regulatory barriers (Cuchet et al. 2007; De Silva et al. 2009). Modern helper-free platforms circumvent these risks by using plasmid-based helper systems and engineered producer cell lines that transiently provide essential viral functions. In the split-helper plasmid strategy, structural and packaging genes are divided across multiple plasmids, each engineered to lack HSV packaging signals and replication origins. This design minimizes the probability of homologous recombination and rcHSV reconstitution (Ingusci et al. 2025a; Ingusci et al. 2025b; De Silva et al. 2009). Furthermore, conditional promoters and regulated expression systems (e.g., Tet-inducible cassettes) have been implemented to restrict expression of potentially cytotoxic immediate-early (IE) proteins, thereby improving producer cell viability and enhancing yields (Toda et al. 1999). For replication-defective HSV (rdHSV) vectors, the availability of bacterial artificial chromosome (BAC)-based cloning and site-specific recombinases (Cre, Flp) has accelerated precise genome engineering. These tools facilitate the rapid construction of deletion mutants, the insertion of therapeutic payloads, and the incorporation of insulators or regulatory sequences, while enabling iterative optimization (Su et al. 2024; Goins et al. 2020). Quality control and analytics play a critical role in validating helper-free production. Sensitive assays such as quantitative PCR (qPCR) and droplet digital PCR (ddPCR) are routinely used to detect residual helper sequences or packaging contamination. In addition, next-generation sequencing (NGS) is increasingly employed to survey recombinant genomes and detect rare recombination events (Cuchet et al. 2007). Infectivity assays in permissive cells, combined with functional potency assays tailored to the therapeutic mechanism-such as neuronal transduction and transgene expression for rdHSV or oncolysis and immune activation for oHSV-are essential components of release testing (De Silva et al. 2009). From a Good Manufacturing Practice (GMP) perspective, helper-free systems have transformed the acceptability of HSV vectors. GMP workflows include adventitious-agent testing, residual host-cell DNA and protein quantification, and lot-release potency assays that reflect the intended clinical use.

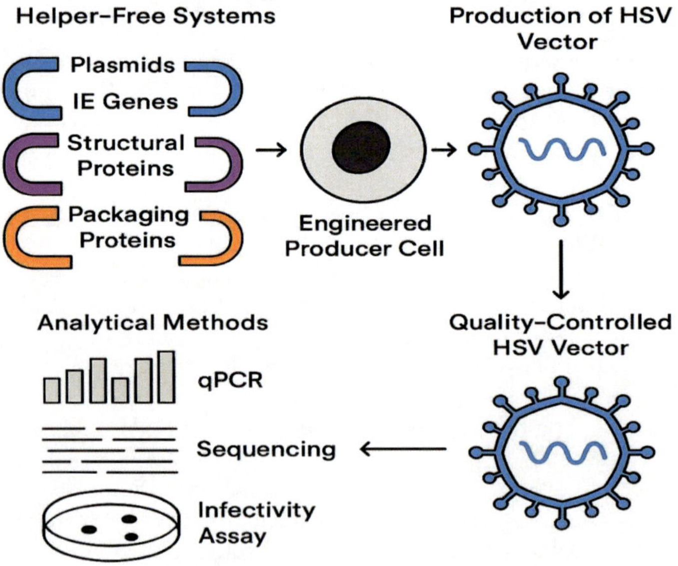

Fig. 8. The development of helper virus–free production systems.

Advances in producer cell line engineering and scalable bioreactor platforms now allow high-titer production under GMP conditions, addressing a historic limitation of HSV vectors (Toda et al. 1999; Su et al.

2024). Collectively, these innovations have established helper virus–free production as the standard for translational HSV vector manufacturing, enabling safe, reproducible, and regulatorily compliant development of both amplicon vectors and rdHSV platforms for clinical applications in neurology, oncology, and regenerative medicine.

Targeted Modifications

The design of targeted HSV vectors has advanced considerably in recent years, driven by the dual needs of precision tropism and controlled payload expression (**Fig. 9**). These innovations are critical for both oncolytic HSV (oHSV) and replication-defective HSV (rdHSV) platforms, as they balance therapeutic potency with safety and specificity.

(i) Glycoprotein retargeting. HSV entry is mediated by multiple glycoproteins, with glycoprotein D (gD) serving as a key determinant of receptor engagement. Modern strategies engineer gD or gB to replace natural receptor-binding domains with tumor- or neuron-specific ligands, antibodies, or designed ankyrin repeat proteins (DARPins), thereby redirecting viral entry toward target cells while reducing off-target infection (Fu & Pan 2025; Campadelli-Fiume et al. 2016). Such modifications are particularly impactful in oHSV, where tumor selectivity can be enhanced by ligand-driven entry restriction.

(ii) MicroRNA (miRNA)-based detargeting. Incorporation of miRNA recognition elements into viral or transgene cassettes restricts expression in off-target tissues. This approach has been adapted in both oHSV and rdHSV to fine-tune tissue specificity without altering capsid tropism.

(iii) Transcriptional and epigenetic logic. Synthetic promoters, enhancers, and epigenetic insulators allow the construction of logic-gated transcriptional programs within HSV genomes. Incorporation of tumor-specific promoters (e.g., hTERT, survivin, nestin) restricts oHSV replication to malignant cells (Toda et al. 1999). In contrast, neuron-specific enhancers (e.g., synapsin, CaMKIIα) sustain long-term, non-immunogenic expression from rdHSV vectors (Ingusci et al. 2025a; Ingusci et al. 2025b). Chromatin insulators (e.g., cHS4, UCOEs) further stabilize transcription, reducing promoter silencing and variegation across neuronal subtypes (Cuchet et al. 2007).

(iv) Payload engineering. Beyond vector targeting, HSV vectors increasingly carry immunomodulatory and functional payloads. oHSV vectors have been armed with GM-CSF, IL-12, CXCL9/10, and checkpoint inhibitor traps, thereby reshaping the tumor microenvironment, enhancing T cell infiltration, and synergizing with systemic immunotherapies (Koch et al. 2020; Shimizu et al. 2023). In rdHSV applications, payloads designed to improve axonal transport and synaptic delivery (e.g., modified neurotrophic factors or transport motifs) facilitate more efficient transgene spread across neuronal networks (Su et al. 2024).

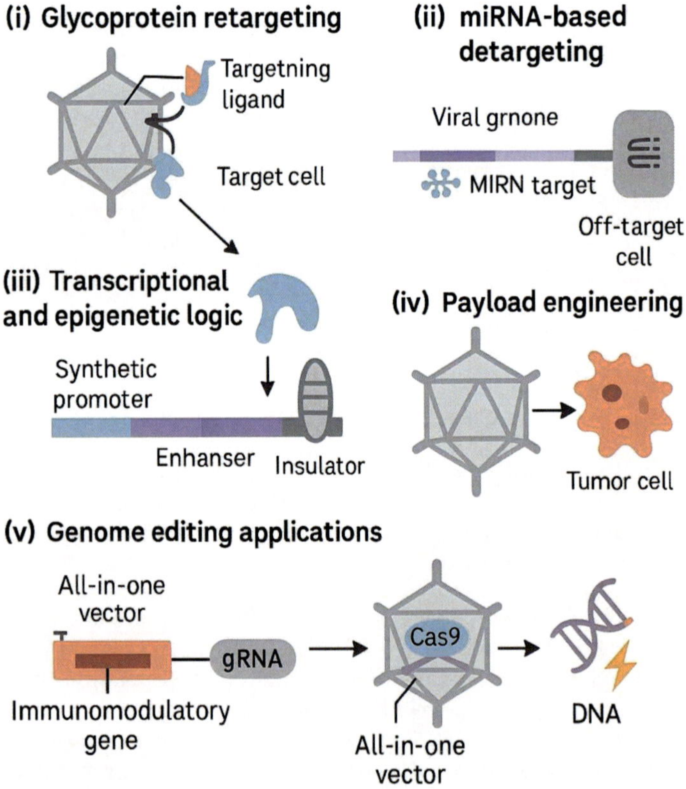

Fig. 9. The design of targeted HSV vectors.

(v) Genome editing applications. With their unparalleled cargo capacity, HSV vectors are uniquely suited to deliver CRISPR-Cas nucleases, meganucleases, or base editors, along with multiplexed gRNA arrays. This enables “all-in-one” genome editing tools that are not feasible with AAV or

LV platforms. Current work focuses on excision or disruption of latent HSV genomes (van Diemen et al., 2016) and on gene correction strategies for large CNS genes, such as DMD or HTT, whose payloads exceed AAV limits-future directions. Expanding the map of promoter-enhancer compatibility across neuronal and glial subtypes using barcoded reporter libraries will allow rational design of subtype-specific vectors. Furthermore, combinatorial glycoprotein engineering and ligand-directed capsids are expected to refine targeting to specific neuronal circuits or glial populations, while minimizing off-target transduction. Collectively, these strategies position HSV vectors as highly modular tools for precision gene therapy, immuno-oncology, and neurogenetic editing.

Attenuation Strategies

The attenuation of HSV vectors is a cornerstone of their safe deployment in both oncolytic virotherapy and CNS-directed gene therapy (**Fig. 10**). The overarching goal is to turn off neurovirulence and uncontrolled replication in healthy tissues while maintaining or enhancing therapeutic activity. A spectrum of molecular, genetic, and translational strategies has been established and refined over the past decade, including canonical genetic deletions. The most widely used attenuation strategy involves deletion of the ICP34.5 (RL1) gene, which normally counteracts the host protein kinase R (PKR) mediated antiviral response by restoring translation by dephosphorylating eIF2α. Removal of ICP34.5 prevents viral neurovirulence while retaining robust replication in many tumor settings (Koch et al. 2020). Similarly, deletion or inactivation of UL39, which encodes the large subunit of ribonucleotide reductase (ICP6), restricts viral DNA synthesis to proliferating cells rich in nucleotide pools, further biasing replication toward tumor tissue (Shimizu et al. 2023). In addition, deletion of ICP47, a viral inhibitor of TAP-mediated antigen presentation, both attenuates immune evasion and enhances the visibility of infected tumor cells to cytotoxic T lymphocytes, thereby augmenting immunotherapeutic synergy (Berkey et al., 2017).

Replication-defective attenuation. For rdHSV vectors, attenuation is achieved by deleting essential immediate-early (IE) genes, such as ICP4 and ICP27, and often ICP22 or ICP0. This strategy abolishes viral gene expression in transduced cells, thereby preventing cytotoxicity and adaptive immune priming (Ingusci et al. 2025a; Ingusci et al. 2025b). Importantly, rdHSV genomes persist as non-replicating episomes capable of supporting large transgene payloads (>30–50 kb), while the absence of viral proteins

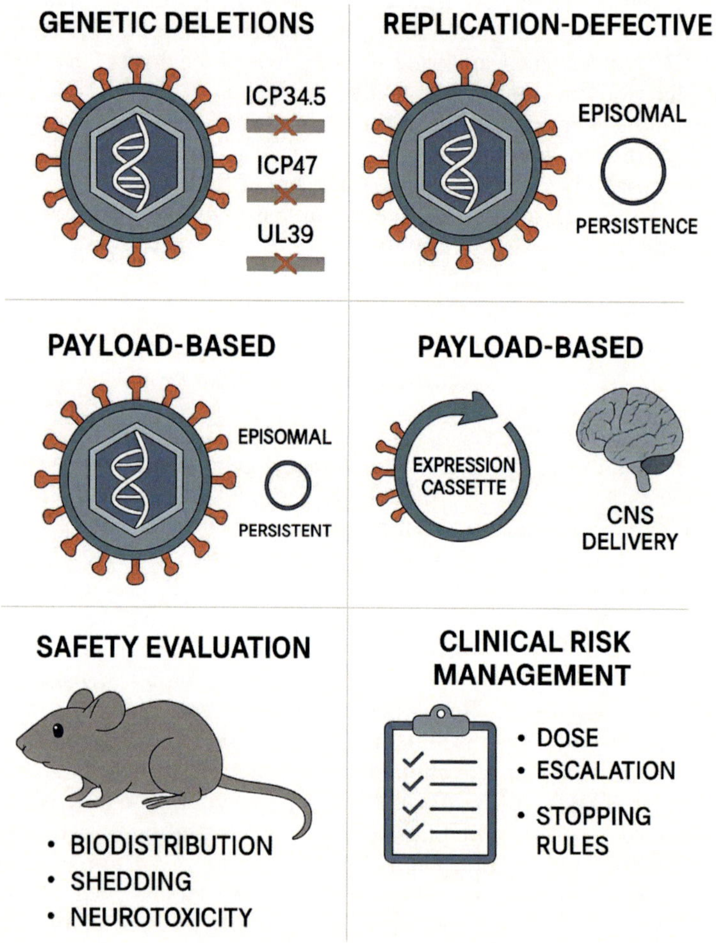

Fig. 10. The attenuation of HSV vectors.

minimizes the risk of neurotoxicity or inflammation-based payload attenuation. The selection of the payload also influences attenuation. In oHSV platforms, expression cassettes frequently encode cytokines (GM-CSF, IL-12), chemokines (CXCL9/10), or immune checkpoint inhibitors, which may intensify local immune activation but require careful dosing to avoid systemic toxicity (Campadelli-Fiume et al. 2016). By contrast, rdHSV payloads prioritize trophic factors, metabolic enzymes, or regulatory proteins with favorable off-target profiles, emphasizing translational safety for long-term CNS applications (Su et al. 2024). Nonclinical safety assessment includes detailed biodistribution, shedding, germline transmission, and neurobehavioral analyses. These studies often use species-specific models that account for differences in HSV immune evasion, such as the reduced potency of ICP47 against murine TAP (Fu & Pan 2025). Advanced safety packages also incorporate neurotoxicity assessments, quantification of viral shedding (qPCR/ddPCR), and long-term monitoring for latent reactivation or horizontal transmission.

Clinical risk management. In line with advanced therapy medicinal product (ATMP) guidelines, dose escalation in clinical trials remains highly conservative. Stopping rules consider early signs of neurotoxicity, herpetic lesions, systemic inflammation, and vector shedding. Regulatory frameworks require validated potency assays that reflect the vector's intended mechanism—cytolytic and immunogenic activity for oHSV, versus neuronal transgene expression for rdHSV (Su et al. 2024). Emerging attenuation strategies integrate synthetic transcriptional circuits, miRNA-based retargeting, and tumor- or neuron-specific promoters to achieve context-dependent restriction of replication or transgene activity. These refinements aim to reduce reliance on broad ICP34.5/UL39 deletions while enabling precision control across distinct therapeutic contexts. Collectively, these attenuation approaches underpin the clinical safety profile of HSV-based vectors, ensuring that therapeutic potency is preserved while minimizing the risks of neurovirulence, off-target replication, and uncontrolled immune activation.

Immune Modulation

The ability of HSV vectors to interact with and remodel host immunity is central to their therapeutic potential, particularly in the context of oncolytic virotherapy and CNS gene delivery (**Fig.11**). Distinct strategies are deployed depending on whether vectors are designed for immunostimulatory anti-tumor responses (oncolytic HSV; oHSV) or for immune evasion and tolerance in the nervous system (replication-defective HSV; rdHSV)-oncolytic immune potentiation. Many oHSV vectors are "armed" with immunomodulatory payloads that amplify both innate and adaptive responses. The prototypical example is alipogene laherparepvec (T-VEC), which expresses GM-CSF to recruit and mature dendritic cells, thereby facilitating cross-presentation of tumor antigens.

Antigens and T cell priming (Andtbacka et al., 2015; Reitmajer et al., 2025). Building on this paradigm, newer vectors encode IL-12, IFN-β, or IL-15 variants, enhancing $CD8^+$ T cell infiltration and promoting durable antitumor immunity (Cheema et al. 2013; Shimizu et al. 2023). Others deploy chemokines such as CXCL9 and CXCL10 to attract effector T and NK cells, or locally expressed checkpoint inhibitors (anti–PD-1, anti–CTLA-4 antibodies) to reverse T cell exhaustion within the tumor microenvironment (Ribas et al. 2018; Thomas et al. 2019). Genetic deletions to enhance immunogenicity. Beyond transgene addition, attenuation strategies themselves contribute to immune modulation. For instance, deletion of ICP47, which normally suppresses MHC-I antigen presentation by inhibiting TAP, restores tumor cell visibility to $CD8^+$ T cells and synergizes with immune checkpoint blockade (Berkey et al. 2017). Immune quietude for CNS applications. By contrast, rdHSV vectors are engineered to minimize immune recognition. The absence of viral gene expression prevents de novo production of viral proteins and limits innate immune activation (Su et al. 2024). Genome design employs insulators, neuron-specific promoters, and chromatin-opening elements to sustain long-term neuronal expression while avoiding glial activation and inflammatory responses (Ingusci et al. 2025a; Ingusci et al. 2025b). This "immunological quietude" is essential for applications in neurodegeneration, metabolic correction, and neuromodulation, where inflammation could exacerbate pathology.

Combination regimens. HSV immune modulation is increasingly explored in combination therapies. Radiation enhances immunogenic cell death and viral replication (Tang et al. 2025). Chemotherapeutic agents such as temozolomide and alkylators remodel the tumor microenvironment to favor viral activity and immune infiltration (Yang et al. 2021). Furthermore, HSV vectors can be combined with adoptive cell therapies, where viral oncolysis releases neoantigens that augment CAR-T or TIL efficacy (Hemminki et al. 2020)-translational immunoprofiling. Recent clinical and translational studies increasingly incorporate spatially resolved immune profiling of injected lesions, alongside CSF cytokine analysis after intrathecal dosing, to quantify immune cascade dynamics and monitor safety (Markert et al. 2014; Friedman et al. 2021). These readouts not only inform mechanisms of action but also guide rational vector design and patient stratification. Collectively, HSV vectors demonstrate a bimodal immunological spectrum: oHSV platforms leverage immune activation to maximize oncolysis and systemic antitumor immunity, whereas rdHSV systems enforce immunological silence to sustain safe, long-term expression in the CNS.

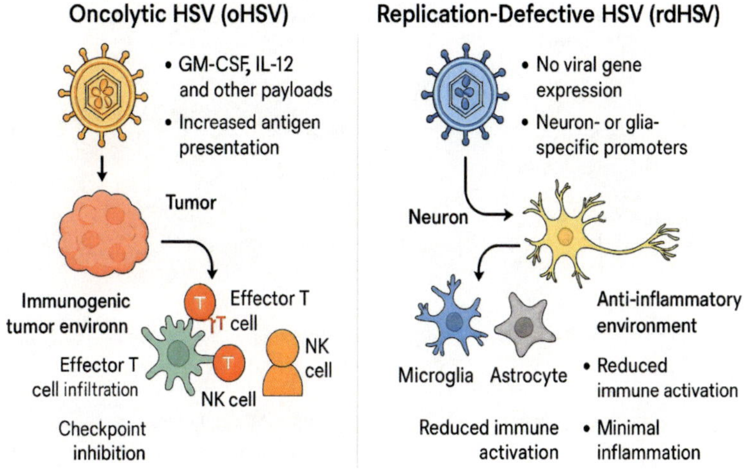

Fig. 11. Immune Modulation of HSV-1.

Genome Integration Avoidance

A fundamental safety feature of HSV-based vectors, including replication-defective HSV (rdHSV) and amplicons, is their design for non-integrative persistence (**Fig. 12**). Unlike retroviral or lentiviral systems, which carry inherent risks of insertional mutagenesis, HSV vectors persist episomally within post-mitotic neurons, enabling long-term transgene expression without genomic disruption (Ingusci et al. 2025a; Ingusci et al. 2025b; Bailer et al. 2017). This property is particularly advantageous for CNS applications, where neurons are largely non-dividing and extremely sensitive to genomic perturbations: epigenetic silencing and transcriptional maintenance. Despite non-integration, episomal HSV genomes are susceptible to heterochromatinization and transcriptional silencing, especially in long-lived neurons. Modern vector design incorporates insulator sequences (e.g., cHS4), CpG dinucleotide minimization, and neuron subtype-specific promoters to stabilize transgene expression (Cuchet et al. 2007; Su et al. 2024). Chromatin-opening elements, such as ubiquitous chromatin opening elements (UCOEs) and scaffold/matrix attachment regions (S/MARs), are also employed to maintain accessible chromatin and prevent variegated expression.

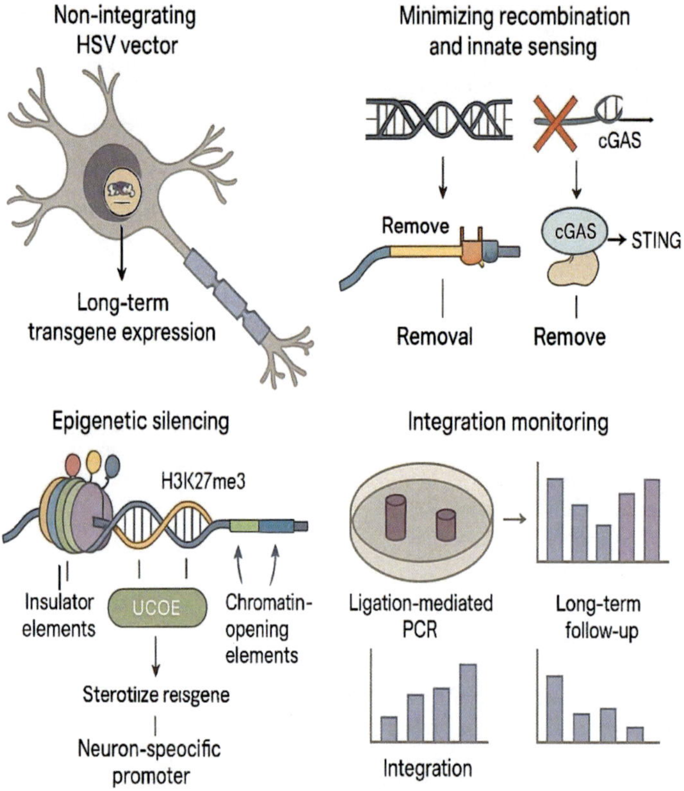

Fig. 12. Fundamental safety feature of HSV-based vectors.

Minimizing recombination and innate sensing. To further reduce genomic instability, HSV vectors omit Cre/Flp recombinase recognition sites, which could mediate unwanted recombination events, and remove bacterial backbone sequences, which may activate innate immune sensors such as cGAS-STING (De Silva et al. 2009). These strategies, when combined, reduce the likelihood of episomal rearrangement or cellular stress responses, supporting both safety and long-term functionality: integration monitoring and translational oversight. Preclinical packages routinely include sensitive integration assays, such as ligation-mediated PCR (LAM-PCR) and integration site sequencing, to detect rare genomic insertions (Bailer et al. 2017). In clinical programs, long-term follow-up protocols aligned with FDA and EMA gene therapy guidance monitor potential late effects, including oncogenic risk, even though integration events are exceedingly rare (FDA 2020)-regulatory and translational implications. The non-integrative nature of HSV vectors offers significant regulatory and clinical advantages, enabling high-capacity gene delivery to neurons without the insertional mutagenesis concerns associated with integrating viral platforms. This feature, combined with careful epigenetic tuning and genome stabilization, positions HSV vectors as a leading platform for long-term CNS gene therapy (Ingusci et al. 2025a; Ingusci et al. 2025b; Cuchet et al. 2007).

Conclusions

Herpes simplex virus (HSV) vectors have emerged as highly versatile platforms for both oncolytic virotherapy and CNS-directed gene therapy, combining large payload capacity, neuronal tropism, and controllable immunogenicity. The breadth of vector architectures—including replication-defective HSV (rdHSV) and amplicons—provides researchers with the flexibility to deliver large genes, multi-cistronic operons, and genome-editing machinery while mitigating the risks of cytotoxicity and insertional mutagenesis. Key advances in genome engineering, latency exploitation, immune modulation, and production methods have enabled HSV vectors to achieve a favorable balance between therapeutic potency and safety. HSV vector platforms exemplify a sophisticated integration of viral biology, engineering, and translational design. Vector design leverages the inherent modularity of HSV, including the UL and US genomic regions, inverted repeats, tegument proteins, and latent genome features, to enable targeted deletions, high-capacity transgene insertion, and neuron-specific expression (Ingusci et al. 2025a; Ingusci et al. 2025b; Fu & Pan 2025). Safety engineering is well established, with attenuation strategies such as deletion of ICP34.5, UL39, and ICP47, and IE gene removal in replication-defective HSV (rdHSV), providing precise control over replication, neurovirulence, and immune recognition. Episomal persistence combined with promoter and insulator design further ensures long-term transgene expression in post-mitotic neurons while minimizing integration risk (Koch et al. 2020; Shimizu et al. 2023; Cuchet et al. 2007). Immune modulation is context-specific, as oncolytic HSV (oHSV) vectors exploit immunostimulatory payloads, including GM-CSF, IL-12, and chemokines, to enhance antitumor immunity. In contrast, rdHSV vectors are engineered for immunological quietude to maintain safe CNS expression. Strategic deletions, such as ICP47, in combination with therapies such as checkpoint blockade or radiochemotherapy, further enhance therapeutic synergy in oncology

(Friedman et al. 2021; Ingusci et al. 2025a; Ingusci et al. 2025b). Finally, manufacturing and translation have matured, with helper virus–free production, BAC-based genome assembly, and precise recombineering enabling scalable, GMP-compliant vector generation with minimal contamination risk, supported by preclinical safety studies and clinical monitoring of biodistribution, immune response, and vector shedding (De Silva et al. 2009; Su et al. 2024). Collectively, these features position HSV vectors as a versatile and clinically viable platform for both CNS gene therapy and oncolytic applications.

Future Directions

The next generation of HSV vectors is poised to leverage enhanced targeting and transcriptional control, enabling precise spatial and temporal regulation of transgene expression (**Fig. 13**). Strategies under development include synthetic promoters, neuron- or tumor-specific enhancers, microRNA retargeting, and combinatorial promoter–insulator architectures, which collectively allow fine-tuned expression in defined cell populations (Toda et al. 1999; Ingusci et al. 2025a; Ingusci et al. 2025b). Barcoded promoter libraries may further accelerate rational design for cell-type-specific applications, optimizing therapeutic outcomes. HSV's unparalleled genome capacity facilitates multiplexed payload delivery, including all-in-one CRISPR/Cas or base-editing systems, multiplexed gRNA arrays, and combinatorial immunomodulatory constructs, surpassing the limits of AAV and lentiviral platforms (van Diemen et al. 2016; Ingusci et al. 2025a; Ingusci et al. 2025b). Coupled with latency-informed vector persistence, which exploits LAT-associated chromatin regulation and epigenetic stabilization, these approaches may improve long-term CNS transgene expression while mitigating immune activation (Yang et al. 2021; Ingusci et al. 2025a; Ingusci et al. 2025b). Integration with combination therapies represents another frontier.

Synergies with radiotherapy, chemotherapy, immune checkpoint blockade, and adoptive cell transfer are likely to enhance oHSV efficacy in oncology, whereas rdHSV vectors may be paired with neuroprotective or neuromodulator interventions for neurodegenerative disorders (Cheema et al. 2013; Ribas et al. 2018). Finally, next-generation clinical translation will benefit from advances in GMP-compliant vector production, sensitive integration and safety assays, immune profiling, and personalized payload design, enabling broader and safer deployment of HSV vectors in both CNS and oncological applications. Regulatory frameworks are evolving to accommodate precision-engineered HSV vectors with defined, non-integrative genomes and controlled immunogenicity. In summary, HSV vectors now constitute a mature, highly adaptable, and translationally ready platform for gene therapy. Future research is poised to harness precision genome engineering, combinatorial payloads, and latency-informed persistence to expand therapeutic impact across oncology and neurology, while maintaining stringent safety and regulatory standards.

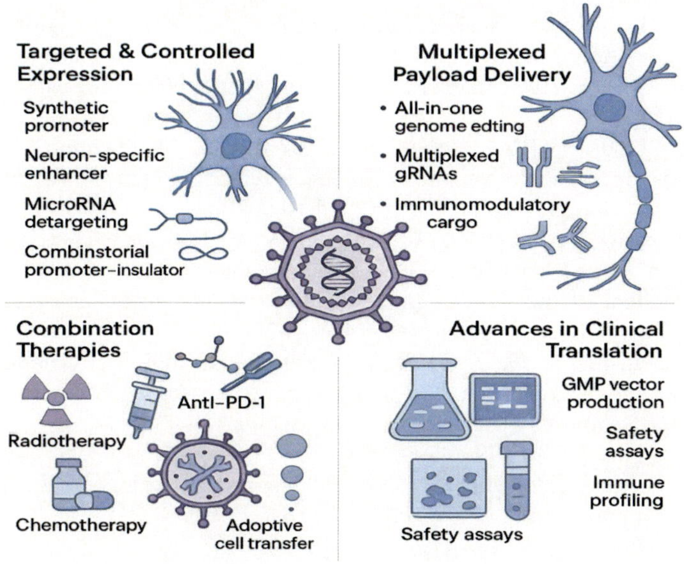

Fig. 13. The next generation of HSV vectors.

References

Andtbacka, R. H. I., Kaufman, H. L., Collichio, F., Amatruda, T., Senzer, N., Chesney, J., … Bommareddy, P. K. (2015). Talimogene laherparepvec improves durable response rate in patients with advanced melanoma. *Journal of Clinical Oncology, 33*(25), 2780–2788. https://doi.org/10.1200/JCO.2014.58.3377

Arbuckle, J. H., Vogel, J. L., Efstathiou, S., & Kristie, T. M. (2023). Deletion of the transcriptional coactivator HCF-1 in vivo impairs the removal of repressive heterochromatin from latent HSV genomes and suppresses the initiation of viral reactivation. *mBio, 14*(1), e0354222.

https://doi.org/10.1128/mbio.03542-22

Aubert, M., Strongin, D. E., Roychoudhury, P., Loprieno, M. A., Haick, A. K., Klouser, L. M., … Jerome, K. R. (2020). Gene editing and elimination of latent herpes simplex virus in vivo. *Nature Communications, 11*(1), 4148. https://doi.org/10.1038/s41467-020-17936-5

Bailer, S. M., Funk, C., Riedl, A., & Ruzsics, Z. (2017). Herpesviral vectors and their application in oncolytic therapy, vaccination, and gene transfer. *Virus Genes, 53*(5), 741–748. https://doi.org/10.1007/s11262-017-1482-7

Berkey, S. E., Thorne, S. H., & Bartlett, D. L. (2017). Oncolytic virotherapy and the tumor microenvironment. *Advances in Experimental Medicine and Biology, 1036*, 157–172. https://doi.org/10.1007/978-3-319-67577-0_11

Bloom, D. C. (2016). Alphaherpesvirus latency: A dynamic state of transcription and reactivation. *Advances in Virus Research, 94*, 53–80. https://doi.org/10.1016/bs.aivir.2015.10.001

Bommareddy, P. K., Patel, A., Hossain, S., & Kaufman, H. L. (2017). Talimogene laherparepvec (T-VEC) and other oncolytic viruses for the treatment of melanoma. *American Journal of Clinical Dermatology, 18*(1), 1–15. https://doi.org/10.1007/s40257-016-0238-9

Campadelli-Fiume, G., Petrovic, B., Leoni, V., Gianni, T., Avitabile, E., Casiraghi, C., & Gatta, V. (2016). Retargeting strategies for oncolytic herpes simplex viruses. *Viruses, 8*(3), 63. https://doi.org/10.3390/v8030063

Cassady, K. A., & Parker, J. N. (2010). Herpesvirus vectors for therapy of brain tumors. *The Open Virology Journal, 4*, 103–108. https://doi.org/10.2174/1874357901004030103

Cheema, T. A., Wakimoto, H., Fecci, P. E., Ning, J., Kuroda, T., Jeyaretna, D. S., Martuza, R. L., & Rabkin, S. D. (2013). Multifaceted oncolytic virus therapy for glioblastoma in an immunocompetent cancer stem cell model. *Proceedings of the National Academy of Sciences of the United States of America, 110*(29), 12006–12011. https://doi.org/10.1073/pnas.1307935110

Canova, P. N., Charron, A. J., & Leib, D. A. (2024). Models of herpes simplex virus latency. *Viruses, 16*(5), 747. https://doi.org/10.3390/v16050747

Cliffe, A. R., Arbuckle, J. H., & Kristie, T. M. (2015). Dynamic changes in HDAC3 occupancy on the latent herpes simplex virus genome during reactivation. *Journal of Virology, 89*(11), 6068–6076. https://doi.org/10.1128/JVI.00443-15

Cuchet, D., Potel, C., Thomas, J., & Epstein, A. L. (2007). HSV-1 amplicon vectors: A promising and versatile tool for gene delivery. *Expert Opinion on Biological Therapy, 7*(7), 975–995. https://doi.org/10.1517/14712598.7.7.975

da Silva, L. F., & Jones, C. (2013). Small non-coding RNAs encoded within the herpes simplex virus type 1 latency associated transcript (LAT) cooperate with the retinoic acid inducible gene I (RIG-I) to induce beta-interferon promoter activity and promote cell survival. *Virus Research, 175*(2), 101–109. https://doi.org/10.1016/j.virusres.2013.04.005

De Silva, S., & Bowers, W. J. (2009). Herpes virus amplicon vectors. *Viruses, 1*(3), 594–629. https://doi.org/10.3390/v1030594

Deng, Y., Lin, Y., Chen, S., Xiang, Y., Chen, H., Qi, S., Oh, H. S., Das, B., Komazin-Meredith, G., Pesola, J. M., Knipe, D. M., Coen, D. M., & Pan, D. (2024). Neuronal miR-9 promotes HSV-1 epigenetic silencing and latency by repressing Oct-1 and Onecut family genes. *Nature Communications, 15*(1), 1991. https://doi.org/10.1038/s41467-024-46057-6

Dolan, A., Jamieson, F. E., Cunningham, C., Barnett, B. C., & McGeoch, D. J. (1998). The genome sequence of herpes simplex virus type 2. *Journal of Virology, 72*(3), 2010–2021. https://doi.org/10.1128/JVI.72.3.2010-2021.1998

Epstein, A. L., & Rabkin, S. D. (2024). Safety of non-replicative and oncolytic replication-selective HSV vectors. *Trends in Molecular Medicine, 30*(8), 781–794. https://doi.org/10.1016/j.molmed.2024.05.014

European Commission. (2018–2025). *EudraLex Volume 4, Part IV: GMP for ATMPs.* Retrieved from https://health.ec.europa.eu/medicinal-products/eudralex/eudralex-volume-4_en

European Commission. (2019). *Medicinal products for human use containing or consisting of genetically modified organisms: Questions and Answers*. European Commission. https://health.ec.europa.eu/system/files/2019-10/gmcells_qa_en_0.pdf

European Commission. (2018). *Guidelines on Good Manufacturing Practice specific to Advanced Therapy Medicinal Products*. EudraLex Volume 4, Part IV. European Commission. https://health.ec.europa.eu/document/download/ad33d9dd-03f0-4bef-af53- 21308ce2187d_en?filename=2017_11_22_guidelines_gmp_for_atmps.pdf

European Commission. (2025). *Advanced therapies*. Public Health, European Commission. https://health.ec.europa.eu/medicinal-products/ product-types/advanced-therapies_en

Frampton, J. E. (2022). Teserpaturev/G47Δ: First approval. *BioDrugs, 36*(5), 667–672. https://doi.org/10.1007/s40259-022-00553-7

Friedman, G. K., Johnston, J. M., Bag, A. K., Bernstock, J. D., Li, R., Aban, I., … Gillespie, G. Y. (2021). Oncolytic HSV-1 G207 immunovirotherapy for pediatric high-grade gliomas. *The New England Journal of Medicine, 384*(17), 1613–1622. https://doi.org/10.1056/NEJMoa2024947

Fu, H., & Pan, D. (2025). Mechanisms of HSV gene regulation during latency and reactivation. *Virology, 602,* 110324. https://doi.org/10.1016/j.virol.2024.110324

Furlan, R., Bergami, A., Brambilla, E., Butti, E., De Simoni, M. G., Campagnoli, M., Marconi, P., Comi, G., & Martino, G. (2007). HSV-1-mediated IL-1 receptor antagonist gene therapy ameliorates MOG(35-55)-induced experimental autoimmune encephalomyelitis in C57BL/6 mice. *Gene Therapy, 14*(1), 93–98. https://doi.org/10.1038/sj.gt.3302805

Gao, Y., Zou, Y., Wu, C., Tao, J., Nie, Z., Yan, J., Wang, P., & Huang, X. (2025). Comparative evaluation of immunomodulatory cytokines for oncolytic therapy based on a high-efficient platform for oHSV1 reconstruction. *Virology Journal, 22*(1), 133. https://doi.org/10.1186/s12985-025-02758-y

Goins, W. F., Huang, S., Hall, B., Marzulli, M., Cohen, J. B., & Glorioso, J. C. (2020). Engineering HSV-1 vectors for gene therapy. *Methods in Molecular Biology, 2060,* 73–90. https://doi.org/10.1007/978-1-4939-9814-2_4

Heldwein, E. E., & Krummenacher, C. (2008). Entry of herpesviruses into mammalian cells. *Cellular and Molecular Life Sciences, 65*(11), 1653–1668. https://doi.org/10.1007/s00018-008-7570-z

Hemminki, O., Dos Santos, J. M., & Hemminki, A. (2020). Oncolytic viruses for cancer immunotherapy. *Journal of Hematology & Oncology, 13*(1), 84. https://doi.org/10.1186/s13045-020-00922-1

Ingusci, S., Goins, W. F., Cohen, J. B., Miyagawa, Y., Knipe, D. M., & Glorioso, J. C. (2025a). Next-generation replication-defective HSV vectors for delivery of large DNA payloads. *Molecular Therapy, 33*(5), 2205–2216. https://doi.org/10.1016/j.ymthe.2025.03.055

Ingusci, S., Cohen, J. B., & Glorioso, J. C. (2025b). Viral and cellular insulators promote sustained HSV vector-mediated transgene expression in brain. *Molecular Therapy, 33*(4), 1420–1433. https://doi.org/10.1016/j.ymthe.2025.02.039

Karpoff, H. M., Kooby, D., D'Angelica, M., Mack, J., Presky, D. H., Brownlee, M. D., Federoff, H., & Fong, Y. (2000). Efficient cotransduction of tumors by multiple herpes simplex vectors: Implications for tumor vaccine production. *Cancer Gene Therapy, 7*(4), 581–588. https://doi.org/10.1038/sj.cgt.7700135

Kaufman, H. L., Shalhout, S. Z., & Iodice, G. (2022). Talimogene laherparepvec: Moving from first-in-class to best-in-class. *Frontiers in Molecular Biosciences, 9,* 834841. https://doi.org/10.3389/fmolb.2022.834841

Kaur, B., Chiocca, E. A., & Cripe, T. P. (2012). Oncolytic HSV-1 virotherapy: Clinical experience and opportunities for progress. *Current Pharmaceutical Biotechnology, 13*(9), 1842–1851. https://doi.org/10.2174/138920112800958814

Koch, M. S., Lawler, S. E., & Chiocca, E. A. (2020). HSV-1 oncolytic viruses from bench to bedside: An overview of current clinical trials. *Cancers, 12*(12), 3514. *https://doi.org/10.3390/cancers12123514*

Le Hars, M., Joussain, C., Jégu, T., & Epstein, A. L. (2025). Non-replicative herpes simplex virus genomic and amplicon vectors for gene therapy—an update. *Gene Therapy, 32*(3), 173–183. https://doi.org/10.1038/s41434-024-00500-x

Markert, J. M., Razdan, S. N., Kuo, H. C., Cantor, A., Knoll, A., Karrasch, M., Nabors, L. B., Markiewicz, M., Agee, B. S., Coleman, J. M., Lakeman, A. D., Palmer, C. A., Parker, J. N., Whitley, R. J., Weichselbaum, R. R., Fiveash, J. B., & Gillespie, G. Y. (2014). A phase 1 trial of oncolytic HSV 1, G207, given in combination with radiation for recurrent GBM demonstrates safety and radiographic responses. *Molecular Therapy, 22*(5), 1048–1055. https://doi.org/10.1038/mt.2014.22

McGeoch, D. J., Rixon, F. J., & Davison, A. J. (2006). Topics in herpesvirus genomics and evolution. *Virus Research, 117*(1), 90–104. https://doi.org/10.1016/j.virusres.2006.01.002

Miyagawa, Y., Marino, P., Verlengia, G., Uchida, H., Goins, W. F., Yokota, S., Geller, D. A., Yoshida, O., Mester, J., Cohen, J. B., & Glorioso, J. C. (2015). Herpes simplex viral-vector design for efficient transduction of nonneuronal cells without cytotoxicity. *Proceedings of the National Academy of Sciences of the United States of America, 112*(13), E1632–E1641. https://doi.org/10.1073/pnas.1423556112

Moralli, D., & Monaco, Z. L. (2020). Gene expressing human artificial chromosome vectors: Advantages and challenges for gene therapy. *Experimental Cell Research, 390*(1), 111931. https://doi.org/10.1016/j.yexcr.2020.111931

Nagy, G., Presley, R., Dhar, S., Jeon, H., Moreira, L., Tull, O., Gupta, A., Chung, D., Tsichlis, P. N., & Parvin, J. D. (2024). Identification of TAP2 protein variants resistant to inhibition by the HSV1 ICP47 protein. *bioRxiv.* https://doi.org/10.1101/2024.11.18.624061

Nicoll, M. P., Proença, J. T., & Efstathiou, S. (2012). The molecular basis of herpes simplex virus latency. *FEMS Microbiology Reviews, 36*(3), 684–705. https://doi.org/10.1111/j.1574-6976.2011.00320.x

Nicoll, M. P., Hann, W., Shivkumar, M., Harman, L. E., Connor, V., Coleman, H. M., Proença, J. T., & Efstathiou, S. (2016). The HSV-1 latency-associated transcript functions to repress latent phase lytic gene expression and suppress virus reactivation from latently infected neurons. *PLOS Pathogens, 12*(4), e1005539. https://doi.org/10.1371/journal.ppat.1005539

Orzalli, M. H., Broekema, N. M., Diner, B. A., Hancks, D. C., Elde, N. C., Cristea, I. M., & Knipe, D. M. (2015). cGAS-mediated stabilization of IFI16 promotes innate signaling during herpes simplex virus infection. *Proceedings of the National Academy of Sciences of the United States of America, 112*(14), E1773–E1781. https://doi.org/10.1073/pnas.1424637112

Packard, J. E., & Dembowski, J. A. (2021). HSV-1 DNA replication-coordinated regulation by viral and cellular factors. *Viruses, 13*(10), 2015. https://doi.org/10.3390/v13102015

Pan, D., Flores, O., Umbach, J. L., Pesola, J. M., Bentley, P., Rosato, P. C., Leib, D. A., Cullen, B. R., & Coen, D. M. (2014). A neuron-specific host microRNA targets herpes simplex virus-1 ICP0 expression and promotes latency. *Cell Host & Microbe, 15*(4), 446–456. https://doi.org/10.1016/j.chom.2014.03.004

PIC/S. (2021–2025). *Annex 2A for ATMPs (PE 009-15).* Retrieved from https://picscheme.org/en/news/revision-of-pics-gmp-guide-pe-009-15

Pierce, C. A., Loh, L. N., Steach, H. R., Cheshenko, N., Preston-Hurlburt, P., Zhang, F., Stransky, S., Kravets, L., Sidoli, S., Philbrick, W., Nassar, M., Krishnaswamy, S., Herold, K. C., & Herold, B. C. (2023). HSV-2 triggers upregulation of MALAT1 in CD4+ T cells and promotes HIV latency reversal. *The Journal of Clinical Investigation, 133*(11), e164317. https://doi.org/10.1172/JCI164317

Praest, P., Luteijn, R. D., Brak-Boer, I. G. J., Lanfermeijer, J., Hoelen, H., Ijgosse, L., Costa, A. I., Gorham, R. D., Jr., Lebbink, R. J., & Wiertz, E. J. H. J. (2018). The influence of TAP1 and TAP2 gene polymorphisms on TAP function and its inhibition by viral immune evasion proteins. *Molecular Immunology, 101,* 55–64. https://doi.org/10.1016/j.molimm.2018.05.025

Reitmajer, M., Nanz, L., Müller, N., Leiter, U., Amaral, T., Aebischer, V., Flatz, L., & Forschner, A. (2025). Comparative real-world outcomes of stage III melanoma patients treated with talimogene laherparepvec or interleukin 2. *Therapeutic Advances in Medical Oncology, 17,* 17588359251324035. https://doi.org/10.1177/17588359251324035

Ribas, A., Dummer, R., Puzanov, I., VanderWalde, A., Andtbacka, R. H. I., Michielin, O., Olszanski, A. J., Malvehy, J., Cebon, J., Fernandez, E., Kirkwood, J. M., Gajewski, T. F., Chen, L., Gorski, K. S., Anderson, A. A., Diede, S. J., Lassman, M. E., Gansert, J., Hodi, F. S., & Long, G. V. (2018). Oncolytic virotherapy promotes intratumoral T cell infiltration and improves anti-PD-1 immunotherapy. *Cell, 174*(4), 1031–1032. https://doi.org/10.1016/j.cell.2018.07.035

Roizman, B., & Whitley, R. J. (2013). An inquiry into the molecular basis of HSV latency and reactivation. *Annual Review of Microbiology, 67,* 355–374. https://doi.org/10.1146/annurev-micro-092412-155654

Sethumadhavan, S., Barth, M., Spaapen, R. M., Schmidt, C., Trowitzsch, S., & Tampé, R. (2022). Viral immune evasins impact antigen presentation by allele-specific trapping of MHC I at the peptide-loading complex. *Scientific Reports, 12*(1), 1516. https://doi.org/10.1038/s41598-022-05000-9

Shimizu, K., Kahramanian, A., Jabbar, M. A. D. A., Turna Demir, F., Gokyer, D., Uthamacumaran, A., Rajan, A., Saad, M. A., Gorham, J., Wakimoto, H., Martuza, R. L., Rabkin, S. D., Hasan, T., & Wakimoto, H. (2023). Photodynamic augmentation of oncolytic virus therapy for central nervous system malignancies. *Cancer Letters, 572,* 216363. https://doi.org/10.1016/j.canlet.2023.216363

Soukupová, M., Zucchini, S., Trempat, P., Ingusci, S., Perrier-Biollay, C., Barbieri, M., Cattaneo, S., Bettegazzi, B., Falzoni, S., Berthommé, H., & Simonato, M. (2021). Improvement of HSV-1 based amplicon vectors for a safe and long-lasting gene therapy in non-replicating cells. *Molecular Therapy—Methods & Clinical Development, 21,* 399–412. https://doi.org/10.1016/j.omtm.2021.03.020

Su, D., Han, L., Shi, C., Li, Y., Qian, S., Feng, Z., & Yu, L. (2024). An updated review of HSV-1 infection-associated diseases and treatment, vaccine development, and vector therapy application. *Virulence, 15*(1), 2425744. https://doi.org/10.1080/21505594.2024.2425744

Tabtieng, T., Lent, R. C., Kaku, M., Monago Sanchez, A., & Gaglia, M. M. (2022). Caspase-mediated regulation and cellular heterogeneity of the cGAS/STING pathway in Kaposi's sarcoma-associated herpesvirus infection. *mBio, 13*(6), e0244622. https://doi.org/10.1128/mbio.02446-22

Takai, S., Majima, T., Reinhart, B., Goins, W. F., Funahashi, Y., Gotoh, M., Tyagi, P., Glorioso, J. C., & Yoshimura, N. (2018). Effects of herpes simplex virus vectors encoding poreless TRPV1 or protein phosphatase 1α in a rat cystitis model induced by hydrogen peroxide. *Gene Therapy, 25*(1), 20–26. https://doi.org/10.1038/gt.2017.94

Tang, S., Yong, L., Cui, Y., Li, H., Bischof, E., & Cai, F. (2025). Harnessing oncolytic viruses for targeted therapy in triple-negative breast cancer. *International Journal of Medical Sciences, 22*(9), 2186–2207. https://doi.org/10.7150/ijms.105683

Thomas, S., Kuncheria, L., Roulstone, V., Kyula, J. N., Mansfield, D., Bommareddy, P. K., Smith, H., Kaufman, H. L., Harrington, K. J., & Coffin, R. S. (2019). Development of a new fusion-enhanced oncolytic immunotherapy platform based on herpes simplex virus type 1. *Journal for Immunotherapy of Cancer, 7*(1), 214. https://doi.org/10.1186/s40425-019-0682-1

Toda, M., Rabkin, S. D., Kojima, H., & Martuza, R. L. (1999). Herpes simplex virus as an in situ cancer vaccine for the induction of specific anti-tumor immunity. *Human Gene Therapy, 10*(3), 385–393. https://doi.org/10.1089/10430349950018832

U.S. Food and Drug Administration. (2020). *Long Term Follow-Up After Administration of Human Gene Therapy Products: Guidance for Industry*. https://www.fda.gov/media/113768/download

U.S. Food and Drug Administration. (2023). *FDA Approves First Topical Gene Therapy for Treatment of Wounds in Patients with Dystrophic Epidermolysis Bullosa*. FDA Press Announcement. May 19, 2023. https://www.fda.gov/news-events/press-announcements/fda-approves-first-topical-gene-therapy-treatment-wounds-patients-dystrophic-epidermolysis-bullosa

van Diemen, F. R., Kruse, E. M., Hooykaas, M. J., Bruggeling, C. E., Schürch, A. C., van Ham, P. M., Imhof, S. M., Nijhuis, M., Wiertz, E. J., & Lebbink, R. J. (2016). CRISPR/Cas9-mediated genome editing of herpesviruses limits productive and latent infections. *PLOS Pathogens, 12*(6), e1005701. https://doi.org/10.1371/journal.ppat.1005701

Wade-Martins, R., Smith, E. R., Tyminski, E., Chiocca, E. A., & Saeki, Y. (2001). An infectious transfer and expression system for genomic DNA loci in human and mouse cells. *Nature Biotechnology, 19*(11), 1067–1070. https://doi.org/10.1038/nbt1101-1067

Wong, B., Birtch, R., Rezaei, R., Jamieson, T., Crupi, M. J. F., Diallo, J. S., & Ilkow, C. S. (2023). Optimal delivery of RNA interference by viral vectors for cancer therapy. *Molecular Therapy, 31*(11), 3127–3145. https://doi.org/10.1016/j.ymthe.2023.09.012

Workenhe, S. T., & Mossman, K. L. (2014). Oncolytic virotherapy and immunogenic cancer cell death: Sharpening the sword for improved cancer treatment strategies. *Molecular Therapy, 22*(2), 251–256. https://doi.org/10.1038/mt.2013.220

Wu, X., & Alvarez-Breckenridge, C. (2023). Moving the pendulum for glioblastoma treatment: One injection at a time. *The Oncologist, 28*(8), 651–653. https://doi.org/10.1093/oncolo/oyad104

Yang, L., Gu, X., Yu, J., Ge, S., & Fan, X. (2021). Oncolytic virotherapy: From bench to bedside. *Frontiers in Cell and Developmental Biology, 9*, 790150. https://doi.org/10.3389/fcell.2021.790150

Yin, D., Ling, S., Wang, D., Dai, Y., Jiang, H., Zhou, X., Paludan, S. R., Hong, J., & Cai, Y. (2021). Targeting herpes simplex virus with CRISPR-Cas9 cures herpetic stromal keratitis in mice. *Nature Biotechnology, 39*(5), 567–577. https://doi.org/10.1038/s41587-020-00781-8

Zhang, J., Zhao, J., Xu, S., Li, J., He, S., Zeng, Y., Xie, L., Xie, N., Liu, T., Lee, K., Seo, G. J., Chen, L., Stabell, A. C., Xia, Z., Sawyer, S. L., Jung, J., Huang, C., & Feng, P. (2018). Species-specific deamidation of cGAS by herpes simplex virus UL37 protein facilitates viral replication. *Cell Host & Microbe, 24*(2), 234–248.e5. https://doi.org/10.1016/j.chom.2018.07.004

Author Biographies

Beyza Aydın graduated from Karadeniz Technical University, Department of Molecular Biology and Genetics. She is currently pursuing her Master's degree in Molecular Biology at Üsküdar University, where she is specializing in translational and applied research. Alongside her graduate studies, she works as an R&D Supervisor at Üsküdar University's NPCELLAB & TRGENMER, contributing to multidisciplinary projects in the fields of advanced therapy medicinal products (ATMPs), immunology, molecular biology, and immunotherapy. Her research focuses on the development of viral vector-based gene delivery systems (AAV and lentivirus), and innovative strategies for cancer immunotherapy including CAR-T cell therapy. In addition, she is engaged in space biology studies, with a particular focus on transcriptomic analyses to investigate cellular responses, immunology and gene expression Dynamics of astronauts under microgravity conditions. By combining expertise in molecular biotechnology, synthetic biology, and immunotherapeutics with space omics research, she aims to bridge terrestrial and space health sciences, advancing next-generation therapeutic strategies for precision medicine both on Earth and beyond.

Cihan Taştan graduated from the METU Molecular Biology and Genetics department in 2011 as a "High Honor" student. In the same year, he was awarded a full scholarship to pursue a PhD in Microbiology-Immunobiology at New York University. He completed his Ph.D. thesis in September 2017, focusing on the relationships between human immune cells and bacterial species in the human body. He received his PhD. In January 2015, he continued his research as a Pre-Doctoral Associate at The Jackson Laboratory-Genomic Medicine Institute. And he took part in the project to develop CRISPR-based genome-modification techniques in human immune cells. Based on these studies, from October 2017 to October 2020, he served as the R&D Unit Manager at Acıbadem LabCell Cell Laboratory, where he led the development of genetically modified CAR-T cell therapies against cancer types and genetic treatments for genetic diseases (for example, Duchenne Muscular Dystrophy). He has continued his studies. He has extensive knowledge and experience in synthetic biology, genetic engineering, and molecular biology, spanning his undergraduate and doctoral periods. He is currently the founding director of the international rare diseases genetic therapy competition and of the hiDNA and Synastra Biotechnology Inc. startups, which develop platforms using Advanced Therapy Medicinal Products (ATMP) technologies. He is the director of CRISPR Valley, where CRISPR gene-engineering technologies are developed and training is provided. He continues to work as a faculty member at Üsküdar University, Department of Molecular Biology and Genetics, and as the director of the Transgenic Cell Technologies Application and Research Center (TRGENMER).

CHAPTER 5

POXVIRUSES

CIHAN INAN

Karadeniz Technical University, Faculty of Science, Department of Molecular Biology and Genetics, Trabzon, Türkiye.

Abstract

Poxviruses (PVs) are double stranded DNA viruses infecting both invertebrate and vertebrate hosts. This family compromised of two subfamilies according to their hosts as Chordopoxvirinae and Entomopoxvirinae. Variola virus is the most known member of the family that infects humans, caused more than 300 million deaths and eradicated by the vaccination campaign conducted by World Health Organisation. Later it was found that PVs especially Vaccinia viruses are oncolytic viruses that infects cancer cells but they do not replicate in healthy cells. Previous studies with PVs showed that it is easy to propagate and recombine this viruses and they have large transgene capacity. Another important fact that makes PVs important is being able to replicate in cytoplasm of the host cell using their own DNA polymerase enzymes while most of the other viruses replicates in the nuclei. While other viral delivery vectors has some drawbacks such as activation in oncogenes and reactions for individuals to have existing immunity, poxviruses have big potential for gene therapy studies.

Studies on vaccinia viruses, which play an active role in the development of vaccines against variola, have revealed that these viruses are important gene therapy agents as well as being oncolytic. Also, interest in other members of the poxvirus family that do not infect humans has led to the emergence of the possibility of using these viruses in non-host organisms. The safe and non-replicative potential of rabbit poxviruses and entomopoxviruses in human cells has recently resulted in increased interest in these viruses including their usage in the vaccine production against SARS-CoV-2. In this chapter, studies on the use of poxviruses as gene therapy agents and potential for future studies are discussed.

Keywords: poxviruses, vacv, poxviral therapy

1. Introduction

Smallpox, caused by the Variola virus, was one of the most devastating diseases in human history, with a 15–45% death rate within a month (Berche 2022; Conrad and Liu 2019). The successful eradication of smallpox in 1977 by the World Health Organization (WHO) marked a historic victory for global vaccination programs. Nonetheless, specific other viruses under the genus Orthopoxvirus have been recorded as infective in humans. These include monkeypox, cowpox, and camelpox viruses, which continue to pose a zoonotic and occasionally epidemic threat, especially in regions with poor surveillance or disrupted ecosystems.

The eradication of smallpox, although complete, has not diminished the scientific and clinical relevance of poxviruses. On the contrary, renewed interest has emerged in the post-eradication era, particularly in the context of bioterrorism preparedness, vaccine platform development, and gene therapy. Variola virus remains a high-concern pathogen under biosafety and national defense strategies, and engineered poxviruses are being studied for potential countermeasures (Jacobs et al., 2009).

The Vaccinia virus (VACV), a member of this family, is acknowledged as the first animal virus to be cultured in cell culture, viewed microscopically, and studied in detail. VACV's historical use as a live vaccine and its biological features have positioned it as a foundational model for poxvirus research and biotechnological development. The Poxviridae family, owing to their distinctive biological characteristics and historical application in human immunization, has emerged as a highly attractive platform for gene delivery vectors (Guo and Bartlett 2004).

Poxviruses are large, double-stranded DNA viruses distinguished by complex structures, which replicate exclusively in the cytoplasm of infected cells, thereby preventing genomic integration (Haddad 2017; Moss 1991; Moss 1996). This replication technique, along with their capacity to incorporate massive transgenic inserts of up to 25 kilobase pairs, renders them optimal candidates for the delivery of intricate genetic payloads (Guo and Bartlett 2004; Smith and Moss 1983). Moreover, their extensive host range and ability for high-titer generation augment their use in both experimental and clinical gene therapy contexts (Haddad 2017).

Unlike many other viral vectors, poxviruses do not rely on the host cell nucleus for replication or gene expression. This attribute minimizes the risk of insertional mutagenesis and avoids issues such as interference with host transcriptional machinery—challenges that have hampered the progress of retroviral and lentiviral gene therapy platforms. Additionally, poxviruses possess their own transcriptional enzymes packaged within the virion, allowing autonomous gene expression upon cytoplasmic entry. The replication cycle of poxviruses, with their distinctive cytoplasmic replication and transcriptional autonomy that eliminates the need for nuclear entry, is shown in Figure 1. This characteristic positions them as excellent candidates for gene therapy, especially in non-dividing or terminally differentiated cells.

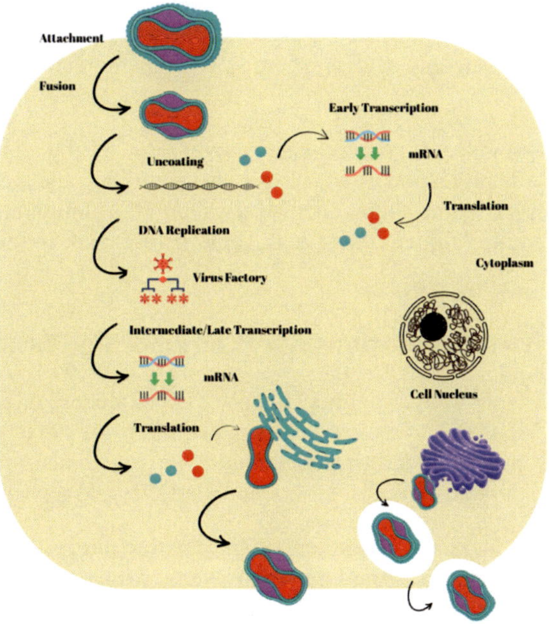

Figure 1. Replication cycle of poxviruses

Vaccinia virus (VACV), the live agent employed in the worldwide eradication of smallpox, has emerged as the model for modified poxviral vectors. The well-characterized genome, established safety profile from widespread historical use, and capacity to induce robust immune responses have been utilized for applications including vaccine production and cancer therapy (Guo and Bartlett 2004; Yaghchi et al., 2015).

Recent advancements in genetic engineering have facilitated the creation of replication-competent and replication-selective poxvirus vectors designed for tumor-specific cytolysis and transgene expression. Oncolytic poxviruses, especially modified VACV strains like JX-594 and GLV-1h68, directly lyse tumor cells while simultaneously stimulating systemic anti-tumor immunity, exemplifying a treatment approach.

Beyond vaccinia, other poxviruses like Myxoma virus (MYXV) and entomopoxviruses (EPV) have also garnered interest. MYXV, while naturally restricted to rabbits, can selectively infect and kill human cancer cells without harming normal human tissues, offering a naturally tumor-selective viral platform (Stanford and McFadden 2007; Rahman and McFadden 2020). EPVs have the ability to enter mammalian cells without causing lethal effects or viral replication. This makes them important candidates in gene therapy studies where safety is paramount (Li, Hall, and Moyer 1997).

This chapter provides a comprehensive overview of the development, engineering, and application of poxviruses as vectors in gene therapy, with particular emphasis on their oncolytic potential, immunomodulatory capabilities, future clinical prospects, and safety and immunological considerations.

2. Poxvirus Generations and Engineering Platforms

The VACV vaccines used throughout history can be categorized into several generations. **Figure 2** summarizes the evolution of VACV vaccine generations from Jennerian cowpox to synthetic constructs, linking each generation to their main features, production platform, and typical use cases.

The first generation, known as the Jennerian vaccines, utilized cowpox virus for immunization against smallpox and were primarily developed by Edward Jenner in the late 1700s. These vaccines were notable for their relative safety compared to earlier methods like variolation. The Wyeth Laboratories, Inc. Dryvax® vaccine represents a significant member of the first generation; it was manufactured from calf lymph using skin-scarification and harvesting techniques and remained the only smallpox vaccine commercially approved for limited use in the United States until

2007. The vaccine production was labor-intensive, based on live animal platforms, and required manual purification and storage under cold-chain conditions.

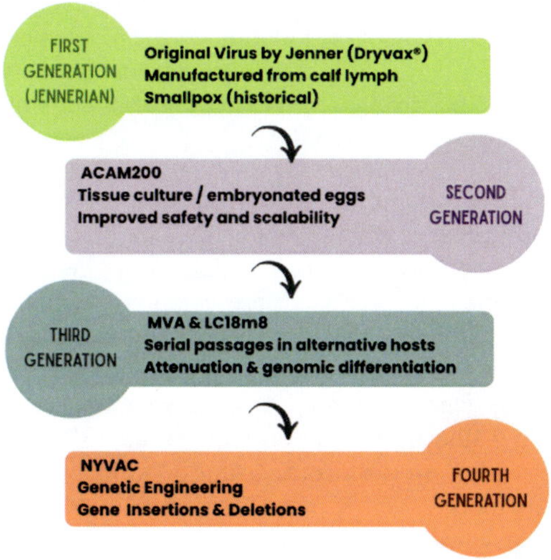

Figure 2. Generations of VACV vaccines and their characteristics

The second-generation vaccines became available through the use of tissue culture systems or embryonated chicken eggs for virus production. This generation was developed primarily to improve safety and scalability of vaccine manufacture. ACAM2000, a virus plaque-purified from Dryvax and propagated in Vero (African green monkey) cells, is a notable example of this generation. Compared to its ancestor, ACAM2000 offered more controlled production and purification. However, it remained a replication-competent virus and required the same dermal inoculation techniques with bifurcated needles, which can occasionally result in localized inflammation, lymphadenopathy, or rare complications such as eczema vaccinatum.

The third generation of VACV vaccines emerged through serial passages in alternative hosts, leading to attenuation and genomic differentiation. Modified Vaccinia Ankara (MVA), one of the best-studied members of this generation, was developed in the late 1950s by passaging the chorioallantois VACV Ankara (CVA) strain in chick embryo fibroblasts over 500 times. This extensive passaging led to the deletion of approximately 30 kb of genomic material and resulted in replication deficiency in most mammalian cells. MVA has been extensively studied for use in both vaccine platforms and gene therapy due to its robust immunogenicity and excellent safety profile in humans, including immunocompromised individuals.

A second member of this generation, LC16m8, was developed in Japan and is characterized by a truncation mutation in the B5R membrane protein, reducing neurovirulence while maintaining immunogenicity. LC16m8 has been approved for use in Japan and demonstrated favorable outcomes during post-licensure surveillance.

Finally, the fourth-generation VACV vaccines involve rational genetic engineering approaches, such as targeted gene deletions or insertions. NYVAC, for instance, was developed by deleting 18 genes involved in viral replication (Tartaglia et al., 1992). These deletions significantly attenuated the virus and eliminated its capacity to replicate in human cells. In addition to deletions, attempts have been made to insert cytokine genes such as IL-2 and IL-12 into the genome, aiming to enhance immunomodulation while further reducing pathogenicity (Kaufman et al., 2002). These modern engineering strategies are performed using homologous recombination or synthetic biology tools, enabling precision control over replication, tropism, and antigen presentation.

3. Vaccinia Virus in Gene Therapy Applications

Vaccinia virus (VACV) stands out as one of the most thoroughly studied viral vectors for gene therapy, primarily due to its historical use in humans, well-characterized genome, large transgene capacity, and cytoplasmic replication strategy. Unlike integrating viral vectors such as lentivirus or retrovirus, VACV does not insert its genome into the host DNA, which greatly reduces the risk of insertional mutagenesis. Additionally, its replication in the cytoplasm ensures rapid gene expression and avoids interference with host nuclear machinery.

VACV's genome can accommodate more than 25 kilobases of foreign DNA, enabling the incorporation of complex therapeutic constructs, including multiple transgenes or regulatory elements (Smith and Moss 1983; Guo and Bartlett 2004). This characteristic is particularly valuable in cancer gene therapy and vaccine development, where simultaneous expression of cytokines, tumor-associated antigens, and reporter genes is often desired. Also, VACV has advantages in effective delivery via intravenous (i.v.) administration (Thorne et al., 2007). These features have made VACV an attractive candidate not only for cancer virotherapy but also for use as a vaccine vector and a platform for delivering therapeutic genes (Haddad 2017; Conrad and Liu 2019; Heo et al., 2013).

A pivotal innovation has been the development of oncolytic VACV vectors, which selectively replicate in and lyse cancer cells. This tumor selectivity is typically achieved through deletion of viral genes involved in nucleotide metabolism, such as thymidine kinase (TK) or viral growth factor (VGF) (Haddad 2017). Because tumor cells often exhibit elevated levels of nucleotide synthesis, TK-deleted viruses can preferentially replicate in malignant tissues while sparing healthy cells.

The best-known example of this approach is JX-594 (Pexa-Vec), a TK-deleted, GM-CSF-expressing VACV strain that has been tested in multiple clinical trials for hepatocellular carcinoma (HCC), colorectal cancer, gastric cancer, renal cell carcinoma and has advanced to Phase 2 trials for some of these indications (Heo et al., 2013; Breitbach et al., 2011; Cousin et al., 2022; Y. Kim et al., 2024; Park et al., 2023; J. H. Kim et al., 2023; Toulmonde et al., 2024). JX-594 combines direct oncolysis with immune stimulation: tumor cells infected by the virus are lysed, releasing tumor antigens, while GM-CSF promotes dendritic cell maturation and T-cell activation. Clinical trials have demonstrated dose-dependent tumor necrosis, systemic immune activation, and prolonged survival in a subset of patients. Notably, JX-594 can be administered both intratumorally and intravenously, and viral replication has been observed specifically within tumors after systemic injection (Breitbach et al., 2011; Cousin et al., 2022).

Another recombinant VACV platform is GLV-1h68, which expresses multiple reporter genes (β-galactosidase, GFP, and luciferase) along with cytosine deaminase to enable gene-directed enzyme prodrug therapy (GDEPT) (Berchtold et al., 2020; Kloker et al., 2020; Pugalenthi et al., 2015). In this strategy, administration of 5-fluorocytosine is converted into the cytotoxic agent 5-fluorouracil specifically in infected tumor cells. GLV-1h68 has demonstrated significant antitumor effects in preclinical models of prostate, pancreatic, and bladder cancer.

Beyond direct tumor lysis, VACV vectors have also been adapted to deliver immunomodulatory payloads. For example, vectors encoding interleukin-12 (IL-12), interferon-beta (IFN-β), or checkpoint blockade antibodies have shown the ability to reshape the tumor microenvironment by enhancing cytotoxic T-cell infiltration and reducing regulatory T-cell populations. VACV expressing VEGFR-1-Fc fusion proteins has also been explored to inhibit angiogenesis, starving tumors of their blood supply (Shakiba et al., 2023).

Another promising application lies in multimodal imaging and treatment monitoring. VACV vectors carrying human sodium iodide symporter (hNIS) or luciferase allow for real-time, non-invasive tracking of viral spread using PET, SPECT, or bioluminescent imaging. This capability supports dose optimization, patient stratification, and therapeutic response assessment (Haddad 2017).

The versatility of VACV has also enabled its integration into combinatorial therapies. Co-administration with immune checkpoint inhibitors such as anti-PD-1 or anti-CTLA-4 has shown synergistic effects, as viral oncolysis releases neoantigens that prime the immune system, while checkpoint blockade sustains T-cell activation. VACV has also been combined with chemotherapy and radiation, with evidence suggesting improved tumor control and reduced metastatic spread.

Chimeric strains such as CF33 further expand VACV's therapeutic scope. CF33 was synthetically constructed using sequences from multiple VACV and RPXV strains to enhance tumor selectivity and safety. Derivatives like CF33-hNIS, CF33-CD19 and CF33-hNIS-antiPDL1 have been tailored to enable targeted imaging and the redirection of CAR-T cells to tumor sites (Y. Woo et al., 2020; Chaurasiya et al., 2020).

In conclusion, Vaccinia virus offers an exceptionally versatile platform for gene therapy applications, particularly in oncology. Its capacity for complex genetic modification, safe replication control, and compatibility with modern immunotherapeutic strategies makes it a leading candidate for future gene-based interventions in both solid and hematologic malignancies.

4. Alternative Poxviruses as Vectors

While Vaccinia virus (VACV) remains the most extensively studied and clinically validated poxvirus vector, it has important limitations. Replication-associated toxicity, preexisting anti-vaccinia immunity in vaccinated populations, and dose-limiting side effects have prompted researchers to explore alternative members of the Poxviridae family. These viruses offer distinct biological advantages—including restricted host tropism, natural tumor selectivity, or replication deficiency in mammalian cells—that may address some of the safety and efficacy concerns encountered with VACV. Their structural and genetic similarity to vaccinia allows the use of established engineering tools and promoter systems, enabling continuity in vector development.

4.1. Myxoma Virus (MYXV)

Myxoma virus (MYXV), a member of the Leporipoxvirus genus, is highly pathogenic in European rabbits but nonpathogenic in other mammalian species, including humans. This unique host restriction, coupled with its ability to selectively replicate in human cancer cells, makes MYXV a compelling candidate for oncolytic virotherapy. Unlike other poxviruses that require attenuation to ensure safety, MYXV is naturally tumor-selective and non-toxic in normal human tissues (Stanford and McFadden 2007; Rahman and McFadden 2020).

MYXV's tumor tropism arises from its exploitation of altered signaling pathways within malignant cells. It can utilize dysregulated PI3K/Akt signaling, commonly seen in transformed cells, to facilitate viral entry and replication. Simultaneously, many cancer cells display defective type I interferon (IFN) responses, which would otherwise restrict viral replication in normal cells. This allows MYXV to evade immune control within tumors, enabling targeted cytolysis(Stanford and McFadden 2007).

MYXV has demonstrated significant therapeutic efficacy in a variety of xenograft and syngeneic tumor models. In glioblastoma, therapy with radiation and temozolomide (TMZ) enhances MYXV replication and reduces cell survival. Also, MYXV and temozolomide injection intratumorally extended survival in mice (Ahmed 2023). In ovarian cancer, MYXV in combination with cisplatin amplified cytotoxic responses and prolonged survival were screened in mouse. In multiple myeloma models, MYXV infection via intravenous injection caused prolonged survival (Rahman and McFadden 2020). In melanoma, MYXV combined with checkpoint inhibitors (e.g., anti-PD-1) showed promise in improving therapeutic outcomes in various cancer models (Valenzuela-Cardenas et al., 2022).

To further enhance its therapeutic potential, MYXV has been engineered to express immune-stimulatory transgenes. MYXV-IL15 promotes NK and CD8+ T cell activation (Tosic et al., 2014). A dual-transgene MYXV encoding a CD47-blocking agent and IFN-γ demonstrated enhanced therapeutic efficacy in murine tumor models by simultaneously promoting phagocytosis and robust $CD8^+$ T cell recruitment, resulting in superior tumor control and extended survival compared to monotherapies (J. H. Kim et al., 2023). These engineered strains show prolonged survival and better tumor control, particularly when administered intravenously or intratumorally in multi-dose regimens.

MYXV has shown synergy with several other therapeutic strategies. In combination with checkpoint inhibitors, MYXV priming increases PD-L1 expression on tumor cells and upregulates neoantigen presentation, making tumors more susceptible to PD-1/PD-L1 blockade. In chemotherapy, by lysing tumor cells and altering the tumor microenvironment, MYXV sensitizes tumors to lower doses of chemotherapeutics (J. K. Woo et al., 2023; Zheng et al., 2022; Wennier et al., 2012). Additionally, there is emerging evidence that MYXV may improve CAR-T cell infiltration and survival within solid tumors, addressing a major limitation of current adoptive cell therapies (Zheng et al., 2022).

Given its non-replicating profile in healthy human tissue, strong immunostimulatory capacity, and compatibility with advanced therapeutic combinations, MYXV continues to be explored in translational settings.

4.2. Avian Poxviruses (FWPV, CNPV/ALVAC)

Avian poxviruses—including Fowlpox virus (FWPV) and Canarypox virus (CNPV, trade name: ALVAC)—belong to the Avipoxvirus genus. These vectors are naturally replication-deficient in mammalian cells, making them exceptionally safe for human applications (Weli and Tryland 2011). Despite their replication block, they retain the ability to express early genes in non-avian cells, enabling them to serve as effective gene delivery platforms for immunization and cancer therapy (Ryan, Harenberg, and Burdin 2007; Kaufman et al., 2014). Also new studies showed that FWPV produce progeny virions in some mammalian cell lines (Weli and Tryland 2011).

When avian poxviruses infect mammalian cells, the viral life cycle is arrested prior to DNA replication. However, early promoter activity is preserved, allowing expression of transgenes inserted under control of early viral promoters. This enables antigen presentation without productive infection or cytotoxicity—a valuable trait for repeated administration or use in immunocompromised individuals.

FWPV has been successfully employed in TRICOM-based cancer vaccines, which include transgenes encoding B7.1 (CD80) for T-cell costimulation, ICAM-1 (CD54) for adhesion and immune synapse formation, and LFA-3 (CD58) for T-cell activation. In one Phase I clinical trial, patients with metastatic colorectal cancer were immunized with recombinant FWPV encoding TRICOM and carcinoembryonic antigen (CEA). The vaccine elicited CEA-specific CD8+ T-cell responses, tumor infiltration, and was well tolerated, with minimal adverse effects (Kaufman et al., 2014). Other tumor-associated antigens (TAAs) such as PSA and MUC1 have also been encoded into FWPV backbones for therapeutic vaccination in prostate, breast and ovarian cancers, respectively (Madan et al., 2012; Mohebtash et al., 2011).

ALVAC has an established track record in infectious disease vaccine trials, including the RV144 HIV vaccine trial in Thailand (Pitisuttithum et al., 2020). The prime-boost regimen using ALVAC-HIV followed by a gp120 protein boost was the first to show partial protection against HIV infection in humans. In addition, ALVAC-based constructs expressing envelope proteins for Zika and Dengue viruses demonstrated immunogenicity and safety in animal models and early-phase clinical trials (Rerks-Ngarm et al., 2009). Also, ALVAC-based vectors have been shown to effectively activate antigen-specific CD4+ and CD8+ T-cell responses in humans, supporting their use in vaccine strategies that require robust cellular immunity (Perreau et al., 2011).

One major advantage of avian poxviruses is their suitability for heterologous prime-boost strategies. ALVAC + MVA or FWPV + VACV combinations are commonly used to avoid anti-vector immunity. As avian vectors are non-cross-reactive with orthopoxviruses, they can be used in alternating regimens to extend the durability of the immune response. Furthermore, the absence of neutralizing antibodies in human populations means multiple booster doses can be administered without loss of efficacy—a major limitation in many other viral vectors (Kaufman et al., 2014).

Avian poxviruses provide several key advantages: they are extremely safe, even in immunocompromised patients; they elicit high immunogenicity without replication; they are already approved for veterinary use (e.g., ALVAC-Rabies, ALVAC-FIV); and there is no preexisting immunity in humans. However, they also carry certain limitations, including lower gene expression compared to replicating vectors, limited systemic immune stimulation unless combined with adjuvants or co-vectors, restriction of transgene expression and creating progeny viruses in mammalian cells, as seen in recent studies.

Despite these limitations, avian poxviruses are one of the most clinically studied poxvirus vectors, with wide applications in both human and veterinary medicine. Their excellent safety profile and compatibility with modern vaccine technologies continue to make them valuable tools in gene therapy and immunotherapy (Weli and Tryland 2011; Kaufman et al., 2014; Ryan, Harenberg, and Burdin 2007).

4.3. Entomopoxviruses (EPVs)

Entomopoxviruses (EPVs) are large double-stranded DNA viruses that naturally infect insects and belong to the Entomopoxvirinae subfamily of Poxviridae. Unlike orthopoxviruses and avipoxviruses, EPVs are completely non-replicative in vertebrate cells, which makes them an exceptionally safe platform for gene delivery—particularly in immunocompromised or pediatric populations. Their biological properties and non-overlapping host range with mammalian cells provide distinct advantages for non-cytolytic gene transfer, vaccine development, and potentially even regenerative medicine.

Although EPVs cannot replicate in mammalian cells, early experiments demonstrated that they could enter vertebrate cells and express transgenes placed under early viral promoters. For instance, Amsacta moorei entomopoxvirus (AmEPV) was engineered to express the lacZ and green fluorescent protein (GFP) genes, successfully producing detectable protein levels in mammalian cell lines (Li, Hall, and Moyer 1997). Transgene expression was transient and non-lethal, providing a useful platform for applications requiring short-term gene expression without immune overactivation or cell lysis. This mechanism makes EPVs especially valuable for temporary modulation of cellular behavior, such as inducing angiogenesis, reprogramming stem cells, or providing growth factors in tissue repair contexts.

Although studies on the clinical use of EPVs have not yet begun, they offer a number of attractive features for future gene therapy applications. In regenerative medicine, EPVs may be proposed as tools for ex vivo modification of stem cells or primary cells prior to transplantation, particularly where immune activation must be minimized. In people with weakened immune systems, EPVs can be given to patients (like those with HIV or who have had transplants) without the risk of spreading throughout the body or causing inflammation, because they do not replicate.

With their importance in gene therapy, EPVs can be compared to other non-replicating/non-integrating vectors like adeno-associated virus (AAV), baculoviruses, and plasmid DNA. EPVs and baculoviruses are insect-origin viruses that can transduce mammalian cells with much higher genome capacity compared to AAV's (Schaly, Ghebretatios, and Prakash 2021). Also, compared to plasmid DNA, EPVs offer higher transfection efficiency and do not require electroporation or chemical delivery methods.

Despite their promise, EPVs face several limitations. These include lower transgene (transient) expression than replicating poxviruses, production challenges such as limited established cell lines and scalable insect hosts, and the fact that no clinical-grade vectors are currently approved or under human trial.

The unique biosafety profile of EPVs may eventually carve out a niche in gene therapy. Their potential lies in applications requiring transitory gene expression where vector elimination is desired post-therapy, dual-vector systems where EPVs deliver helper functions alongside immunostimulatory viruses, and gene therapy—especially for genetic diseases that require gene transfer without lasting inflammation or toxicity. In summary, entomopoxviruses, despite being in the early phases of development, signify a promising family of gene therapy vectors that provide unmatched safety, substantial cargo capacity, and a physiologically compatible platform that enhances current viral vectors.

5. From Safety to Immunity: Host-Virus Interactions

The development of poxvirus-based vectors for gene therapy requires a precise equilibrium between therapeutic effectiveness and clinical safety. Poxviruses, particularly Vaccinia virus (VACV), have shown notable immunostimulatory and oncolytic capabilities. However, these same properties—especially their replication competency and immunogenic nature—necessitate sophisticated control strategies to minimize off-target effects. Understanding host–virus interactions is therefore vital in optimizing poxviral vectors for safe and efficient therapeutic applications.

VACV's ability to replicate in mammalian cells brings both therapeutic promise and potential hazards. On the beneficial side, viral replication within tumor tissues results in direct cell lysis, immunogenic death, and the self-amplification of the therapeutic payload. This mechanism underpins the success of several oncolytic VACV strains, such as JX-594 (Pexa-Vec), which has shown clinical activity in hepatocellular carcinoma. However, if replication occurs outside the tumor microenvironment—particularly in immunocompromised patients—it can provoke serious systemic inflammation, hepatotoxicity, and unintended viral dissemination. These findings underscore the necessity for attenuation strategies that retain tumor-specific efficacy while limiting pathogenicity in healthy tissues.

To address safety concerns, genetic modifications such as deletions in the thymidine kinase (TK) gene, viral growth factor (VGF), and SPI-1/SPI-2 protease inhibitors have been introduced. These deletions limit viral replication to metabolically active tumor cells and mitigate virulence. For instance, double-deleted VACV strains lacking both TK and VGF maintain oncolytic activity while demonstrating improved safety in preclinical models (Thorne et al., 2007). In parallel, highly attenuated strains such as Modified Vaccinia Ankara (MVA), ALVAC, and Fowlpox virus (FWPV) have been developed, which are replication-deficient in human cells and have been successfully used in immunocompromised populations.

A critical factor influencing the clinical application of poxvirus vectors is their interaction with the host immune system. Poxvirus particles are recognized by various pattern recognition receptors (PRRs), including Toll-like receptors and cytoplasmic DNA sensors (Lu and Zhang 2020). This recognition activates robust innate immune responses characterized by the release of interferons (IFN-α/β), TNF-α, and IL-6. These cytokines promote dendritic cell maturation and the recruitment of natural killer (NK) cells and cytotoxic T lymphocytes.

Another immunological barrier is the presence of preexisting immunity to VACV, particularly in individuals vaccinated against smallpox. This immunity can lead to rapid vector neutralization upon re-administration, thereby limiting treatment durability. To overcome this, researchers have employed heterologous prime–boost strategies involving non-cross-reactive vectors such as MVA, ALVAC, or FWPV. Additional approaches include PEGylation or transient immune evasion mechanisms to prolong vector persistence, as well as direct intratumoral injection to bypass systemic immune surveillance.

Replication-deficient vectors such as MVA and FWPV offer several advantages. They are safe in immunocompromised hosts, permit multiple doses with minimal toxicity, and maintain strong immunogenicity—particularly in prime–boost regimens. In HIV and cancer vaccine trials, these vectors have proven safe even in patients with AIDS or undergoing chemotherapy, further confirming their utility across diverse clinical populations (Harrer et al., 2005; Blomquist et al., 2004).

Entomopoxviruses (EPVs) represent a new frontier in ultra-safe vector design. These insect-origin viruses are incapable of replicating in mammalian cells, yet they can express transgenes without triggering cytopathic effects or genome integration. Their unique biosafety profile may make them particularly suitable for pediatric, regenerative, or immunologically fragile settings. While their transgene expression levels are currently lower than VACV, advancements in promoter engineering and delivery systems are expected to close this gap in the near future.

6. Barriers to Clinical Translation

Despite the promising therapeutic potential of poxvirus vectors in gene therapy and oncolytic virotherapy, several biological, immunological, technical, and regulatory challenges continue to constrain their clinical translation. These barriers must be addressed systematically to fully unlock the potential of poxviruses in routine therapeutic settings.

One of the major challenges is preexisting immunity, especially to Vaccinia virus (VACV). In populations previously vaccinated against smallpox, the presence of neutralizing antibodies and memory T cells can rapidly eliminate the viral vector before it reaches target tissues. This premature clearance diminishes therapeutic gene expression and weakens the vector's efficacy, particularly in treatment regimens requiring multiple administrations. Various strategies have been explored to overcome this hurdle, including the use of heterologous prime-boost regimens with non-cross-reactive vectors such as MVA, ALVAC, or FWPV. Additionally, transient immune evasion strategies, such as PEGylation and pseudotyping, are under development to reduce immune recognition.

Another significant barrier is immunotoxicity, especially in systemically administered or high-dose settings. While the inherent immunogenicity of poxviruses can be leveraged to stimulate antitumor responses, it may also result in systemic inflammation, cytokine release syndrome, and dose-limiting side effects. The development of attenuated strains, such as MVA and TK-/VGF- VACV, has improved safety profiles, but often at the cost of reduced intratumoral replication and therapeutic gene expression.

Compared to other viral vectors, poxviruses offer a distinctive combination of large transgene capacity, cytoplasmic replication, and immunogenicity. These features are summarized in Table 1 and highlight the unique advantages that support their continued development, especially in cancer gene therapy and immuno-oncology.

Table 1. Comparative features of viral vectors in gene therapy.

Feature	Poxvirus (Vacv, Mva, Etc.)	Adenovirus	Adeno associated virus	Lentivirus
Genome Type	dsDNA (cytoplasmic replication)	dsDNA (nuclear)	ssDNA (nuclear)	ssRNA (reverse transcribed)
Genome Size (Kb)	170-250	~36	~4-6	~8–10
Transgene Capacity	High (up to 25–30 kb)	Moderate (~8 kb)	Limited (~5 kb)	Moderate (~8 kb)
Integration	No (cytoplasmic, episomal)	No	No	Yes
Immunogenicity	High	High	Low to Moderate	Moderate
Cell Tropism	Broad	Broad	Broad (tissue-specific serotypes)	Dividing & non-dividing cells
Replication Competence	Depends on strain	Mostly non-replicating	Non-replicating	Replication-defective
Clinical Use Cases	Oncolytic virotherapy, vaccines	Vaccines, cancer therapy	Monogenic disorders, retina/ muscle	Hematopoietic diseases
Risk Of Insertional Mutagenesis	None	None	None	Present
Production Complexity	High (esp. for replicating strains)	Moderate	High purity, complex	High (GMP required)
Re-Dosing Feasibility	Limited due to immune memory	Limited	Possible	Difficult (integration)

Although poxviruses are known for their large genome capacity, this feature is not without limitations. Overloading the genome with multiple or large transgenes can compromise replication efficiency and vector stability. Strongly immunogenic or cytotoxic transgenes may also impair viral fitness. Additionally, careful attention must be given to promoter selection, transgene positioning, and the interaction between payloads and the viral backbone to ensure consistent expression. Long-term propagation of engineered vectors can also lead to genetic instability, necessitating rigorous quality control during vector manufacturing.

Finally, production and regulatory challenges represent a critical bottleneck. The manufacture of poxvirus vectors, particularly replication-competent strains, requires high-containment facilities and stringent biosafety protocols. Ensuring consistency in viral titers, genome integrity, and transgene expression adds further complexity. Regulatory agencies demand comprehensive documentation regarding biodistribution, shedding, recombination risks, and environmental safety. These requirements can prolong development timelines and increase costs, especially for early-phase translational studies or small-scale biotech companies.

7. Conclusion

Poxviruses have emerged as one of the most versatile platforms for gene therapy and oncolytic virotherapy. Their unique attributes—including large genome capacity, cytoplasmic replication, strong immunogenicity, and extensive clinical history—position them at the forefront of modern virotherapeutics.

Vaccinia virus (VACV) remains the most extensively studied and clinically validated poxvirus vector. Engineered VACV strains such as JX-594 (Pexa-Vec) and GLV-1h68 have demonstrated dual mechanisms of action by directly lysing tumor cells and stimulating systemic antitumor immunity. Genetic modifications, including deletions of TK, VGF, and SPI-1/SPI-2, have significantly improved safety while retaining therapeutic efficacy. Furthermore, VACV's compatibility with systemic delivery and multimodal imaging techniques enhances its clinical appeal and facilitates treatment monitoring.

Beyond VACV, alternative poxviruses bring new possibilities to the field. Myxoma virus (MYXV), for instance, naturally exhibits tumor selectivity and does not cause disease in humans, making it a promising candidate for cancer treatment. Avian poxviruses like Fowlpox (FWPV) and Canarypox (ALVAC) are non-replicative in human cells but can still express transgenes, offering a safe and effective option for prime-boost vaccination strategies. Entomopoxviruses (EPVs), though still in early development, represent an ultra-safe vector class for non-replicating gene delivery, especially in sensitive or immunocompromised populations.

Despite these advances, several hurdles remain. These include preexisting immunity, immunotoxicity, limited tumor penetration, and the complexity of manufacturing and regulatory compliance. Overcoming these challenges will require an integrated approach that combines advanced vector engineering with tailored delivery systems and synergistic therapeutic combinations. Approaches such as tumor-specific promoters, synthetic biology tools, and immune-evasive coatings are currently under investigation to enhance the precision and safety of poxvirus vectors.

As summarized in Table 1, poxviruses compare favorably with other viral vectors such as adenoviruses, AAV, and lentiviruses, particularly in settings that demand high cargo capacity, strong immune activation, and non-integrating expression. Looking ahead, the convergence of synthetic biology, immunogenomics, and artificial intelligence-driven vector design may further accelerate the development of next-generation poxvirus vectors.

With a robust foundation of preclinical and clinical research, and an expanding toolbox of genetic and immunological strategies, poxviruses are poised to play a central role in the future of precision medicine, especially in the treatment of complex cancers and infectious diseases.

References

Ahmed, T. (2023). Oncolytic virotherapy using neural stem cells as a novel treatment option for glioblastoma multiforme. *MedComm – Oncology*, *2*(1), e23. https://doi.org/10.1002/MOG2.23

Berche, P. (2022). Life and death of smallpox. *La Presse Médicale*, *51*(3), 104117. https://doi.org/10.1016/j.lpm.2022.104117

Berchtold, S., Beil, J., Raff, C., Smirnow, I., Schell, M., D'alvise, J., Gross, S., & Lauer, U. M. (2020). Assessing and Overcoming Resistance Phenomena against a Genetically Modified Vaccinia Virus in Selected Cancer Cell Lines. *International Journal of Molecular Sciences 2020, Vol. 21, Page 7618*, *21*(20), 7618. https://doi.org/10.3390/IJMS21207618

Blomquist, D. V., Green, P., Laidlaw, S. M., Skinner, M. A., Borrow, P., & Duarte, C. A. (2004). Induction of a Strong HIV-Specific CD8+ T Cell Response in Mice Using a Fowlpox Virus Vector Expressing an HIV-1 Multi-CTL-Epitope Polypeptide. https://doi.org/10.1089/08828240260066260

Breitbach, C. J., Burke, J., Jonker, D., Stephenson, J., Haas, A. R., Chow, L. Q. M., Nieva, J., Hwang, T.-H., Moon, A., Patt, R., Pelusio, A., Le Boeuf, F., Burns, J., Evgin, L., De Silva, N., Cvancic, S., Robertson, T., Je, J.-E., Lee, Y.-S., … Kirn, D. H. (2011). Intravenous delivery of a multi-mechanistic cancer-targeted oncolytic poxvirus in humans. *Nature*, *477*(7362), 99–102. https://doi.org/10.1038/nature10358

Chaurasiya, S., Chen, N. G., Lu, J., Martin, N., Shen, Y., Kim, S.-I., Warner, S. G., Woo, Y., & Fong, Y. (2020). A chimeric poxvirus with J2R (thymidine kinase) deletion shows safety and anti-tumor activity in lung cancer models. *Cancer Gene Therapy*, *27*(3–4), 125–135. https://doi.org/10.1038/s41417-019-0114-x

Conrad, S. J., & Liu, J. (2019). Poxviruses as Gene Therapy Vectors: Generating Poxviral Vectors Expressing Therapeutic Transgenes. In *Methods in Molecular Biology* (Vol. 1937, pp. 189–209). https://doi.org/10.1007/978-1-4939-9065-8_11

Cousin, S., Toulmonde, M., Kind, M., Guegan, J. P., Bessede, A., Cantarel, C., Bellera, C., & Italiano, A. (2022). Phase 2 trial of intravenous oncolytic virus JX-594 combined with low-dose cyclophosphamide in patients with advanced breast cancer. *Experimental Hematology and Oncology*, *11*(1), 1–4. https://doi.org/10.1186/S40164-022-00338-2

Guo, Z. S., & Bartlett, D. L. (2004). Vaccinia as a vector for gene delivery. *Expert Opinion on Biological Therapy*, *4*(6), 901–917. https://doi.org/10.1517/14712598.4.6.901

Haddad, D. (2017). Genetically engineered vaccinia viruses as agents for cancer treatment, imaging, and transgene delivery. *Frontiers in Oncology*, *7*(MAY), 1–12. https://doi.org/10.3389/fonc.2017.00096

Harrer, E., Bäuerle, M., Ferstl, B., Chaplin, P., Petzold, B., Mateo, L., Handley, A., Tzatzaris, M., Vollmar, J., Bergmann, S., Rittmaier, M., Eismann, K., Müller, S., Kalden, J. R., Spriewald, B., Willbold, D., & Harrer, T. (2005). Therapeutic vaccination of HIV-1-infected patients on HAART with a recombinant HIV-1 nef-expressing MVA: Safety, immunogenicity and influence on viral load during treatment interruption. *Antiviral Therapy*, *10*(2), 285–300. https://doi.org/10.1177/135965350501000212

Heo, J., Reid, T., Ruo, L., Breitbach, C. J., Rose, S., Bloomston, M., Cho, M., Lim, H. Y., Chung, H. C., Kim, C. W., Burke, J., Lencioni, R., Hickman, T., Moon, A., Lee, Y. S., Kim, M. K., Daneshmand, M., Dubois, K., Longpre, L., … Kirn, D. H. (2013). Randomized dose-finding clinical trial of oncolytic immunotherapeutic vaccinia JX-594 in liver cancer. *Nature Medicine*, *19*(3), 329–336. https://doi.org/10.1038/nm.3089

Jacobs, B. L., Langland, J. O., Kibler, K. V., Denzler, K. L., White, S. D., Holechek, S. A., Wong, S., Huynh, T., & Baskin, C. R. (2009). Vaccinia virus vaccines: Past, present and future. *Antiviral Research*, *84*(1), 1–13. https://doi.org/10.1016/j.antiviral.2009.06.006

Kaufman, H. L., Flanagan, K., Lee, C. S. D., Perretta, D. J., & Horig, H. (2002). Insertion of interleukin-2 (IL-2) and interleukin-12 (IL-12)

genes into vaccinia virus results in effective anti-tumor responses without toxicity. *Vaccine*, *20*(13–14), 1862–1869. https://doi.org/10.1016/S0264-410X(02)00032-4

Kaufman, H. L., Kim, D. W., Kim-Schulze, S., DeRaffele, G., Jagoda, M. C., Broucek, J. R., & Zloza, A. (2014). Results of a Randomized Phase I Gene Therapy Clinical Trial of Nononcolytic Fowlpox Viruses Encoding T Cell Costimulatory Molecules. *Human Gene Therapy*, *25*(5), 452–460. https://doi.org/10.1089/hum.2013.217

Kim, J. H., Kim, Y., Shin, Y., Oh, D., Kwon, W. S., Kim, T. S., Lee, N., Oh, K., Chung, H. C., Jeung, H.-C., & Rha, S. Y. (2023). Abstract 2685: Synergistic antitumor effect of oncolytic virus and cytotoxic chemotherapy in gastric cancer. *Cancer Research*, *83*(7_Supplement), 2685–2685. https://doi.org/10.1158/1538-7445.AM2023-2685

Kim, Y., Song, Y., Choi, Y., Jang, J., Kim, S., Liu, T.-L., Baek, K., Oh, K., Ma, S., Kim, T. S., Kwon, W. S., Yoo, S., Kim, J. H., & Rha, S. Y. (2024). Abstract 5396: Vascularized gastric cancer 3D co-culture model using a microphysiological system as an oncolytic virus testing platform. *Cancer Research*, *84*(6_Supplement), 5396–5396. https://doi.org/10.1158/1538-7445.AM2024-5396

Kloker, L. D., Berchtold, S., Smirnow, I., Beil, J., Krieg, A., Sipos, B., & Lauer, U. M. (2020). Oncolytic vaccinia virus GLV-1h68 exhibits profound antitumoral activities in cell lines originating from neuroendocrine neoplasms. *BMC Cancer*, *20*(1). https://doi.org/10.1186/S12885-020-07121-8,

Li, Y., Hall, R. L., & Moyer, R. W. (1997). Transient, nonlethal expression of genes in vertebrate cells by recombinant entomopoxviruses. *Journal of Virology*, *71*(12), 9557–9562. https://doi.org/10.1128/jvi.71.12.9557-9562.1997

Lu, Y., & Zhang, L. (2020). DNA-Sensing Antiviral Innate Immunity in Poxvirus Infection. *Frontiers in Immunology*, *11*, 552225. https://doi.org/10.3389/FIMMU.2020.01637

Madan, R. A., Mohebtash, M., Arlen, P. M., Vergati, M., Rauckhorst, M., Steinberg, S. M., Tsang, K. Y., Poole, D. J., Parnes, H. L., Wright, J. J., Dahut, W. L., Schlom, J., & Gulley, J. L. (2012). Ipilimumab and a poxviral vaccine targeting prostate-specific antigen in metastatic castration-resistant prostate cancer: a phase 1 dose-escalation trial. *The Lancet Oncology*, *13*(5), 501–508. https://doi.org/10.1016/S1470-2045(12)70006-2

Mohebtash, M., Tsang, K. Y., Madan, R. A., Huen, N. Y., Poole, D. J., Jochems, C., Jones, J., Ferrara, T., Heery, C. R., Arlen, P. M., Steinberg, S. M., Pazdur, M., Rauckhorst, M., Jones, E. C., Dahut, W. L., Schlom,

J., & Gulley, J. L. (2011). A pilot study of MUC-1/CEA/TRICOM poxviral-based vaccine in patients with metastatic breast and ovarian cancer. *Clinical Cancer Research*, *17*(22), 7164–7173. https://doi.org/10.1158/1078-0432.CCR-11-0649

Moss, B. (1991). Vaccinia Virus: A Tool for Research and Vaccine Development. *Science*, *252*(5013), 1662–1667. https://doi.org/10.1126/science.2047875

Moss, B. (1996). Genetically engineered poxviruses for recombinant gene expression, vaccination, and safety. *Proceedings of the National Academy of Sciences of the United States of America*, *93*(21), 11341–11348. https://doi.org/10.1073/pnas.93.21.11341

Park, J. S., Lee, M. E., Jang, W. S., Kim, J., Lee, N., Oh, K., & Ham, W. S. (2023). Anti-PD1 plus oncolytic virus as first-line treatment option for metastatic renal cell carcinomas. *Journal of Clinical Oncology*, *41*(6_suppl), 675–675. https://doi.org/10.1200/JCO.2023.41.6_SUPPL.675

Perreau, M., Welles, H. C., Harari, A., Hall, O., Martin, R., Maillard, M., Dorta, G., Bart, P.-A., Kremer, E. J., Tartaglia, J., Wagner, R., Esteban, M., Levy, Y., & Pantaleo, G. (2011). DNA/NYVAC Vaccine Regimen Induces HIV-Specific CD4 and CD8 T-Cell Responses in Intestinal Mucosa. *Journal of Virology*, *85*(19), 9854–9862. https://doi.org/10.1128/JVI.00788-11

Pitisuttithum, P., Nitayaphan, S., Chariyalertsak, S., Kaewkungwal, J., Dawson, P., Dhitavat, J., Phonrat, B., Akapirat, S., Karasavvas, N., Wieczorek, L., Polonis, V., Eller, M. A., Pegu, P., Kim, D., Schuetz, A., Jongrakthaitae, S., Zhou, Y., Sinangil, F., Phogat, S., … Chinaworapong, S. (2020). Late boosting of the RV144 regimen with AIDSVAX B/E and ALVAC-HIV in HIV-uninfected Thai volunteers: a double-blind, randomised controlled trial. *The Lancet HIV*, *7*(4), e238–e248. https://doi.org/10.1016/S2352-3018(19)30406-0

Pugalenthi, A., Mojica, K., Ady, J. W., Johnsen, C., Love, D., Chen, N. G., Aguilar, R. J., Szalay, A. A., & Fong, Y. (2015). Recombinant vaccinia virus GLV-1h68 is a promising oncolytic vector in the treatment of cholangiocarcinoma. *Cancer Gene Therapy*, *22*(12), 591–596. https://doi.org/10.1038/CGT.2015.60,

Rahman, M. M., & McFadden, G. (2020). Oncolytic Virotherapy with Myxoma Virus. *Journal of Clinical Medicine*, *9*(1), 171. https://doi.org/10.3390/jcm9010171

Rerks-Ngarm, S., Pitisuttithum, P., Nitayaphan, S., Kaewkungwal, J., Chiu, J., Paris, R., Premsri, N., Namwat, C., de Souza, M., Adams, E., Benenson, M., Gurunathan, S., Tartaglia, J., McNeil, J. G., Francis, D.

P., Stablein, D., Birx, D. L., Chunsuttiwat, S., Khamboonruang, C., … Kim, J. H. (2009). Vaccination with ALVAC and AIDSVAX to Prevent HIV-1 Infection in Thailand. *New England Journal of Medicine*, *361*(23), 2209–2220. https://doi.org/10.1056/NEJMOA0908492

Ryan, E. J., Harenberg, A., & Burdin, N. (2007). The Canarypox-virus vaccine vector ALVAC triggers the release of IFN-γ by Natural Killer (NK) cells enhancing Th1 polarization. *Vaccine*, *25*(17), 3380–3390. https://doi.org/10.1016/J.VACCINE.2006.12.048

Schaly, S., Ghebretatios, M., & Prakash, S. (2021). Baculoviruses in gene therapy and personalized medicine. *Biologics: Targets and Therapy*, *15*, 115–132. https://doi.org/10.2147/BTT.S292692

Shakiba, Y., Vorobyev, P. O., Mahmoud, M., Hamad, A., Kochetkov, D. V., Yusubalieva, G. M., Baklaushev, V. P., Chumakov, P. M., & Lipatova, A. V. (2023). Recombinant Strains of Oncolytic Vaccinia Virus for Cancer Immunotherapy. *Biochemistry (Moscow) 2023 88:6*, *88*(6), 823–841. https://doi.org/10.1134/S000629792306010X

Smith, G. L., & Moss, B. (1983). Infectious poxvirus vectors have capacity for at least 25 000 base pairs of foreign DNA. *Gene*, *25*(1), 21–28. https://doi.org/10.1016/0378-1119(83)90163-4

Stanford, M. M., & McFadden, G. (2007). Myxoma virus and oncolytic virotherapy: a new biologic weapon in the war against cancer. *Expert Opinion on Biological Therapy*, *7*(9), 1415–1425. https://doi.org/10.1517/14712598.7.9.1415

Tartaglia, J., Cox, W. I., Taylor, J., Perkus, M., Riviere, M., Meignier, B., & Paoletti, E. (1992). Highly Attenuated Poxvirus Vectors. *AIDS Research and Human Retroviruses*, *8*(8), 1445–1447. https://doi.org/10.1089/AID.1992.8.1445,

Thorne, S. H., Hwang, T. H. H., O'Gorman, W. E., Bartlett, D. L., Sei, S., Kanji, F., Brown, C., Werier, J., Cho, J. H., Lee, D. E., Wang, Y., Bell, J., & Kirn, D. H. (2007). Rational strain selection and engineering creates a broad-spectrum, systemically effective oncolytic poxvirus, JX-963. *The Journal of Clinical Investigation*, *117*(11), 3350. https://doi.org/10.1172/JCI32727

Tosic, V., Thomas, D. L., Kranz, D. M., Liu, J., McFadden, G., Shisler, J. L., MacNeill, A. L., & Roy, E. J. (2014). Myxoma virus expressing a fusion protein of interleukin-15 (IL15) and IL15 receptor alpha has enhanced antitumor activity. *PLoS ONE*, *9*(10). https://doi.org/10.1371/JOURNAL.PONE.0109801,

Toulmonde, M., Guegan, J. P., Spalato-Ceruso, M., Peyraud, F., Kind, M., Vanhersecke, L., Le Loarer, F., Perret, R., Cantarel, C., Bellera, C., Bessede, A., & Italiano, A. (2024). Reshaping the tumor microenvironment of cold soft-tissue sarcomas with oncolytic viral therapy: a phase 2 trial of intratumoral JX-594 combined with avelumab and low-dose cyclophosphamide. *Molecular Cancer*, *23*(1), 1–7. https://doi.org/10.1186/S12943-024-01946-8

Valenzuela-Cardenas, M., Gowan, C., Dryja, P., Bartee, M. Y., & Bartee, E. (2022). TNF blockade enhances the efficacy of myxoma virus-based oncolytic virotherapy. *J Immunother Cancer*, *10*, 4770. https://doi.org/10.1136/jitc-2022-004770

Weli, S. C., & Tryland, M. (2011). Avipoxviruses: Infection biology and their use as vaccine vectors. *Virology Journal*, *8*(1), 1–15. https://doi.org/10.1186/1743-422X-8-49

Wennier, S. T., Liu, J., Li, S., Rahman, M. M., Mona, M., & McFadden, G. (2012). Myxoma virus sensitizes cancer cells to gemcitabine and is an effective oncolytic virotherapeutic in models of disseminated pancreatic cancer. *Molecular Therapy*, *20*(4), 759–768. https://doi.org/10.1038/mt.2011.293

Woo, J. K., Kim, T. G., Im, N. Y., Son, K. Y., Cho, M., Jeong, Y. J., Hong, J. I., Kang, B. R., Enkhtaivan, G., Cho, N. H., Alain, T., Park, D. G., & Lee, Y. S. (2023). Dual-Armed Oncolytic Myxoma Virus Encoding IFN-γ and CD47 Promotes Lymphocyte Infiltration and Tumor Suppression of Syngeneic Murine Melanoma. *Cancers*, *15*(19), 4703. https://doi.org/10.3390/CANCERS15194703/S1

Woo, Y., Zhang, Z., Yang, A., Chaurasiya, S., Park, A. K., Lu, J., Kim, S. I., Warner, S. G., Von Hoff, D., & Fong, Y. (2020). Novel Chimeric Immuno-Oncolytic Virus CF33-hNIS-antiPDL1 for the Treatment of Pancreatic Cancer. *Journal of the American College of Surgeons*, *230*(4), 709–717. https://doi.org/10.1016/J.JAMCOLLSURG.2019.12.027

Yaghchi, C. Al, Zhang, Z., Alusi, G., Lemoine, N. R., & Wang, Y. (2015). Vaccinia virus, a promising new therapeutic agent for pancreatic cancer. *Immunotherapy*, *7*(12), 1249–1258. https://doi.org/10.2217/imt.15.90

Zheng, N., Fang, J., Xue, G., Wang, Z., Li, X., Zhou, M., Jin, G., Rahman, M. M., McFadden, G., & Lu, Y. (2022). Induction of tumor cell autosis by myxoma virus-infected CAR-T and TCR-T cells to overcome primary and acquired resistance. *Cancer Cell*, *40*(9), 973. https://doi.org/10.1016/J.CCELL.2022.08.001

Author Biography

Asst. Prof. Cihan INAN; is a faculty member in the Department of Molecular Biology and Genetics at Karadeniz Technical University (Türkiye), specializing in Molecular Virology. His research focuses on host–virus interactions of DNA viruses; the potential use of entomopoxviruses as gene therapy agents; and the antimicrobial, antiviral, antiproliferative effects of various compounds.

CHAPTER 6

RETROVIRAL DELIVERY SYSTEMS IN GENE THERAPY

BERRAK KURT

General Directorate of Agricultural Research and Policies, Ankara, Türkiye.

Abstract

Over the past two decades, gene therapy has revolutionized medicine by emerging as an effective strategy for treating various diseases. It has been shown that gene therapy offers promising outcomes not only for genetic disorders but also for acquired diseases such as cancer, neurodegenerative disorders, and Acquired Immune Deficiency Syndrome (AIDS). The success of gene therapy critically depends on the efficient delivery of genetic molecules into the nucleus of the host cell and their stable maintenance within the host genome. Various viral and non-viral gene delivery systems have been developed to achieve this.

Viral gene delivery systems exploit the inherent ability of viruses to integrate their genetic material into the host cell genome. Among these, replication-deficient retroviral vectors, engineered to prevent autonomous replication, facilitate the stable transfer of therapeutic genes into the host genome, thereby enabling the expression of the desired protein. The potential of retroviruses for genetic material transfer was first recognized in the 1980s. As the first family of viruses to be modified for gene delivery, retroviruses are enveloped RNA viruses with a circular structure, measuring 80–120 nm in diameter and possessing a genetic material carrying capacity of approximately 9 kb. In retroviral vectors, the viral genes gag (capsid), pol (reverse transcriptase), and env (envelope glycoprotein), which are essential for viral replication, are deleted to prevent viral propagation. Instead, a therapeutic gene is added, so that the vector consists only of the sequences necessary for RNA replication and integration and the therapeutic gene.

Retroviral gene delivery systems offer a significant advantage in the treatment of chronic diseases due to their ability to ensure the stable integration of viral sequences. However, these systems also exhibit certain limitations, including low transfection efficiency in vitro studies, inefficiency in non-dividing post-mitotic cells, and particle instability. Therefore, retroviral gene delivery systems are recommended for ex vivo gene therapy applications.

Introduction

Gene therapy is an innovative method based on the transfer of therapeutic genetic material (DNA or RNA) into the patient's cells for the treatment of hereditary or acquired diseases or for the alleviation of their symptoms. In this process, the transferred genetic material may enhance the expression of the targeted gene, suppress it, or directly edit the genetic sequence. The foundations of gene therapy were laid in the 1960s, and it reached a significant milestone in 1990 with a phase I clinical trial conducted on patients with adenosine deaminase (ADA) deficiency (Blaese et al., 1995). Following this development, gene therapy has taken its place as a promising treatment method for diseases with poor prognosis and rare disorders such as cancer, cardiovascular diseases, HIV/AIDS, cystic fibrosis, and hemoglobinopathies.

The efficient and safe delivery of genetic material to the target cell is of critical importance for the success of gene therapy. The carrier systems used for this purpose are referred to as "vectors" and are generally classified into two main groups: viral and non-viral.

Viral vectors are frequently used for the transfer of the desired gene into the cell. In order to ensure their safe delivery to the target cell, the replication ability of viral vectors is eliminated by various methods, while maintaining high transduction efficiency and sustainability. In this section, retroviral vectors, which are among the main viral vectors used for gene transfer, and their gene delivery mechanisms will be examined.

Retroviral Vectors

Retroviral vectors provide higher transduction efficiency because the designed transgenes integrate into the genome of the target cell and are transferred to new generations of cells, thereby continuing to express the transgene, allowing for the long-term treatment of genetic diseases (Shimotohno and Temin, 1981). Viral vectors have been used in approximately 75% of clinical studies involving gene therapy, and retroviral vectors are the most frequently used tools for gene delivery. According to the Journal of Gene Medicine databases, 35% of gene therapy protocols employ retroviruses, while adenoviral vectors account for 27% and pox viral vectors for 6%. The most commonly used type in clinical applications is the well-characterized Moloney murine leukemia virus (MMLV). The genome of this virus encodes the gag, pol, and env polyproteins, which are necessary for replication and packaging (Edelstein et al., 2007).

Thanks to the extensive improvements made in the new-generation models of retroviral vectors, safer and more efficient vectors have been developed. When designing a vector, the aim is to minimize the potential risks that may be observed in the long term and to maximize the gene silencing efficiency of the gene therapy system. A more comprehensive and mechanistic understanding of retroviral integration models is thought to be beneficial for creating safer and more effective platforms.

1. General Structure of Retroviruses

Retroviruses are enveloped viruses characterized by a single-stranded RNA (ssRNA) genome with diploid nature (Coffin, 1979). They possess capsids measuring approximately 80–100 nm in diameter and contain a linear single-stranded RNA (ssRNA) genome of 7–12 kb in length. According to the classification of the International Committee on Taxonomy of Viruses (ICTV), the family Retroviridae consists of two subfamilies: Orthoretrovirinae and Spumaretrovirinae. The Orthoretrovirinae subfamily includes the genera Alpharetrovirus, Betaretrovirus, Gammaretrovirus, Deltaretrovirus, Epsilonretrovirus, and Lentivirus. The Spumaretrovirinae includes Simianfoamy virus, Humanfoamy virus and Felinefoamy virus (Lochelt et al., 1993).

In all retroviruses, the genetic regions required for the structural and functional integrity of the viral particle are conserved. The gag, pol, and env genes located within the genome encode, respectively, the capsid proteins, the essential enzymes (reverse transcriptase, RNase H, integrase), and the envelope glycoproteins. The retroviral genome is positive-sense ssRNA; however, after entering the host cell, it does not function directly as mRNA and requires host-derived tRNA for replication (Varmus, 1982).

From the perspective of genome organization, retroviruses are classified as simple or complex. Both groups contain the gag, pro, and pol genes, while complex retroviruses additionally encode various regulatory genes (Ruben et al., 1989).

The lipid envelope of retroviruses plays a critical role in the replication cycle. The Env glycoproteins embedded within the viral lipid envelope bind to specific receptors on the surface of target cells, initiating the first step of infection. Interaction with receptors such as CD4 induces conformational changes in the Env protein, which facilitate subsequent interaction with chemokine receptors. This process mediates the fusion of the viral envelope with the host cell membrane and the transfer of the viral core into the cytoplasm. Once in the cytoplasm, the ssRNA is converted into double-stranded DNA through the activity of reverse transcriptase. This DNA then enters the nucleus, assumes a circular form, and integrates into the host genome to form a provirus. Such integration ensures the long-term and stable expression of retroviral genes (Bowerman et al., 1989; Roe et al., 1993; Li et al., 2006).

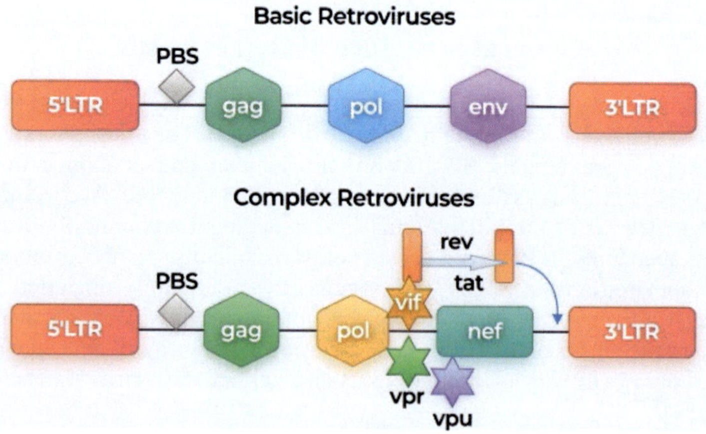

Figure 1: Basic and Complex Retroviruses (Created by the authors using https://www.canva.com and https://illustrae.co/)

The packaging signal required for retroviral genome encapsidation is most often located between the start codon of the gag gene and the donor site (SD). This region is directly associated with genome dimerization, and mutations occurring in dimer initiation regions significantly decrease packaging efficiency (Zhou et al., 2014).

2. Life Cycle of Retroviruses

The life cycle of retroviruses proceeds in two stages, defined as early and late phases.

Early phase: In the early phase, viral entry into the host cell, reverse transcription of the RNA genome, and nuclear transport of the resulting cDNA take place. In oncoretroviruses, integration occurs during cell division through the temporary breakdown of the nuclear envelope, whereas lentiviruses can infect non-dividing cells via active transport mechanisms (Bowerman et al., 1989; Roe et al., 1993; Li et al., 2006).

Late phase: In the late phase, new viral proteins are synthesized through transcription and translation from the provirus integrated into the host genome. These proteins, together with full-length viral RNAs, assemble to form mature virions, and viral particles are released from the host cell by budding through the plasma membrane (Bowerman et al., 1989; Roe et al., 1993; Li et al., 2006).

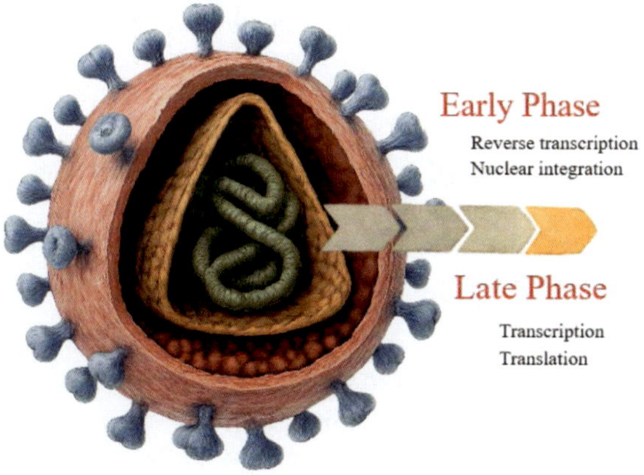

Figure 2: Life Cyle of Retroviruses (Created by the authors using https://www.canva.com and https://illustrae.co/)

3. Gene Therapy and the History of Retroviral Vectors

Gene therapy research based on retroviral vectors was initiated by Howard M. Temin et al. using the alpharetroviral Rous sarcoma virus. According to the provirus hypothesis proposed by Temin and his collaborators, genetic information can be transferred not only from DNA to RNA, but also from

RNA to DNA, and replication requires cellular DNA. In addition, mutations induced by viral infection may exhibit heritable characteristics (Temin, 1976). Subsequently, Moloney murine leukemia virus (MoMLV), which is still widely used today, was employed in the packaging of genomic RNA into virions (D'Souza and Summers, 2005). By the 1990s, HIV-1 retroviral systems had come into use. Following these preclinical studies, the first clinical trial was conducted by Rosenberg et al., in which tumor-infiltrating lymphocytes (TILs) isolated from patients with advanced melanoma were transduced with the neomycin phosphotransferase and tumor necrosis factor (TNF) genes in an attempt to expand the therapeutic window (Rosenberg et al., 1990).

However, gene therapies based on retroviral systems have not always yielded favorable outcomes. In the 2000s, during a clinical trial performed on pediatric patients with severe combined immunodeficiency (SCID), where $CD34^+$ hematopoietic progenitor cells were transduced ex vivo, five out of twenty children developed T-cell leukemia and two of them died (Fischer et al., 2010). This incident was regarded as a major safety concern in gene therapy studies employing viral delivery systems, and since then, numerous strategies have been developed to enhance safety. Today, gene therapies continue with both viral and non-viral delivery systems that have been improved in terms of safety and efficacy.

4. Production of Retroviral Vectors

Retroviral vectors are obtained by arranging proviral retroviral sequences on a plasmid using recombinant DNA methods. In retroviral vectors, all trans-acting elements in the genome are removed in order to eliminate the replication ability of the virus, and instead only long terminal repeats (LTRs), the psi (ψ) packaging signal, and the necessary regions for transgene expression are added. This design significantly reduces the possibility of generating retroviruses with replicative capacity (Zhou et al., 2014).

For the purpose of increasing safety, retroviral gene contents have generally been divided into three separate plasmid systems: the first plasmid carries the gag and pol genes; the second plasmid carries the env gene; and the third plasmid carries the gene to be transferred (transgene) together with the LTRs and ψ packaging signal surrounding it (Zhou et al., 2014). Retroviral entry and tropism are regulated by the retroviral envelope protein (Env). In addition, for the purpose of expanding tropism, heterologous envelope proteins such as VSV-G are used, and pseudotyping is performed (Yee et al., 1994).

Self-inactivating (SIN) vectors, which eliminate the promoter activity of viral promoters in the U3 region of the LTRs, have also been developed. In these vectors, a large part of the U3 region, which contains the promoter/enhancer elements in the 3′-LTR, is deleted, thus preventing the integrated provirus from carrying viral LTR promoter/enhancer activity. Transgene expression, on the other hand, is maintained through a heterologous internal promoter (for example, CMV type) in order to reduce the risk of insertional oncogenesis (Yu et al., 1986; Zufferey et al., 1998).

The gene carrying capacity of retroviral vectors can reach up to approximately 10 kb; however, since an increase in gene size can decrease vector expression level and transduction efficiency, such sizes are generally not preferred.

4.1. Strategies to Increase the Efficiency of Retroviral Vectors

The low viral titer and insufficient transduction efficiency observed in the early forms of retroviral vectors, as well as the technical difficulties encountered in in vivo applications, have made it necessary to develop new strategies. In this context, various methods have been adopted, such as optimizing the choice of promoter in vector designs, improving the functional properties of packaging cell lines, and using pseudotyping approaches.

4.1.1. Suspension Packaging Cell Lines

As a result of studies aimed at increasing the safety and transduction capacity of MLV-derived retroviral vectors, suspension packaging cell lines derived from human T- and B-lymphoblastoid cells have been developed. These cell lines significantly increase both the production amount and stability of recombinant viruses, making it possible to produce retroviruses with high stability reaching levels of 10^7–10^8 IU/ml. In addition, these cell lines have prevented the formation of replication-competent retroviruses (RCR), which is a critical safety issue in retroviral gene transfer systems, and have provided a reliable alternative for high-capacity vector production (Wysocki et al., 2001; Chan et al., 2001; Pizzato et al., 2001).

4.1.2. Macrophage-derived Packaging Cells

Macrophage-derived packaging cell lines, originating from murine macrophage cells, like suspension packaging cell lines, enable the production of recombinant retroviruses at high titers (10^8 IU/ml). The recombinant viruses contained in these cell lines transduce immune cells in intratumoral injection, modulating the tumor microenvironment and enhancing therapeutic efficacy (Wysocki et al., 2001; Pastorino et al., 2001).

4.1.3. Targeting PiT1 and PiT2 Retroviral Receptors

PiT1 and PiT2 retroviral receptors play a critical role in enhancing the entry mechanism and targeting capacity of retroviral vectors, and in developing the ability to transfer genes to more cells. The env proteins of gibbon ape leukemia virus (GaLV) and amphotropic murine leukemia virus (A-MuLV), which are widely used in gene therapy, transform human cells via the PiT1 and PiT2 receptors, which are sodium-dependent phosphate symporters. There are studies showing that the expression of these receptors directly and indirectly affects the transduction efficiency of retroviral vectors.

In a model system using Chinese hamster ovary (CHO) cells lacking retroviral receptors, where functional PiT2 expression was induced by the removal of tetracycline analogs, it was demonstrated that there is a linear relationship between virus binding and transduction efficiency at different levels of receptor expression. Similarly, in murine hematopoietic stem cells, subpopulations with higher PiT2 mRNA levels were found to be more efficiently transduced. However, some studies on a series of human cell lines have revealed that there is more than a 400-fold difference in infectivity between cells expressing similar levels of PiT1 and PiT2 (Uckert et al., 1998; Grabarczyk et al., 2001).

These data indicate that receptor level is not the only factor limiting transduction, but various receptor-based interventions must do to increase transduction efficiency. For this purpose, induction of receptors with phosphate-depleted medium and temporary overexpression of receptors using different carriers have increased transduction rates, and the range of cells that can be effectively modified with retroviral vectors has been expanded. In addition, a >4-fold increase in transduction efficiency of human primary lymphocytes resistant to retroviral vectors has been achieved by using a combination of the 10A1-MuLV env protein, which uses both receptors, and vectors pseudotyped with GaLV and A-MuLV envelopes (Uckert et al., 2000).

4.1.4. Pseudotyping

In order to overcome limitations related to stability, MLV-derived vectors produced in suspension packaging cell lines were pseudotyped with a spleen necrosis virus (SNV) envelope protein, thus developing a strategy to take advantage of the benefits provided by different viral species. The pseudotyped viral particles obtained by this method were able to infect SNV-sensitive cell lines at titers up to 10^5 IU/ml and showed resistance to inactivation by the human complement system. Such vectors have the potential to selectively target and effectively transduce human T-cell lines. In addition, this strategy combined the "high efficiency but low specificity" property of MLV-based vectors with a targeted therapeutic approach. As a result, MLV vectors pseudotyped with SNV envelope protein, resistant to human serum, have been shown to be a suitable tool for targeted gene transfer in humans under in vivo conditions (Logg et al., 2001).

In order to increase the efficiency of gene therapy, pseudotyping has also been performed with gibbon ape leukemia virus (GALV). GALV pseudotyping has been found to have the potential to modify one-fifth of bone marrow and peripheral blood cells for long periods. In gene therapy studies targeting human stem cells, GALV pseudotyping has enabled more effective outcomes (Williams et al., 2000).

Pseudotyping with the RD114 envelope protein of feline endogenous retrovirus has been found to be highly effective in efficiently transducing $CD34^+$ T lymphocytes. In some studies including RD114 pseudotyping, proviral genomes were detected in up to 90% of the myeloid and lymphoid cells of recipients, even in long-term follow-up (Kelly et al., 2000).

Pseudotyping with the vesicular stomatitis virus G (VSV-G) envelope protein, despite high vector titers and stability, did not yield the expected results. VSV-G was found to exert toxic effects on repopulating cells and showed low transduction efficiency in $CD34^+/CD38^-$ cells (Yam et al., 1998; Rebel et al., 1999; Evans et al., 1999).

As a different strategy, pseudotyping was also performed with chimeric envelopes containing interleukin-2 (IL-2) peptide sequences. This pseudotyping effectively transduced target cells through cytokine-mediated receptor signaling (Akkina et al., 1996).

5. Advantages of Retroviral Vectors in Gene Therapy

5.1. Ability of Permanent Gene Transfer

The most important advantage of retroviruses is their ability to convert their single-stranded RNA genomes into double-stranded DNA molecules and to integrate this DNA stably into the genome of the target cell. This ability provides retroviral vectors with the option of permanently altering the nuclear genome of the host cell (Zhou et al., 2014).

5.2. Manipulation of Genetic Structures

The simplicity of isolating the proviral form of retroviruses significantly facilitates the application of molecular modifications on the genome. In the original structure of the retroviral genome, cis elements, which are biologically active nucleic acid sequences, and trans elements, which are protein-coding regions, are functionally completely independent from each other. This functional difference allows these two factors to be kept entirely separate in recombinant vector systems, ensuring that a single RNA molecule containing the cis signals required for packaging, reverse transcription, and integration is expressed from the transfer vector, thereby guaranteeing the production of replication-deficient viral particles. Through this mechanism, the transfer of any viral gene to infected cells is prevented, the provirus remains functionally deficient in terms of replication, and viral proliferation is avoided (Yu et al., 1986; Zufferey et al., 1998).

6. Potential Risks of Retroviral Vectors in Gene Therapy and Current Technological Approaches for Risk Reduction

6.1. Insertional Mutagenesis and Oncogene Activation

The most critical safety problem that retroviral vectors may cause in gene transfer systems is insertional mutagenesis and the subsequent activation of oncogenes. This phenomenon has long been recognized as a mechanism in the interactions of wild-type retroviruses with the host genome. In a clinical study conducted for the treatment of X-linked severe combined immunodeficiency (X-SCID), where replication-deficient retroviral vectors were used, the development of T-cell leukemia was reported in 2 out of 10 treated patients (Anson, 2004).

When the mechanisms underlying oncogene activation are examined, it has been determined that if the provirus integrates into the upstream region of the target gene in the "sense" orientation, the transcription process initiated by the viral long terminal repeats (LTRs) leads to excessive expression of the respective oncogene. To reduce this risk, SIN (self-inactivating) vectors, in which the U3 regions in the proviral LTRs are deleted, have been developed to abolish transcriptional activity, thereby significantly decreasing the risk of LTR-mediated oncogene activation (Yu et al., 1986; Zufferey et al., 1998).

Another safety issue is that the strong enhancer elements in the proviral LTRs can activate neighboring cellular promoters, thereby disrupting transcriptional balance. This situation may occur even in large genomic regions, independent of the orientation of integration. For this reason, the selection of promoters that do not contain strong enhancer regions is considered an important strategy in terms of safety (Shin and Steffen, 1993; Lazo et al., 1990; Selten et al., 1984; Bartholomew and Ihle, 1991).

Retroviral integration can also damage oncogenes or regulatory regions of tumor suppressor genes, thereby triggering uncontrolled gene expression. Applications targeting non-dividing cells or requiring minimal proliferative stimulation reduce the likelihood of integration occurring in risky genomic regions. Lentiviral and spumaviral vectors within the retrovirus family enable effective transduction of hematopoietic stem cells with lower levels of cytokine stimulation. HIV-1 and similar lentiviral vectors, due to their ability to infect non-dividing cells and their different integration preferences, are considered advantageous in terms of safety. Compared to gammaretroviruses such as MoMLV, these vectors carry a lower risk of oncogene activation (Miyoshi, 2004).

6.2. Formation of Replication-Competent Retroviruses (RCR)

The formation of RCRs has been regarded as one of the most significant safety issues since the beginning of retroviral vector technology. This situation may result from recombination among vector components themselves or with endogenous retroviral sequences present in the cell lines used during production. In addition, activation of dormant endogenous proviral sequences can also lead to RCR.

To reduce the risk of RCR formation, strategies such as encoding helper functions on different plasmids, decreasing sequence homology among plasmids, removing or mutating unnecessary cis elements, employing self-inactivating (SIN) vector designs, and selecting production cell lines that do not carry endogenous retroviral sequences are used. Thanks to these methods, the probability of RCR formation has been reduced to very low levels in modern vector systems (Otto et al., 1994; Chong et al., 1998).

7. Types of Retroviral Vectors

7.1. Gammaretroviral Vectors

Gammaretroviral vectors have a simple organization that does not require accessory genes. Their packaging systems are designed in such a way that only the sequences encoding gag and pol need to be added. The transduction efficiency of these vectors is dependent on the cell cycle. The most commonly used gammaretroviral vectors (γ-RVs) in clinical and research applications are based on Murine Leukemia Virus (MLV), which can be produced at high titers. Moloney Murine Leukemia Virus (MoMLV) can only integrate viral DNA during mitosis, as it cannot transport therapeutic genes into the nucleus outside of cell division; therefore, it can only transduce dividing cells. The viral genome integrates into the host genome through a pre-integration complex (PIC), consisting of proviral DNA (with two long terminal repeats [LTRs]), host proteins, integrase, p12, and capsid protein (Katz et al., 2005; Kim and Robin, 2007).

MoMLV-based systems can be organized in both replication-competent and replication-deficient vector forms. In replication-deficient versions, the regions containing gag and env genes are deleted, the desired gene is cloned into these sites, and the vector is designed to include the packaging signal (Ψ), primer binding site (PBS), and LTRs. This gene cassette must not contain intron sequences, internal polyadenylation signals, or large secondary structures that may interfere with reverse transcriptase. The deleted gag, pol, and env genes are provided through helper plasmids and co-transferred into packaging cells. For this purpose, stable helper cell lines expressing gag/pol (GP) and env have been developed. For example, the GP+E-86 and GP+envAM-12 packaging cell lines were generated by electroporating two plasmids into NIH-3T3 fibroblast cells. The GP+E-86 line produces ecotropic particles that can infect only mouse and rat cells, whereas the GP+envAM-12 line produces amphotropic particles capable of infecting other mammalian cells, including human cells. Xenotropic MoMLV represents the form with the broadest cellular tropism, being able to infect a wide variety of cell types, including those of mice (Markowitz, 1988).

The tropism of vectors can be altered by pseudotyping strategies. One of the most commonly used envelopes for this purpose is the Vesicular Stomatitis Virus glycoprotein (VSV-G). VSV-G has the capacity to infect both mammalian and non-mammalian cells, while also increasing particle stability and allowing purification through ultracentrifugation. However, the VSV-G protein can be recognized by the complement system, which may decrease in vivo transduction efficiency (Hu et al., 2016; Gutierrez-Guerrero et al., 2020; Dautzenberg et al., 2021).

7.2. Foamyviral (Spumaviral) Vectors

Although foamyviruses are complex retroviruses with accessory gene structures, foamyvirus-based vectors can function without requiring these accessory genetic components. These vectors are considered safer for gene delivery because they are non-pathogenic and do not spread horizontally in humans. Reverse transcription is completed in the virion-producing cells, and the genomes enabling transduction are in cDNA form. This allows foamyviral vectors to remain in a passive state in non-dividing cells and to become active once the cells begin to proliferate (Zhou et al., 2014). The long terminal repeats (LTRs) are regulated by the Bel1 transactivator. The Bel1 protein ensures that the LTRs remain silent in cells transduced with foamyviral vectors (Hill et al., 1999).

Preclinical studies conducted with foamyviral vectors have demonstrated that these vectors can be particularly useful for gene transfer into hematopoietic stem cells (Zhou et al., 2014).

7.3. Lentiviral Vectors

Lentiviruses, which are complex retroviruses, contain not only the gag, pol, and env proteins but also the "tat" gene, which provides transcriptional activation, and the "rev" gene, which ensures the export of unspliced viral RNA from the nucleus (Bieniasz et al., 1999). In addition, HIV-1, a member of the lentivirus family, includes vif, vpr, vpu, and nef genes, which further enhance viral pathogenicity (Basmaciogullari et al., 2014; Seissler et al., 2017). Similar to murine oncoviruses, lentiviruses can easily cross the nuclear membrane with their pre-integration complex (PIC) and can transduce quiescent cells (Naldini et al., 1996; Zhou et al., 2014).

Lentiviral vectors resemble other retroviruses in terms of integration into the host cell genome. However, unlike simple retroviruses that are effective only in dividing cells, lentiviruses can efficiently transduce non-dividing cells such as hematopoietic stem cells (HSCs) and neurons (Zhou et al., 2014).

The most important advantage of lentiviral systems is that the integrated genomic copies can provide long-term and stable transgene expression.

Furthermore, these vectors have a transgene packaging capacity of approximately 8–10 kb. Unlike gammaretroviruses such as MLV, lentiviral integration occur more frequently in intronic regions and at sites distant from promoters, which contributes to reducing potential oncogenic risk and immune responses (Zhou et al., 2014). However, lentiviral integration is still dependent on the cell cycle. Pseudotyping with VSV-G, which has been employed to enhance transduction efficiency in other vector types, has not been found effective in lentiviral vectors (Korin and Zack, 1998).

In recent years, some improvements have been made to increase the safety and efficacy of lentiviral vector systems. By deleting vif, vpu, vpr, nef, tat, rev genes and the TATA box and transcription factor binding sites in the 3′-LTR, and by adding regulatory elements such as MAR, WPRE, and cppt, transduction efficiency has been enhanced (Bulcha et al., 2021).

8. Preclinical and Clinical Applications of Retroviral Vectors

8.1. Treatment of Corneal Opacity

Effective treatment options for corneal opacity are quite limited, and experimental gene therapies appear as a promising alternative. Preclinical studies were conducted with a retroviral vector carrying the antiproliferative dominant negative mutant cyclin G1 (dnG1) for the prevention of corneal opacity, which develops after phototherapeutic keratectomy (PTK) and can cause severe complications impairing visual acuity in up to 15% of patients. High-titer retroviral vectors were produced using a transient three-plasmid co-transfection system, in which packaging components such as gag-pol, the amphotropic CAE envelope (env), or chimeric env containing a collagen-binding motif derived from von Willebrand factor (vWF) were placed on separate plasmids. In this study, collagen-targeted retroviral vectors were developed by exploiting the high binding affinity between vWF and collagen. It was shown that gene delivery with collagen-targeted vectors (Mx-nBg) in laser-injured corneas was significantly increased compared to untargeted vectors (CAE-nBg) (Behrens et al., 2002).

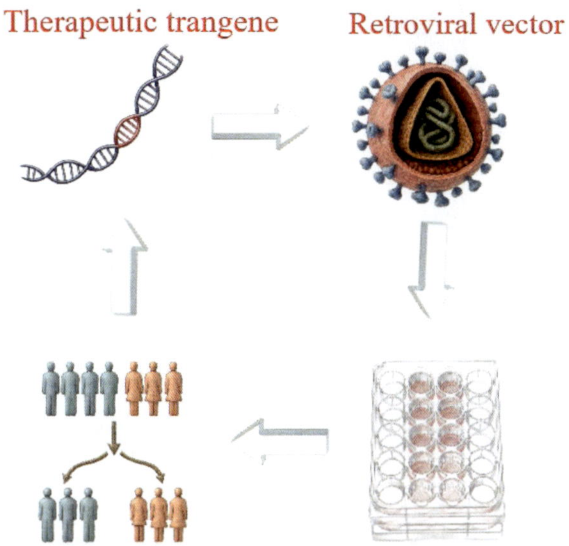

Figure 3: Schematic Representation of Retroviral Vector-Mediated Gene Therapy (Created by the authors using https://www.canva.com and https://illustrae.co/)

As a result of the study, topical application of dnG1 retroviral vector-containing eye drops was found to be safe and effective for preventing the development of corneal opacity after PTK. The data obtained demonstrated that collagen-targeted dnG1 retroviral vectors may represent an effective therapeutic option to prevent excimer laser-induced corneal opacity (Behrens et al., 2002).

8.2. Cancer Therapy

Retroviral vectors have become important tools in the field of cancer therapy, particularly in RNA interference (RNAi)-based approaches, for the functional analysis of genes and the development of therapeutic strategies for diseases. Moloney Murine Leukemia Virus (MoMLV)-based retroviral systems have been used in the creation of short hairpin RNA (shRNA) libraries for screening purposes. In addition, retrovirally delivered shRNAs have been reported to provide long-term suppression of HIV-1 transcription. Lentiviral vectors derived from HIV, on the other hand, are widely applied in advanced biotechnological applications such as stable gene silencing and stem cell engineering (Aruleba et al., 2004; Berns et al., 2004; Yamagishi et al., 2009).

In breast cancer models, RNAi triggers delivered via lentiviral vectors have been shown to suppress leptin/leptin receptor (ObR) signaling and associated pathway factors (ERα, VEGF), which are involved in tumor cell proliferation, migration, invasion, angiogenesis, and metastasis, thereby decreasing tumor progression. Moreover, this approach has also been effective in the long-term silencing of genes that are difficult to target pharmacologically, such as Hsp25/Hsp27 (Kaur et al., 2011).

In cervical cancer, lentiviral-based RNAi systems developed against the E6 and E7 oncogenes of papillomavirus have been reported at the preclinical level to suppress tumor growth and progression. Similarly, in small cell lung cancer, lentiviral vector-mediated RNAi applications have been shown to be effective in inhibiting cell proliferation and bone metastasis (Gu et al., 2006).

A phase II clinical trial is ongoing in patients with stage III and IV orthotopic glioblastoma, in which a retroviral vector (MoMLV) containing cytosine deaminase is being used. Preclinical results of this study showed that the vector spreads the transgene by infecting neighboring cells through a bystander effect (Hlavaty et al., 2011; Perez et al., 2012). In another clinical trial conducted in glioblastoma patients, PA317 cells transduced with an MLV vector containing herpes simplex virus thymidine kinase (HSV-tk), which phosphorylates and activates ganciclovir (GCV), were implanted intratumorally in fifteen patients. Partial success was achieved, with significant tumor size reduction observed in one-third of the patients (Oldfield et al., 1993).

Retroviral-based gene therapy has also been tested in graft-versus-host disease (GVHD), a complication that develops after allogeneic bone marrow transplantation and can lead to death in a very short period of time. Lymphocytes transduced with a retroviral vector containing HSV-tk were transferred to patients, and the cytotoxic effect of GCV was enhanced. This therapy suppressed the immune response-inducing cells in patients who developed GVHD, leading to clinical improvement (Bonini et al., 1997).

Retroviral and lentiviral vectors have also come to prominence in chimeric antigen receptor T cell (CAR-T) therapy, which has emerged as a novel approach in cancer treatment. In ex vivo and autologous therapies, retroviral and lentiviral vectors are successfully used for the transduction of hematopoietic stem cells. The chimeric receptor consists of a single-chain antibody externally and a T cell receptor (TCR) signaling domain intracellularly, and it recognizes the hematopoietic surface protein CD19. In a clinical study, a lentiviral vector expressing this receptor efficiently transduced tumor-targeted T cells, demonstrated activation in all patients regardless of HLA compatibility, and no cases of insertional oncogenesis were detected (Maus et al., 2014). In pediatric B-cell acute lymphoblastic leukemia (B-ALL), lentiviral vector-based CAR-T cell therapy (Kymriah) and in B-cell lymphoma, gammaretroviral vector-based CAR-T cell therapy (Yescarta) have both received FDA approval (Kochenderfer et al., 2009). Table 1 presents FDA-approved retroviral vector-mediated gene and cell therapy agents used in various cancer types.

8.3. Treatment of Human Immunodeficiency Virus (HIV)

Although highly active antiretroviral therapy (HAART) currently provides an effective therapeutic option against HIV-1 infections, which represent a serious health problem, the emergence of drug resistance and the risk of toxicity over time necessitate the development of alternative therapeutic approaches. Lentiviral vector strategies based on shRNA and inhibitory agents have emerged as an alternative for suppressing drug resistance and enabling more effective viral control. For this purpose, a lentiviral vector was designed combining an shRNA targeting HIV-1 tat/rev mRNA, a nucleolus-specific decoy suppressing the HIV tat protein, and a ribozyme suppressing the CCR5 receptor that regulates HIV-1 entry into the cell (lentiviral vector rHIV7-shI-TAR-CCR5RZ). This therapy inhibited viral replication more effectively and for a longer period (+42 days) compared to monotherapies in primary hematopoietic cells (Li et al., 2005).

Alongside successful retroviral approaches in HIV therapy, there have also been unsuccessful trials based on lentiviral vectors. In one clinical study, a lentiviral vector was used for ex vivo gene transfer into $CD34^+$ hematopoietic stem cells, yet no clinical response was observed. However, expression of anti-tat/rev shRNA-CCR5 ribozyme in peripheral blood was detected for up to three years (DiGiusto et al., 2010).

Product	Company	Therapy	Vector	Disease
Abecma	Celgene	Cell-based gene therapy	Lentiviral	Multiple Myeloma
Aucatzyl	Autolus	Cell-based gene therapy	Lentiviral	Acute Lymphoblastic Leukemia
Breyanzi	Juno Therapeutics	Cell-based gene therapy	Lentiviral	Large B-Cell Lymphoma
Carvykti	Janssen Biotech	Cell-based gene therapy	Lentiviral	Multiple Myeloma
Fucaso	Nanjing IASO Bio.	Cell-based gene therapy	Lentiviral	Multiple Myeloma
Kymriah	Novartis	Cell-based gene therapy	Lentiviral	Follicular Lymphoma
Lenmeldy	Orchard Therapeutics	Cell-based gene therapy	Lentiviral	M. Leukodystrophy
Libmeldy	Orchard Therapeutics	Cell-based gene therapy	Lentiviral	M. Leukodystrophy
Lyfgenia	Bluebird Bio	Cell-based gene therapy	Lentiviral	Sickle Cell Disease
Relma-cel	JW Therapeutics	Cell-based gene therapy	Lentiviral	Lymphoma
Skysona	Bluebird Bio	Gene therapy	Lentiviral	CAD
Tecelra	Adaptimmune	Cell-based gene therapy	Lentiviral	Synovial Sarcoma
Zevor-cel	CARsgen Therapeutics	Cell-based gene therapy	Lentiviral	Multiple Myeloma
Zynteglo	Bluebird Bio	Cell-based gene therapy	Lentiviral	ß-Thalassemia
Strimvelis	Orchard Therapeutics	Cell-based gene therapy	Retroviral	ADA-SCID
Tecartus	Kite Pharma	Cell-based gene therapy	Retroviral	Lymphoma
Yescarta	Kite Pharma	Cell-based gene therapy	Retroviral	Lymphoma

Table 1: Approved viral-vector–mediated gene and cell therapies (https://www.fda.gov/vaccines-blood-biologics/cellular-and-gene-therapy-products/approved-cellular-and-gene-therapy-products)

8.4. Treatment of Rare Diseases

In recent years, retroviral-based gene therapy approaches targeting hereditary, rare, and otherwise untreatable diseases have also been developed. In metachromatic leukodystrophy (MLD), a lysosomal storage disease caused by a deficiency of the arylsulfatase A (ARSA) enzyme, attempts have been made to correct the defect by ex vivo transfer of the ARSA gene via a lentiviral vector (Biffi et al., 2013). In progressive neurodegenerative MLD, ARSA deficiency results in sulfatide accumulation, leading to multi-organ failure and death within a few years (Platt et al., 2018). Biffi et al. transplanted ARSA gene-transduced HSCs into three pediatric MLD patients. In follow-ups up to 24 months, significant ARSA activity was detected in both cerebrospinal fluid (CSF) and hematopoietic cells (Biffi et al., 2013).

Lentiviral vector-based approaches have also been tested in Wiskott-Aldrich Syndrome, a rare X-linked disorder characterized by immunodeficiency, thrombocytopenia, and eczema. In a clinical trial involving three patients, the WAS gene was delivered into autologous $CD34^+$ HSCs via a lentiviral vector. Following transplantation, thrombocytopenia and eczema improved in all patients, and resistance to infections was observed (Aiuti et al., 2013; Malik and Masab, 2023).

Adenosine deaminase (ADA) deficiency causes severe combined immunodeficiency (SCID), leaving the body unable to defend itself against infections and predisposing patients to opportunistic infections. In a gene therapy trial including ADA-SCID patients, a retroviral vector containing the ADA enzyme was transferred into two pediatric patients, resulting in clinical success (Giblett et al., 1972; Blaese et al., 1995). Since LTR-driven gammaretroviral vectors expressing ADA had been used for a long time in ADA-SCID patients without major adverse events, the ATMP Strimvelis gene therapy gained clinical approval. However, because one patient developed T-cell leukemia during Strimvelis treatment, its use was temporarily suspended to assess the risk of insertional mutagenesis (Morgan et al., 2021).

In X-linked SCID (SCID-X1), characterized by multiple mutations in the interleukin-2 receptor gamma (IL2RG) gene, lentiviral vector-based approaches achieved T-cell activation and clinical improvement (Noguchi et al., 1993; Sauer et al., 2014). In SCID-X1 patients, a lentiviral SIN vector containing elongation factor 1 alpha has been shown to enhance therapeutic efficacy by reconstructing T and B lymphocytes as well as natural killer (NK) cells (De Ravin et al., 2016; Macarz et al., 2019).

In epidermolysis bullosa, a disease caused by mutations in the COL7A1 gene and characterized by skin fragility, retroviral and lentiviral vectors containing the gene enabled expression of collagen VII, alleviating symptoms. In another retroviral vector-based study, epidermal stem cell grafts containing the laminin-5 (LAMP-5) gene were applied to patients with epidermolysis bullosa, restoring epidermal integrity (Mavilio et al., 2006; Perdoni et al., 2015).

Gene therapy approaches have also been tested in familial hypercholesterolemia caused by mutations in the LDL receptor. Recombinant retroviral vectors containing the LDL receptor were transferred into patient-derived hepatocytes and subsequently reinfused into the patients as an autologous treatment. In the patients included in this study, LDL/HDL balance was maintained for 18 months (Grossman et al., 1994).

In cerebral adrenoleukodystrophy (CALD), a lysosomal storage disease inherited in an X-linked manner and characterized by peroxisomal metabolic dysfunction, deficiency of the ALDP enzyme leads to the accumulation of long-chain fatty acids in the nervous system, adrenal glands, and plasma, resulting in inflammatory demyelination. In this highly fatal disease, gene therapy approaches are being explored alongside standard protocols. Lenti-D™ gene therapy, based on lentiviral vectors, was tested in 32 CALD patients, and during an average follow-up of 30 months, no significant adverse reactions were detected. Moreover, gene-marked cells were identified in the patients (Morgan et al., 2021). This therapy is considered a candidate for clinical approval in CALD patients.

Beta thalassemia major is a severe blood disorder caused by the inability to synthesize the beta-globin chain of hemoglobin, characterized by microcytic hypochromic anemia, anisopoikilocytosis, low or absent HbA levels, and elevated HbA_2 levels (Langer, 2000). Patients with beta thalassemia major who do not undergo transfusion therapy typically die within an average of twenty years. Gene therapy studies have provided an alternative therapeutic option for beta thalassemia major patients. Lentiviral-based gene therapy ensured stable gene expression throughout treatment. Furthermore, no leukemia development or significant adverse reactions were observed, and patients did not require transfusion for a long time (Cavazzana-Calvo et al., 2010).

Retroviral-based gene therapy approaches have been explored not only in humans but also in other species for the treatment of rare diseases. In canine leukocyte adhesion deficiency, foamy viral vectors were applied in vivo and clinical success was achieved (Burtner et al., 2014).

9. Legal Regulations in Gene Therapy Studies

The legal regulations governing clinical studies in the field of gene therapy began in the 1970s and have undergone changes over the years, reaching their current form. Today, gene therapies, which are evaluated within the framework of both health risks and ethical principles, are supervised by international organizations. All clinical studies involving gene therapies are carried out in compliance with Good Clinical Practice (GCP) guidelines, CFR, FDA 1572, International Conference on Harmonisation (ICH) guidelines, and informed consent regulations (Williams et al., 2000). Institutions and committees authorized for the supervision and regulation of gene therapies are presented in Table 2.

The National Institutes of Health (NIH) has established guidelines that include oversight and adverse event reporting for studies that receive NIH institutional funding or are supported by the NIH. According to these guidelines, all studies in which recombinant DNA is transferred into humans are subject to review by the Food and Drug Administration (FDA), the Office of Biotechnology Activities (OBA), and the Recombinant DNA Advisory Committee (RAC). The FDA, within the scope of an Investigational New Drug (IND) application, holds full authority over clinical trials involving gene therapy, including clinical holds at Phase I and the authority to terminate studies when necessary. The RAC is authorized to review studies in terms of scientific content, ethical issues, preliminary safety data, and adverse events. All serious adverse events (SAEs) that occur during studies, including cases where the relationship to the study has not been fully established, must be reported to the Office of Biotechnology Activities. In addition to adverse event reporting, the OBA is also responsible for the review of modifications made within the study and the evaluation of new findings (Williams et al., 2000).

The Office for Human Research Protections (OHRP), an independent body operating under the Department of Health and Human Services (DHHS), imposes various obligations on institutions and investigators conducting clinical research involving gene therapies regarding the protection of human subjects, the informed consent process, and the establishment of an Institutional Review Board (IRB). In cases where these obligations are not fulfilled, the OHRP has the authority to impose sanctions on both institutions and investigators. The oversight and suspension authority of Institutional Review Boards (IRBs) resides with both the OHRP and the FDA (Williams et al., 2000).

Agencies and Commitees	
Department of Health and Human Services	DHHS
Office for Human Research Protection	OHRP
Office for Protection of Research Risks	OPRP
Food and Drug Administration	FDA
Office for Biologics Evalution and Research	CBER
National Institute of Health	NIH
Office of Biotechnology Activities	OBA
Office of Recombinant DNA Activities	ORDA
Recombinant DNA Advisory Commitee	RAC
Institutional Biosafety Commitee	IBC

Table 2: Agencies and committees with authority to review and regulate clinical therapy involving gene therapies (Williams et al., 2000).

Conclusion

It has been demonstrated that, through the permanent gene transfer capability and high transduction efficiency of retroviral systems, long-term therapeutic effects can be achieved, while risks such as insertional mutagenesis and the formation of replication-competent retroviruses (RCRs) can be mitigated by various strategies. The outcomes obtained in rare diseases such as SCID, Wiskott–Aldrich syndrome, MLD, and CALD, as well as in HIV infection and oncological diseases, provide evidence that the efficacy–safety balance of these platforms can be optimized.

The future is being shaped along three main axes: (i) safer vector architectures (integration-prone designs that minimize genotoxicity), (ii) more refined control in cell and tissue targeting (advanced pseudotyping), and (iii) combined strategies incorporating gene editing (CRISPR).

In conclusion, retroviral and lentiviral vectors have proven their translational success; across a broad spectrum ranging from rare hereditary disorders to hematological malignancies, they have become complementary—and, in certain contexts, alternative—to standard care. Conducting scientific progress in harmony with ethical and regulatory frameworks, along with transparent sharing of long-term follow-up and real data, will reinforce the safety and accessibility of these therapies. In the coming period, personalized targeting, combined designs (gene transfer + gene editing), and production–economic optimization will be the key to providing durable, safe, and sustainable benefits of gene therapies to broader patient populations.

References

1. Aiuti, A., Biasco, L., Scaramuzza, S., Ferrua, F., Cicalese, M. P., Baricordi, C., Dionisio, F., Calabria, A., Giannelli, S., Castiello, M. C., Bosticardo, M., Evangelio, C., Assanelli, A., Casiraghi, M., Di Nunzio, S., Callegaro, L., Benati, C., Rizzardi, P., Pellin, D., Di Serio, C., Naldini, L. (2013). Lentiviral hematopoietic stem cell gene therapy in patients with Wiskott-Aldrich syndrome. Science (New York, N.Y.), 341(6148), 1233151. https://doi.org/10.1126/science.1233151
2. Akkina, R. K., Walton, R. M., Chen, M. L., Li, Q. X., Planelles, V., & Chen, I. S. (1996). High-efficiency gene transfer into CD34+ cells with a human immunodeficiency virus type 1-based retroviral vector pseudotyped with vesicular stomatitis virus envelope glycoprotein G. Journal of virology, 70(4), 2581–2585. https://doi.org/10.1128/JVI.70.4.2581-2585.1996
3. Anson D. S. (2004). The use of retroviral vectors for gene therapy-what are the risks? A review of retroviral pathogenesis and its relevance to retroviral vector-mediated gene delivery. Genetic vaccines and therapy, 2(1), 9. https://doi.org/10.1186/1479-0556-2-9
4. Approved Cellular and Gene Therapy Products. Published May 2025. Accessed May 2025. https://www.fda.gov/vaccines-blood-biologics/cellular-and-gene-therapy-products/approved-cellular-and-gene-therapy-products
5. Bartholomew, C., & Ihle, J. N. (1991). Retroviral insertions 90 kilobases proximal to the Evi-1 myeloid transforming gene activate transcription from the normal promoter. Molecular and cellular biology, 11(4), 1820–1828. https://doi.org/10.1128/mcb.11.4.1820-1828.1991
6. Basmaciogullari, S., & Pizzato, M. (2014). The activity of Nef on HIV-1 infectivity. Frontiers in microbiology, 5, 232. https://doi.org/10.3389/fmicb.2014.00232

7. Behrens, A., Gordon, E. M., Li, L., Liu, P. X., Chen, Z., Peng, H., La Bree, L., Anderson, W. F., Hall, F. L., & McDonnell, P. J. (2002). Retroviral gene therapy vectors for prevention of excimer laser-induced corneal haze. Investigative ophthalmology & visual science, 43(4), 968–977.
8. Berns, K., Hijmans, E. M., Mullenders, J., Brummelkamp, T. R., Velds, A., Heimerikx, M., … Bernards, R. (2004). A large-scale RNAi screen in human cells identifies new components of the p53 pathway. Nature, 428(6981), 431–437. https://doi.org/10.1038/nature02371
9. Bieniasz, P. D., Grdina, T. A., Bogerd, H. P., & Cullen, B. R. (1999). Recruitment of cyclin T1/P-TEFb to an HIV type 1 long terminal repeat promoter proximal RNA target is both necessary and sufficient for full activation of transcription. Proceedings of the National Academy of Sciences of the United States of America, 96(14), 7791–7796. https://doi.org/10.1073/pnas.96.14.7791
10. Biffi, A., Montini, E., Lorioli, L., Cesani, M., Fumagalli, F., Plati, T., Baldoli, C., Martino, S., Calabria, A., Canale, S., Benedicenti, F., Vallanti, G., Biasco, L., Leo, S., Kabbara, N., Zanetti, G., Rizzo, W. B., Mehta, N. A., Cicalese, M. P., Casiraghi, M., Naldini, L. (2013). Lentiviral hematopoietic stem cell gene therapy benefits metachromatic leukodystrophy. Science (New York, N.Y.), 341(6148), 1233158. https://doi.org/10.1126/science.1233158
11. Blaese RM, Culver KW, Miller AD, Carter CS, Fleisher T, Clerici M, et al. (1995) T lymphocyte-directed gene therapy for ADA-SCID: initial trial results after 4 years. Science 270(5235): 475–480.
12. Blaese, R. M., Culver, K. W., Miller, A. D., Carter, C. S., Fleisher, T., Clerici, M., Shearer, G., Chang, L., Chiang, Y., Tolstoshev, P., Greenblatt, J. J., Rosenberg, S. A., Klein, H., Berger, M., Mullen, C. A., Ramsey, W. J., Muul, L., Morgan, R. A., & Anderson, W. F. (1995). T lymphocyte-directed gene therapy for ADA- SCID: initial trial results after 4 years. Science (New York, N.Y.), 270(5235), 475–480. https://doi.org/10.1126/science.270.5235.475
13. Bonini, C., Ferrari, G., Verzeletti, S., Servida, P., Zappone, E., Ruggieri, L., Ponzoni, M., Rossini, S., Mavilio, F., Traversari, C., & Bordignon, C. (1997). HSV-TK gene transfer into donor lymphocytes for control of allogeneic graft-versus-leukemia. Science (New York, N.Y.), 276(5319), 1719–1724. https://doi.org/10.1126/science.276.5319.1719

14. Bowerman B, Brown PO, Bishop JM, Varmus HE. (1989) A nucleoprotein complex mediates the integration of retroviral DNA. Genes and Development 3(4): 469–478.
15. Bulcha, J. T., Wang, Y., Ma, H., Tai, P. W. L., & Gao, G. (2021). Viral vector platforms within the gene therapy landscape. Signal transduction and targeted therapy, 6(1), 53. https://doi.org/10.1038/s41392-021-00487-6
16. Burtner, C. R., Beard, B. C., Kennedy, D. R., Wohlfahrt, M. E., Adair, J. E., Trobridge, G. D., Scharenberg, A. M., Torgerson, T. R., Rawlings, D. J., Felsburg, P. J., & Kiem, H. P. (2014). Intravenous injection of a foamy virus vector to correct canine SCID-X1. Blood, 123(23), 3578–3584. https://doi.org/10.1182/blood-2013-11-538926
17. Cavazzana-Calvo, M., Payen, E., Negre, O., Wang, G., Hehir, K., Fusil, F., Down, J., Denaro, M., Brady, T., Westerman, K., Cavallesco, R., Gillet-Legrand, B., Caccavelli, L., Sgarra, R., Maouche-Chrétien, L., Bernaudin, F., Girot, R., Dorazio, R., Mulder, G. J., Polack, A., … Leboulch, P. (2010). Transfusion independence and HMGA2 activation after gene therapy of human β-thalassaemia. Nature, 467(7313), 318–322. https://doi.org/10.1038/nature09328
18. Chan, L. M., Coutelle, C., & Themis, M. (2001). A novel human suspension culture packaging cell line for production of high-titre retroviral vectors. Gene therapy, 8(9), 697–703. https://doi.org/10.1038/sj.gt.3301456
19. Chong, H., Starkey, W., & Vile, R. G. (1998). A replication-competent retrovirus arising from a split-function packaging cell line was generated by recombination events between the vector, one of the packaging constructs, and endogenous retroviral sequences. Journal of virology, 72(4), 2663–2670. https://doi.org/10.1128/JVI.72.4.2663-2670.1998
20. Coffin JM. (1979) Structure, replication, and recombination of retrovirus genomes: some unifying hypotheses. Journal of General Virology 42(1): 1–26
21. Dautzenberg, I.J.C., Rabelink, M.J.W.E. & Hoeben, R.C. The stability of envelope-pseudotyped lentiviral vectors. Gene Ther 28, 89–104 (2021). https://doi.org/10.1038/s41434-020-00193-y
22. De Ravin, S. S., Wu, X., Moir, S., Anaya-O'Brien, S., Kwatemaa, N., Littel, P., Theobald, N., Choi, U., Su, L., Marquesen, M., Hilligoss, D., Lee, J., Buckner, C. M., Zarember, K. A., O'Connor, G., McVicar, D., Kuhns, D., Throm, R. E., Zhou, S., Notarangelo, L. D., Kardava, L. (2016). Lentiviral hematopoietic stem cell gene

therapy for X-linked severe combined immunodeficiency. Science translational medicine, 8(335), 335ra57. https://doi.org/10.1126/scitranslmed.aad8856
23. DiGiusto, D. L., Krishnan, A., Li, L., Li, H., Li, S., Rao, A., Mi, S., Yam, P., Stinson, S., Kalos, M., Alvarnas, J., Lacey, S. F., Yee, J. K., Li, M., Couture, L., Hsu, D., Forman, S. J., Rossi, J. J., & Zaia, J. A. (2010). RNA-based gene therapy for HIV with lentiviral vector-modified CD34(+) cells in patients undergoing transplantation for AIDS-related lymphoma. Science translational medicine, 2(36), 36ra43. https://doi.org/10.1126/scitranslmed.300093
24. D'Souza, V., & Summers, M. F. (2005). How retroviruses select their genomes. Nature reviews. Microbiology, 3(8), 643–655. https://doi.org/10.1038/nrmicro1210
25. Edelstein ML, Abedi MR, Wixon J. (2007) Gene therapy clinical trials worldwide to 2007–an update. Journal of Gene Medicine 9(10): 833–842.
26. Evans, J. T., Kelly, P. F., O'Neill, E., & Garcia, J. V. (1999). Human cord blood CD34+CD38- cell transduction via lentivirus-based gene transfer vectors. Human gene therapy, 10(9), 1479–1489. https://doi.org/10.1089/10430349950017815
27. Fischer A, Hacein-Bey-Abina S, Cavazzana-Calvo M. (2010) 20 years of gene therapy for SCID. Nature Immunology 11(6): 457–460.
28. Giblett, E. R., Anderson, J. E., Cohen, F., Pollara, B., & Meuwissen, H. J. (1972). Adenosine-deaminase deficiency in two patients with severely impaired cellular immunity. Lancet (London, England), 2(7786), 1067–1069. https://doi.org/10.1016/s0140-6736(72)92345-8
29. Grabarczyk, P., Gryska, K., Wysocki, P. J., Izycki, D., & Mackiewicz, A. (2001). Improving the retroviral vector (RV) systems for immunotherapy of cancer. Advances in experimental medicine and biology, 495, 389–392. https://doi.org/10.1007/978-1-4615-0685-0_57
30. Grossman, M., Raper, S. E., Kozarsky, K., Stein, E. A., Engelhardt, J. F., Muller, D., Lupien, P. J., & Wilson, J. M. (1994). Successful ex vivo gene therapy directed to liver in a patient with familial hypercholesterolaemia. Nature genetics, 6(4), 335–341. https://doi.org/10.1038/ng0494-335
31. Gu, W., Putral, L., Hengst, K., Minto, K., Saunders, N. A., Leggatt, G., & McMillan, N. A. (2006). Inhibition of cervical cancer cell growth in vitro and in vivo with lentiviral-vector delivered short

hairpin RNA targeting human papillomavirus E6 and E7 oncogenes. Cancer gene therapy, 13(11), 1023–1032. https://doi.org/10.1038/sj.cgt.7700971
32. Gutierrez-Guerrero, A., Cosset, F. L., & Verhoeyen, E. (2020). Lentiviral Vector Pseudotypes: Precious Tools to Improve Gene Modification of Hematopoietic Cells for Research and Gene Therapy. Viruses, 12(9), 1016. https://doi.org/10.3390/v12091016
33. Hill, C. L., Bieniasz, P. D., & McClure, M. O. (1999). Properties of human foamy virus relevant to its development as a vector for gene therapy. The Journal of general virology, 80 (Pt 8), 2003–2009. https://doi.org/10.1099/0022-1317-80-8-2003
34. Hlavaty, J., Jandl, G., Liszt, M., Petznek, H., König-Schuster, M., Sedlak, J., Egerbacher, M., Weissenberger, J., Salmons, B., Günzburg, W. H., & Renner, M. (2011). Comparative evaluation of preclinical in vivo models for the assessment of replicating retroviral vectors for the treatment of glioblastoma. Journal of neuro-oncology, 102(1), 59–69. https://doi.org/10.1007/s11060-010-0295-5
35. Hu, S., Mohan Kumar, D., Sax, C., Schuler, C., & Akkina, R. (2016). Pseudotyping of lentiviral vector with novel vesiculovirus envelope glycoproteins derived from Chandipura and Piry viruses. Virology, 488, 162–168. https://doi.org/10.1016/j.virol.2015.11.012
36. Katz, R. A., Greger, J. G., & Skalka, A. M. (2005). Effects of cell cycle status on early events in retroviral replication. Journal of cellular biochemistry, 94(5), 880–889. https://doi.org/10.1002/jcb.20358
37. Kaur, P., Nagaraja, G. M., & Asea, A. (2011). Combined lentiviral and RNAi technologies for the delivery and permanent silencing of the hsp25 gene. In A. Asea & P. Kaur (Eds.), Methods in Molecular Biology (Vol. 787, pp. 121–136). Humana Press. https://doi.org/10.1007/978-1-61779-295-3_10
38. Kelly, P. F., Vandergriff, J., Nathwani, A., Nienhuis, A. W., & Vanin, E. F. (2000). Highly efficient gene transfer into cord blood nonobese diabetic/severe combined immunodeficiency repopulating cells by oncoretroviral vector particles pseudotyped with the feline endogenous retrovirus (RD114) envelope protein. Blood, 96(4), 1206–1214.
39. Kim, SH., Robbins, P.D. (2007). Retroviral Vectors for Gene Therapy. In: Lysosomal Storage Disorders. Springer, Boston, MA. https://doi.org/10.1007/978-0-387-70909-3_5
40. Kochenderfer, J. N., Feldman, S. A., Zhao, Y., Xu, H., Black, M. A., Morgan, R. A., Wilson, W. H., & Rosenberg, S. A. (2009).

Construction and preclinical evaluation of an anti-CD19 chimeric antigen receptor. Journal of immunotherapy (Hagerstown, Md. : 1997), 32(7), 689–702. https://doi.org/10.1097/CJI.0b013e3181ac6138
41. Korin, Y. D., & Zack, J. A. (1998). Progression to the G1b phase of the cell cycle is required for completion of human immunodeficiency virus type 1 reverse transcription in T cells. Journal of virology, 72(4), 3161–3168. https://doi.org/10.1128/JVI.72.4.3161-3168.1998
42. Langer AL. Beta-Thalassemia. 2000 Sep 28 [Updated 2024 Feb 8]. In: Adam MP, Feldman J, Mirzaa GM, et al., editors. GeneReviews® [Internet]. Seattle (WA): University of Washington, Seattle; 1993-2025. Available from: https://www.ncbi.nlm.nih.gov/books/NBK1426/
43. Lazo, P. A., Lee, J. S., & Tsichlis, P. N. (1990). Long-distance activation of the Myc protooncogene by provirus insertion in Mlvi-1 or Mlvi-4 in rat T-cell lymphomas. Proceedings of the National Academy of Sciences of the United States of America, 87(1), 170–173. https://doi.org/10.1073/pnas.87.1.170
44. Li M, Mizuuchi M, Burke TR, Jr., Craigie R. (2006) Retroviral DNA integration: reaction pathway and critical intermediates. EMBO Journal 25(6): 1295–1304.
45. Li, M. J., Kim, J., Li, S., Zaia, J., Yee, J. K., Anderson, J., Akkina, R., & Rossi, J. J. (2005). Long-term inhibition of HIV-1 infection in primary hematopoietic cells by lentiviral vector delivery of a triple combination of anti-HIV shRNA, anti-CCR5 ribozyme, and a nucleolar-localizing TAR decoy. Molecular therapy : the journal of the American Society of Gene Therapy, 12(5), 900–909. https://doi.org/10.1016/j.ymthe.2005.07.524
46. Lochelt M, Muranyi W, Flugel RM. (1993) Human foamy virus genome possesses an internal, Bel-1-dependent and functional promoter. Proceedings of the National Academy of Sciences USA 90(15): 7317–7321.
47. Logg, C. R., Tai, C. K., Logg, A., Anderson, W. F., & Kasahara, N. (2001). A uniquely stable replication-competent retrovirus vector achieves efficient gene delivery in vitro and in solid tumors. Human gene therapy, 12(8), 921–932. https://doi.org/10.1089/104303401750195881
48. MacKenzie, K. L., Hackett, N. R., Crystal, R. G., & Moore, M. A. (2000). Adenoviral vector-mediated gene transfer to primitive

human hematopoietic progenitor cells: assessment of transduction and toxicity in long-term culture. Blood, 96(1), 100–108.

49. Malik MA, Masab M. Wiskott-Aldrich Syndrome. [Updated 2023 Jun 26]. In: StatPearls [Internet]. Treasure Island (FL): StatPearls Publishing; 2025 Jan-. Available from: https://www.ncbi.nlm.nih.gov/books/NBK539838/

50. Mamcarz, E., Zhou, S., Lockey, T., Abdelsamed, H., Cross, S. J., Kang, G., Ma, Z., Condori, J., Dowdy, J., Triplett, B., Li, C., Maron, G., Aldave Becerra, J. C., Church, J. A., Dokmeci, E., Love, J. T., da Matta Ain, A. C., van der Watt, H., Tang, X., Janssen, W., Sorrentino, B. P. (2019). Lentiviral Gene Therapy Combined with Low-Dose Busulfan in Infants with SCID-X1. The New England journal of medicine, 380(16), 1525–1534. https://doi.org/10.1056/NEJMoa1815408

51. Markowitz, D., Goff, S., & Bank, A. (1988). Construction and use of a safe and efficient amphotropic packaging cell line. Virology, 167(2), 400–406.

52. Maus, M. V., Grupp, S. A., Porter, D. L., & June, C. H. (2014). Antibody-modified T cells: CARs take the front seat for hematologic malignancies. Blood, 123(17), 2625–2635. https://doi.org/10.1182/blood-2013-11-492231

53. Mavilio, F., Pellegrini, G., Ferrari, S., Di Nunzio, F., Di Iorio, E., Recchia, A., Maruggi, G., Ferrari, G., Provasi, E., Bonini, C., Capurro, S., Conti, A., Magnoni, C., Giannetti, A., & De Luca, M. (2006). Correction of junctional epidermolysis bullosa by transplantation of genetically modified epidermal stem cells. Nature medicine, 12(12), 1397–1402. https://doi.org/10.1038/nm1504

54. Miyoshi H. (2004). Gene delivery to hematopoietic stem cells using lentiviral vectors. Methods in molecular biology (Clifton, N.J.), 246, 429–438. https://doi.org/10.1385/1-59259-650-9:429

55. Morgan, M. A., Galla, M., Grez, M., Fehse, B., & Schambach, A. (2021). Retroviral gene therapy in Germany with a view on previous experience and future perspectives. Gene therapy, 28(9), 494–512. https://doi.org/10.1038/s41434-021-00237-x

56. Naldini, L., Blömer, U., Gallay, P., Ory, D., Mulligan, R., Gage, F. H., Verma, I. M., & Trono, D. (1996). In vivo gene delivery and stable transduction of nondividing cells by a lentiviral vector. Science (New York, N.Y.), 272(5259), 263–267. https://doi.org/10.1126/science.272.5259.263

57. Nathwani, A. C., Persons, D. A., Stevenson, S. C., Frare, P., McClelland, A., Nienhuis, A. W., & Vanin, E. F. (1999). Adenovirus-

mediated expresssion of the murine ecotropic receptor facilitates transduction of human hematopoietic cells with an ecotropic retroviral vector. Gene therapy, 6(8), 1456–1468. https://doi.org/10.1038/sj.gt.3300974

58. Noguchi, M., Yi, H., Rosenblatt, H. M., Filipovich, A. H., Adelstein, S., Modi, W. S., McBride, O. W., & Leonard, W. J. (1993). Interleukin-2 receptor gamma chain mutation results in X-linked severe combined immunodeficiency in humans. Cell, 73(1), 147–157. https://doi.org/10.1016/0092-8674(93)90167-o
59. Oldfield, E. H., Ram, Z., Culver, K. W., Blaese, R. M., DeVroom, H. L., & Anderson, W. F. (1993). Gene therapy for the treatment of brain tumors using intra-tumoral transduction with the thymidine kinase gene and intravenous ganciclovir. Human gene therapy, 4(1), 39–69. https://doi.org/10.1089/hum.1993.4.1-39
60. Otto, E., Jones-Trower, A., Vanin, E. F., Stambaugh, K., Mueller, S. N., Anderson, W. F., & McGarrity, G. J. (1994). Characterization of a replication-competent retrovirus resulting from recombination of packaging and vector sequences. Human gene therapy, 5(5), 567–575. https://doi.org/10.1089/hum.1994.5.5-567
61. Paddison, P. J., Silva, J. M., Conklin, D. S., Schlabach, M., Li, M., Aruleba, S., Balija, V., O'Shaughnessy, A., Gnoj, L., Scobie, K., Chang, K., Westbrook, T., Cleary, M., Sachidanandam, R., McCombie, W. R., Elledge, S. J., & Hannon, G. J. (2004). A resource for large-scale RNA-interference-based screens in mammals. Nature, 428(6981), 427–431. https://doi.org/10.1038/nature02370
62. Pastorino, S., Massazza, S., Cilli, M., Varesio, L., & Bosco, M. C. (2001). Generation of high-titer retroviral vector-producing macrophages as vehicles for in vivo gene transfer. Gene therapy, 8(6), 431–441. https://doi.org/10.1038/sj.gt.3301405
63. Perdoni C, Osborn MJ, Tolar J. Gene editing toward the use of autologous therapies in recessive dystrophic epidermolysis bullosa. Transl Res. 2016 Feb;168:50-58. doi: 10.1016/j.trsl.2015.05.008. Epub 2015 May 27. PMID: 26073463; PMCID: PMC4662628.
64. Perez, O. D., Logg, C. R., Hiraoka, K., Diago, O., Burnett, R., Inagaki, A., Jolson, D., Amundson, K., Buckley, T., Lohse, D., Lin, A., Burrascano, C., Ibanez, C., Kasahara, N., Gruber, H. E., & Jolly, D. J. (2012). Design and selection of Toca 511 for clinical use: modified retroviral replicating vector with improved stability and gene expression. Molecular therapy : the journal of the American Society of Gene Therapy, 20(9), 1689–1698. https://doi.org/10.1038/mt.2012.83

65. Pizzato, M., Merten, O. W., Blair, E. D., & Takeuchi, Y. (2001). Development of a suspension packaging cell line for production of high titre, serum-resistant murine leukemia virus vectors. Gene therapy, 8(10), 737–745. https://doi.org/10.1038/sj.gt.3301457
66. Platt, F. M., d'Azzo, A., Davidson, B. L., Neufeld, E. F., & Tifft, C. J. (2018). Lysosomal storage diseases. Nature reviews. Disease primers, 4(1), 27. https://doi.org/10.1038/s41572-018-0025-4
67. Rebel, V. I., Tanaka, M., Lee, J. S., Hartnett, S., Pulsipher, M., Nathan, D. G., Mulligan, R. C., & Sieff, C. A. (1999). One-day ex vivo culture allows effective gene transfer into human nonobese diabetic/severe combined immune-deficient repopulating cells using high-titer vesicular stomatitis virus G protein pseudotyped retrovirus. Blood, 93(7), 2217–2224.
68. Roe T, Reynolds TC, Yu G, Brown PO. (1993) Integration of murine leukemia virus DNA depends on mitosis. EMBO Journal 12(5): 2099–2108.
69. Rosenberg, S. A., Aebersold, P., Cornetta, K., Kasid, A., Morgan, R. A., Moen, R., Karson, E. M., Lotze, M. T., Yang, J. C., & Topalian, S. L. (1990). Gene transfer into humans--immunotherapy of patients with advanced melanoma, using tumor-infiltrating lymphocytes modified by retroviral gene transduction. The New England journal of medicine, 323(9), 570–578. https://doi.org/10.1056/NEJM199008303230904
70. Ruben S, Perkins A, Purcell R, Joung K, Sia R, Burghoff R, et al. (1989) Structural and functional characterization of human immunodeficiency virus tat protein. Journal of Virology 63(1): 1–8.
71. Sauer, A. V., Di Lorenzo, B., Carriglio, N., & Aiuti, A. (2014). Progress in gene therapy for primary immunodeficiencies using lentiviral vectors. Current opinion in allergy and clinical immunology, 14(6), 527–534. https://doi.org/10.1097/ACI.0000000000000114
72. Seissler, T., Marquet, R., & Paillart, J. C. (2017). Hijacking of the Ubiquitin/Proteasome Pathway by the HIV Auxiliary Proteins. Viruses, 9(11), 322. https://doi.org/10.3390/v9110322
73. Selten, G., Cuypers, H. T., Zijlstra, M., Melief, C., & Berns, A. (1984). Involvement of c-myc in MuLV-induced T cell lymphomas in mice: frequency and mechanisms of activation. The EMBO journal, 3(13), 3215–3222. https://doi.org/10.1002/j.1460-2075.1984.tb02281.x

74. Shimotohno K, Temin HM. (1981) Formation of infectious progeny virus after insertion of herpes simplex thymidine kinase gene into DNA of an avian retrovirus. Cell 26(1 Pt 1): 67–77.
75. Shin, S., & Steffen, D. L. (1993). Frequent activation of the lck gene by promoter insertion and aberrant splicing in murine leukemia virus-induced rat lymphomas. Oncogene, 8(1), 141–149.
76. Temin H. M. (1976). The DNA provirus hypothesis. Science (New York, N.Y.), 192(4244), 1075–1080. https://doi.org/10.1126/science.58444
77. Uckert, W., Becker, C., Gladow, M., Klein, D., Kammertoens, T., Pedersen, L., & Blankenstein, T. (2000). Efficient gene transfer into primary human CD8+ T lymphocytes by MuLV-10A1 retrovirus pseudotype. Human gene therapy, 11(7), 1005–1014. https://doi.org/10.1089/10430340050015310
78. Uckert, W., Willimsky, G., Pedersen, F. S., Blankenstein, T., & Pedersen, L. (1998). RNA levels of human retrovirus receptors Pit1 and Pit2 do not correlate with infectibility by three retroviral vector pseudotypes. Human gene therapy, 9(17), 2619–2627. https://doi.org/10.1089/hum.1998.9.17-2619
79. Varmus HE. (1982) Form and function of retroviral proviruses. Science 216(4548): 812–820.
80. Williams, D. A., Nienhuis, A. W., Hawley, R. G., & Smith, F. O. (2000). Gene Therapy 2000. Hematology. American Society of Hematology. Education Program, 376–393. https://doi.org/10.1182/asheducation-2000.1.376
81. Wysocki, P. J., Grabarczyk, P., & Mackiewicz, A. (2001). Recent developments in retroviral gene delivery systems. Expert opinion on biological therapy, 1(6), 911–913. https://doi.org/10.1517/14712598.1.6.911
82. Yam, P. Y., Yee, J. K., Ito, J. I., Sniecinski, I., Doroshow, J. H., Forman, S. J., & Zaia, J. A. (1998). Comparison of amphotropic and pseudotyped VSV-G retroviral transduction in human CD34+ peripheral blood progenitor cells from adult donors with HIV-1 infection or cancer. Experimental hematology, 26(10), 962–968.
83. Yamagishi, M., Ishida, T., Miyake, A., Cooper, D. A., Kelleher, A. D., Suzuki, K., … Watanabe, T. (2009). Retroviral delivery of promoter-targeted shRNA induces long-term silencing of HIV-1 transcription. Microbes and Infection, 11(4), 500–508. https://doi.org/10.1016/j.micinf.2009.01.002

84. Yee, J. K., Friedmann, T., & Burns, J. C. (1994). Generation of high-titer pseudotyped retroviral vectors with very broad host range. Methods in cell biology, 43 Pt A, 99–112. https://doi.org/10.1016/s0091-679x(08)60600-7
85. Yu, S. F., von Rüden, T., Kantoff, P. W., Garber, C., Seiberg, M., Rüther, U., Anderson, W. F., Wagner, E. F., & Gilboa, E. (1986). Self-inactivating retroviral vectors designed for transfer of whole genes into mammalian cells. Proceedings of the National Academy of Sciences of the United States of America, 83(10), 3194–3198. https://doi.org/10.1073/pnas.83.10.3194
86. Zhou, J., Ding, Y., Burnett, J.C. and Rossi, J. (2014). Retroviruses for Cancer Therapy. In Cancer Gene Therapy by Viral and Non-viral Vectors (eds M.K. Brenner and M.-C. Hung). https://doi.org/10.1002/9781118501665.ch2
87. Zufferey, R., Dull, T., Mandel, R. J., Bukovsky, A., Quiroz, D., Naldini, L., & Trono, D. (1998). Self-inactivating lentivirus vector for safe and efficient in vivo gene delivery. Journal of virology, 72(12), 9873–9880. https://doi.org/10.1128/JVI.72.12.9873-9880.1998

Author Biography

Dr. Berrak Kurt received her DVM (Doctor of Veterinary Medicine) degree from Ankara University Faculty of Veterinary Medicine in 2009. She completed her Ph.D. in Department of Biochemistry at the same faculty in 2024. Her doctoral thesis investigated the inhibition of MDM2/MDMX expression under radiofrequency exposure using the dual inhibitor RO-5963 in chronic lymphocytic leukemia. She has also led national projects about p53 modulation, dual inhibitors, and the biochemical and functional properties of royal jelly. Dr. Kurt has expertise in molecular and cellular techniques, including CRISPR-Cas9, flow cytometry, exosome biology, nanoparticle studies, gene delivery, and plasma-based therapies. Her research interests focus on cancer biology, gene regulation, exosome-based therapeutics, and gene delivery systems, with a particular emphasis on retroviral gene delivery.

PART II:

NONVIRAL DELIVERY SYSTEMS

CHAPTER 7

RECENT DEVELOPMENTS IN EXTRACELLULAR VESICLE-BASED NANOMEDICINES, HIGHLIGHTING TECHNOLOGICAL IMPROVEMENTS AND CLINICAL PROSPECTS

ZOI KARDASI[1,2],
EFSTATHIA TRIANTAFYLLOPOULOU[3,#],
NATASSA PIPPA[3], MARIA G. ROUBELAKIS[1,2],
MARIA GAZOULI[1]

[1]Department of Basic Medical Sciences, Laboratory of Biology, Medical School, National and Kapodistrian University of Athens, 11527 Athens, Greece
[2]Cell and Gene Therapy Laboratory, Centre of Basic Research, BRFAA, 11527, Athens, Greece.
[3]Section of Pharmaceutical Technology, Department of Pharmacy, School of Health Sciences, National and Kapodistrian University of Athens, Panepistimioupolis Zografou, 15771 Athens, Greece.
(#) equal contribution to this work

Abstract

Extracellular vesicles (EVs) are nanoscale, lipid-bilayered structures secreted by nearly all cell types into the extracellular environment. They are classified into various subtypes, including microvesicles/ectosomes, apoptotic bodies, and exosomes. EVs are key players in cellular communication, impacting interactions between cells, tissues, and organs, both in health and disease. This emerging multidisciplinary field of EV research is reflected in the growing body of literature, with over 45,000 publications in the past two decades, according to the PubMed database. This chapter aims to highlight the recent progress in the application of EVs within the realm of nanomedicines. It will first delve into the physicochemical and biological properties of EVs, with a particular focus on the methods for isolating these vesicles and their role in enhancing characterization techniques. The concept of Critical Quality Attributes (CQAs) will be introduced, alongside the application of the Quality by Design (QbD) approach to the development of EV-based nanomedicines. Additionally, the chapter will cover the use of EVs in drug delivery and targeting, as well as their role in regenerative medicine and cell-free tissue engineering, illustrated by examples from recent research. The various applications of EVs in treating diverse diseases will be discussed, emphasizing their ability to improve the therapeutic index of encapsulated active pharmaceutical ingredients (APIs), minimize adverse drug reactions, enhance targeting, and enable early disease detection. One notable application of EVs is their involvement in cancer nanomedicine. EVs derived from tumor cells are known to influence the tumor microenvironment and promote cancer progression. Recent data from our laboratory, along with other studies, indicate that secretome and EVs derived from stromal cells have the potential to alleviate inflammation in human intestinal subepithelial myofibroblasts and promote regenerative effects in liver diseases. Furthermore, circulating EVs are already being explored as biomarkers and drug delivery vehicles in cardiovascular diseases. In conclusion, this chapter seeks to summarize the latest advancements in EV applications within nanomedicine, with a focus on their rapid clinical translation for the detection, prevention, and treatment of various diseases.

Keywords: Extracellular vesicles; Exosomes; Nanomedicine; Drug delivery; Regenerative medicine; Biomarkers; Clinical translation

Introduction

Extracellular vesicles (EVs) are nano to micro-sized membrane-bound vesicles, surrounded by a phospholipid bilayer that is actively secreted by almost all cell types in both normal or diseased conditions (Fais et al., 2016) and found in most body fluids (Du et al., 2023; Tong et al., 2025; Wu et al., 2021). They can be categorized into three major groups: micro-vesicles, apoptotic bodies and exosomes, primarily based on their biogenesis, secretion pathways, size, cargo, and function (Zaborowski et al., 2015). Initially, EVs were considered merely a means for cells to dispose of unnecessary materials, such as proteins or lipids; however, they are now acknowledged as essential mediators of intercellular communication, either in proximal or distant sites (Stavrou et al., 2022; Vader et al., 2016). EVs participate in intercellular communication by carrying biological information, such as proteins, lipids, nucleic acids and metabolites as internal cargo alongside surface-associated molecules that form or are integrated within the protein corona, from parent cells to recipient cells. The protein corona on EVs critically influences their function by affecting cell targeting, uptake, and stability. It carries bioactive molecules that contribute to therapeutic effects like immunomodulation and tissue repair. Altering the corona can significantly impact EV efficacy, making it a key factor in EV-based therapies (Wolf et al., 2022). Furthermore, EVs modulate various physiological processes, such as immune responses, tissue repair, neuronal communication, organ development, and reproduction (Wu et al., 2021; Yáñez-Mó et al., 2015), while also influencing pathological conditions, including cardiovascular diseases, neurodegeneration, cancer and inflammation (Gurung et al., 2021) in recipient cells (Du et al., 2023; Tong et al., 2025; Wang et al., 2020).

EVs have generated great potential for clinical application in nanomedicine, as a novel, alternative, cell-free strategy for disease diagnosis and therapy (Fais et al., 2016; Gurung et al., 2021). EVs are highly suitable for application as biomarkers, drug-delivery vehicles and mediators in a range of therapeutic approaches, including cancer, immunotherapy or regenerative medicine (Fais et al., 2016; Lener et al., 2015). The dual potential of EVs as diagnostic tools and therapeutic agents supports their use in the early detection of diseases, the monitoring of therapeutic responses, and the targeted delivery of therapeutic agents, due to their unique physiological and biochemical characteristics (Fais et al., 2016; Wu et al., 2021). Accumulating evidence have indicated that these vesicles have therapeutic effects on many diseases, such as cardiac repair, liver diseases, kidney diseases, wound healing, autoimmune and neurodegenerative disorders and diabetes. Due to their highly promising potential, EV research has now advanced to the clinical level for therapeutic applications in humans (Fan et al., 2022).

The persistent challenges in developing an optimal artificial drug delivery system have highlighted the necessity for exploring naturally derived approaches (Vader et al., 2016). EVs have been utilized as drug-delivery vehicle for therapeutic small-molecules because of its unique properties that allow them to survive in the extracellular space, bypass biological barriers, including the blood brain barrier (BBB), and deliver their biologically active molecular cargo (de Abreu et al., 2020; Haney et al., 2015; Kim et al., 2021; Klyachko et al., 2020; Vader et al., 2016). Similar to artificial nanocarriers, EVs can enhance the properties of a free drug, including its stability and solubility, and the protection of the drug against degradation (Klyachko et al., 2020). However, these natural nanocarriers provide significant benefits over conventional synthetic nanosystems with respect to drug delivery, including enhanced biocompatibility, high-stability, long systemic circulation time, low degradation rate, low systemic toxicity and immunogenicity, strong cargo preservation, pathogen capture characteristics and easy absorption by target cells (Fan et al., 2022; Haney et al., 2015; Kim et al., 2021). The therapeutic molecules contained within EVs, along with their associated protein corona, contributes synergistically to therapeutic outcomes, enhancing the overall efficacy of encapsulated agents (Klyachko et al., 2020). Moreover, EVs can be bioengineered to enhance their stability, bioactivity and targeting capacity for specific cell types and tissues (Abreu et al., 2020; Villata et al., 2020). Despite these advantages, EV isolation, characterization, low drug loading efficiency, functional heterogenicity and limited production yields represent difficulties that must be overcome for their future applications (Klyachko et al., 2020; Manno et al., 2025; Meng et al., 2020; Wu et al., 2021).

This book chapter aims to provide a comprehensive overview of the most recent breakthroughs in the application of extracellular vesicles (EVs) in nanomedicine, highlighting their accelerating clinical translation for the early detection, prevention, and treatment of a wide range of diseases, as well as the challenges it encounters.

Methods of literature review

An extensive literature review was performed in the electronic databases PubMed, Google Scholar, and Scopus for English-language peer-reviewed publications. The publications from the past fifteen years (2010–2025) served as a comprehensive guide for the systematic investigation of EVs. The chapter's research was focused on intrinsic properties, methods of isolation, characterization techniques, and their applications in drug delivery, targeting, regenerative medicines, and diagnostics. The authors performed the literature search, excluding the studies with full text unavailable, publication language other than English, and conference abstracts. After the screening of applications in the aforementioned electronic databases, 79 full-text studies were included in all the sections of the chapter.

Intrinsic properties of Extracellular vesicles (EVs)

Typically, EVs are categorized into three main types based on their size: exosomes (~30–200 nm), microvesicles (~200–1000 nm), and apoptotic bodies (~1–5 μm); however, ongoing research has identified, additional sub-populations, including exomeres (<50 nm) and large oncosomes (~1–10 μm) (Du et al., 2023; Y. Wang et al., 2020; Wu et al., 2021). The formation of these diverse EV sub-populations is influenced by various culture conditions, isolation methods, and purification protocols (Du et al., 2023). More specifically, apoptotic bodies represent membrane-bound vesicular structures generated during the late stages of apoptosis. These vesicles encapsulate fragmented DNA and other cellular components within a membrane. They produce specific signals, which actively recruit phagocytes to the site of cell death and mediate the efficient clearance of apoptotic cells, thereby maintaining tissue homeostasis and preventing inflammation.

Microvesicles are generated through a process involving the outward budding and subsequent fission of the plasma membrane, a tightly regulated process involving actin cytoskeletal remodeling and alterations in membrane lipid composition (Meng et al., 2020). In contrast, exosomes originate from the endocytic endosomal pathway, where the plasma membrane invaginates, leading to the internalization of extracellular and membrane-associated components that form early endosomes (Du et al., 2023). These early endosomes subsequently mature into multivesicular bodies (MVBs), within which intraluminal vesicles are generated through inward budding of the endosomal membrane, capturing cytosolic proteins, lipids, and RNAs destined for secretion.

Due to their biological origin, EVs have good histocompatibility and stability and have unique physiological regulatory functions. The proteins and their post-translational modifications of EVs indicate their localization, cellular origin and mechanism of secretion. These vesicles are isolated and characterized based on various techniques, including differential centrifugation, density gradient ultracentrifugation, immunocapture, ultrafiltration, polymer precipitation, size-exclusion chromatography, and membrane affinity chromatography (Fan et al., 2022; Yáñez-Mó et al., 2015). Due to the minimal differences in biophysical properties and molecular cargo among extracellular vesicle sub-populations, accurate post-release discrimination and classification of these remains technically challenging (Yáñez-Mó et al., 2015). In nanomedicine exosomes and microvesicles are most commonly used, because of their smaller size (Fan et al., 2022).

To exert their biological functions, EVs, must bind to and be recognized by their recipient cells. This selective binding and accumulation in specific tissues or organs, suggests that EVs have targeting capabilities towards certain cell types (Wu et al., 2021). Such interactions not only foster communication between cells but also play crucial role in guiding the EVs to their targeted cells (Kumar et al., 2024). Notably, the regulation of the molecular mechanisms governing the targeting of EVs to specific cells, along with the subsequent fate of EVs upon attachment to the cell surface, plays a vital role in modulating the biological responses of recipient cells (Wu et al., 2021). It is well-established that EVs exhibit intrinsic targeting capabilities, suggesting that EVs from different cell sources possess different targeting characteristics (Murphy et al., 2019; Vader et al., 2016). Even when EVs are derived from the same cell type, variations in their properties can occur, influenced by factors such as the developmental stage of the cells of origin, their function, and the extent of cellular activation or stimulation (Prada et al., 2016).

The interaction between EVs and their target cells involves intricate regulatory mechanisms, including the recognition, receptor-mediated binding, cellular internalization, and subsequent intracellular trafficking of EVs (Kumar et al., 2024). The targeting mechanism of EVs is mediated by receptors and ligands present on their surface, which exhibit a natural affinity for receptors that are abundantly expressed on the surface of the target cells (Song et al., 2022).

Among these receptors-ligand molecules are tetraspanin proteins, integrins, immunoglobulins, and proteoglycans (Yáñez-Mó et al., 2015). The process of cellular uptake can occur through multiple mechanisms, such as protein interactions, direct membrane fusion and endocytosis (Dang et al., 2020; Y. Wang et al., 2020; Wu et al., 2021). Factors that influence the targeting specificity of EVs include their protein and lipid composition as well as glycan composition and negative charge (Murphy et al., 2019). Additionally, the composition of the phospholipid bilayer of EVs, which consists of phosphatidylserine, cholesterol and sphingolipids, plays a significant role in EV targeting. Furthermore, EVs exhibit a preference for targeting cells histogenetically close to them; tumor cells preferentially interact with homologous tumor cells, Schwann cells target peripheral nerve tissue, and microglia are directed towards cells within the central nervous system. Moreover, the acidic microenvironment characteristic of injured tissue enhances the targeting efficiency of EVs, as the lower pH facilitates interactions between EV surface components and specific receptors on the target cells.

Targeting by specific adhesion molecules determines EV biodistribution (Yáñez-Mó et al., 2015). For the effective therapeutic application of EVs, a thorough understanding of their biodistribution and tissue-specific targeting upon exogenous administration is imperative, as these factors critically influence both their therapeutic efficacy and safety profiles (Murphy et al., 2019; Vader et al., 2016). Research indicated that EVs tend to accumulate primarily in organs such as liver, spleen, lungs and gastrointestinal tract of mice, which could be advantageous for targeted therapies (Murphy et al., 2019).

For instance, a biodistribution study of EVs derived from red blood cells demonstrated a preferential uptake by the liver (44.9%), bone (22.5%), skin (9.7%), muscle (5.8%), spleen (3.4%), kidney (2.7%), and lungs (1.8%). In contrast, EVs derived from melanoma cells predominantly localized to the lungs and spleen (Yáñez-Mó et al., 2015). The significant accumulation of EVs in the brain has not been observed under normal physiological conditions; however, this distribution may be altered during ischemic stroke (Murphy et al., 2019). The biodistribution of EVs is likely influenced by various factors such as the origin of the parent cell, the EV dose, route of administration, and the presence of various target cell types capable of internalizing circulating EVs (Vader et al., 2016; Yáñez-Mó et al., 2015). Studies comparing intraperitoneal (i.p.), subcutaneous (s.c.), and intravenous (i.v.) injections revealed that certain routes (i.p. and s.c). led to lower accumulation in the liver and spleen, while enhancing EV presence in the pancreas and gastrointestinal tract. Notably, higher doses of EV may reduce liver accumulation, potentially due to saturation of the mononuclear phagocyte system (MPS), which may limit the ability of the liver to further uptake EVs at elevated concentrations (Vader et al., 2016).

Multiple independent studies have shown that the half-life of purified exogenous EVs, when systemically administered into circulation, is notably short, as they are swiftly recognized and internalized by the MPS, particularly within the liver and spleen. However, one study revealed that human platelet concentrate-derived EVs remained in the circulation with a half-life of 5.5 hours. While EVs may resist complement-mediated lysis due to the presence of glycosylphosphatidylinositol-anchored CD55 and CD59, their clearance from circulation is predominantly attributed to their retention and subsequent uptake by target organs (Yáñez-Mó et al., 2015). Bioengineering approaches such as attaching polyethylene glycol to the surface of EVs, can significantly extend their circulation time, and promote targeted accumulation in sites of interest, like tumors or inflamed tissues (Vader et al., 2016).

Critical Quality Attributes and characterization techniques of EVs

Methods of isolation

Given the intrinsic properties of extracellular vesicles (EVs), this section discusses their key characteristics that are fundamental to their application in nanomedicine and precision medicine. Firstly, the methods of their isolation are presented briefly. Several methods for the isolation of EVs have appeared in the literature. Each technique exhibits several advantages and limitations, taking into account the simplicity, cost, time, and scalability. Ultracentrifugation (differential and density gradient) is high-speed sequential centrifugation to remove cells and debris. It is the most frequently used technique due to its simplicity and low cost. On the other hand, to the high-speed forces, EV damage is observed. The low purity of EVs is another limitation of this method. Schematic representation of the centrifugation-based protocol is visualized in Figure 1-1. A higher degree of purity can be achieved by density gradient ultracentrifugation, but it is a time-consuming method needing high expertise. Immunoaffinity isolation is a technique with high specification, using antibodies targeting EV surface markers, but its usage is limited due to the limited salability and high cost. Commercial kits and/or polyethylene glycol (PEG) are used for the EVs isolation by precipitation-based techniques, which are fast and easy, but further purification is required due to the presence of lipoproteins and other contaminants. Filtration-based methods are also fast, but sometimes damage to EVs is observed. Recently, microfluidics also appeared in literature as a promising methodology for the preparation of EVs in low volumes with high precision in their physicochemical characteristics. Namely, according to Mousavi et al. (2022), the microfluidic devices provide ameliorated detection and monitoring of EVs due to increased efficiency in sieving, trapping, and immunological separation of low volumes (Mousavi et al., 2022). A novel microfluidic device has developed fast filtration of exosomes from small volumes of patient plasma with double filtration for isolation of purified exosomes (Ramnauth et al., 2023). Comparisons of EV enrichment, separation, and purification methods are summarized in Table 1-1.

Characterization techniques

The physicochemical and biological characteristics of the EVs are of paramount importance for their applications, safety, effectiveness, route of administration, and stability both in biological media and storage. According to the ICH Q8 guideline for the design and development of pharmaceutical products, these characteristics are named Critical Quality Attributes (CQAs). In this section of the chapter, the CQAs of EVs are presented, along with the analytical techniques employed for their evaluation and monitoring. The size and the size distribution of the EVs are of the most important physicochemical characteristics of all the nanoparticles, including EVs, because they can influence the absorption, metabolism, distribution, excretion, and toxicology (ADMET) profile of the encapsulated active pharmaceutical ingredients (APIs) and, consequently, their pharmacokinetics. They can be evaluated by dynamic light scattering (DLS) and nanoparticle tracking analysis (NTA).

Most of the published data about EVs include the above techniques for the characterization of the mean size and size distribution of the EVs (Peng et al., 2022). Their size ranges between 30nm and 1000 nm, expressed in diameter (Saludas et al., 2021). It should be noted that slight variations in the size and size distribution of EVs may be observed for the same sample when using the aforementioned techniques. These differences arise due to the underlying physical principles of each method. The route of administration of EVs is strongly dependent on the size of the EVs, meaning that i.v. administration can be achieved for those EVs with sizes below 100nm. The zeta potential and the surface charge are also crucial CQAs of EVs, affecting the interaction with plasma proteins and the colloidal and storage stability. The interaction with plasma proteins can influence the clearance of EVs, and for this reason, the zeta potential and surface charge are important physical properties. The zeta potential can be evaluated by electrophoretic light scattering (ELS). The morphological characterization usually is done by imaging techniques including SEM, TEM, and cryo-TEM (Jayasinghe et al., 2022; Peng et al., 2022). The shape can be identified by these techniques, and other characteristics such as the lamellarity, membrane thickness, membrane curvature, size, and size distribution can also be evaluated. Surface functionalization is strongly associated with specific targeting to cells, tissues, and organs. Jayasinghe et al. (2022) functionalized EVs with an enzyme. They incubated the EVs in a solution containing the enzyme, followed by incubation in a streptavidin solution. The streptavidin was used to prevent cross-linking of biotin probes between EVs (Jayasinghe et al., 2022).

The presence of dyes, antibodies, lipids, proteins, glycoproteins, and/or peptides is responsible for specific functionalization and targeting strategies. The surface functionalization is also referred to in the literature as the surface marker profile (Pham et al., 2021; Mondal et al., 2023). Several techniques are used for the identification of markers: mass spectroscopy, flow cytometry, and Western blot (Jayasinghe et al., 2022; Pham et al., 2021).

Colloidal stability is synonymous with the physicochemical stability over time in storage conditions. The maintenance of the above CQAs during time is crucial to the effectiveness of EVs as pharmaceutical dosage forms. The temperature, pH, light, oxidative stress and other environmental factors can influence the stability of EVs and lead to aggregation and sedimentation phenomena causing also problems in clinical use. Furthermore, the leakage of the encapsulated API can also take place during instability phenomena. The concentration of EVs also should be determined and is considered as CQAs. The concentration of EVs strongly affects their dose. The concentration can be quantified by flow cytometry and/or enzyme-linked immunosorbent assays (ELISA) (Tang et al., 2023). Purity and endotoxin levels are also crucial for their effectiveness in preclinical and clinical applications. EVs should be free of contaminants, in order to avoid adverse effects and immunogenicity (Jayasinghe et al., 2022; Pham et al., 2021). The endoxins and pyrogens are synonymous with bacterial contamination and should be quantified according to the requirements of the route of administration.

Last but not least, the encapsulation and loading efficiency are CQAs, which are strongly related to the therapeutic index of the EV-based platform. Several APIs can be encapsulated, such as small pharmaceuticals, proteins and/or peptides, and nucleic acids (DNA, RNA, siRNA, etc.) (Mondal et al., 2023; Saludas et al., 2021). Exogenous and endogenous loading are the main techniques for the encapsulation of APIs into EVs. Exogenous loading includes the co-incubation, chemical transfection, electroporation, and sonication techniques, while endogenous cell engineering and co-incubation of small pharmaceuticals (Tang et al., 2020). It should be noted that chemical transfections are widely used for the loading of nucleic acids/genetic material in EVs. All the other techniques are used for loading small molecular weight therapeutic agents or proteins or nucleic acids. Each technique exhibited several advantages and limitations that are visualized in Figure 1-2.

According to the recent literature, the fast clinical translation of EV-based therapeutic approaches is strongly dependent on the imaging techniques, especially for the diseases of the CNS. With Magnetic Resonance Imaging (MRI) and combined PET/CT, the medical doctors can diagnose the diseases, monitor the pharmacokinetics of the EVs, and help precision medicine. Additionally, the visualization of EVs in vivo can give information on their accumulation and targeting to specific tissues and organs. For this reason, labeling and radiolabeling are used for the MRI and nuclear imaging with EVs, respectively (Gao et al., 2021).

Summarizing all the above, it can be concluded that the controlling and monitoring of the CQAs of EVs is crucial and necessary to guarantee the Quality by Design (QbD) approach of engineering of EVs-based nanotherapeutics with added value for fast clinical translation with added value for the patients.

Regulatory perspectives

Regulatory agencies in the US and Europe are working to prepare the regulatory framework for the development and approval of EV-based medicinal products. Currently, the Food and Drug Administration (FDA) requires an Investigational New Drug (IND) and clinical trials. In Europe, the European Medicines Agency (EMA) categorized EVs under the Committee of Advanced Therapies (CAT), i.e., Advanced Therapy Medicinal Products (ATMP).

Namely, the EMA/CAT considers that the product composed of exosomes carrying recombinant mRNA encoding for the cystic fibrosis transmembrane conductance regulator protein and microRNA-17 falls within the definition of a gene therapy medicinal product. This medicinal product is a suspension for aerosol delivery via a nebulizer device for the treatment of cystic fibrosis.

The intended use and the therapeutic claim are of paramount importance to the categorization of EVs as biological, medicinal products, medical devices, and cosmeceutical/nutraceutical products. The uncertainty of their categorization is still under discussion in regulatory agencies. There is a scientific and regulatory debate about whether the EV-based products are biopharmaceuticals, advanced therapies, or medicinal products. Additionally, some EV-based products are medical devices because they are used for diagnostic purposes (Lee et al., 2024). The isolation and the production method are also crucial, because the medicinal products should be prepared under the guidelines and requirements of Good Manufacturing Practices (GMP). Furthermore, the scale-up of the production of EV-based products remains a technological challenge. The technology transfer from a laboratory to the industrial scale is mandatory for their fast clinical translation. There is also a lack of knowledge if there is batch-to-batch variability, which is observed very often in biological and nanomedicine products that are already marketed products in clinical use (Yadav et al., 2024). Quality control is another challenge that should be considered since the purity, contamination, and physicochemical/morphological characterization, as well as stability during storage and use, are not clear for large quantities and scales. Universal guidelines are not available for manufacturers in comparison to other medicinal products or medical devices, where ISO guidelines and regulations are widely used for design, development, and manufacturing stages.

Last but not least, for the completion of the technical dossier, the ADMET profile and pharmacokinetic data should be available. Immunogenicity and carcinogenicity should be clarified in preclinical studies, too. No data has been available for long-term toxicity until today (Lee et al., 2024). These aforementioned considerations are discussed in the FDA's last decade (i.e., the Public Safety Notification on Exosome Products available on December 6th, 2019).

Table 1-1. Comparison of EV Enrichment, Separation, and Purification Methods. [Adapted from (Tang et al., 2023)].

Isolation Methods	Working Principle	Advantage	Drawback
Ultracentrifugation	Based on the size of EVs. Large ones precipitate earlier, while small ones require greater centrifugal force to precipitate easily.	The most commonly used method; Less reagent consumption; EVs can be isolated from a large number of samples.	High equipment cost; Time-consuming; High speed centrifugation may damage EVs.
Density-gradient ultracentrifugation	Based on EV density	High purity; Good to maintain the activity of EVs.	Complexity; Time-consuming.
Co-precipitation	Polymer-based precipitators bind to hydrophobic proteins and lipid molecules for co-precipitation to separate EVs.	Easy and simple to handle; Low time requirement.	Low purity and recovery; More heteroprotein; Produces polymers that are difficult to remove.

Size-Exclusion Chromatography	Based on the size of EV molecules, a porous gel matrix causes separation.	High purity	Needs special equipment; Time-consuming and laborious.
Ultrafiltration	Relative division using different interceptions; a sub-mass ultrafiltration membrane is used for selective separation of samples.	Simple and efficient; No sample size limitation; Does not affect EVs' biological activity.	Low yields; protein contamination; deformation of vesicles
Immunoaffinity Enrichment	EV surface-specific marker, coated with corresponding antibody; EVs can be isolated by incubating the magnetic beads with EVs.	Simple operation; Does not affect EVs' morphological integrity; High specificity.	Low efficiency; Not suitable for large quantities; Antibodies are expensive.
Field-flow fractionation	Macromolecules flow through flat channels, applying force fields perpendicular to the sample flow to achieve separation based on different sizes and molecular weights.	Broad separation range; Wide variety of eluents.	Lengthy duration; Requires fractionation equipment.

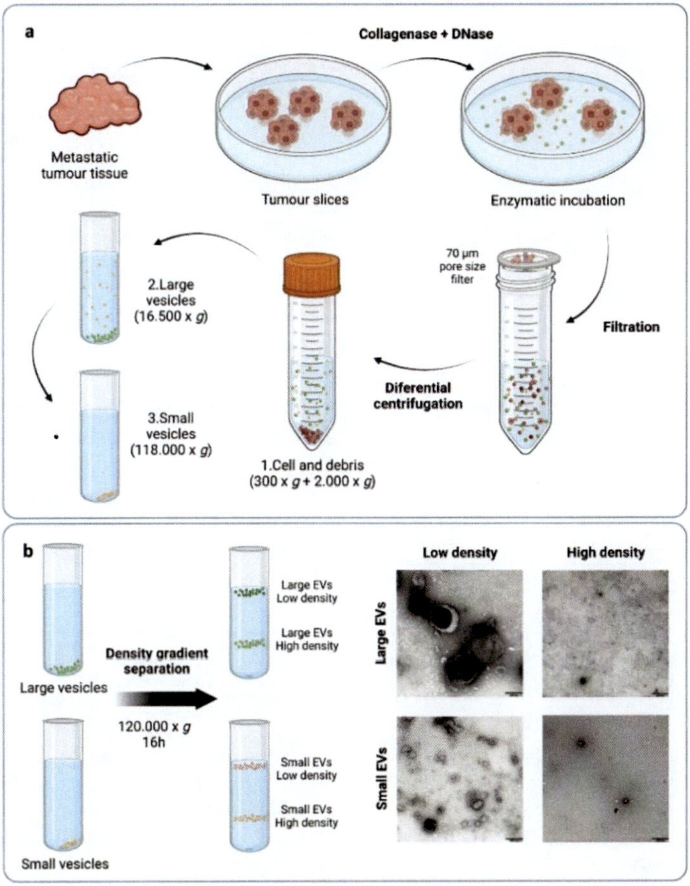

Figure 1-1. Schematic overview of the centrifugation-based protocol used to isolate vesicles from metastatic melanoma tissues, and posterior vesicle isolation through a density gradient separation. a. The tumour tissues were dissected into smaller pieces that were incubated in cell culture media containing collagenase D and DNase I for 30 min allowing the tissue EVs to be released into the media. EVs were isolated from the media by differential centrifugation resulting in two subpopulations of EVs (large EVs (16,500 × g_{avg} pellet) and small EVs (118,000 × g_{avg} pellet)). b. Isolated large and small EVs were bottom loaded on an iodixanol gradient (45–20%). From both populations of vesicles, two fractions were visible after the separation, with one fraction containing high density EVs (1.16–19 g/cm^3) and one containing low density EVs (1.11–1.12 g/cm^3). Ten micrograms of low and high density vesicles from both large and small EVs were loaded onto grids, negative stained and evaluated by transmission electron microscopy. Scale bars are 200 nm [Adapted from (Gonzalez-Melero et al., 2023)].

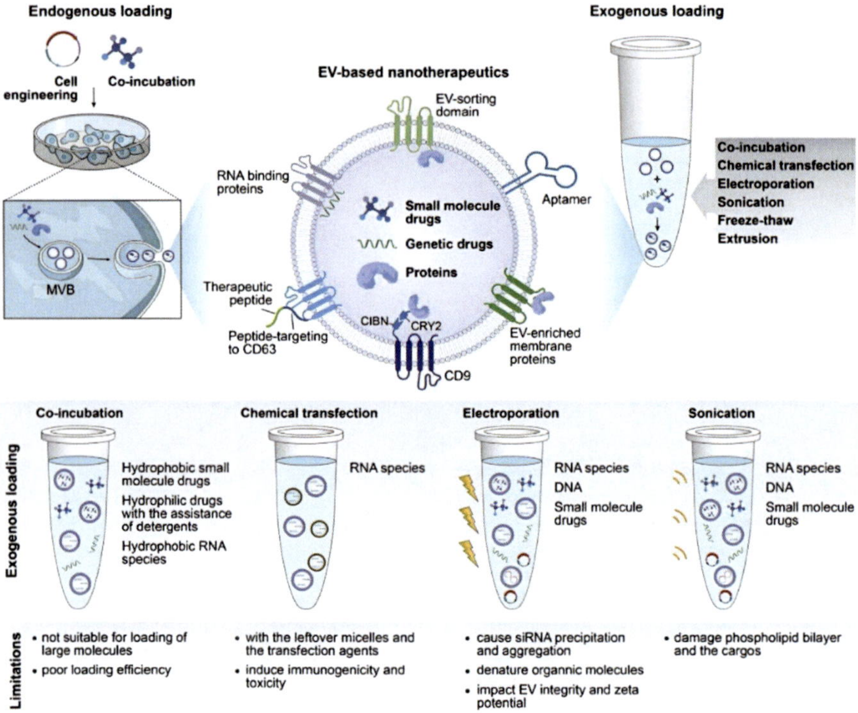

Figure 1-2. Illustration of cargo-loading techniques to produce EV-based nanotherapeutics. Cargo-loading can be carried out either endogenously (pre-loading parental cells with the cargo followed by inducing EV production) or exogenously (directly loading the EVs after their production and isolation) [Adapted from (Tang et al., 2020)].

Applications of EVs in Nanomedicine

Drug delivery and targeting

It is well known that EVs have potency in vivo due to their composition. However, they could be ideal as drug delivery systems as well. Their biocompatibility, their size and capacity are characteristics that favor their usage as drug or gene delivery carriers. In this manner, their payload could be either small molecules, such as Active Pharmaceutical Ingredients (APIs) or macromolecules such as proteins, peptides, or nucleic acids (Mondal et al., 2023)

Considering their applications as drug delivery systems, they could be useful in the treatment of several diseases including cardiovascular ones. Chi and colleagues (2023) selected empagliflozin, which is an antidiabetic API, for the recovery after myocardial infarction. They demonstrated the synergistic effect of the drug with EVs mediated from mesenchymal stem cells in the repair of the cardiac function. Utilizing TEM, NTA, and western blot analysis, they characterize the loaded and unloaded EVs showing similar morphology and size. In vitro and in vivo assays advocated the superiority of loaded EVs in cardiac recovery ameliorating the cell viability and multiplication (Chi et al., 2023). Dapagliflozin loaded nanoparticles derived from human induced pluripotent stem cells (hiPSCs) after differentiation were fabricated via extrusion method. The spherical nanostructures had a particle size of 200 nm and a negative surface charge being promising candidates for wound repair of diabetic patients. SDS-PAGE and FTIR techniques confirmed the maintenance of the initial cellular proteins and the successful drug encapsulation respectively, which was indicated equal to 45%. Considering the API's in vitro release profile, it was demonstrated the stimuli-responsive release in the wound's microenvironment. More importantly, in vivo experiments exhibited significant wound repair in nine days (Figure 1-3) compared to unloaded nanoparticles or free dapagliflozin (Zhang et al., 2023).

Except for EVs that originate from human cells, they could be derived from bacteria as well. These outer membrane vesicles could be excellent candidates for pharmacotherapy. Such an example comes from Huang et al. (2020) that utilized such EVs from bacteria species, namely Acinetobacter baumannii for antibacterial treatment. They formed EVs loaded with antibiotics via adding a small dose of different types of antibiotic molecules into the culture medium of bacteria leading to intact EVs with different characteristics comprising of proteins that were differentially expressed. Their results indicate the importance of the preparation protocol and the utilized drug dose for good encapsulation efficiency as well as the EVs capability to protect their cargo under different environmental conditions. They also declared the ability for efficient antibacterial activity in vitro in different pathogenic species. Biocompatibility in low doses by oral administration enabled further experiments exhibiting effectiveness in vivo in lower dosage than the free drug (Huang et al., 2020).

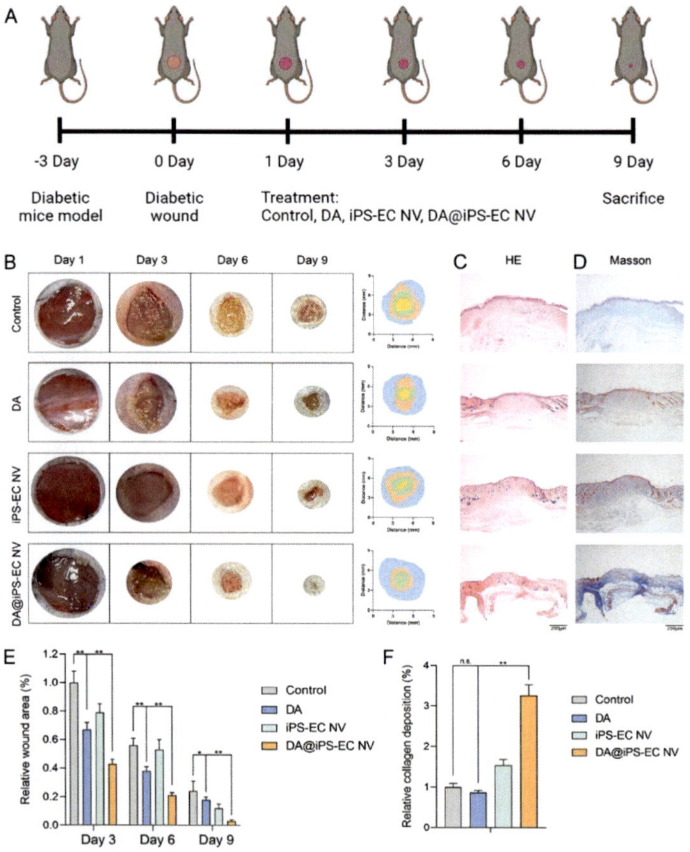

Figure 1-3. Exosome mimetics promote diabetic wound healing. A) Schematic diagram of the therapeutic strategy in vivo. B, E) The macroscopic images of wounds, wound closure traces, and the corresponding quantitative size of the wound area at different time points (**$p < 0.01$, *$p < 0.05$). C) The H&E images showed the formation of epidermis and dermis tissue in diabetic wounds. D, F) The Masson staining images showed the collagen deposition level of diabetic wounds (**$p < 0.01$, n.s.: no significance) [Adapted from (Zhang et al., 2023)].

Keeping in mind the necessity for innovative and effective treatment in the battle of cancer, there are several studies giving prominence to the value of EVs as drug delivery vectors in cancer treatment. Some examples are discussed below. EVs derived from milk encapsulating cis-platin were formed to defeat drug-resistant carcinoma. The loaded systems had a similar morphology, but a larger size compared to unloaded ones, whereas they were examined for their effectiveness in drug-resistant cancer cells in contrast to free drug. Even though encapsulation efficiency was only 18%, EVs permitted the efficient delivery of cis-platin avoiding endosomes due to the cell internalization via specific mechanism according to preclinical data (Figure 1-4) (Zhou et al., 2022).

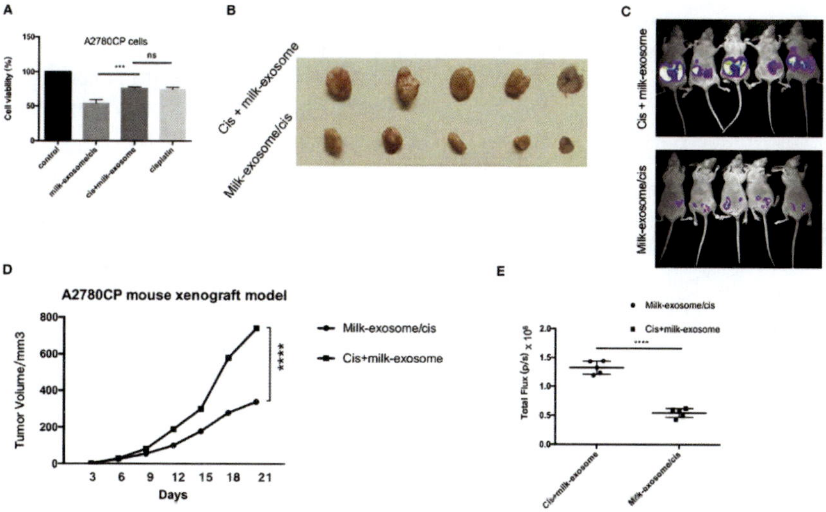

Figure 1-4. Effect of milk-exosome loaded cisplatin on cisplatin-resistant ovarian cancer in vitro and in vivo. A) The cisplatin-resistant ovarian cancer A2780CP cells were treated with cisplatin (5 μg/mL), milk-exosome/cis (5 μg exosomal cisplatin/mL), milk-exosome, and PBS. CCK8 assays were conducted after 24h. Three independent experiments with biological repeats. B) Milk-exosome/cis enhanced the anti-cancer effect in vivo. Nude mice were subcutaneously injected with A2780CP cells. Mixture of cisplatin (4 mg/kg b.wt.) with milk-exosomes, and milk-exosome/cis (4 mg exosomal cisplatin/kg b.wt.) were injected every 3 days. Gross appearance of the tumors. C) The size of the tumors was measured every 3 days. D) Milk-exosome/cis enhanced the anti-cancer effect in bioluminescent ovarian cancer model in vivo. E) Bioluminescent images were visualized and calculated. ****$P<0.0001$ and ***$P<0.001$, n.s.: no significance [Adapted from (Zhou et al., 2022)].

Active targeting via surface modifications is the selected strategy for several developments. Normal cell lines were modified to express iRGD peptide and KRAS siRNA in order EVs to be formed for gene delivery showing lung tumor selectivity. The functionalized EVs had an average size of 180 nm, while their capability for targeting cancer cells as well as gene silencing and thus limiting tumor growth was confirmed in vitro and in vivo (Zhou et al., 2019). Additionally, EVs coming from red blood cells were modified to be able to deliver peptides or nucleic acids in specific cancer cell lines. The authors highlighted the biocompatibility and short-term non-immunogenicity of the functionalized EVs by in vitro and in vivo protocols. Their innovation regards the utilization of in-house methods for altering successfully the surface of EVs by adding intact peptides and antibodies acting as ligands or respective ligands conjugated with therapeutic peptides. The loaded systems seem to have good targeting ability and efficient antitumor activity according to in vivo assays. Their results are promising for the formation of tailor-made EVs as targeting therapeutics (Jayasinghe et al., 2022).

Another interesting work involves the engineering of the EVs surface derived from fibroblastic cells of mice with a ligand for efficient brain targeting and the co-delivery of methotrexate and a functional peptide; in particular Lys-Leu-Ala (KLA). The ligand is a synthetic peptide that incorporated the therapeutic one, while the modifications and loading of EVs did not change much their physicochemical properties showing an average size approximately equal to 320 nm. In vitro, ex vivo, and in vivo models indicated effective and selective accumulation in brain tumor sites and a prolongation of the survival of mice compared to free drug or unmodified loaded EVs (Ye et al., 2018).

Exploiting the peculiar solid tumor microenvironment, Guo et al. (2021) formed a multifunctional drug delivery system comprised of EVs mediated from Gram negative bacteria, an anticancer drug, a PEGylated mannose as the ligand, and a nucleic acid. The ligand:EVs ratio was optimized at 1:5 for targeted uptake by macrophages, so that the expression of the siRNA to differentiate tumor's metabolism, while the drug was modified properly to be specifically released in the tumor pH area before the phagocytosis. The preclinical results highlighted the anticancer efficiency of the drug delivery system inhibiting tumor growth via multiple mechanisms (Guo et al., 2021). A multifunctional system was also proposed by Li et al. (2023) against breast cancer. In this case, the intrinsic immunogenic activity of the bacteria-based EVs was used for their encapsulation into macrophages enabling tumor targeting. Furthermore, doxorubicin and a compound with photothermal properties were incorporated into the system as well. The multifunctional therapeutics had a positive impact on tumor inhibition and could prevent potential metastatic incidents, whereas no toxicity issues arose in vivo (Li et al., 2023).

Considering hybrid EVs, there are a lot of works regarding their functionality as drug delivery systems. A typical example regards the formation of liposomes amalgamated with EVs for synergistic treatment against large metastatic tumors. The hybrid nanoparticles were prepared via freeze-thaw cycles having similar physicochemical characteristics to liposomes, and their hybrid nature was confirmed via several techniques including microscopic ones. The capability of liposomes to release their cargo in a temperature dependent manner was investigated as well. Synergistic therapy included hyperthermia and simultaneous intravenous delivery of hybrid EVs loaded with an anticancer API and membrane proteins useful in immunotherapy. Their preclinical results advocated targeted delivery in tumor sites and promising anticancer effect via multiple mechanisms (Lv et al., 2020).

Regenerative Medicine

In recent years, an increasing amount of evidence has highlighted EVs as promising carriers for drug and gene delivery within the realm of regenerative medicine. These vesicles possess an intrinsic capacity to modulate cellular functions (Lee et al., 2021; Moghassemi et al., 2024; Ramasubramanian et al., 2020) and are able to reduce inflammation, apoptosis, while promoting proliferation and angiogenesis, positioning them as a promising therapeutic option for tissue regeneration.

EVs from various cellular sources transfer tissue-specific remodeling molecules and mediate distinct metabolic pathways to promote repair and regeneration. Notably, EVs derived from stem or progenitor cells, particularly mesenchymal stromal cells (MSCs), have displayed exceptional efficacy in promoting regeneration (Moghassemi et al., 2024; Ramasubramanian et al., 2020; Lamichhane et al., 2015). For example, exosomes from placenta-derived MSCs exhibit neuroprotective and immunomodulatory effects, while those derived from bone marrow- MSCs contribute to bone regeneration. Furthermore, exosomes from endothelial progenitor cells deliver microRNAs that enhance angiogenesis, aiding in the vascularization of damaged tissue (Ramasubramanian et al., 2020). Furthermore, exosomes have been incorporated into scaffolds engineered for tissue regeneration applications, demonstrating the ability to modulate cellular responses such as proliferation, migration, and differentiation, resulting in enhanced tissue regeneration and restoration (Moghassemi et al., 2024). The application of EVs in regenerative medicine has been explored for the treatment of diseases affecting various organ systems and tissues, including cardiovascular system, respiratory system, nervous system, bone and cartilage, skin, liver and kidney (Table 1-2, Figure 1-4). Three molecular components within the cargo of EVs, derived from diverse progenitor cell types, have emerged as pivotal players in EV-mediated tissue repair and regeneration: proteins, mRNAs and miRNAs. EVs can deliver essential proteins directly or modulate their signaling pathways by regulating gene expression via mRNAs or miRNAs. Proteomic analyses of MSC-derived exosomes have revealed the presence of proteins implicated in angiogenesis, coagulation, apoptosis, inflammation, and extracellular matrix remodeling, contributing to the ultimate goal of tissue repair and regeneration. Regarding miRNAs (miR), numerous studies have proved their involvement in the regulation of cell proliferation, differentiation, and apoptosis during tissue regeneration (Figure 1-5).

For instance, miR-124 and miR-9/9* facilitate the direct reprogramming of fibroblasts into neuron-like cells by regulating the chromatin remodeling complex (Yoo et al., 2011), while miR-1 and miR-133a protect the myocardium from apoptosis, oxidative stress, and fibrosis, enhancing cardiac regeneration (Izarra et al., 2014). In a rat model of infarcted heart, the EVs derived from cardiac progenitor cells have shown the ability to decrease cardiomyocyte apoptosis and promote vascular remodeling, through the modulation of miRNA-target gene expression (miR-210, miR-132, and miR-146a-3p) (Moghiman et al., 2021).

Moreover, mRNAs act as crucial molecular messengers within EVs, significantly contributing to tissue regeneration. In a study involving a mouse model of acute renal ischemia, MSC-EVs, which promoted the proliferation of peritubular capillary endothelial cells were found to contain mRNAs of vascular endothelial growth factor (VEGF-A), basic fibroblast growth factor (bFGF), and insulin-like growth factor 1 (IGF-1) (Figliolini et al., 2020). The regenerative therapeutic effects of EVs are primarily mediated through their interactions with target cell surfaces and subsequent cargo transfer, activating a cascade of signaling pathways, such as MAPK, pAkt/mTOR, Wnt/b-catenin, PI3K/Akt, Notch, TGF- β/Smad, STAT, Erk1/2, CaMKII, Efna3 and Hedgehog signaling (Lee et al., 2021; Li et al., 2022). These critical signaling pathways modulate various physiological functions, including immune responses, inflammation reduction, apoptosis inhibition, angiogenesis promotion, and oxidative stress alleviation, ultimately improving disease-related complications and enhancing regenerative processes (Li et al., 2022). Among the aforementioned, the key focus areas in regenerative medicine are cell viability and apoptosis, angiogenesis and immunomodulation.

Table 1-2. Extracellular Vesicle in Regenerative medicine: Cellular Sources, Effective Components, and Therapeutic Applications in various organ systems and tissues.

Target tissue	Cellular Sources	Effective components	Therapeutic effect/Disease	Reference
Cardiovascular system	Human umbilical cord (hUC)-derived MSCs	Not investigated	Acute myocardial infarction	(Bian et al., 2014)
	Adipose-derived stromal cells	miR-93-5p	Acute myocardial Infarction	(Liu et al., 2018)
	Fibroblasts-derived Induced Pluripotent Stem Cells (iPSCs)	miR-145, let-7 family, miR-302a-5p, miR-19b, miR-20a, miR-126-3p, miR-130a-3p, miR-210-3p, miR-17-92, miR-290-295	Myocardial Infarction	(Adamiak et al., 2018)
	BM-derived MSCs	microRNA-210	Myocardial infarction	(Zhu et al., 2018)
	human Umbilical cord blood (hUCB)-derived Endothelial progenitor cells	Not investigated	Vascular injury	(Li et al., 2016)
	hUC-derived MSCs	miR-181a	Myocardial ischemia-reperfusion injury	(Wei et al., 2019)

Respiratory system	BM-derived MSCs	Not investigated	Acute lung injury	(Khatri et al., 2018)
	hUCB-derived MSCs	VEGF siRNA	Neonatal hyperoxic lung injury	(Ahn et al., 2018)
	hUC-derived MSCs	tumor necrosis factor α stimulated gene-6 (TSG-6)	Bronchopulmonary dysplasia	(Chaubey et al., 2018)
	hBM-derived MSCs	keratinocyte growth factor (KGF)	Severe Pneumonia	(Monsel et al., 2015)
Nervous system	BM-derived MSCs	miR-133b	Stroke (middle cerebral artery occlusion)	(Xin et al., 2012; Xin et al., 2013)
	Schwann Cells	p75-neurotrophin receptor, GTPase RhoA	Sciatic nerve injury	(Lopez-Verrilli et al., 2013)
	Human embryonic stem cells (H9 cell line)	TGF-β, Smad2, Smad4	Ischemic Stroke	(Xia et al., 2021)
	BM-derived MSCs	Not investigated	Traumatic brain injury	(Kim et al., 2016)
	BM-derived MSCs	miR-124	Traumatic brain Injury	(Yang et al., 2019)
	hUC-derived MSCs	NF-κb suppresion	Traumatic brain Injury	(Zhang et al., 2022)

Bone and Cartilage	BM-derived MSCs	miR-532–5p	Intervertebral disc degeneration	(Zhu et al., 2020)
	human Placental-derived MSCs	AntagomiR-4450, zinc finger protein-121 (ZNF121)	Intervertebral Disc Degeneration	(Yuan et al., 2020)
	MSCs differentiated from hiPSCs	Not investigated	Osteoporosis	(Qi et al., 2016)
Skin	human Urine-derived Stem cells	deleted in malignant brain tumors 1 (DMBT1)	Diabetes mellitus acute skin wounds	(Chen et al., 2018)
	hUC-derived MSCs	miR-150-5p	Skin wounds	(Xiu et al., 2022)
	hUC-derived MSCs	Wnt4	Skin wounds	(Zhang et al., 2015)
	BM-derived macrophages	C-C motif chemokine ligand 24 (CCL24), C-C motif chemokine ligand 22 (CCL22), and milk fat globule-epidermal growth factor factor 8 protein (MFG-E8)	Skin wounds	(Kim et al., 2019)

Liver	hUC-derived MSCs	Chaperonin containing TCP1 subunit 2 (CCT2)	Liver Ischemia/ Reperfusion Injury	(Zheng et al., 2020)
	BM-derived MSCs and fibroblasts	Not investigated	concanavalin A-induced Liver injury	(Tamura et al., 2016)
	BM-derived MSCs	Y-RNA-1 non-coding RNA	Lethal Hepatic Failure	(Haga et al., 2017)
Kidneys	MSCs differentiated from hiPSCs	Specificity protein (SP1)	Renal ischemia/ reperfusion injury	(Yuan et al., 2017)
	hUC-MSCs	Not investigated	Acute kidney injury	(Zhou et al., 2013)
	Adipose tissue–derived autologous MSCs	IL-10	Renal injury	(Eirin et al., 2017)

Cell proliferation and apoptosis

Given their ability to regulate cell proliferation and apoptosis EVs demonstrate promising therapeutic potential for regenerative medicine (Li et al., 2022). For instance, treatment with human umbilical cord MSC-derived microvesicles has been shown to inhibit cisplatin-induced apoptosis and enhance cell proliferation via the ERK 1/2 and MAPK pathways (Barile et al., 2014). Similarly, in an acute kidney injury model, bone marrow MSC-derived exosomes have demonstrated the ability to decrease apoptosis and increase induced proximal tubular epithelial cell proliferation, as a result of exosome-mediated RNA transfer (Tomasoni et al., 2013). Furthermore, umbilical cord MSC-derived exosomes enhanced the proliferation and migration of skin cells *in vitro* following heat stress, mediated by Wnt signaling through the delivery of Wnt4 (Zhang et al., 2015). Additionally, bone marrow-MSC exosomes effectively reduce neuronal cell apoptosis and inhibit the activation of A1 neurotoxic reactive astrocytes, which results in suppressing glial scar formation, alleviating inflammation, promoting axonal regeneration, and eventually improving functional behavioral recovery in spinal cord injury (SCI) rat model (Liu et al., 2019). Furthermore, exosomes from hypoxia-stimulated tubular epithelial cells activated fibroblasts via TGF-β1 signaling, leading to enhanced fibroblast proliferation and potentially contributing to accelerated tissue repair (Borges et al., 2013).

Angiogenesis

Effective vascularization is essential for engineering large tissues ensuring adequate nutrient and oxygen delivery, as well as waste removal. EV-induced angiogenesis is increasingly recognized as a key therapeutic mechanism in regenerative applications, with various types of EVs capable of promoting angiogenesis through multiple pathways, including the transfer of mRNAs, miRNAs, and proteins (De Jong et al., 2014; Li et al., 2022). Endothelial cell-derived EVs have been demonstrated to promote angiogenic activity in recipient endothelial cells by stimulating Notch-dependent tip-cell formation and initiating pro-angiogenic action, alongside miR-214-mediated inhibition of cellular senescence (van Balkom et al., 2013). MSC-derived exosomes can activate the signaling pathways AKT, ERK, and STAT3 during wound healing, and upregulate growth factors including HGF, NGF, IGF-1, and SDF-1. This promotes vascular endothelial cell proliferation and migration, facilitating neovascularization and ultimately enhancing skin repair (Shabbir et al., 2015).

Immunomodulation

While an excessive immune response may lead to tissue damage, encapsulation, or rejection of a tissue-engineered construct, controlled immune activation acts as a key regulator of regenerative processes such as cell recruitment, proliferation, and angiogenesis—critical factors for successful tissue engineering (De Jong et al., 2014). Numerous research groups have elucidated the immunomodulatory effects of EVs, exerting either immunosuppressive or immunostimulatory actions, depending on the specific bioactive molecules they carry and the pathological features of the diseases. Specific miRNAs, such as miR-142-3p and miR-126-3p (Reis et al., 2018), and certain enriched proteins in EVs, play key immunomodulatory roles, promoting dendritic cell maturation and anti-inflammatory effects, while miR-21a-5p and miR-223 reduce inflammatory factors and induce macrophage polarization towards the anti-inflammatory M2 phenotype (Lo Sicco et al., 2017). In a mouse model of acute lung injury EVs derived from human bone marrow-MSCs can effectively reduce the inflammation, by suppressing macrophage inflammatory protein-2 expression, a process potentially linked to the upregulation of keratinocyte growth factor (KGF)-mRNA at the injury site (Zhu et al., 2014). Moreover, MSC-EVs promoted the differentiation of monocytes into an M2-like phenotype in vitro, thereby inducing the reprogramming of activated $CD4^+$ T-cells into regulatory T-cells (Zhang et al., 2014). Exosomes derived from fetal liver MSCs facilitate the transfer of latency-associated peptides, TGF-β, and thrombospondin 1, thereby activating TGF-β/Smad2/3 signaling in natural killer (NK) cells. Additionally, these exosomes attenuate NK cell cytotoxicity in vitro, indicating their potential therapeutic application in autoimmune diseases (Fan et al., 2019).

Diagnostics

EVs have gained attention as promising tools for clinical diagnostics, biomarker identification, and the potential advancement of targeted therapies (Roy et al., 2018). The analysis of EVs in liquid biopsies has become a novel approach to better understand their involvement in various diseases (Sanz-Ros et al., 2023). EV-based diagnostics offer a practical alternative to conventional methods such as tissue biopsies or imaging, due to several noteworthy advantages (Jia et al., 2014).

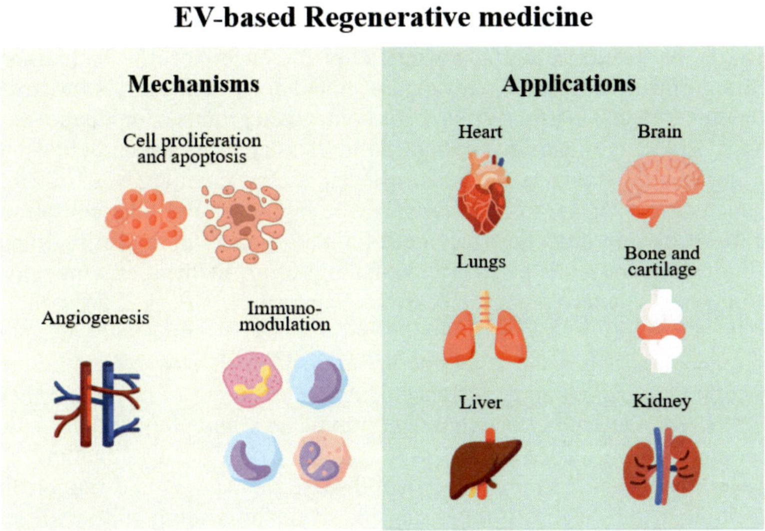

Figure 1-5. Mechanisms and therapeutic targets of extracellular vesicle-based regenerative medicine.

Most importantly, the release rate of EVs is significantly increased from diseased cells, coupled with distinct alterations in their molecular cargo that mirror the underlying pathological conditions. Notably, EVs are abundantly present in the bloodstream and other body fluids, enabling their collection through minimally invasive procedures (Jia et al., 2014; Kanninen et al., 2016; Sanz-Ros et al., 2023). This non-invasive accessibility supports their potential use in the early detection of various diseases. Moreover, the encapsulation of EV contents within a lipid bilayer confers protection against enzymatic degradation, offering a significant advantage over conventional specimens by preserving the integrity of potential biomarkers. Another significant advantage of EV-based diagnostics is attributed to their high structural stability, allowing prolonged sample storage before analysis and supporting longitudinal monitoring of therapeutic response (Jia et al., 2014; Kanninen et al., 2016). Equally important, the cellular origin of EVs can be identified through their surface marker profiles, providing valuable insight into the tissue of origin (Kanninen et al., 2016). Lastly, EVs may offer a more comprehensive reflection of the disease landscape than fine-needle biopsies, especially in the context of intra-tumoral heterogeneity. Their analysis also supports real-time evaluation and monitoring of treatment efficacy (Jia et al., 2014).

EV-based diagnostics is now predominantly focused on detecting and characterizing cancer-specific biomarkers (Sanz-Ros et al., 2023), directed towards the detection and characterization of cancer-specific biomarkers, with significant progress already demonstrated in the context of brain cancer (Kanninen et al., 2016). While EVs hold great promise for diagnostics, several challenges persist. Technical hurdles such as standardizing and scaling up the isolation methods, as well as the complexity of reliably characterizing EV cargo. Additionally, the high cost and time-consuming nature of current analytical techniques hinder their routine use in clinical settings. Patient-related factors, including prior medication, may also influence exosomal content and affect diagnostic accuracy. Furthermore, the heterogeneity of EV populations and the lack of universally accepted reference standards make result interpretation difficult. However, continued research and technological advancements are expected to overcome these barriers, enabling the effective integration of EVs into clinical diagnostics (Kanninen et al., 2016; Urabe et al., 2020). Consequently, ongoing EV research is expected to uncover novel disease biomarkers and support the development of diagnostic tools capable of distinguishing and stratifying disease subpopulations, ultimately facilitating personalized therapeutic strategies (Roy et al., 2018). Consequently, ongoing investigations into EVs are expected to unveil novel disease biomarkers and propel the development of diagnostic tools that can distinguish and stratify disease subpopulations. This, in turn, will pave the way for personalized therapeutic strategies, marking a significant advance in the field of medicine.

Biomarkers

EVs have recently gained attention as a novel form of liquid biopsy due to their ability to carry disease-specific molecules that accurately reflect the current pathological state of an individual (Mathew et al., 2020; Urabe et al., 2020). This capability makes them a promising source of biomarkers for minimally invasive disease assessment. The abundance and diverse molecular cargo of EVs—including proteins, miRNAs, mRNAs, long noncoding RNAs (lncRNAs), and lipids— have been extensively investigated as potential diagnostic indicators across a wide array of human pathologies (Bernardi et al., 2020; Kanninen et al., 2016; Urabe et al., 2020; Zamani et al., 2019). Circulating EVs have been consistently recognized for their stability and ease of isolation from a variety of body fluids, including plasma, serum, blood, saliva, urine, amniotic fluid, bronchoalveolar fluid, breast milk, and semen (Mathew et al., 2020; Urabe et al., 2020), and they can be dynamically monitored to reflect the physiological and pathological states of their parent cells (Bernardi et al., 2020; Ciferri et al., 2021). EVs have shown prognostic value in a wide range of clinical conditions, such as cancers, cardiovascular disorders, neurological and neurodegenerative diseases, as well as liver dysfunctions (Bernardi et al., 2020).

Cancer

In the realm of oncology, EVs isolated from patients with head and neck cancers have been shown to carry oncogenic miRNA molecules, tumor-derived DNA fragments and RNA molecules, as well as tumor-specific proteins (Mathew et al., 2020). Additionally, exosomal DNA contains the entire genome and reflects the mutational profile of parental tumor cells, highlighting its translational potential as a circulating biomarker for the early detection of cancer and metastasis (Thakur et al., 2014). For instance, serum EV-associated miR-19a-3p has been identified as a potential prognostic biomarker for predicting colorectal cancer (Matsumura et al., 2015), while elevated levels of miR-1290 and miR-375 in EVs have been correlated with decreased survival rate in advanced prostate cancer (Huang et al., 2015). Furthermore, miR-21 and the long noncoding RNA activated by transforming growth factor β, detected in serum-derived extracellular vesicles, have emerged as potential prognostic biomarkers for hepatocellular carcinoma (Lee et al., 2019). Proteomic analyses have identified glypican-1, a specific marker enriched in cancer derived EVs, through studies involving breast cancer cells, fibroblasts, and non-tumorigenic cells (Sadovska et al., 2015). Comparative analyses have shown that EVs derived from cancer stem cells are enriched in angiogenesis-related mRNAs (e.g., VEGF, FGF, MMP-2/9) and exhibit distinct miRNA molecules, targeting pathways related to proliferation, transcription, adhesion, and metabolism. Specifically, $CD105^+$ MVs are enriched with miRNAs associated with renal carcinomas and tumor progression, including miR-29c, miR-19b, miR-151, miR-92, miR-141, miR-200c, and miR-650 (Nawaz et al., 2014).

Cardiovascular system

Flow Cytometry studies have revealed correlations between a population of endothelial-derived microparticles and disease activity, glomerulonephritis, and vascular dysfunction. This suggests that the endothelial microparticle phenotype holds significant potential as a specific biomarker for vascular pathology in systemic lupus erythematosus (SLE) (Nielsen et al., 2011), with an observed increase in endothelial microparticles during active SLE compared to controls (Parker et al., 2014). Elevated levels of miR-26a in exosomes from lupus nephritis (LN) patients have been observed, showing a positive correlation with urinary protein levels, indicating its potential as a predictive biomarker of podocyte injury. Likewise, reduced levels of miR-29c in LN patients have been reported compared to healthy controls (Ichii et al., 2014). Following myocardial injury, cardiomyocyte-derived exosomes enriched with cardiac-specific miRNAs, such as miR-1 and miR-133a, lead to elevated circulating levels observed in patients with acute coronary syndromes and myocardial infarction, with particularly increased serum miR-133a in unstable angina pectoris, supporting its potential as a biomarker for cardiovascular diseases (Kuwabara et al., 2011). Additionally, exosomal p53-responsive microRNAs, including miR-34a, miR-192, and miR-194 were found to be significantly elevated in patients who developed heart failure (HF) following acute myocardial infarction (AMI), indicating that these miRNAs may serve as predictive biomarkers for ischemic HF post-AMI (Matsumoto et al., 2013).

Nervous system

Since direct access to diseased brain tissue is rarely possible, EV from neural and non-neural cells are seen as potential carriers of clinical and biological information in central nervous system disorders. EV markers such as $CD62E^+$ for extracranial and $CD31^+/CD42b^-$ for intracranial stenosis have been identified in stroke and stroke mimics, enabling improved estimation of stroke timing and clinical severity (Jung et al., 2009). Notably, proteomic enrichment analysis of urinary EVs associated with neurological disorders has revealed the presence of proteins such as DJ-1, ApoE, Syntaxin-7, tyrosine-protein kinases (Yes, Lyn, FRK, and HCK), proteasome subunit alpha type-7, all seven isoforms of 14–3-3 proteins, casein kinase I, and a diverse set of Rab proteins (Wang et al., 2019). In another study, a highly accurate diagnostic approach for traumatic brain injury (TBI) was developed by isolating GluR2-positive brain-derived EVs from plasma. By employing RNA sequencing combined with machine learning, researchers identified a panel of seven miRNAs (miR-129-5p, miR-212-5p, miR-9-5p, miR-152-5p, miR-21, miR-374b-5p, and miR-664-3p) capable of distinguishing TBI cases from healthy controls (Ko et al., 2018).

Liver

In hepatology, elevated levels of hepatocyte-derived EVs have been observed in both pre-cirrhotic and cirrhotic NASH patients compared to healthy controls, with asialoglycoprotein receptor 1 (ASGPR1) and long-chain fatty acid transport protein 5 (FATP-5) employed as specific markers for hepatocyte-derived EVs (Povero et al., 2020). Also, high levels of EV-associated $ASGPR1^{+}$ and $CD34^{+}$ also serve as markers of non-response to corticosteroid therapy in severe alcoholic hepatitis (Sukriti et al., 2018). Another study showed reduced $ASGR2^{+}$ and cytochrome P450 2E1 ($CYP2E1^{+}$) EVs after bariatric surgery in NAFLD patients (Nakao et al., 2021). Furthermore, plasma concentrations of EVs and EV-associated cytokeratin-18 fragments (M30 and M65) are reliable non-invasive biomarkers for alcoholic hepatitis (Bissonnette et al., 2017), while plasma EV concentration and EV-associated sphingolipid content correlate with the severity and mortality of alcoholic steatohepatitis (Sehrawat et al., 2021). Patients with cirrhosis exhibit elevated levels of endothelial-derived extracellular vesicles ($CD31^{+}/41^{-}$, $CD31^{+}/42b^{-}$, or CD62e) compared to healthy individuals, which positions them as potential biomarkers for cirrhosis (Rautou et al., 2012).

In summary, the potential of EVs as biomarkers across various clinical domains is increasingly recognized, paving the way for innovative diagnostic and therapeutic approaches in the management of diverse diseases.

Conclusions and future perspectives

Extracellular vesicles constitute a promising scientific field in biomedicine and drug development. This chapter presents the properties of the EVs, their preparation methods, as well as their critical quality attributes and characterization methods. An extensive literature review was performed for their applications in drug delivery and regenerative medicine. EVs can encapsulate a wide range of APIs, including anticancer ones and nucleic acids and peptides for gene therapy and targeting, respectively. They have recently gained attention as a novel form of liquid biopsy due to their ability to carry disease-specific active ingredients that accurately reflect the current pathological state of an individual. Several publications showed that EVs can be used as biomarkers in several diseases, especially in cancer and liver diseases. EVs are potential candidates for diagnostic kits, nanomedicines, and cell-free alternatives to stem cells, as the great number of publications worldwide reveal. On the other hand, the need for standardized protocols for their isolation, characterization, and scale-up are the main challenges that the scientific community, in collaboration with regulatory agencies, should overcome. The added value of their use in clinical practice is the driving force for the design and development of EV-based medicines without adverse drug reactions and with a high therapeutic index.

References

Adamiak, M., Cheng, G., Bobis-Wozowicz, S., Zhao, L., Kedracka-Krok, S., Samanta, A., Karnas, E., Xuan, Y.-T., Skupien-Rabian, B., Chen, X., Jankowska, U., Girgis, M., Sekula, M., Davani, A., Lasota, S., Vincent, R. J., Sarna, M., Newell, K. L., Wang, O.-L., … Zuba-Surma, E. K. (2018). Induced Pluripotent Stem Cell (iPSC)–Derived Extracellular Vesicles Are Safer and More Effective for Cardiac Repair Than iPSCs. *Circulation Research*, *122*(2), 296–309. https://doi.org/10.1161/CIRCRESAHA.117.311769

Ahn, S. Y., Park, W. S., Kim, Y. E., Sung, D. K., Sung, S. I., Ahn, J. Y., & Chang, Y. S. (2018). Vascular endothelial growth factor mediates the therapeutic efficacy of mesenchymal stem cell-derived extracellular vesicles against neonatal hyperoxic lung injury. *Experimental & Molecular Medicine*, *50*(4), 1–12. https://doi.org/10.1038/s12276-018-0055-8

Barile, L., Lionetti, V., Cervio, E., Matteucci, M., Gherghiceanu, M., Popescu, L. M., Torre, T., Siclari, F., Moccetti, T., & Vassalli, G. (2014). Extracellular vesicles from human cardiac progenitor cells inhibit cardiomyocyte apoptosis and improve cardiac function after myocardial infarction. *Cardiovascular Research*, *103*(4), 530–541. https://doi.org/10.1093/cvr/cvu167

Bernardi, S., & Balbi, C. (2020). Extracellular Vesicles: From Biomarkers to Therapeutic Tools. *Biology*, *9*(9), 258. https://doi.org/10.3390/biology9090258

Bian, S., Zhang, L., Duan, L., Wang, X., Min, Y., & Yu, H. (2014). Extracellular vesicles derived from human bone marrow mesenchymal stem cells promote angiogenesis in a rat myocardial infarction model. *Journal of Molecular Medicine*, *92*(4), 387–397. https://doi.org/10.1007/s00109-013-1110-5

Bissonnette, J., Altamirano, J., Devue, C., Roux, O., Payancé, A., Lebrec, D., Bedossa, P., Valla, D., Durand, F., Ait-Oufella, H., Sancho-Bru, P., Caballeria, J., Ginès, P., Boulanger, C. M., Bataller, R., & Rautou, P. (2017). A prospective study of the utility of plasma biomarkers to diagnose alcoholic hepatitis. *Hepatology*, *66*(2), 555–563. https://doi.org/10.1002/hep.29080

Borges, F. T., Melo, S. A., Özdemir, B. C., Kato, N., Revuelta, I., Miller, C. A., Gattone, V. H. I., LeBleu, V. S., & Kalluri, R. (2013). TGF-β1–Containing Exosomes from Injured Epithelial Cells Activate Fibroblasts to Initiate Tissue Regenerative Responses and Fibrosis. *Journal of the American Society of Nephrology*, *24*(3), 385.

https://doi.org/10.1681/ASN.2012101031

Chaubey, S., Thueson, S., Ponnalagu, D., Alam, M. A., Gheorghe, C. P., Aghai, Z., Singh, H., & Bhandari, V. (2018). Early gestational mesenchymal stem cell secretome attenuates experimental bronchopulmonary dysplasia in part via exosome-associated factor TSG-6. *Stem Cell Research & Therapy*, *9*(1), 173. https://doi.org/10.1186/s13287-018-0903-4

Chen, C.-Y., Rao, S.-S., Ren, L., Hu, X.-K., Tan, Y.-J., Hu, Y., Luo, J., Liu, Y.-W., Yin, H., Huang, J., Cao, J., Wang, Z.-X., Liu, Z.-Z., Liu, H.-M., Tang, S.-Y., Xu, R., & Xie, H. (2018). Exosomal DMBT1 from human urine-derived stem cells facilitates diabetic wound repair by promoting angiogenesis. *Theranostics*, *8*(6), 1607–1623. https://doi.org/10.7150/thno.22958

Chi, B., Zou, A., Mao, L., Cai, D., Xiao, T., Wang, Y., Wang, Q., Ji, Y., & Sun, L. (2023). Empagliflozin-Pretreated Mesenchymal Stem Cell-Derived Small Extracellular Vesicles Attenuated Heart Injury. *Oxidative Medicine and Cellular Longevity*, *2023*, 1–17. https://doi.org/10.1155/2023/7747727

Ciferri, M. C., Quarto, R., & Tasso, R. (2021). Extracellular Vesicles as Biomarkers and Therapeutic Tools: From Pre-Clinical to Clinical Applications. *Biology*, *10*(5), 359. https://doi.org/10.3390/biology10050359

Dang, X. T. T., Kavishka, J. M., Zhang, D. X., Pirisinu, M., & Le, M. T. N. (2020). Extracellular Vesicles as an Efficient and Versatile System for Drug Delivery. *Cells*, *9*(10), 2191. https://doi.org/10.3390/cells9102191

de Abreu, R. C., Fernandes, H., da Costa Martins, P. A., Sahoo, S., Emanueli, C., & Ferreira, L. (2020). Native and bioengineered extracellular vesicles for cardiovascular therapeutics. *Nature Reviews Cardiology*, *17*(11), 685–697. https://doi.org/10.1038/s41569-020-0389-5

De Jong, O. G., Van Balkom, B. W. M., Schiffelers, R. M., Bouten, C. V. C., & Verhaar, M. C. (2014). Extracellular Vesicles: Potential Roles in Regenerative Medicine. *Frontiers in Immunology*, *5*. https://doi.org/10.3389/fimmu.2014.00608

Du, S., Guan, Y., Xie, A., Yan, Z., Gao, S., Li, W., Rao, L., Chen, X., & Chen, T. (2023). Extracellular vesicles: A rising star for therapeutics and drug delivery. *Journal of Nanobiotechnology*, *21*(1), 231. https://doi.org/10.1186/s12951-023-01973-5

Eirin, A., Zhu, X.-Y., Puranik, A. S., Tang, H., McGurren, K. A., van Wijnen, A. J., Lerman, A., & Lerman, L. O. (2017). Mesenchymal stem cell–derived extracellular vesicles attenuate kidney inflammation. *Kidney International*, *92*(1), 114–124. https://doi.org/10.1016/j.kint.2016.12.023

Fais, S., O'Driscoll, L., Borras, F. E., Buzas, E., Camussi, G., Cappello, F., Carvalho, J., Cordeiro da Silva, A., Del Portillo, H., El Andaloussi, S., Ficko Trček, T., Furlan, R., Hendrix, A., Gursel, I., Kralj-Iglic, V., Kaeffer, B., Kosanovic, M., Lekka, M. E., Lipps, G., … Giebel, B. (2016). Evidence-Based Clinical Use of Nanoscale Extracellular Vesicles in Nanomedicine. *ACS Nano*, *10*(4), 3886–3899. https://doi.org/10.1021/acsnano.5b08015

Fan, Y., Herr, F., Vernochet, A., Mennesson, B., Oberlin, E., & Durrbach, A. (2019). Human Fetal Liver Mesenchymal Stem Cell-Derived Exosomes Impair Natural Killer Cell Function. *Stem Cells and Development*, *28*(1), 44–55. https://doi.org/10.1089/scd.2018.0015

Fan, Z., Jiang, C., Wang, Y., Wang, K., Marsh, J., Zhang, D., Chen, X., & Nie, L. (2022). Engineered extracellular vesicles as intelligent nanosystems for next-generation nanomedicine. *Nanoscale Horizons*, *7*(7), 682–714. https://doi.org/10.1039/D2NH00070A

Figliolini, F., Ranghino, A., Grange, C., Cedrino, M., Tapparo, M., Cavallari, C., Rossi, A., Togliatto, G., Femminò, S., Gugliuzza, M. V., Camussi, G., & Brizzi, M. F. (2020). Extracellular Vesicles From Adipose Stem Cells Prevent Muscle Damage and Inflammation in a Mouse Model of Hind Limb Ischemia. *Arteriosclerosis, Thrombosis, and Vascular Biology*, *40*(1), 239–254. https://doi.org/10.1161/ATVBAHA.119.313506

Gao, Y., Chu, C., Jablonska, A., Bulte, J. W. M., Walczak, P., & Janowski, M. (2021). Imaging as a tool to accelerate the translation of extracellular vesicle-based therapies for central nervous system diseases. *WIREs Nanomedicine and Nanobiotechnology*, *13*(3), e1688. https://doi.org/10.1002/wnan.1688

Gonzalez-Melero, L., Hernandez, R. M., Santos-Vizcaino, E., & Igartua, M. (2023). Tumour-derived extracellular vesicle based vaccines for melanoma treatment. *Drug Delivery and Translational Research*, *13*(5), 1520–1542. https://doi.org/10.1007/s13346-023-01328-5

Guo, Q., Li, X., Zhou, W., Chu, Y., Chen, Q., Zhang, Y., Li, C., Chen, H., Liu, P., Zhao, Z., Wang, Y., Zhou, Z., Luo, Y., Li, C., You, H., Song, H., Su, B., Zhang, T., Sun, T., & Jiang, C. (2021). Sequentially Triggered Bacterial Outer Membrane Vesicles for Macrophage Metabolism Modulation and Tumor Metastasis Suppression. *ACS Nano*, *15*(8), 13826–13838. https://doi.org/10.1021/acsnano.1c05613

Gurung, S., Perocheau, D., Touramanidou, L., & Baruteau, J. (2021). The exosome journey: From biogenesis to uptake and intracellular signalling. *Cell Communication and Signaling*, *19*(1), 47. https://doi.org/10.1186/s12964-021-00730-1

Haga, H., Yan, I. K., Takahashi, K., Matsuda, A., & Patel, T. (2017). Extracellular Vesicles from Bone Marrow-Derived Mesenchymal Stem Cells Improve Survival from Lethal Hepatic Failure in Mice. *Stem Cells Translational Medicine*, *6*(4), 1262–1272. https://doi.org/10.1002/sctm.16-0226

Haney, M. J., Klyachko, N. L., Zhao, Y., Gupta, R., Plotnikova, E. G., He, Z., Patel, T., Piroyan, A., Sokolsky, M., Kabanov, A. V., & Batrakova, E. V. (2015). Exosomes as drug delivery vehicles for Parkinson's disease therapy. *Journal of Controlled Release*, *207*, 18–30. https://doi.org/10.1016/j.jconrel.2015.03.033

Hingert, D., Ekström, K., Aldridge, J., Crescitelli, R., & Brisby, H. (2020). Extracellular vesicles from human mesenchymal stem cells expedite chondrogenesis in 3D human degenerative disc cell cultures. *Stem Cell Research & Therapy*, *11*(1), 323. https://doi.org/10.1186/s13287-020-01832-2

Huang, W., Zhang, Q., Li, W., Yuan, M., Zhou, J., Hua, L., Chen, Y., Ye, C., & Ma, Y. (2020). Development of novel nanoantibiotics using an outer membrane vesicle-based drug efflux mechanism. *Journal of Controlled Release*, *317*, 1–22. https://doi.org/10.1016/j.jconrel.2019.11.017

Huang, X., Yuan, T., Liang, M., Du, M., Xia, S., Dittmar, R., Wang, D., See, W., Costello, B. A., Quevedo, F., Tan, W., Nandy, D., Bevan, G. H., Longenbach, S., Sun, Z., Lu, Y., Wang, T., Thibodeau, S. N., Boardman, L., … Wang, L. (2015). Exosomal miR-1290 and miR-375 as prognostic markers in castration-resistant prostate cancer. *European Urology*, *67*(1), 33–41. https://doi.org/10.1016/j.eururo.2014.07.035

Ichii, O., Otsuka-Kanazawa, S., Horino, T., Kimura, J., Nakamura, T., Matsumoto, M., Toi, M., & Kon, Y. (2014). Decreased miR-26a expression correlates with the progression of podocyte injury in autoimmune glomerulonephritis. *PloS One*, *9*(10), e110383. https://doi.org/10.1371/journal.pone.0110383

Izarra, A., Moscoso, I., Levent, E., Cañón, S., Cerrada, I., Díez-Juan, A., Blanca, V., Núñez-Gil, I.-J., Valiente, I., Ruíz-Sauri, A., Sepúlveda, P., Tiburcy, M., Zimmermann, W.-H., & Bernad, A. (2014). miR-133a Enhances the Protective Capacity of Cardiac Progenitors Cells after Myocardial Infarction. *Stem Cell Reports*, *3*(6), 1029–1042. https://doi.org/10.1016/j.stemcr.2014.10.010

Jayasinghe, M. K., Pirisinu, M., Yang, Y., Peng, B., Pham, T. T., Lee, C. Y., Tan, M., Vu, L. T., Dang, X. T., Pham, T. C., Chen, H., Leung, A. Y. H., Cho, W. C., Shi, J., & Le, M. T. (2022). Surface-engineered extracellular vesicles for targeted delivery of therapeutic RNAs and peptides for cancer therapy. *Theranostics*, *12*(7), 3288–3315. https://doi.org/10.7150/thno.68667

Jia, S., Zocco, D., Samuels, M. L., Chou, M. F., Chammas, R., Skog, J., Zarovni, N., Momen-Heravi, F., & Kuo, W. P. (2014). Emerging technologies in extracellular vesicle-based molecular diagnostics. *Expert Review of Molecular Diagnostics*, *14*(3), 307–321. https://doi.org/10.1586/14737159.2014.893828

Jung, K.-H., Chu, K., Lee, S.-T., Park, H.-K., Bahn, J.-J., Kim, D.-H., Kim, J.-H., Kim, M., Kun Lee, S., & Roh, J.-K. (2009). Circulating endothelial microparticles as a marker of cerebrovascular disease. *Annals of Neurology*, *66*(2), 191–199. https://doi.org/10.1002/ana.21681

Kanninen, K. M., Bister, N., Koistinaho, J., & Malm, T. (2016). Exosomes as new diagnostic tools in CNS diseases. *Biochimica et Biophysica Acta (BBA) - Molecular Basis of Disease*, *1862*(3), 403–410. https://doi.org/10.1016/j.bbadis.2015.09.020

Khatri, M., Richardson, L. A., & Meulia, T. (2018). Mesenchymal stem cell-derived extracellular vesicles attenuate influenza virus-induced acute lung injury in a pig model. *Stem Cell Research & Therapy*, *9*(1), 17. https://doi.org/10.1186/s13287-018-0774-8

Kim, D., Nishida, H., An, S. Y., Shetty, A. K., Bartosh, T. J., & Prockop, D. J. (2016). Chromatographically isolated $CD63^{+}CD81^{+}$ extracellular vesicles from mesenchymal stromal cells rescue cognitive impairments after TBI. *Proceedings of the National Academy of Sciences*, *113*(1), 170–175. https://doi.org/10.1073/pnas.1522297113

Kim, H., Wang, S. Y., Kwak, G., Yang, Y., Kwon, I. C., & Kim, S. H. (2019). Exosome-Guided Phenotypic Switch of M1 to M2 Macrophages for Cutaneous Wound Healing. *Advanced Science*, *6*(20), 1900513. https://doi.org/10.1002/advs.201900513

Kim, J.-K., Youn, Y.-J., Lee, Y.-B., Kim, S.-H., Song, D.-K., Shin, M., Jin, H. K., Bae, J., Shrestha, S., & Hong, C.-W. (2021). Extracellular vesicles from dHL-60 cells as delivery vehicles for diverse therapeutics. *Scientific Reports*, *11*(1), 8289. https://doi.org/10.1038/s41598-021-87891-8

Klyachko, N. L., Arzt, C. J., Li, S. M., Gololobova, O. A., & Batrakova, E. V. (2020). Extracellular Vesicle-Based Therapeutics: Preclinical and Clinical Investigations. *Pharmaceutics*, *12*(12), 1171.

https://doi.org/10.3390/pharmaceutics12121171

Ko, J., Hemphill, M., Yang, Z., Sewell, E., Na, Y. J., Sandsmark, D. K., Haber, M., Fisher, S. A., Torre, E. A., Svane, K. C., Omelchenko, A., Firestein, B. L., Diaz-Arrastia, R., Kim, J., Meaney, D. F., & Issadore, D. (2018). Diagnosis of traumatic brain injury using miRNA signatures in nanomagnetically isolated brain-derived extracellular vesicles. *Lab on a Chip*, *18*(23), 3617–3630. https://doi.org/10.1039/c8lc00672e

Kumar, M. A., Baba, S. K., Sadida, H. Q., Marzooqi, S. A., Jerobin, J., Altemani, F. H., Algehainy, N., Alanazi, M. A., Abou-Samra, A.-B., Kumar, R., Al-Shabeeb Akil, A. S., Macha, M. A., Mir, R., & Bhat, A. A. (2024). Extracellular vesicles as tools and targets in therapy for diseases. *Signal Transduction and Targeted Therapy*, *9*(1), 1–41. https://doi.org/10.1038/s41392-024-01735-1

Kuwabara, Y., Ono, K., Horie, T., Nishi, H., Nagao, K., Kinoshita, M., Watanabe, S., Baba, O., Kojima, Y., Shizuta, S., Imai, M., Tamura, T., Kita, T., & Kimura, T. (2011). Increased MicroRNA-1 and MicroRNA-133a Levels in Serum of Patients With Cardiovascular Disease Indicate Myocardial Damage. *Circulation: Cardiovascular Genetics*, *4*(4), 446–454. https://doi.org/10.1161/CIRCGENETICS.110.958975

Lamichhane, T. N., Sokic, S., Schardt, J. S., Raiker, R. S., Lin, J. W., & Jay, S. M. (2015). Emerging Roles for Extracellular Vesicles in Tissue Engineering and Regenerative Medicine. *Tissue Engineering Part B: Reviews*, *21*(1), 45–54. https://doi.org/10.1089/ten.teb.2014.0300

Lee, J. Y., & Kim, H.-S. (2021). Extracellular Vesicles in Regenerative Medicine: Potentials and Challenges. *Tissue Engineering and Regenerative Medicine*, *18*(4), 479–484. https://doi.org/10.1007/s13770-021-00365-w

Lee, K. W. A., Chan, L. K. W., Hung, L. C., Phoebe, L. K. W., Park, Y., & Yi, K.-H. (2024). Clinical Applications of Exosomes: A Critical Review. *International Journal of Molecular Sciences*, *25*(14), 7794. https://doi.org/10.3390/ijms25147794

Lee, Y. R., Kim, G., Tak, W. Y., Jang, S. Y., Kweon, Y. O., Park, J. G., Lee, H. W., Han, Y. S., Chun, J. M., Park, S. Y., & Hur, K. (2019). Circulating exosomal noncoding RNAs as prognostic biomarkers in human hepatocellular carcinoma. *International Journal of Cancer*, *144*(6), 1444–1452. https://doi.org/10.1002/ijc.31931

Lener, T., Gimona, M., Aigner, L., Börger, V., Buzas, E., Camussi, G., Chaput, N., Chatterjee, D., Court, F. A., Portillo, H. A. del, O'Driscoll, L., Fais, S., Falcon-Perez, J. M., Felderhoff-Mueser, U., Fraile, L., Gho, Y. S., Görgens, A., Gupta, R. C., Hendrix, A., … Giebel, B. (2015).

Applying extracellular vesicles based therapeutics in clinical trials – an ISEV position paper. *Journal of Extracellular Vesicles*, *4*(1), 30087. https://doi.org/10.3402/jev.v4.30087

Li, M., Fang, F., Sun, M., Zhang, Y., Hu, M., & Zhang, J. (2022). Extracellular vesicles as bioactive nanotherapeutics: An emerging paradigm for regenerative medicine. *Theranostics*, *12*(11), 4879–4903. https://doi.org/10.7150/thno.72812

Li, X., Chen, C., Wei, L., Li, Q., Niu, X., Xu, Y., Wang, Y., & Zhao, J. (2016). Exosomes derived from endothelial progenitor cells attenuate vascular repair and accelerate reendothelialization by enhancing endothelial function. *Cytotherapy*, *18*(2), 253–262. https://doi.org/10.1016/j.jcyt.2015.11.009

Li, Y., Wu, J., Qiu, X., Dong, S., He, J., Liu, J., Xu, W., Huang, S., Hu, X., & Xiang, D.-X. (2023). Bacterial outer membrane vesicles-based therapeutic platform eradicates triple-negative breast tumor by combinational photodynamic/chemo-/immunotherapy. *Bioactive Materials*, *20*, 548–560. https://doi.org/10.1016/j.bioactmat.2022.05.037

Liu, J., Jiang, M., Deng, S., Lu, J., Huang, H., Zhang, Y., Gong, P., Shen, X., Ruan, H., Jin, M., & Wang, H. (2018). miR-93-5p-Containing Exosomes Treatment Attenuates Acute Myocardial Infarction-Induced Myocardial Damage. *Molecular Therapy Nucleic Acids*, *11*, 103–115. https://doi.org/10.1016/j.omtn.2018.01.010

Liu, W., Wang, Y., Gong, F., Rong, Y., Luo, Y., Tang, P., Zhou, Z., Zhou, Z., Xu, T., Jiang, T., Yang, S., Yin, G., Chen, J., Fan, J., & Cai, W. (2019). Exosomes Derived from Bone Mesenchymal Stem Cells Repair Traumatic Spinal Cord Injury by Suppressing the Activation of A1 Neurotoxic Reactive Astrocytes. *Journal of Neurotrauma*, *36*(3), 469–484. https://doi.org/10.1089/neu.2018.5835

Liu, X., Li, Q., Niu, X., Hu, B., Chen, S., Song, W., Ding, J., Zhang, C., & Wang, Y. (2017). Exosomes Secreted from Human-Induced Pluripotent Stem Cell-Derived Mesenchymal Stem Cells Prevent Osteonecrosis of the Femoral Head by Promoting Angiogenesis. *International Journal of Biological Sciences*, *13*(2), 232–244. https://doi.org/10.7150/ijbs.16951

Lo Sicco, C., Reverberi, D., Balbi, C., Ulivi, V., Principi, E., Pascucci, L., Becherini, P., Bosco, M. C., Varesio, L., Franzin, C., Pozzobon, M., Cancedda, R., & Tasso, R. (2017). Mesenchymal Stem Cell-Derived Extracellular Vesicles as Mediators of Anti-Inflammatory Effects: Endorsement of Macrophage Polarization. *Stem Cells Translational Medicine*, *6*(3), 1018–1028. https://doi.org/10.1002/sctm.16-0363

Lopez-Verrilli, M. A., Picou, F., & Court, F. A. (2013). Schwann cell-derived exosomes enhance axonal regeneration in the peripheral nervous system. *Glia*, *61*(11), 1795–1806. https://doi.org/10.1002/glia.22558

Lu, K., Li, H., Yang, K., Wu, J., Cai, X., Zhou, Y., & Li, C. (2017). Exosomes as potential alternatives to stem cell therapy for intervertebral disc degeneration: In-vitro study on exosomes in interaction of nucleus pulposus cells and bone marrow mesenchymal stem cells. *Stem Cell Research & Therapy*, *8*(1), 108. https://doi.org/10.1186/s13287-017-0563-9

Lv, Q., Cheng, L., Lu, Y., Zhang, X., Wang, Y., Deng, J., Zhou, J., Liu, B., & Liu, J. (2020). Thermosensitive Exosome–Liposome Hybrid Nanoparticle-Mediated Chemoimmunotherapy for Improved Treatment of Metastatic Peritoneal Cancer. *Advanced Science*, *7*(18), 2000515. https://doi.org/10.1002/advs.202000515

Manno, M., Bongiovanni, A., Margolis, L., Bergese, P., & Arosio, P. (2025). The physico-chemical landscape of extracellular vesicles. *Nature Reviews Bioengineering*, *3*(1), 68–82. https://doi.org/10.1038/s44222-024-00255-5

Mathew, M., Zade, M., Mezghani, N., Patel, R., Wang, Y., & Momen-Heravi, F. (2020). Extracellular Vesicles as Biomarkers in Cancer Immunotherapy. *Cancers*, *12*(10), 2825. https://doi.org/10.3390/cancers12102825

Matsumoto, S., Sakata, Y., Suna, S., Nakatani, D., Usami, M., Hara, M., Kitamura, T., Hamasaki, T., Nanto, S., Kawahara, Y., & Komuro, I. (2013). Circulating p53-Responsive MicroRNAs Are Predictive Indicators of Heart Failure After Acute Myocardial Infarction. *Circulation Research*, *113*(3), 322–326. https://doi.org/10.1161/CIRCRESAHA.113.301209

Matsumura, T., Sugimachi, K., Iinuma, H., Takahashi, Y., Kurashige, J., Sawada, G., Ueda, M., Uchi, R., Ueo, H., Takano, Y., Shinden, Y., Eguchi, H., Yamamoto, H., Doki, Y., Mori, M., Ochiya, T., & Mimori, K. (2015). Exosomal microRNA in serum is a novel biomarker of recurrence in human colorectal cancer. *British Journal of Cancer*, *113*(2), 275–281. https://doi.org/10.1038/bjc.2015.201

Meng, W., He, C., Hao, Y., Wang, L., Li, L., & Zhu, G. (2020). Prospects and challenges of extracellular vesicle-based drug delivery system: Considering cell source. *Drug Delivery*, *27*(1), 585–598. https://doi.org/10.1080/10717544.2020.1748758

Moghassemi, S., Dadashzadeh, A., Sousa, M. J., Vlieghe, H., Yang, J., León-Félix, C. M., & Amorim, C. A. (2024). Extracellular vesicles in nanomedicine and regenerative medicine: A review over the last decade. *Bioactive Materials*, *36*, 126–156. https://doi.org/10.1016/j.bioactmat.2024.02.021

Moghiman, T., Barghchi, B., Esmaeili, S.-A., Shabestari, M. M., Tabaee, S. S., & Momtazi-Borojeni, A. A. (2021). Therapeutic angiogenesis with exosomal microRNAs: An effectual approach for the treatment of myocardial ischemia. *Heart Failure Reviews*, *26*(1), 205–213. https://doi.org/10.1007/s10741-020-10001-9

Mondal, J., Pillarisetti, S., Junnuthula, V., Saha, M., Hwang, S. R., Park, I., & Lee, Y. (2023). Hybrid exosomes, exosome-like nanovesicles and engineered exosomes for therapeutic applications. *Journal of Controlled Release*, *353*, 1127–1149. https://doi.org/10.1016/j.jconrel.2022.12.027

Monsel, A., Zhu, Y., Gennai, S., Hao, Q., Hu, S., Rouby, J.-J., Rosenzwajg, M., Matthay, M. A., & Lee, J. W. (2015). Therapeutic Effects of Human Mesenchymal Stem Cell-derived Microvesicles in Severe Pneumonia in Mice. *American Journal of Respiratory and Critical Care Medicine*, *192*(3), 324–336. https://doi.org/10.1164/rccm.201410-1765OC

Mousavi, S. M., Amin Mahdian, S. M., Ebrahimi, M. S., Taghizadieh, M., Vosough, M., Sadri Nahand, J., Hosseindoost, S., Vousooghi, N., Javar, H. A., Larijani, B., Hadjighassem, M. R., Rahimian, N., Hamblin, M. R., & Mirzaei, H. (2022). Microfluidics for detection of exosomes and microRNAs in cancer: State of the art. *Molecular Therapy - Nucleic Acids*, *28*, 758–791. https://doi.org/10.1016/j.omtn.2022.04.011

Murphy, D. E., de Jong, O. G., Brouwer, M., Wood, M. J., Lavieu, G., Schiffelers, R. M., & Vader, P. (2019). Extracellular vesicle-based therapeutics: Natural versus engineered targeting and trafficking. *Experimental & Molecular Medicine*, *51*(3), 1–12. https://doi.org/10.1038/s12276-019-0223-5

Nakao, Y., Amrollahi, P., Parthasarathy, G., Mauer, A. S., Sehrawat, T. S., Vanderboom, P., Nair, K. S., Nakao, K., Allen, A. M., Hu, T. Y., & Malhi, H. (2021). Circulating extracellular vesicles are a biomarker for NAFLD resolution and response to weight loss surgery. *Nanomedicine: Nanotechnology, Biology and Medicine*, *36*, 102430. https://doi.org/10.1016/j.nano.2021.102430

Nawaz, M., Camussi, G., Valadi, H., Nazarenko, I., Ekström, K., Wang, X., Principe, S., Shah, N., Ashraf, N. M., Fatima, F., Neder, L., & Kislinger, T. (2014). The emerging role of extracellular vesicles as biomarkers for urogenital cancers. *Nature Reviews Urology*, *11*(12), 688–701. https://doi.org/10.1038/nrurol.2014.301

Nielsen, C. T., Østergaard, O., Johnsen, C., Jacobsen, S., & Heegaard, N. H. H. (2011). Distinct features of circulating microparticles and their relationship to clinical manifestations in systemic lupus erythematosus. *Arthritis and Rheumatism*, *63*(10), 3067–3077. https://doi.org/10.1002/art.30499

Parker, B., Al-Husain, A., Pemberton, P., Yates, A. P., Ho, P., Gorodkin, R., Teh, L. S., Alexander, M. Y., & Bruce, I. N. (2014). Suppression of inflammation reduces endothelial microparticles in active systemic lupus erythematosus. *Annals of the Rheumatic Diseases*, *73*(6), 1144–1150. https://doi.org/10.1136/annrheumdis-2012-203028

Peng, B., Nguyen, T. M., Jayasinghe, M. K., Gao, C., Pham, T. T., Vu, L. T., Yeo, E. Y. M., Yap, G., Wang, L., Goh, B. C., Tam, W. L., Luo, D., & Le, M. T. (2022). Robust delivery of RIG-I agonists using extracellular vesicles for anti-cancer immunotherapy. *Journal of Extracellular Vesicles*, *11*(4), e12187. https://doi.org/10.1002/jev2.12187

Pham, T. C., Jayasinghe, M. K., Pham, T. T., Yang, Y., Wei, L., Usman, W. M., Chen, H., Pirisinu, M., Gong, J., Kim, S., Peng, B., Wang, W., Chan, C., Ma, V., Nguyen, N. T. H., Kappei, D., Nguyen, X., Cho, W. C., Shi, J., & Le, M. T. N. (2021). Covalent conjugation of extracellular vesicles with peptides and nanobodies for targeted therapeutic delivery. *Journal of Extracellular Vesicles*, *10*(4), e12057. https://doi.org/10.1002/jev2.12057

Povero, D., Yamashita, H., Ren, W., Subramanian, M. G., Myers, R. P., Eguchi, A., Simonetto, D. A., Goodman, Z. D., Harrison, S. A., Sanyal, A. J., Bosch, J., & Feldstein, A. E. (2020). Characterization and Proteome of Circulating Extracellular Vesicles as Potential Biomarkers for NASH. *Hepatology Communications*, *4*(9), 1263–1278. https://doi.org/10.1002/hep4.1556

Prada, I., & Meldolesi, J. (2016). Binding and Fusion of Extracellular Vesicles to the Plasma Membrane of Their Cell Targets. *International Journal of Molecular Sciences*, *17*(8), 1296. https://doi.org/10.3390/ijms17081296

Qi, X., Zhang, J., Yuan, H., Xu, Z., Li, Q., Niu, X., Hu, B., Wang, Y., & Li, X. (2016). Exosomes Secreted by Human-Induced Pluripotent Stem Cell-Derived Mesenchymal Stem Cells Repair Critical-Sized Bone Defects through Enhanced Angiogenesis and Osteogenesis in Osteoporotic Rats. *International Journal of Biological Sciences*, *12*(7), 836–849. https://doi.org/10.7150/ijbs.14809

Ramasubramanian, L., Kumar, P., & Wang, A. (2020). Engineering Extracellular Vesicles as Nanotherapeutics for Regenerative Medicine. *Biomolecules*, *10*(1), 48. https://doi.org/10.3390/biom10010048

Ramnauth, N., Neubarth, E., Makler-Disatham, A., Sher, M., Soini, S., Merk, V., & Asghar, W. (2023). Development of a Microfluidic Device for Exosome Isolation in Point-of-Care Settings. *Sensors*, *23*(19), 8292. https://doi.org/10.3390/s23198292

Rautou, P., Bresson, J., Sainte–Marie, Y., Vion, A., Paradis, V., Renard, J., Devue, C., Heymes, C., Letteron, P., Elkrief, L., Lebrec, D., Valla, D., Tedgui, A., Moreau, R., & Boulanger, C. M. (2012). Abnormal Plasma Microparticles Impair Vasoconstrictor Responses in Patients With Cirrhosis. *Gastroenterology*, *143*(1), 166-176.e6. https://doi.org/10.1053/j.gastro.2012.03.040

Reis, M., Mavin, E., Nicholson, L., Green, K., Dickinson, A. M., & Wang, X.-N. (2018). Mesenchymal Stromal Cell-Derived Extracellular Vesicles Attenuate Dendritic Cell Maturation and Function. *Frontiers in Immunology*, *9*, 2538. https://doi.org/10.3389/fimmu.2018.02538

Roy, S., Hochberg, F. H., & Jones, P. S. (2018). Extracellular vesicles: The growth as diagnostics and therapeutics; a survey. *Journal of Extracellular Vesicles*, *7*(1), 1438720. https://doi.org/10.1080/20013078.2018.1438720

Sadovska, L., Eglītis, J., & Linē, A. (2015). "Extracellular Vesicles as Biomarkers and Therapeutic Targets in Breast Cancer". *Anticancer Research*, *35*(12), 6379–6390.

Saludas, L., Oliveira, C. C., Roncal, C., Ruiz-Villalba, A., Prósper, F., Garbayo, E., & Blanco-Prieto, M. J. (2021). Extracellular Vesicle-Based Therapeutics for Heart Repair. *Nanomaterials*, *11*(3), 570. https://doi.org/10.3390/nano11030570

Sanz-Ros, J., Mas-Bargues, C., Romero-García, N., Huete-Acevedo, J., Dromant, M., & Borrás, C. (2023). The Potential Use of Mitochondrial Extracellular Vesicles as Biomarkers or Therapeutical Tools. *International Journal of Molecular Sciences*, *24*(8), 7005. https://doi.org/10.3390/ijms24087005

Sehrawat, T. S., Arab, J. P., Liu, M., Amrollahi, P., Wan, M., Fan, J., Nakao, Y., Pose, E., Navarro-Corcuera, A., Dasgupta, D., Liao, C., He, L., Mauer, A. S., Avitabile, E., Ventura-Cots, M., Bataller, R. A., Sanyal, A. J., Chalasani, N. P., Heimbach, J. K., … Malhi, H. (2021). Circulating Extracellular Vesicles Carrying Sphingolipid Cargo for the Diagnosis and Dynamic Risk Profiling of Alcoholic Hepatitis. *Hepatology*, *73*(2), 571–585. https://doi.org/10.1002/hep.31256

Shabbir, A., Cox, A., Rodriguez-Menocal, L., Salgado, M., & Van Badiavas, E. (2015). Mesenchymal Stem Cell Exosomes Induce Proliferation and Migration of Normal and Chronic Wound Fibroblasts, and Enhance Angiogenesis In Vitro. *Stem Cells and Development*, *24*(14), 1635–1647. https://doi.org/10.1089/scd.2014.0316

Song, H., Chen, X., Hao, Y., Wang, J., Xie, Q., & Wang, X. (2022). Nanoengineering facilitating the target mission: Targeted extracellular vesicles delivery systems design. *Journal of Nanobiotechnology*, *20*(1), 431. https://doi.org/10.1186/s12951-022-01638-9

Stavrou, A., & Ortiz, A. (2022). Extracellular Vesicles: A Novel Tool in Nanomedicine and Cancer Treatment. *Cancers*, *14*(18), 4450. https://doi.org/10.3390/cancers14184450

Sukriti, S., Maras, J. S., Bihari, C., Das, S., Vyas, A. K., Sharma, S., Hussain, S., Shasthry, S., Choudhary, A., Premkumar, M., Kumar, D., Kumar, G., Mukhopadhyay, C., Kumar, A., Trehanpati, N., Rautou, P. E., Moreau, R., & Sarin, S. K. (2018). Microvesicles in hepatic and peripheral vein can predict nonresponse to corticosteroid therapy in severe alcoholic hepatitis. *Alimentary Pharmacology & Therapeutics*, *47*(8), 1151–1161. https://doi.org/10.1111/apt.14564

Tamura, R., Uemoto, S., & Tabata, Y. (2016). Immunosuppressive effect of mesenchymal stem cell-derived exosomes on a concanavalin A-induced liver injury model. *Inflammation and Regeneration*, *36*(1), 26. https://doi.org/10.1186/s41232-016-0030-5

Tang, T.-T., Wang, B., Lv, L.-L., & Liu, B.-C. (2020). Extracellular vesicle-based Nanotherapeutics: Emerging frontiers in anti-inflammatory therapy. *Theranostics*, *10*(18), 8111–8129. https://doi.org/10.7150/thno.47865

Tang, Y., Liu, X., Sun, M., Xiong, S., Xiao, N., Li, J., He, X., & Xie, J. (2023). Recent Progress in Extracellular Vesicle-Based Carriers for Targeted Drug Delivery in Cancer Therapy. *Pharmaceutics*, *15*(7), 1902. https://doi.org/10.3390/pharmaceutics15071902

Thakur, B. K., Zhang, H., Becker, A., Matei, I., Huang, Y., Costa-Silva, B., Zheng, Y., Hoshino, A., Brazier, H., Xiang, J., Williams, C., Rodriguez-Barrueco, R., Silva, J. M., Zhang, W., Hearn, S., Elemento, O., Paknejad, N., Manova-Todorova, K., Welte, K., … Lyden, D. (2014). Double-stranded DNA in exosomes: A novel biomarker in cancer detection. *Cell Research*, *24*(6), 766–769. https://doi.org/10.1038/cr.2014.44

Tomasoni, S., Longaretti, L., Rota, C., Morigi, M., Conti, S., Gotti, E., Capelli, C., Introna, M., Remuzzi, G., & Benigni, A. (2013). Transfer of Growth Factor Receptor mRNA Via Exosomes Unravels the Regenerative Effect of Mesenchymal Stem Cells. *Stem Cells and Development*, *22*(5), 772–780. https://doi.org/10.1089/scd.2012.0266

Tong, Y., Sun, J., Jiang, X., Jia, X., Xiao, H., Wang, H., & Yang, G. (2025). A study on the production of extracellular vesicles derived from novel immortalized human placental mesenchymal stromal cells. *Scientific Reports*, *15*(1), 3568. https://doi.org/10.1038/s41598-025-87371-3

Urabe, F., Kosaka, N., Ito, K., Kimura, T., Egawa, S., & Ochiya, T. (2020). Extracellular vesicles as biomarkers and therapeutic targets for cancer. *American Journal of Physiology-Cell Physiology*, *318*(1), C29–C39. https://doi.org/10.1152/ajpcell.00280.2019

Vader, P., Mol, E. A., Pasterkamp, G., & Schiffelers, R. M. (2016). Extracellular vesicles for drug delivery. *Advanced Drug Delivery Reviews*, *106*, 148–156. https://doi.org/10.1016/j.addr.2016.02.006

van Balkom, B. W. M., de Jong, O. G., Smits, M., Brummelman, J., den Ouden, K., de Bree, P. M., van Eijndhoven, M. A. J., Pegtel, D. M., Stoorvogel, W., Würdinger, T., & Verhaar, M. C. (2013). Endothelial cells require miR-214 to secrete exosomes that suppress senescence and induce angiogenesis in human and mouse endothelial cells. *Blood*, *121*(19), 3997–4006. https://doi.org/10.1182/blood-2013-02-478925

Villata, S., Canta, M., & Cauda, V. (2020). EVs and Bioengineering: From Cellular Products to Engineered Nanomachines. *International Journal of Molecular Sciences*, *21*(17), 6048. https://doi.org/10.3390/ijms21176048

Wang, S., Kojima, K., Mobley, J. A., & West, A. B. (2019). Proteomic analysis of urinary extracellular vesicles reveal biomarkers for neurologic disease. *eBioMedicine*, *45*, 351–361. https://doi.org/10.1016/j.ebiom.2019.06.021

Wang, Y., Zhao, M., Liu, S., Guo, J., Lu, Y., Cheng, J., & Liu, J. (2020). Macrophage-derived extracellular vesicles: Diverse mediators of pathology and therapeutics in multiple diseases. *Cell Death & Disease*, *11*(10), 1–18. https://doi.org/10.1038/s41419-020-03127-z

Wei, Z., Qiao, S., Zhao, J., Liu, Y., Li, Q., Wei, Z., Dai, Q., Kang, L., & Xu, B. (2019). miRNA-181a over-expression in mesenchymal stem cell-derived exosomes influenced inflammatory response after myocardial ischemia-reperfusion injury. *Life Sciences*, *232*, 116632. https://doi.org/10.1016/j.lfs.2019.116632

Wolf, M., Poupardin, R. W., Ebner-Peking, P., Andrade, A. C., Blöchl, C., Obermayer, A., Gomes, F. G., Vari, B., Maeding, N., Eminger, E., Binder, H.-M., Raninger, A. M., Hochmann, S., Brachtl, G., Spittler, A., Heuser, T., Ofir, R., Huber, C. G., Aberman, Z., … Strunk, D. (2022). A functional corona around extracellular vesicles enhances angiogenesis, skin regeneration and immunomodulation. *Journal of Extracellular Vesicles*, *11*(4), e12207.

https://doi.org/10.1002/jev2.12207

Wu, P., Zhang, B., Ocansey, D. K. W., Xu, W., & Qian, H. (2021). Extracellular vesicles: A bright star of nanomedicine. *Biomaterials*, *269*, 120467. https://doi.org/10.1016/j.biomaterials.2020.120467

Xia, Y., Hu, G., Chen, Y., Yuan, J., Zhang, J., Wang, S., Li, Q., Wang, Y., & Deng, Z. (2021). Embryonic Stem Cell Derived Small Extracellular Vesicles Modulate Regulatory T Cells to Protect against Ischemic Stroke. *ACS Nano*, *15*(4), 7370–7385. https://doi.org/10.1021/acsnano.1c00672

Xin, H., Li, Y., Buller, B., Katakowski, M., Zhang, Y., Wang, X., Shang, X., Zhang, Z. G., & Chopp, M. (2012). Exosome-mediated transfer of miR-133b from multipotent mesenchymal stromal cells to neural cells contributes to neurite outgrowth. *Stem Cells*, *30*(7), 1556–1564. https://doi.org/10.1002/stem.1129

Xin, H., Li, Y., Liu, Z., Wang, X., Shang, X., Cui, Y., Zhang, Z. G., & Chopp, M. (2013). MiR-133b Promotes Neural Plasticity and Functional Recovery After Treatment of Stroke with Multipotent Mesenchymal Stromal Cells in Rats Via Transfer of Exosome-Enriched Extracellular Particles. *Stem Cells*, *31*(12), 2737–2746. https://doi.org/10.1002/stem.1409

Xiong, Y.-Y., Gong, Z.-T., Tang, R.-J., & Yang, Y.-J. (2021). The pivotal roles of exosomes derived from endogenous immune cells and exogenous stem cells in myocardial repair after acute myocardial infarction. *Theranostics*, *11*(3), 1046–1058. https://doi.org/10.7150/thno.53326

Xiu, C., Zheng, H., Jiang, M., Li, J., Zhou, Y., Mu, L., & Liu, W. (2022). MSCs-Derived miR-150-5p-Expressing Exosomes Promote Skin Wound Healing by Activating PI3K/AKT Pathway through PTEN. *International Journal of Stem Cells*, *15*(4), 359–371. https://doi.org/10.15283/ijsc21135

Yadav, A., Xuan, Y., Sen, C. K., & Ghatak, S. (2024). Standardized Reporting of Research on Exosomes to Ensure Rigor and Reproducibility. *Advances in Wound Care*, *13*(11), 584–599. https://doi.org/10.1089/wound.2024.0093

Yáñez-Mó, M., Siljander, P. R.-M., Andreu, Z., Bedina Zavec, A., Borràs, F. E., Buzas, E. I., Buzas, K., Casal, E., Cappello, F., Carvalho, J., Colás, E., Cordeiro-da Silva, A., Fais, S., Falcon-Perez, J. M., Ghobrial, I. M., Giebel, B., Gimona, M., Graner, M., Gursel, I., … De Wever, O. (2015). Biological properties of extracellular vesicles and their physiological functions. *Journal of Extracellular Vesicles*, *4*(1), 27066. https://doi.org/10.3402/jev.v4.27066

Yang, Y., Ye, Y., Kong, C., Su, X., Zhang, X., Bai, W., & He, X. (2019). MiR-124 Enriched Exosomes Promoted the M2 Polarization of Microglia and Enhanced Hippocampus Neurogenesis After Traumatic Brain Injury by Inhibiting TLR4 Pathway. *Neurochemical Research*, *44*(4), 811–828. https://doi.org/10.1007/s11064-018-02714-z

Ye, Z., Zhang, T., He, W., Jin, H., Liu, C., Yang, Z., & Ren, J. (2018). Methotrexate-Loaded Extracellular Vesicles Functionalized with Therapeutic and Targeted Peptides for the Treatment of Glioblastoma Multiforme. *ACS Applied Materials & Interfaces*, *10*(15), 12341–12350. https://doi.org/10.1021/acsami.7b18135

Yoo, A. S., Sun, A. X., Li, L., Shcheglovitov, A., Portmann, T., Li, Y., Lee-Messer, C., Dolmetsch, R. E., Tsien, R. W., & Crabtree, G. R. (2011). MicroRNA-mediated conversion of human fibroblasts to neurons. *Nature*, *476*(7359), 228–231. https://doi.org/10.1038/nature10323

Yuan, Q., Wang, X., Liu, L., Cai, Y., Zhao, X., Ma, H., & Zhang, Y. (2020). Exosomes Derived from Human Placental Mesenchymal Stromal Cells Carrying AntagomiR-4450 Alleviate Intervertebral Disc Degeneration Through Upregulation of ZNF121. *Stem Cells and Development*, *29*(16), 1038–1058. https://doi.org/10.1089/scd.2020.0083

Yuan, X., Li, D., Chen, X., Han, C., Xu, L., Huang, T., Dong, Z., & Zhang, M. (2017). Extracellular vesicles from human-induced pluripotent stem cell-derived mesenchymal stromal cells (hiPSC-MSCs) protect against renal ischemia/reperfusion injury via delivering specificity protein (SP1) and transcriptional activating of sphingosine kinase 1 and inhibiting necroptosis. *Cell Death & Disease*, *8*(12), 3200. https://doi.org/10.1038/s41419-017-0041-4

Zaborowski, M. P., Balaj, L., Breakefield, X. O., & Lai, C. P. (2015). Extracellular Vesicles: Composition, Biological Relevance, and Methods of Study. *BioScience*, *65*(8), 783–797. https://doi.org/10.1093/biosci/biv084

Zamani, P., Fereydouni, N., Butler, A. E., Navashenaq, J. G., & Sahebkar, A. (2019). The therapeutic and diagnostic role of exosomes in cardiovascular diseases. *Trends in Cardiovascular Medicine*, *29*(6), 313–323. https://doi.org/10.1016/j.tcm.2018.10.010

Zhai, M., Zhu, Y., Yang, M., & Mao, C. (2020). Human Mesenchymal Stem Cell Derived Exosomes Enhance Cell-Free Bone Regeneration by Altering Their miRNAs Profiles. *Advanced Science*, *7*(19), 2001334. https://doi.org/10.1002/advs.202001334

Zhang, B., Wang, M., Gong, A., Zhang, X., Wu, X., Zhu, Y., Shi, H., Wu, L., Zhu, W., Qian, H., & Xu, W. (2015). HucMSC-Exosome Mediated-

Wnt4 Signaling Is Required for Cutaneous Wound Healing. *Stem Cells*, *33*(7), 2158–2168. https://doi.org/10.1002/stem.1771

Zhang, B., Yin, Y., Lai, R. C., Tan, S. S., Choo, A. B. H., & Lim, S. K. (2014). Mesenchymal Stem Cells Secrete Immunologically Active Exosomes. *Stem Cells and Development*, *23*(11), 1233–1244. https://doi.org/10.1089/scd.2013.0479

Zhang, W., Wang, L., Guo, H., Chen, L., & Huang, X. (2023). Dapagliflozin-Loaded Exosome Mimetics Facilitate Diabetic Wound Healing by HIF-1 α -Mediated Enhancement of Angiogenesis. *Advanced Healthcare Materials*, *12*(7), 2202751. https://doi.org/10.1002/adhm.202202751

Zhang, Z.-W., Wei, P., Zhang, G.-J., Yan, J.-X., Zhang, S., Liang, J., & Wang, X.-L. (2022). Intravenous infusion of the exosomes derived from human umbilical cord mesenchymal stem cells enhance neurological recovery after traumatic brain injury via suppressing the NF-κB pathway. *Open Life Sciences*, *17*(1), 189–201. https://doi.org/10.1515/biol-2022-0022

Zheng, J., Lu, T., Zhou, C., Cai, J., Zhang, X., Liang, J., Sui, X., Chen, X., Chen, L., Sun, Y., Zhang, J., Chen, W., Zhang, Y., Yao, J., Chen, G., & Yang, Y. (2020). Extracellular Vesicles Derived from Human Umbilical Cord Mesenchymal Stem Cells Protect Liver Ischemia/Reperfusion Injury by Reducing CD154 Expression on $CD4^+$ T Cells via CCT2. *Advanced Science*, *7*(18), 1903746. https://doi.org/10.1002/advs.201903746

Zhou, G., Gu, Y., Zhu, Z., Zhang, H., Liu, W., Xu, B., Zhou, F., Zhang, M., Hua, K., Wu, L., & Ding, J. (2022). Exosome Mediated Cytosolic Cisplatin Delivery Through Clathrin-Independent Endocytosis and Enhanced Anti-cancer Effect via Avoiding Endosome Trapping in Cisplatin-Resistant Ovarian Cancer. *Frontiers in Medicine*, *9*, 810761. https://doi.org/10.3389/fmed.2022.810761

Zhou, Y., Xu, H., Xu, W., Wang, B., Wu, H., Tao, Y., Zhang, B., Wang, M., Mao, F., Yan, Y., Gao, S., Gu, H., Zhu, W., & Qian, H. (2013). Exosomes released by human umbilical cord mesenchymal stem cells protect against cisplatin-induced renal oxidative stress and apoptosis in vivo and in vitro. *Stem Cell Research & Therapy*, *4*(2), 34. https://doi.org/10.1186/scrt194

Zhou, Y., Yuan, Y., Liu, M., Hu, X., Quan, Y., & Chen, X. (2019). Tumor-specific delivery of KRAS siRNA with iRGD-exosomes efficiently inhibits tumor growth. *ExRNA*, *1*(1), 28. https://doi.org/10.1186/s41544-019-0034-9

Zhu, G., Yang, X., Peng, C., Yu, L., & Hao, Y. (2020). Exosomal miR-532–5p from bone marrow mesenchymal stem cells reduce intervertebral disc degeneration by targeting RASSF5. *Experimental Cell Research*, *393*(2), 112109. https://doi.org/10.1016/j.yexcr.2020.112109

Zhu, J., Kai, L., Zhang, N., Zhao, Y., Ma, Q., Shen, J., Lin, Y., Xiang, P., Tang, Y., Hu, X., Chen, J., Zhu, W., Webster, K. A., Wang, J., & Yu, H. (2018). Myocardial reparative functions of exosomes from mesenchymal stem cells are enhanced by hypoxia treatment of the cells via transferring microRNA-210 in an nSMase2-dependent way. *Artificial Cells, Nanomedicine, and Biotechnology*, *46*(8), 1659–1670. https://doi.org/10.1080/21691401.2017.1388249

Zhu, Y.-G., Feng, X.-M., Abbott, J., Fang, X.-H., Hao, Q., Monsel, A., Qu, J.-M., Matthay, M. A., & Lee, J. W. (2014). Human mesenchymal stem cell microvesicles for treatment of Escherichia coli endotoxin-induced acute lung injury in mice. *Stem Cells*, *32*(1), 116–125. https://doi.org/10.1002/stem.1504

Author Biographies

Maria Gazouli: Professor of Biology – Genetics – Nanomedicine, Laboratory of Biology, Department of Basic Medical Sciences, Medical School of Athens, National and Kapodistrian University of Athens, Greece.

Zoi Kardasi: PhD student at Laboratory of Biology, Department of Basic Medical Sciences, Medical School of Athens, National and Kapodistrian University of Athens, Greece.

Natassa Pippa: Assistant Professor, Section of Pharmaceutical Technology, Department of Pharmacy, School of Health Sciences, National and Kapodistrian University of Athens, Greece.

Maria G. Roubelakis: Professor of Biology and applications of Regenerative Medicine, Laboratory of Biology, Department of Basic Medical Sciences, Medical School of Athens, National and Kapodistrian University of Athens, Greece.

Efstathia Triantafyllopoulou: PhD student at Section of Pharmaceutical Technology, Department of Pharmacy, School of Health Sciences, National and Kapodistrian University of Athens, Greece.

CHAPTER 8

EXOSOMES

NIHAN ÖRÜKLÜ

Gazi University, Faculty of Medicine, Department of Immunology, Ankara, Türkiye

Abstract

Gene therapy holds vast therapeutic promise, but its widespread clinical success is hampered by the limitations of current delivery systems. While viral vectors are highly efficient, they pose significant risks related to immunogenicity and restricted packaging capacity, and non-viral systems often lack sufficient transduction efficiency and targeting specificity. This has led to the emergence of exosomes (30–150 nm), naturally secreted extracellular vesicles, as a superior, next-generation delivery platform. Exosomes offer key biological advantages, including intrinsic low immunogenicity, high biocompatibility, stability for fragile genetic cargo and a unique ability to cross biological barriers. Their unique properties stem from their origin via endosomal biogenesis, a process strictly regulated by molecular machinery proteins. For clinical viability, rigorous quality control and characterization are mandatory, guided by MISEV guidelines, utilizing size analysis and validation with specific markers. To optimize therapeutic effect, exosomes must be engineered, involving strategies such as endogenous modification and exogenous modification using techniques such as electroporation, sonication, or extrusion. Exosomes serve as powerful carriers for a diverse range of nucleic acids, messenger RNAs (mRNAs) for protein translation, microRNAs (miRNAs) and small interfering RNAs (siRNAs) for RNA interference (RNAi) therapy, as well as complex tools like plasmid DNA and CRISPR/Cas9 components. This versatility allows them to deliver therapeutic genes and silence pathogenic genes. Exosomes are currently being actively developed across major disease areas, including cancer gene therapy, the treatment of neurodegenerative diseases, regenerative medicine and immune modulation. Ultimately, the inherent biological properties and customizable nature of exosomes position them as a transformative technology in gene therapy, although addressing remaining challenges in scalability and standardization is critical for their eventual translation from bench to bedside.

Keywords: exosome, gene therapy, immunotherapy

Introduction

Gene therapy represents a powerful therapeutic approach that involves the delivery of genetic material into patient cells to correct or modulate disease-causing genes. In recent years, this field has witnessed significant milestones, with therapies such as *onasemnogene abeparvovec* for spinal muscular atrophy and *voretigene neparvovec* for Leber congenital amaurosis gaining regulatory approval (Chongmelaxme et al., 2025; Henderson et al., 2024). These advancements underscore the therapeutic potential of gene-based interventions. However, a persistent and critical challenge in gene therapy is the development of delivery systems that are both efficient and safe (Cetin et al., 2024).

Viral vectors, including adeno-associated viruses (AAVs), lentiviruses, and adenoviruses, have been the mainstay of gene delivery due to their high transduction efficiency and stable gene expression profiles (De Haan et al., 2021). Nonetheless, their clinical application is hindered by several limitations, including immunogenicity, restricted packaging capacity, risks of insertional mutagenesis, and manufacturing complexity (Yudaeva et al., 2024). Non-viral vectors, such as lipid nanoparticles (LNPs), cationic polymers, and dendrimers, offer a safer alternative but often lack sufficient cellular uptake, endosomal escape, or tissue specificity. These limitations underscore the need for novel delivery vehicles that combine the safety profile of non-viral systems with the targeting efficiency of biological carriers. While these have improved safety profiles, they often suffer from lower transfection efficiency and challenges in targeted delivery. Among the most promising of these is a class of naturally occurring nanoparticles known as exosomes (Khan, 2024; Shtykalova et al., 2023).

Exosomes, a subtype of extracellular vesicles (EVs) ranging from 30 to 150 nanometers (nm) in diameter, have recently emerged as promising candidates for gene delivery (Doyle & Wang, 2019). Derived from the endosomal compartment of virtually all cell types, exosomes are naturally equipped to mediate intercellular communication through the transfer of functional proteins, lipids, and nucleic acids. Their endogenous origin grants them several advantageous properties, including low immunogenicity, high biocompatibility, capacity for systemic circulation, and intrinsic targeting capabilities—especially when derived from specific parental cell types (Chen et al., 2023; Isaac et al., 2021; Lopes et al., 2023).

Exosomes can encapsulate and carry a diverse and biologically active cargo of proteins, lipids, and nucleic acids, including messenger RNAs (mRNAs), microRNAs (miRNAs), small interfering RNAs (siRNAs), antisense oligonucleotides (ASOs), and CRISPR/Cas9 components (Zhu et al., 2023). Recent innovations have made it possible to load these cargoes into exosomes through various strategies such as electroporation, lipid-based transfection, parental cell engineering, and mechanical extrusion (Ferreira et al., 2022).

The unique biological properties of exosomes make them a highly attractive alternative to traditional gene delivery systems. Their low immunogenicity and high biocompatibility significantly reduce the risk of adverse immune reactions, a major concern with viral vectors. Furthermore, their endogenous origin and ability to cross biological barriers, notably the blood-brain barrier (BBB), offer unprecedented potential for targeted gene delivery to hard-to-reach tissues (Szwedowicz et al., 2022). Despite these promising features, challenges remain. The heterogeneity of exosomes, low isolation yields, and lack of standardized manufacturing protocols pose barriers to clinical translation. Moreover, rigorous regulatory frameworks are still under development for exosome-based therapeutics, especially those involving gene editing tools (J. Li et al., 2025). This chapter will delve into the fundamental biology of exosomes and their growing role as a sophisticated and efficient delivery platform in modern gene therapy.

Classification and Nomenclature According to MISEV

The field of extracellular vesicle (EV) research has grown exponentially, but with this growth came a proliferation of inconsistent terminology. To address this challenge and enhance research rigor, reproducibility and transparency, the International Society for Extracellular Vesicles (ISEV) developed the Minimal information for studies of extracellular vesicles (MISEV) guidelines, with the latest version being MISEV2023 (Saint-Pol & Culot, 2025). A key principle of these guidelines is a move away from using biogenesis-based terms like "exosome" as a primary unless their intracellular origin is proven. Instead, the MISEV guidelines propose a more precise, evidence-based classification system using operational terms like physical characteristics (size), biochemical composition (molecular markers), cellular origin and context and state of the parent cell (Welsh et al., 2024).

EVs can be classified by size, with small EVs (sEVs) defined as those under 200 nm in diameter, which often corresponds to the operational range for exosomes, and medium/large EVs (m/lEVs) being larger than 200 nm (Lee et al., 2023). Density-based classification is also used, with exosomes typically exhibiting a density between 1.10 to 1.19 g/mL in sucrose or iodixanol gradients. Biochemically, exosomes are enriched in specific protein markers, including tetraspanins (CD9, CD63, CD81), ESCRT-related proteins (TSG101, Alix), and flotillin, while negative markers such as calnexin, GM130, and cytochrome C should be absent in purified EV preparations. This marker profile helps to distinguish exosomes from other EV types (Zhang et al., 2020). EVs can be classified by the cell type from which they were isolated. This is a very useful descriptor, as it provides important context for their function. For example, EVs can be described as "platelet-derived EVs" or "cancer cell-derived EVs." Context and state of the parent cell describes the condition under which the EVs were produced, such as a state of stress, hypoxia, or inflammation (Salomon et al., 2022). From a practical perspective, MISEV guidelines recommend reporting isolation methods, including ultracentrifugation, size-exclusion chromatography, or density gradient separation, and require comprehensive characterization using at least two positive protein markers, one negative marker, and size distribution analysis via nanoparticle tracking analysis, dynamic light scattering, or electron microscopy (Zhang et al., 2024).

Table 1: Comparison of Exosomes, Microvesicles, and Apoptotic Bodies

Feature	Exosomes	Microvesicles	Apoptotic Bodies
Biogenesis	MVB fusion with plasma membrane	Outward budding of plasma membrane	Apoptotic cell disassembly
Size (nm)	30–150	100–1000	500–2000
Density (g/mL)	1.10–1.19	Broader, often lower	Variable
Markers	CD63, CD81, TSG101, Alix	Integrins, selectins, annexins	DNA, histones, organelles

Biogenesis and Biology of Exosomes

Among the heterogeneous population of EVs, exosomes are distinguished not only by their relatively small size and specific buoyant density, but more fundamentally by their unique endosomal biogenesis, which represents the most definitive criterion for discriminating them from microvesicles and apoptotic bodies. The formation of exosomes begins within the endosomal system through a multi-step, highly regulated process (Doyle & Wang, 2019; Xie et al., 2022). Unlike apoptotic bodies or microvesicles, which are generated through direct outward budding of the plasma membrane or during cell death, exosomes originate from the endosomal compartment of viable cells. They are nanosized vesicles and are secreted by almost all eukaryotic cells into the extracellular environment (Battistelli & Falcieri, 2020; Gregory & Rimmer, 2023).

The biogenesis of exosomes begins with the invagination of the plasma membrane to form early endosomes. These early endosomes then mature into late endosomes, which are also referred to as multivesicular bodies (MVBs), through a second round of inward budding of their limiting membrane. Within these MVBs, the inward budding of the limiting membrane leads to the formation of intraluminal vesicles (ILVs). When MVBs fuse with the plasma membrane, these ILVs are released into the extracellular space as exosomes (Palomar-Alonso et al., 2024; Xu et al., 2023). This process is tightly regulated by molecular machinery, including the endosomal sorting complex required for transport (ESCRT), which plays a key role in cargo sorting and vesicle scission. The ESCRT complex is composed of four multi-protein subcomplexes (ESCRT-0, -I, -II, and -III) that work sequentially to recognize, cluster, and sort ubiquitinated cargo proteins into budding vesicles (Ahmed et al., 2019). Proteins such as Tumor Susceptibility Gene 101 (TSG101) and ALIX are key components of the ESCRT machinery and are often used as markers for exosome purification. TSG101, a core component of the ESCRT-I complex, plays a central role in exosome biogenesis by recognizing ubiquitinated cargo proteins and initiating the inward budding of the endosomal membrane. Alix functions as an adaptor protein that bridges ESCRT-I/II with ESCRT-III, thereby facilitating membrane scission and assisting in the selective loading of cargo into intraluminal vesicles. Together, TSG101 and Alix coordinate the proper formation of multivesicular bodies and ensure the efficient release of exosomes upon fusion with the plasma membrane (Larios et al., 2020; Lee et al., 2024).

In addition to the canonical ESCRT-dependent mechanism, exosome biogenesis can also proceed via ESCRT-independent pathways. These involve lipid-driven mechanisms in which bioactive lipids like ceramide promote membrane curvature and budding, as well as tetraspanin-enriched microdomains that facilitate vesicle formation without the requirement for the ESCRT complex (Elsherbini & Bieberich, 2018). The existence of both ESCRT-dependent and -independent pathways highlights the biological diversity and redundancy in exosome production, suggesting that cells may utilize different mechanisms depending on context and cell type (Komori & Fukuda, 2024).

The fusion of the MVBs with the cell's plasma membrane releases these ILVs into the extracellular space, at which point they are known as exosomes. This highly controlled process results in a cargo that is not a random sampling of the cell's contents but rather a selective and biologically active mixture (Zhao et al., 2021). The composition of exosomes reflects the cell of origin and contains proteins, lipids, nucleic acids. Proteins commonly found in exosomes include the tetraspanins (CD9, CD63 and CD81). They are integral membrane proteins which regulate membrane organization, cargo sorting, and intraluminal vesicle formation. Beyond their role in biogenesis, they mediate target cell recognition, adhesion, and uptake, thereby shaping exosome tropism and function, while also serving as widely used biomarkers due to their abundance and stability (Jankovicova et al., 2020). Other enriched proteins include ALIX and TSG101, which are involved in vesicle formation. HSP70 and HSP90, two major heat shock proteins enriched in exosomes, function as molecular chaperones that maintain protein stability and prevent aggregation under stress conditions. They are actively involved in exosomal cargo sorting and trafficking, thereby influencing the molecular composition of exosomes. In addition, these proteins contribute to intercellular communication by enhancing exosome uptake and modulating signaling pathways in recipient cells, with exosomal HSP70 also implicated in immune activation. Owing to their abundance and stability, HSP70 and HSP90 are widely recognized as canonical markers for exosome identification (Cordonnier et al., 2017).

Exosomes possess a lipid composition that is distinct from the plasma membrane of their parental cells, reflecting their specialized biogenesis and functional roles. They are enriched in lipids such as cholesterol, sphingomyelin, ceramide, glycosphingolipids and phosphatidylserine, giving their membranes raft-like properties, stability, and resistance to degradation (Ghadami & Dellinger, 2023). Ceramide, generated through the action of neutral sphingomyelinases, is particularly important because it drives

ESCRT-independent exosome biogenesis, facilitating inward budding of the endosomal membrane and the formation of intraluminal vesicles (Elsherbini & Bieberich, 2018). Another key feature is the exposure of phosphatidylserine on the outer leaflet of the exosomal membrane. This lipid not only contributes to the curvature and budding of membranes but also serves as a recognition signal that enhances binding, uptake, and fusion with recipient cells. Additionally, the asymmetrical distribution of lipids within the bilayer plays an active role in sorting and packaging of molecular cargo into exosomes. This unique lipid composition provides mechanical stability, protects exosomes in circulation, regulates vesicle formation pathways, and mediates their interactions with target cells, thereby making lipids critical bioactive determinants of exosomal function (Donoso-Quezada et al., 2021).

Exosomes serve as powerful carriers of genetic information by transporting a wide variety of nucleic acids. They contain messenger RNA (mRNA), which can be delivered to recipient cells and subsequently translated into functional proteins, thereby transferring cellular traits and influencing processes such as tissue regeneration, immune modulation, and tumor progression (Chavda et al., 2023). Exosomes are also particularly enriched in microRNAs (miRNAs), which are selectively packaged and act as post-transcriptional regulators by binding to target mRNAs to suppress translation or promote degradation. Through this mechanism, exosomal miRNAs play pivotal roles in regulating gene expression, modulating the immune system, promoting angiogenesis, and driving cancer metastasis, often by reprogramming stromal or immune cells in the tumor microenvironment (Fazio et al., 2025). In addition to mRNA and miRNA, exosomes also carry long non-coding RNAs (lncRNAs), transcripts longer than 200 nucleotides that lack protein-coding potential but regulate gene expression through diverse mechanisms such as chromatin remodeling, transcriptional regulation, and miRNA sponging. Exosomal lncRNAs are increasingly recognized for their involvement in cancer progression, drug resistance, and immune regulation, and are being explored as novel diagnostic biomarkers (Kolat et al., 2019). Recent studies have also revealed that exosomes can carry DNA, including single-stranded DNA (ssDNA), double-stranded DNA (dsDNA), and mitochondrial DNA (mtDNA). The presence of dsDNA and ssDNA often mirrors the mutational status of the parental cell, making them promising tools for liquid biopsy–based diagnostics, especially in cancer. Meanwhile, mtDNA within exosomes can modulate bioenergetic functions and inflammatory signaling in recipient cells (Pan & Wang, 2025). Together, these findings highlight that exosomes are not simply RNA carriers but versatile vehicles of genetic material, capable of regulating protein synthesis, gene expression, and genomic signaling across diverse physiological and pathological contexts (Lee et al., 2024). These nucleic acids are not randomly packaged but are selectively incorporated based on cell-type-specific and stimulus-dependent mechanisms. Notably, the RNA cargo contained within exosomes is protected from extracellular RNases by the lipid bilayer, allowing for stable and functional delivery to recipient cells. This endogenous mechanism of horizontal gene transfer is one of the foundational principles that underlies the potential of exosomes as natural gene delivery vehicles in therapeutic applications (Janas et al., 2015).

The physiological roles of exosomes are diverse and context-dependent. In the immune system, exosomes derived from antigen-presenting cells can carry MHC class I and II molecules, co-stimulatory proteins, and cytokines, enabling them to modulate T cell activation or suppression, influence B cell behavior, and contribute to the induction of immune tolerance (Li et al., 2019). In cancer biology, tumor-derived exosomes have been shown to promote angiogenesis, metastasis, immune evasion, and drug resistance through the transfer of oncogenic proteins and RNA molecules to surrounding stromal and immune cells (Aakel et al., 2025). In the central nervous system, neuronal and glial exosomes participate in the regulation of synaptic plasticity, myelination, and neuroinflammatory signaling (Spinelli et al., 2025).

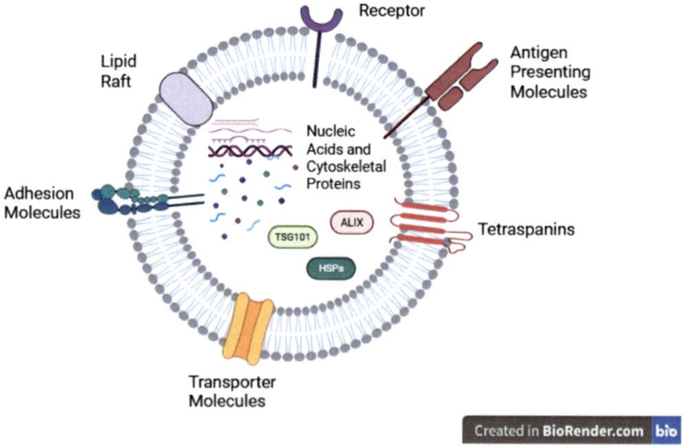

The natural ability of exosomes to transport genetic material across cellular barriers in a stable, specific, and minimally immunogenic manner has laid the foundation for their use in gene therapy. Unlike viral vectors, which may elicit strong immune responses or pose insertional mutagenesis risks, exosomes offer a safer and more versatile platform. Their biological origin allows for extended circulation times, biocompatibility, and even the capacity to traverse the blood–brain barrier, making them particularly valuable for neurological applications. Moreover, exosomes can be engineered to enhance their tropism toward specific cell types, increase cargo loading efficiency, or incorporate synthetic modifications that improve therapeutic outcomes (Pofali et al., 2020).

Sources of Exosomes for Gene Therapy

Exosomes can be harvested from a wide range of cell types, both physiological and engineered, depending on their intended therapeutic application. Commonly used sources include mesenchymal stem cells (MSCs), dendritic cells (DCs), tumor cells, T cells, macrophages, and immortalized cell lines such as HEK293 or B16-F10. MSCs are particularly attractive due to their immunomodulatory properties and low immunogenicity, and they are widely used in regenerative medicine. Exosomes derived from dendritic cells can carry immunologically active molecules, making them useful in vaccine development. Additionally, patient-derived or autologous exosomes are increasingly being explored to reduce immune rejection risks. The choice of source cell is critical, as it not only determines the surface protein and lipid composition of the exosomes, but also affects their targeting ability, bio-distribution, and therapeutic cargo compatibility. In gene therapy, engineered donor cells are often transfected or transduced with plasmids, mRNA, or CRISPR constructs prior to exosome harvesting, ensuring the vesicles contain the desired genetic cargo (Chen et al., 2025; J. Li et al., 2025).

Isolation Techniques for Exosomes

Isolating a pure, functional, and consistent population of exosomes from complex biological fluids or cell culture media is a critical and challenging first step in their therapeutic development. No single method is perfect; therefore, researchers often combine techniques to balance the need for high purity, yield, and scalability (Yakubovich et al., 2022).

1. Differential Ultracentrifugation (UC)

This is the oldest and most widely used method, often considered the conventional standard. It separates particles based on their size and buoyant density using a series of sequential centrifugation steps. The process begins with low-speed centrifugation (e.g., 2,000 x g) to pellet large cellular debris. The supernatant is then centrifuged at higher speeds (e.g., 10,000-20,000 x g) to remove larger microvesicles. Finally, the resulting supernatant is subjected to very high-speed ultracentrifugation (e.g., 100,000 x g or higher) to pellet the smaller exosomes. It's a well-established method, widely available, and relatively cost-effective. Despite its advantages, the final preparation is often heterogeneous and contaminated with non-vesicular particles like proteins and lipoproteins. The high centrifugal forces can also cause exosome aggregation or physical damage, which may affect their biological activity. It is a very time-consuming and labor-intensive process (Clos-Sansalvador et al., 2022).

2. Size-Based Isolation

These methods separate exosomes based on their physical size, offering a gentler alternative to UC.

2.1. Size-Exclusion Chromatography (SEC)

This technique uses a column packed with porous beads. A sample is passed through the column, and particles are separated based on their hydrodynamic radius. Larger particles are unable to enter the pores and elute first, while smaller particles like exosomes enter the beads, increasing their path length and delaying their elution. This method provides a cleaner and more intact preparation than UC, as it separates exosomes from contaminating protein aggregates. It is also a very gentle method but can be difficult to scale for large sample volumes and has relatively low throughput (Clos-Sansalvador et al., 2022).

2.2. Density Gradient Ultracentrifugation

This method is often used after a pre-enrichment step to achieve very high purity. The sample is layered on a continuous or discontinuous density gradient (e.g., sucrose or iodixanol). During ultracentrifugation, particles separate and sediment to a position that matches their density. Since exosomes have a characteristic density of 1.13–1.19 g/mL, this method allows for a highly specific separation. While excellent for obtaining high purity exosomes and for analytical purposes, it is very time-consuming, labor-intensive, and not suitable for large-scale therapeutic production. (Konoshenko et al., 2018).

3. Immunoaffinity-Based Isolation

This is the most specific isolation method, relying on the unique surface markers of exosomes. Antibodies against common exosome markers, such as tetraspanins (CD9, CD63, CD81), are immobilized on a solid support, such as magnetic beads or a chromatography column. The exosome-containing sample is passed over the support, allowing for specific binding and capture. Unbound contaminants are washed away, and the exosomes are then eluted. This method provides the highest purity, allowing for the isolation of specific exosome subpopulations but can have a low yield, as not all exosomes express the chosen markers. The elution step can also be harsh, potentially damaging the exosomes. This method is also expensive (Khanabdali et al., 2024).

4. Polymer-Based Precipitation

This method uses polymers, such as polyethylene glycol (PEG), to precipitate exosomes out of solution. Mechanism is based on adding a polymer to the sample "crowds out" the exosomes, reducing their solubility and causing them to aggregate and precipitate at the bottom of the tube. It is a fast, simple, and relatively inexpensive method that does not require specialized equipment. But it yields a very impure preparation, as the polymer precipitates proteins and other large non-exosomal particles along with the exosomes. This method is generally not recommended for therapeutic applications (Marzouk et al., 2025).

5. Ultrafiltration and Tangential Flow Filtration (TFF)

Membrane-based ultrafiltration relies on size-selective membranes to concentrate and purify exosomes. Typically, 100 kDa molecular weight cut-off (MWCO) filters are used. TFF offers better scalability and reproducibility than batch ultrafiltration and is frequently used in large-scale GMP-compliant exosome manufacturing. However, membrane clogging and vesicle loss can occur, necessitating optimization (Kim et al., 2024).

6. Microfluidic Technologies

Microfluidic platforms integrate immunoaffinity, filtration, and electrophoresis techniques on chip-scale devices for rapid exosome isolation. These are ideal for diagnostic or point-of-care applications and allow single-vesicle analysis. However, their throughput is currently insufficient for therapeutic-scale production. In clinical and GMP settings, tangential flow filtration combined with SEC or density gradient ultracentrifugation is commonly employed to achieve a balance between yield, purity, and scalability (Raju et al., 2022).

Engineering Exosomes for Gene Delivery

While exosomes naturally possess several features that make them attractive carriers for gene delivery—such as nanoscale size, biocompatibility, and intrinsic ability to transport RNA between cells—their native properties are not always sufficient to meet therapeutic needs. Engineering exosomes for gene delivery involves modifying their content and surface to improve their therapeutic efficacy. The primary goals of exosome engineering are to enhance cargo loading efficiency, improve targeted delivery to specific cells or tissues, and increase their stability and circulation time in the body (L. Li et al., 2025). Exosome engineering can broadly be categorized into two main strategies: the modification of donor cells prior to exosome production (endogenous engineering) and direct modification of exosomes after isolation (exogenous engineering) (Chen et al., 2024).

Endogenous loading, or pre-loading, is a sophisticated method of engineering exosomes by modifying their parent cells before the exosomes are secreted. This approach takes advantage of the cell's natural biogenesis and cargo sorting mechanisms to ensure the therapeutic genetic material is efficiently packaged. Parental cells are genetically or chemically manipulated to influence the characteristics of the exosomes they produce. This is often achieved by transfecting donor cells with plasmids encoding the nucleic acids or proteins of interest (X. Wang et al., 2024). For instance, to enhance RNA cargo loading, cells may be engineered to overexpress therapeutic mRNAs, microRNAs, or short interfering RNAs (siRNAs), which are then selectively packaged into exosomes through naturally occurring sorting pathways. These include RNA-binding proteins such as hnRNPA2B1 and YBX1, which recognize specific sequence motifs and facilitate the incorporation of RNA into exosomal lumens (Fabbiano et al., 2020). Moreover, fusing the cargo molecules with protein domains known to be enriched in exosomes—such as the C1C2 domain of lactadherin or the N-terminus of Lamp2b—has been shown to significantly enhance their exosomal loading efficiency (Choi et al., 2022).

Targeting specificity is another major focus of exosome engineering. Although exosomes display some degree of natural tropism based on their cell of origin, this property is typically insufficient for selective delivery to specific tissues or pathological sites *in vivo*. To overcome this limitation, membrane proteins on exosomes can be modified to include targeting ligands (He et al., 2022; L. Li et al., 2025). One well-characterized method involves the fusion of targeting peptides to exosomal membrane proteins such as Lamp2b. For example, Alvarez-Erviti and colleagues demonstrated that dendritic cell-derived exosomes engineered to express Lamp2b fused to a rabies virus glycoprotein (RVG) peptide could specifically deliver siRNA across the blood-brain barrier to neurons, microglia, and oligodendrocytes in mice—a significant milestone in targeted central nervous system (CNS) gene delivery (Alvarez-Erviti et al., 2011).

Exogenous engineering, in contrast, refers to the direct modification of exosomes after they have been isolated from producer cells. This strategy offers the advantage of flexibility, as it allows researchers to work with already-purified vesicles, avoiding the need for donor cell genetic manipulation (Sadeghi et al., 2023). Various physical and chemical techniques have been employed to load genetic cargo into exosomes post-isolation (Luan et al., 2017).

These include electroporation, which uses short electrical pulses to create temporary pores in the exosomal membrane, facilitating the entry of negatively charged molecules such as siRNAs or plasmid DNA. By applying an electrical current to exosomes suspended in a conductive solution, the phospholipid bilayer is disrupted, forming small, temporary openings. This process enables drugs or nucleotides to diffuse into the exosome's interior. After the loading is complete, the exosome membrane's integrity is restored. This method is particularly effective for delivering larger molecules, like siRNA or miRNA, which are too big to spontaneously enter the exosome on their own. In fact, electroporation has shown superior loading efficiency for siRNA compared to chemical transfection methods. Despite its effectiveness, electroporation can cause RNA aggregation and lead to exosome instability, which can limit the amount of cargo that can be loaded. To mitigate these issues, researchers have found that using optimized buffers, such as trehalose disaccharide, can help preserve the structural integrity of exosomes and prevent aggregation (Zeng et al., 2023). Alternative methods such as sonication, extrusion, or saponin-mediated membrane permeabilization have also been developed. Each of these techniques aims to transiently disrupt the exosomal membrane, enabling cargo diffusion into the vesicle lumen (Luan et al., 2017).

The sonication method uses a probe sonicator to apply ultrasonic energy. The sound waves generate mechanical forces and cavitation (the formation and rapid collapse of tiny bubbles) that disrupt the exosome's lipid bilayer. This disruption creates transient, microscopic pores in the membrane. The therapeutic cargo, which is in the solution, can then diffuse through these temporary openings into the exosome's core. After the sonication is stopped, the exosome membrane's integrity is restored, trapping the cargo inside. The process is often performed in an ice bath to prevent damage from heat generated by the sonication (Fu et al., 2020; Lai et al., 2025).

Extrusion is a mechanical method for loading therapeutic cargo into exosomes by forcing them through porous membranes. This process is designed to disrupt the exosome membrane and facilitate the mixing of the cargo and the exosomes. In this method, exosomes and the desired drug or nucleic acid are mixed and then passed through a syringe-based lipid extruder containing porous membranes, typically with pore sizes between 100 and 400 nanometers. As the mixture is forced through the tiny pores, the intense mechanical pressure and shear forces disrupt the exosome membranes. This allows the therapeutic cargo to become encapsulated within the exosomes as the membranes re-form (Zeng et al., 2023).

The freeze-thaw cycle method is a straightforward technique for loading genetic material into exosomes. The process involves first incubating exosomes with the desired cargo at room temperature. The mixture is then subjected to rapid freezing, typically at -80°C or in liquid nitrogen, followed by thawing at room temperature. This cycle is usually repeated at least three times to ensure the cargo is encapsulated within the exosomes (Nowak et al., 2023).

Chemical approaches like copper-catalyzed azide alkyne cycloaddition, known as click chemistry, have been employed for covalent attachment of targeting ligands, imaging agents, or nucleic acids to the exosomal surface or interior, thereby expanding the functional utility of these vesicles (Mukerjee et al., 2025). Moreover, recent innovations in bio-orthogonal labeling and lipid fusion techniques have allowed for the integration of synthetic liposomes or nanoparticles with exosomes, creating hybrid systems that combine the strengths of biological and synthetic platforms (Rodriguez & Vader, 2022).

Despite these advances, several challenges persist in exosome engineering. One major hurdle is the limited standardization and scalability of loading techniques, particularly for clinical-grade production. Electroporation and chemical transfection may affect exosome integrity or introduce residual contaminants that are difficult to remove. Furthermore, the efficiency of cargo incorporation and the stability of the loaded material can vary widely depending on the size, polarity, and secondary structure of the nucleic acids being delivered. Another concern is the potential alteration of surface protein profiles during engineering, which may inadvertently affect biodistribution or immunogenicity (Kimiz-Gebologlu & Oncel, 2022; Pan et al., 2023).

Table 2. Exosome Cargo Loading Methods for Gene Therapy

Loading Method	Mechanism	Cargo Type	Advantages	Limitations
Parental Cell Engineering	Transfecting donor cells to endogenously package genetic material	miRNA, mRNA, proteins	Biologically relevant, stable incorporation	Low efficiency, indirect control over cargo
Electroporation	Electric field-induced pore formation	siRNA, miRNA, mRNA, CRISPR	Widely used, relatively efficient for small RNAs	RNA aggregation, possible damage to exosome structure
Sonication	Membrane disruption by ultrasound waves	siRNA, mRNA, protein	Higher loading than electroporation	Membrane deformation, protein denaturation
Extrusion	Forceful passage through filters	Plasmid DNA, RNA, proteins	Uniform size distribution	Physicochemical alteration of vesicles
Saponin Permeabilization	Pore formation using saponin	Small RNAs, drugs	Gentle, scalable	Potential toxicity if not removed
Transfection Reagents	Lipid-mediated fusion or endocytosis	siRNA, mRNA, plasmid DNA	Convenient, reproducible	Chemical contaminants, variable efficiency
Freeze-Thaw Cycles	Physical membrane disruption	Various (RNAs, proteins)	Simple, no reagents required	Low reproducibility, aggregation

Therapeutic Cargos Delivered by Exosomes

Exosomes have proven to be highly effective vehicles for delivering a wide range of therapeutic cargos, particularly for gene therapy applications. Their intrinsic ability to carry nucleic acids and proteins between cells, coupled with their biocompatibility and capacity to evade immune detection, make them ideal candidates for the delivery of genetic materials (J. Li et al., 2025). This section explores in detail six major classes of cargos that have been successfully loaded into exosomes: siRNAs, miRNAs, mRNAs, antisense oligonucleotides (ASOs), plasmid/minicircle DNA, and CRISPR/Cas9 systems.

Messenger RNA (mRNA) represents a powerful platform for transient gene expression, allowing for therapeutic protein production without altering the host genome. Unlike DNA-based therapies, mRNA does not require nuclear localization for expression and avoids the risk of insertional mutagenesis, making it a safer modality for clinical translation (Aslan et al., 2021). However, free mRNA is unstable and susceptible to degradation by extracellular RNases. Exosomes offer a protective environment that enhances the stability of mRNA and facilitates its delivery to the cytoplasm of target cells, where translation can occur efficiently. Endogenous packaging of mRNA into exosomes occurs via mechanisms involving specific 3′-UTR motifs and binding proteins such as YBX1 and FMR1. Additionally, donor cells can be engineered to overexpress therapeutic mRNAs, which are then naturally sorted into exosomes (Iqbal et al., 2024). For example, Haney et al. reported the successful delivery of catalase mRNA via exosomes to neurons and microglia, resulting in reduced oxidative stress in a Parkinson's disease model (Haney et al., 2015). Similar approaches have been used to deliver mRNA encoding brain-derived neurotrophic factor (BDNF), VEGF, and other therapeutics. As the success of mRNA vaccines against SARS-CoV-2 has demonstrated, mRNA is a potent therapeutic cargo, and exosomes may help extend its applications to new frontiers (Gote et al., 2023).

MicroRNAs (miRNAs) are small, non-coding RNA molecules (~22 nucleotides) that regulate gene expression by binding to the 3' untranslated regions (3' UTRs) of target mRNAs, leading to translational repression or mRNA degradation. miRNAs play critical roles in regulating cell proliferation, differentiation, immune responses, and apoptosis. Dysregulation of specific miRNAs has been linked to the pathogenesis of cancer, cardiovascular disease, autoimmune disorders, and neurodegeneration (O'Brien et al., 2018). Exosomes are natural carriers of miRNAs and mediate intercellular communication in both physiological and pathological contexts. The presence of RNA-binding proteins such as hnRNPA2B1, YBX1, and SYNCRIP facilitates selective miRNA sorting into exosomes (Fabbiano et al., 2020). In therapeutic applications, exosomes can be engineered to deliver specific miRNAs to alter gene expression in target cells. For example, exosomes enriched in miR-126 have been used to restore endothelial function and promote angiogenesis in ischemic heart disease models (Moeinabadi-Bidgoli et al., 2023). In neurodegenerative disease models such as Huntington's disease, exosomal miR-124 delivery has demonstrated neuroprotective effects (Lee et al., 2017), while exosomal miR-21 and miR-146a have shown anti-inflammatory and anti-fibrotic activities in lung and liver injury models (Lang et al., 2023). These examples underscore the utility of exosomes as both diagnostic biomarkers and delivery tools for miRNA-based therapeutics.

Small interfering RNAs (siRNAs) are double-stranded RNA molecules approximately 20–25 nucleotides in length that mediate post-transcriptional gene silencing through the RNA interference (RNAi) pathway. After cellular uptake, siRNAs are incorporated into the RNA-induced silencing complex (RISC), where they guide the complex to degrade target messenger RNAs (mRNAs) with sequence complementarity, effectively reducing gene expression (Hu et al., 2020). Despite their therapeutic potential, siRNAs are vulnerable to rapid degradation in the bloodstream, and efficient intracellular delivery remains a major challenge. Exosomes have emerged as natural delivery vehicles capable of overcoming these limitations. Their lipid bilayer structure protects siRNAs from nuclease degradation and facilitates their endocytosis by recipient cells (Shahabipour et al., 2016). Exosomes derived from mesenchymal stem cells (MSCs), dendritic cells, or cancer cells have been successfully loaded with siRNAs targeting genes involved in oncogenesis, inflammation, or fibrosis. A prominent example is the use of exosomes loaded with siRNAs against the oncogenic KRAS^G12D^ mutation in pancreatic ductal adenocarcinoma (PDAC) (Kalluri et al., 2025). Researchers demonstrated that these exosomes selectively delivered siRNA to tumor tissues and effectively suppressed KRAS expression in vivo, reducing tumor burden without apparent toxicity. Such results illustrate the potential of exosome-siRNA therapies as a safer alternative to synthetic nanoparticles or viral vectors.

Antisense oligonucleotides (ASOs) are short, chemically modified single-stranded DNA or RNA molecules that bind to complementary RNA targets, modulating gene expression by blocking translation, altering splicing, or inducing RNase H-mediated degradation (Collotta et al., 2023). Several ASO therapies have been approved for genetic disorders such as spinal muscular atrophy (e.g., nusinersen) and Duchenne muscular dystrophy (e.g., eteplirsen) (Krey-Grauert et al., 2025). Despite their therapeutic promise, ASOs face limitations related to poor cellular uptake, off-target effects, and rapid renal clearance. Exosomes offer a promising solution by encapsulating ASOs within their lipid bilayer, which protects the cargo and enhances intracellular delivery (Fu et al., 2020). *In vitro* and *in vivo* studies have shown that exosome-mediated ASO delivery leads to higher bioavailability and sustained gene knockdown compared to free oligonucleotides (Yang et al., 2021). Recent preclinical efforts have focused on optimizing ASO loading into exosomes through electroporation, chemical transfection, or by engineering donor cells. For example, exosomes carrying ASOs targeting exon 51 of the dystrophin gene have been proposed as a treatment strategy for Duchenne muscular dystrophy, offering a non-immunogenic and targeted delivery alternative (Oppeneer et al., 2025).

DNA vectors, including plasmids and minicircles, are widely used for gene therapy because they enable sustained expression of therapeutic genes. Minicircles, which are derived from plasmids but lack bacterial backbone sequences, offer improved transgene expression and reduced immunogenicity. However, delivering large, negatively charged DNA molecules across the plasma membrane and into the nucleus remains a formidable challenge (Do et al., 2025). Exosomes provide a biocompatible platform for non-viral DNA delivery. Several studies have demonstrated the successful incorporation of plasmid or minicircle DNA into exosomes using electroporation, lipofection, or calcium chloride precipitation. Once internalized by target cells, the DNA must be released from endosomes and trafficked to the nucleus to achieve expression. While the efficiency of exosome-mediated DNA transfection is currently lower than that of viral vectors, the significantly reduced risk of insertional mutagenesis and immune activation makes this strategy highly attractive (Wallen et al., 2023). Advanced approaches are exploring the use of nuclear localization signals, exosome–liposome hybrids, or exosome surface modification with cell-penetrating peptides to enhance the efficiency of DNA vector delivery. These innovations may eventually make exosome-based DNA therapy a viable clinical alternative for diseases requiring long-term gene expression (Lee et al., 2025).

The CRISPR/Cas9 system has revolutionized the field of genome editing due to its unprecedented precision, efficiency, and programmability. Derived from the adaptive immune defense mechanism of *Streptococcus pyogenes*, CRISPR (Clustered Regularly Interspaced Short Palindromic Repeats) functions through the Cas9 endonuclease, which is guided by a short RNA molecule—known as a guide RNA (gRNA)—to introduce double-strand breaks (DSBs) at specific genomic loci. These DSBs are then repaired by the host cell through either non-homologous end joining (NHEJ) or homology-directed repair (HDR), leading to targeted gene disruption or sequence correction (Li et al., 2023). Despite its transformative potential, the delivery of CRISPR/Cas9 components into target cells remains one of the biggest challenges limiting its therapeutic application. Exosomes have emerged as a promising non-viral delivery system for CRISPR/Cas9 gene editing tools, combining biocompatibility with efficient cargo transfer and the ability to cross physiological barriers (Sanadgol et al.). A number of strategies exist for loading exosomes with CRISPR/Cas9 components, each with its own advantages. One of the most straightforward methods involves packaging Cas9 messenger RNA (mRNA) and a separate guide RNA (gRNA) into the exosomes. Once delivered to a target cell's cytoplasm, the Cas9 mRNA is translated into a protein that then complexes with the gRNA to initiate gene editing (Dara et al., 2024). A different, often preferred, strategy is to deliver a pre-assembled Cas9 ribonucleoprotein (RNP) complex, which consists of the Cas9 protein already bound to its gRNA. This approach provides immediate and transient gene editing, significantly reducing the risk of off-target effects that can occur with prolonged nuclease activity (S. Zhang et al., 2021). While less common due to safety concerns, it's also possible to load exosomes with plasmid DNA that contains the genetic instructions for both the Cas9 protein and the gRNA. This method is less favored because the plasmid must travel to the nucleus and has the potential to integrate into the host cell's genome, which can lead to unpredictable changes.

To improve the efficiency of CRISPR/Cas9 loading and targeting, exosome engineering has been employed. For instance, fusion of exosomal membrane proteins (like CD63 or Lamp2b) with Cas9-binding peptides or RNA-binding motifs has enabled selective packaging of genome-editing components (Bahadorani et al., 2024). One notable application involved exosomes delivering CRISPR components to silence oncogenic *KRAS* in pancreatic cancer models, resulting in significant tumor suppression (McAndrews et al., 2021). While issues such as loading efficiency and off-target effects remain, exosome-mediated CRISPR delivery represents a cutting-edge approach for the treatment of cardiovascular, neurological, renal, genetic, optical, and stem cell, as well as blood disorders and muscular degeneration (Aslan et al., 2024).

Quality Control and Characterization of Exosomes

Ensuring the identity, purity, potency, and safety of exosomes is essential for their application in gene therapy. According to the MISEV 2018 guidelines, a comprehensive quality control framework is required to verify that isolated extracellular vesicles (EVs) are indeed exosomes and to confirm that they possess the expected physicochemical and functional properties (Saint-Pol & Culot, 2025). The first step in exosome characterization involves determining their size distribution and particle concentration. This is commonly achieved using techniques such as nanoparticle tracking analysis (NTA), dynamic light scattering (DLS), or tunable resistive pulse sensing (TRPS). Exosomes typically fall within the 30–150 nm range, with a peak around 100 nm in diameter. NTA not only allows visualization of Brownian motion but also quantifies vesicle concentration in particles per milliliter, a crucial parameter for dosage standardization in therapeutic applications (Wu et al., 2024).

To confirm their morphology, transmission electron microscopy (TEM) or cryo-electron microscopy (Cryo-EM) is used to visualize the characteristic cup-shaped or spherical structures of exosomes. These imaging methods help differentiate exosomes from other membrane fragments or non-vesicular contaminants. Additionally, atomic force microscopy (AFM) can be used to examine topographical and mechanical features of vesicles, though it is less frequently applied in routine quality assessments (Dilsiz, 2024). Another critical component of exosome validation is the identification of specific surface and internal markers. Canonical exosome proteins such as CD63, CD81, and CD9 are typically detected by Western blot, flow cytometry, or immunocapture-based mass spectrometry. Internal markers such as TSG101 and Alix are also used to confirm endosomal origin (Akdeniz et al., 2025). To ensure purity, negative markers like calnexin (endoplasmic reticulum) and GM130 (Golgi) are simultaneously assessed, since their absence suggests minimal contamination by cellular organelles or debris. Mass Spectrometry offers a more comprehensive approach to proteomic analysis, identifying both positive markers and potential contaminants from the isolation process (Chavda et al., 2023).

Exosomes intended for gene delivery must also be analyzed for nucleic acid and protein cargo content. RNA analysis is often conducted using qRT-PCR, Bioanalyzer, or RNA sequencing, providing information about the presence and integrity of therapeutic mRNA, siRNA, or miRNA cargo (Miceli et al., 2024). On the protein side, liquid chromatography–mass spectrometry (LC-MS/MS) offers in-depth characterization of the proteome and helps evaluate whether bioactive or immune-modulatory molecules are present (Bi et al., 2025). Bicinchoninic Acid Assay (BCA) is a common method for measuring the total protein concentration in a sample. The ratio of the number of particles (from NTA or TRPS) to the amount of total protein is a useful indicator of purity, with a higher ratio suggesting fewer protein contaminants (Escudero-Cernuda et al., 2025). Importantly, exosomes must undergo functional assays to validate their therapeutic efficacy and confirm that the intended genetic modifications are achieved. These assays may include *in vitro* gene knockdown, protein expression, cytokine release, or cell migration analyses, depending on the therapeutic context. Such evaluations are vital to demonstrate biological activity after exosome loading and target cell uptake (Nguyen et al., 2020). For clinical applications, exosomes must also be confirmed to be sterile and endotoxin-free. Sterility is assessed by conventional microbiological tests, while endotoxin levels are measured using the Limulus Amebocyte Lysate (LAL) assay. Exosomes prepared for human administration are required to have endotoxin levels below accepted regulatory thresholds to avoid inflammatory responses (Mendt et al., 2018).

Overall, exosome characterization is not a single-step process but a multilayered assessment of physical properties, molecular signatures, and biological functions. Quality control must be performed both before and after therapeutic cargo loading to ensure that the engineering process does not compromise exosome integrity, cargo stability, or targeting ability. Only through such rigorous profiling can exosomes be reliably translated from bench to bedside as gene delivery vectors (Chen & Li, 2025).

Applications of Exosomes in Gene Therapy

The unique biological properties of exosomes -including their low immunogenicity, natural targeting, and ability to traverse biological barriers- have positioned them as a versatile and potent delivery platform for gene therapy across a wide spectrum of diseases. Their application is rapidly expanding, with ongoing research demonstrating their efficacy in delivering various therapeutic cargoes, from single genes to complex RNA molecules (Chen et al., 2021).

1. Exosomes in Cancer Gene Therapy

Exosomes are being explored in cancer gene therapy through two primary strategies: direct delivery of therapeutic genes to kill malignant cells and modulation of the tumor microenvironment to inhibit growth and metastasis (Javdani-Mallak et al., 2025).

Therapeutic Gene and Suicide Gene Delivery: Exosomes can be engineered to deliver tumor suppressor genes, such as the p53 gene, which is frequently mutated in human cancers. By packaging and delivering functional p53 mRNA or plasmid DNA to tumor cells, exosomes can restore a cell's ability to undergo apoptosis by activating key downstream pathways like Bax and Bak (Cesur-Ergun & Demir-Dora, 2023). Another powerful approach involves delivering suicide genes that convert a non-toxic prodrug into a toxic compound, leading to localized cell death. For example, exosomes derived from mesenchymal stem cells have been successfully engineered to carry the gene for TRAIL (Tumor Necrosis Factor-Related Apoptosis-Inducing Ligand), which selectively induces programmed cell death by activating its death receptors (DR4 and DR5) on the surface of cancer cells without harming healthy tissue (Shamili et al., 2018).

RNA Interference (RNAi) Therapy: Exosomes are highly effective carriers for RNAi-based therapeutics, offering a way to silence oncogenes or genes that confer drug resistance (Chen et al., 2018). For example, exosomes can be loaded with specific microRNAs (miRNAs), such as miR-143 and miR-145, which are known to be downregulated in various cancers. Delivering these miRNAs can inhibit key oncogenic pathways by targeting genes like KRAS and MYC, reversing drug resistance and sensitizing tumor cells to conventional chemotherapy (Wang et al., 2025). Additionally, exosomes can be engineered to deliver small interfering RNAs (siRNAs) to silence genes like Bcl-2, an anti-apoptotic protein often overexpressed in cancer, thereby promoting cell death and improving treatment efficacy (Zhang et al., 2025).

2. Exosomes in Neurodegenerative Diseases

The ability of exosomes to efficiently cross the blood-brain barrier (BBB)—a highly restrictive barrier that prevents the vast majority of drugs and gene therapy vectors from reaching the central nervous system—makes them an exceptional platform for treating neurodegenerative disorders. The proposed mechanisms for their BBB penetration include transcytosis and direct fusion with the brain endothelial cells (Ramos-Zaldivar et al., 2022).

Delivery of Neurotrophic Factors: Exosomes can be engineered to carry genes encoding crucial neurotrophic factors that support neuronal survival and function (Dehghani et al., 2025). For example, in Parkinson's disease, which is characterized by the loss of dopamine-producing neurons, exosomes can deliver the gene for Glial Cell-Derived Neurotrophic Factor (GDNF). The delivered GDNF can then be expressed in brain cells, promoting the survival and maintenance of dopaminergic neurons in the substantia nigra. Similarly, the delivery of the gene for Brain-Derived Neurotrophic Factor (BDNF) via exosomes holds immense promise for treating Alzheimer's disease by promoting neuronal health and synaptic plasticity (Yang et al., 2025).

Gene Silencing: Exosomes are an ideal vehicle for delivering nucleic acids to silence genes responsible for the toxic protein aggregation that is a hallmark of many neurodegenerative disorders. For instance, in Huntington's disease, which is caused by a mutant huntingtin gene, exosomes can be loaded with siRNAs to specifically reduce the expression of the mutant allele in brain cells. This approach aims to lower the production of the toxic huntingtin protein, potentially halting or reversing disease progression. Research has even shown that exosomes can be surface-modified with a RVG peptide to enhance their specific targeting of neurons (Nouri et al., 2024; L. Zhang et al., 2021).

3. Exosomes in Regenerative Medicine and Tissue Repair

Exosomes are a natural vehicle for tissue regeneration, carrying a cargo of pro-regenerative molecules. This function can be amplified by engineering them to deliver specific genes to injured tissues (McMullan et al., 2025).

Cardiac Repair: Following a myocardial infarction (heart attack), the delivery of pro-angiogenic genes is critical for restoring blood flow to damaged cardiac tissue. Exosomes can be loaded with plasmids encoding Vascular Endothelial Growth Factor (VEGF-A) or Hepatocyte Growth Factor (HGF). Upon delivery, these exosomes promote the formation of new blood vessels (angiogenesis) and reduce fibrotic scarring, leading to improved oxygen supply to cardiomyocytes and enhanced cardiac function (Chae et al., 2025).

Bone and Cartilage Regeneration: Exosomes can be utilized to deliver genes for growth factors essential for bone and cartilage repair (Huber et al., 2022). For example, the genes for Bone Morphogenetic Protein 2 (BMP-2) and BMP-7 can be packaged into exosomes. Upon delivery to a fracture site, these exosomes promote the differentiation of mesenchymal stem cells into osteoblasts (bone-forming cells) and inhibit osteoclast activity, thereby accelerating bone healing and regeneration (Du et al., 2025).

4. Exosomes for Immune Modulation

Exosomes are not merely passive delivery vehicles; they are intrinsic players in the body's immune system, constantly mediating communication between immune cells and other cell types. This inherent biological function can be therapeutically harnessed to either suppress an overactive immune response or to boost an anti-tumor immune response, positioning them as a promising tool for treating a wide array of immune-related diseases (Zou et al., 2021).

Exosomes as Immunosuppressants for Autoimmune Diseases: In autoimmune diseases, the immune system attacks the body's own tissues, leading to chronic inflammation and tissue damage. Conventional immunosuppressants often have broad, systemic side effects (Song et al., 2025). Exosomes offer a targeted alternative by delivering a payload of anti-inflammatory and tolerogenic molecules to modulate the immune response locally. The immunosuppressive potential of exosomes is largely derived from those secreted by mesenchymal stem cells (MSCs) and tolerogenic dendritic cells (tDCs). These exosomes can actively suppress the proliferation of pro-inflammatory effector T-cells (Th1 and Th17) and promote the differentiation of regulatory T-cells (Tregs), which are crucial for maintaining self-tolerance (Yi et al., 2025). The mechanisms of this effect are multifaceted and may be through protein and cytokine delivery or miRNA-mediated gene regulation.

Protein and Cytokine Delivery: Exosomes can transfer immunosuppressive proteins, such as Fas ligand (FasL) and Programmed Death-Ligand 1 (PD-L1), to T-cells. The interaction between FasL on the exosome and its receptor on activated T-cells can trigger apoptosis, thus eliminating the T-cells responsible for the autoimmune attack. Similarly, the PD-L1 on exosomes can bind to the PD-1 receptor on T-cells, leading to T-cell inactivation and anergy (Li et al., 2022; Wang & Shi, 2022).

miRNA-Mediated Gene Regulation: Exosomes carry a rich cargo of microRNAs (miRNAs) that can reprogram immune cells. For example, exosomes from MSCs have been shown to transfer miR-155 to dendritic cells, which subsequently reduces their pro-inflammatory cytokine production (Nail et al., 2023). Conversely, exosomes can deliver miRNAs that upregulate anti-inflammatory pathways. The transfer of genes encoding key anti-inflammatory cytokines, such as Interleukin-10 (IL-10) and Transforming Growth Factor-beta (TGF-β), via exosomes can also be used to locally dampen the immune response at the site of inflammation, as seen in models of rheumatoid arthritis and inflammatory bowel disease (Y. Wang et al., 2024).

Exosomes as Immunostimulants in Cancer Immunotherapy: The use of exosomes in cancer immunotherapy is a dynamic field, with two main strategies emerging: using native tumor-derived exosomes and using engineered exosomes as vaccines (Cao et al., 2022).

Tumor-Derived Exosomes as Cancer Vaccines: Tumor cells naturally release exosomes that contain a variety of tumor-associated antigens (TAAs). While these native tumor exosomes often possess immunosuppressive properties that help the tumor evade the immune system, they can be modified to become potent immunostimulants. By isolating these exosomes from a patient, they can be processed and loaded with immune-activating molecules. When re-administered, these modified exosomes can be taken up by antigen-presenting cells (APCs), such as dendritic cells. The APCs then process the tumor antigens and present them to cytotoxic T-cells, leading to a robust and targeted anti-tumor immune response (Jiale Li et al., 2025).

Engineered Exosomes for Targeted Immunotherapy: A more controlled approach involves engineering exosomes from non-cancerous cells to carry specific payloads. These exosomes can be loaded with specific tumor antigens to serve as a cellular-free vaccine platform. Additionally, they can be engineered to carry genes encoding immunostimulatory cytokines, such as Granulocyte-Macrophage Colony-Stimulating Factor (GM-CSF) or Interferon-gamma (IFN-γ). When these exosomes are administered, they are specifically taken up by APCs, which become activated and present the antigens to T-cells. This results in the proliferation of tumor-specific cytotoxic T-cells that can effectively seek out and destroy cancer cells. This method avoids the risks associated with using live cells for immunotherapy, such as off-target effects and potential toxicity (Liu et al., 2023; Lyu et al., 2024).

Advantages of Exosomes for Gene Therapy

The inherent biological properties of exosomes make them a highly promising and attractive alternative to conventional viral and synthetic gene delivery systems. Their advantages are multifaceted, addressing many of the limitations associated with existing methods and offering new possibilities for therapeutic applications (Rajput et al., 2022).

1. Low Immunogenicity and High Biocompatibility

A major limitation of viral vectors, particularly adeno-associated viruses (AAVs) and adenoviruses, is their potential to elicit a strong host immune response. The viral capsid proteins are recognized as foreign antigens, triggering both innate and adaptive immune responses. This can lead to the rapid clearance of the vector by macrophages and a significant risk of systemic inflammation. Furthermore, the development of neutralizing antibodies by B-cells limits the possibility of repeat dosing, as subsequent administrations of the same viral serotype become ineffective (Keeler et al., 2025). As naturally occurring vesicles secreted by the body's own cells, exosomes possess an intrinsic low immunogenicity. They are recognized by the immune system as part of the body's natural communication network, which allows them to circulate for longer periods in the bloodstream without triggering a significant inflammatory or adaptive immune response. This makes repeat dosing more feasible and significantly enhances their safety profile, a critical consideration for clinical translation (Araujo-Abad et al., 2025).

2. Natural Targeting and "Homing" Abilities

Unlike many synthetic nanoparticles that require complex surface modifications for targeted delivery, exosomes have a natural "homing" ability. The surface proteins on an exosome, such as integrins, tetraspanins, and various adhesion molecules, facilitate their selective binding to specific receptors on the surface of recipient cells. This inherent tropism allows exosomes to be preferentially taken up by certain cell types, tissues, or even organs (He et al., 2022). For example, studies have shown that exosomes derived from a particular cancer cell line express a specific integrin that enables them to home to a metastatic site, such as the liver or lungs (Izraely & Witz, 2021). Similarly, exosomes from mesenchymal stem cells (MSCs) are enriched with surface markers that guide them to sites of inflammation and tissue damage (Abid et al., 2024). This natural targeting mechanism provides a significant advantage for delivering therapeutic genes to hard-to-reach or specific sites of disease without the need for extensive and potentially immunogenic surface engineering (He et al., 2022).

3. Ability to Cross Biological Barriers

Exosomes are uniquely suited to traverse biological barriers that are impermeable to most other delivery systems. Most notably, they have been shown to efficiently cross the blood-brain barrier (BBB), a highly restrictive barrier composed of tightly connected endothelial cells, astrocytes, and pericytes that prevents the vast majority of drugs and gene therapy vectors from reaching the central nervous system. The small size and unique membrane composition of exosomes are believed to facilitate their passage through the BBB via mechanisms such as transcytosis, or even direct fusion with the endothelial cell membrane. The ability of exosomes to bypass the BBB makes them an exceptional candidate for treating neurodegenerative diseases like Alzheimer's, Parkinson's, and Huntington's, as well as brain tumors like glioblastoma, for which effective delivery methods are desperately needed. Their unique characteristics also allow them to cross the blood-placenta barrier and the intestinal barrier, broadening their potential therapeutic reach for systemic or oral gene therapy applications (Nouri et al., 2024; Ravichandiran et al., 2024).

4. High Stability and Protection of Cargo

The lipid bilayer membrane of exosomes provides a robust protective shell for their fragile cargo, such as mRNA and other nucleic acids, from degradation by circulating enzymes (e.g., ribonucleases) in the bloodstream. The exosomal membrane is rich in specific lipids like sphingomyelin and cholesterol, which contribute to its structural integrity and resistance to enzymatic breakdown. This encapsulation ensures that the therapeutic genetic material remains intact and functional until it reaches the target cell (Skotland et al., 2017). In contrast, "naked" or poorly protected nucleic acids are quickly degraded in the extracellular environment, often within minutes, which severely limits their therapeutic efficacy. The stability of exosomes contributes to a longer half-life in circulation and a greater chance of successful delivery to the target site (Zeng et al., 2023).

5. Biocompatibility and Inherent Biological Function

Beyond simply acting as passive carriers, exosomes possess an inherent biological activity that can be therapeutically beneficial. The exosome itself is a biologically active particle that carries its own native cargo of proteins and nucleic acids, which can modulate the recipient cell's behavior. This creates a synergistic effect, where the exosome not only delivers a therapeutic gene but also contributes to the treatment through its native contents (Huang et al., 2023). For example, MSC-derived exosomes carry an array of anti-inflammatory and pro-regenerative proteins and miRNAs. When these exosomes are used to deliver a therapeutic gene for tissue repair, their native cargo can simultaneously reduce inflammation and stimulate cellular growth, thus enhancing the overall therapeutic outcome in a way that purely synthetic delivery systems cannot (Sadeghi et al., 2023).

References

Aakel, N., Mohammed, R., Fathima, A., Kerzabi, R., Abdallah, A., & Ibrahim, W. N. (2025). Role of Exosome in Solid Cancer Progression and Its Potential Therapeutics in Cancer Treatment. *Cancer Med*, *14*(9), e70941. https://doi.org/10.1002/cam4.70941

Abid, A. I., Conzatti, G., Toti, F., Anton, N., & Vandamme, T. (2024). Mesenchymal stem cell-derived exosomes as cell free nanotherapeutics and nanocarriers. *Nanomedicine*, *61*, 102769. https://doi.org/10.1016/j.nano.2024.102769

Ahmed, I., Akram, Z., Iqbal, H. M. N., & Munn, A. L. (2019). The regulation of Endosomal Sorting Complex Required for Transport and accessory proteins in multivesicular body sorting and enveloped viral budding - An overview. *Int J Biol Macromol*, *127*, 1-11. https://doi.org/10.1016/j.ijbiomac.2019.01.015

Akdeniz, M., Al-Shaebi, Z., & Aydin, O. (2025). A Solution for Exosome-Based Analysis: Surface-Enhanced Raman Spectroscopy and Artificial Intelligence. *Advanced Intelligent Discovery*, *n/a*(n/a), 202500040. https://doi.org/https://doi.org/10.1002/aidi.202500040

Alvarez-Erviti, L., Seow, Y., Yin, H., Betts, C., Lakhal, S., & Wood, M. J. (2011). Delivery of siRNA to the mouse brain by systemic injection of targeted exosomes. *Nat Biotechnol*, *29*(4), 341-345. https://doi.org/10.1038/nbt.1807

Araujo-Abad, S., Berna, J. M., Lloret-Lopez, E., Lopez-Cortes, A., Saceda, M., & de Juan Romero, C. (2025). Exosomes: from basic research to clinical diagnostic and therapeutic applications in cancer. *Cell Oncol (Dordr)*, *48*(2), 269-293. https://doi.org/10.1007/s13402-024-00990-2

Aslan, C., Kiaie, S. H., Zolbanin, N. M., Lotfinejad, P., Ramezani, R., Kashanchi, F., & Jafari, R. (2021). Exosomes for mRNA delivery: a novel biotherapeutic strategy with hurdles and hope. *BMC Biotechnol*, *21*(1), 20. https://doi.org/10.1186/s12896-021-00683-w

Aslan, C., Zolbanin, N. M., Faraji, F., & Jafari, R. (2024). Exosomes for CRISPR-Cas9 Delivery: The Cutting Edge in Genome Editing. *Mol Biotechnol*, *66*(11), 3092-3116. https://doi.org/10.1007/s12033-023-00932-7

Bahadorani, M., Nasiri, M., Dellinger, K., Aravamudhan, S., & Zadegan, R. (2024). Engineering Exosomes for Therapeutic Applications: Decoding Biogenesis, Content Modification, and Cargo Loading Strategies. *Int J Nanomedicine*, *19*, 7137-7164. https://doi.org/10.2147/IJN.S464249

Battistelli, M., & Falcieri, E. (2020). Apoptotic Bodies: Particular Extracellular Vesicles Involved in Intercellular Communication. *Biology (Basel)*, *9*(1). https://doi.org/10.3390/biology9010021
Bi, Y., Wang, L., Li, C., Shan, Z., & Bi, L. (2025). Unveiling exosomal biomarkers in neurodegenerative diseases: LC-MS-based profiling. *Extracellular Vesicle*, *5*, 100071. https://doi.org/https://doi.org/10.1016/j.vesic.2025.100071
Cao, Y., Xu, P., Shen, Y., Wu, W., Chen, M., Wang, F., Zhu, Y., Yan, F., Gu, W., & Lin, Y. (2022). Exosomes and cancer immunotherapy: A review of recent cancer research. *Front Oncol*, *12*, 1118101. https://doi.org/10.3389/fonc.2022.1118101
Cesur-Ergun, B., & Demir-Dora, D. (2023). Gene therapy in cancer. *J Gene Med*, *25*(11), e3550. https://doi.org/10.1002/jgm.3550
Cetin, B., Erendor, F., Eksi, Y. E., Sanlioglu, A. D., & Sanlioglu, S. (2024). Gene and cell therapy of human genetic diseases: Recent advances and future directions. *J Cell Mol Med*, *28*(17), e70056. https://doi.org/10.1111/jcmm.70056
Chae, C. W., Choi, G., Yoon, T., & Kwon, Y. W. (2025). Exosome-Based Therapy in Cardiovascular Diseases: A New Frontier in Cardiovascular Disease Treatment. *Korean Circ J*, *55*(6), 461-480. https://doi.org/10.4070/kcj.2025.0022
Chavda, V. P., Pandya, A., Kumar, L., Raval, N., Vora, L. K., Pulakkat, S., Patravale, V., Salwa, Duo, Y., & Tang, B. Z. (2023). Exosome nanovesicles: A potential carrier for therapeutic delivery. *Nano Today*, *49*, 101771. https://doi.org/https://doi.org/10.1016/j.nantod.2023.101771
Chen, H., & Li, Q. (2025). Recent advances in scalable exosome production: Challenges and innovations. *Chinese Journal of Plastic and Reconstructive Surgery*, *7*(3), 149-163. https://doi.org/https://doi.org/10.1016/j.cjprs.2025.05.001
Chen, H., Wang, L., Zeng, X., Schwarz, H., Nanda, H. S., Peng, X., & Zhou, Y. (2021). Exosomes, a New Star for Targeted Delivery. *Front Cell Dev Biol*, *9*, 751079. https://doi.org/10.3389/fcell.2021.751079
Chen, J., Zhang, G., Wan, Y., Xia, B., Ni, Q., Shan, S., Hu, Z., & Liang, X. J. (2023). Immune cell-derived exosomes as promising tools for cancer therapy. *J Control Release*, *364*, 508-528. https://doi.org/10.1016/j.jconrel.2023.11.003
Chen, X., Mangala, L. S., Rodriguez-Aguayo, C., Kong, X., Lopez-Berestein, G., & Sood, A. K. (2018). RNA interference-based therapy and its delivery systems. *Cancer Metastasis Rev*, *37*(1), 107-124. https://doi.org/10.1007/s10555-017-9717-6

Chen, Y., Qi, W., Wang, Z., & Niu, F. (2025). Exosome Source Matters: A Comprehensive Review from the Perspective of Diverse Cellular Origins. *Pharmaceutics*, *17*(2). https://doi.org/10.3390/pharmaceutics17020147

Chen, Z., Xiong, M., Tian, J., Song, D., Duan, S., & Zhang, L. (2024). Encapsulation and assessment of therapeutic cargo in engineered exosomes: a systematic review. *J Nanobiotechnology*, *22*(1), 18. https://doi.org/10.1186/s12951-023-02259-6

Choi, H., Yim, H., Park, C., Ahn, S. H., Ahn, Y., Lee, A., Yang, H., & Choi, C. (2022). Targeted Delivery of Exosomes Armed with Anti-Cancer Therapeutics. *Membranes (Basel)*, *12*(1). https://doi.org/10.3390/membranes12010085

Chongmelaxme, B., Yodsurang, V., Vichayachaipat, P., Srimatimanon, T., & Sanmaneechai, O. (2025). Gene-based therapy for the treatment of spinal muscular atrophy types 1 and 2 : a systematic review and meta-analysis. *Gene Ther*, *32*(4), 301-330. https://doi.org/10.1038/s41434-024-00503-8

Clos-Sansalvador, M., Monguio-Tortajada, M., Roura, S., Franquesa, M., & Borras, F. E. (2022). Commonly used methods for extracellular vesicles' enrichment: Implications in downstream analyses and use. *Eur J Cell Biol*, *101*(3), 151227. https://doi.org/10.1016/j.ejcb.2022.151227

Collotta, D., Bertocchi, I., Chiapello, E., & Collino, M. (2023). Antisense oligonucleotides: a novel Frontier in pharmacological strategy. *Front Pharmacol*, *14*, 1304342. https://doi.org/10.3389/fphar.2023.1304342

Cordonnier, M., Chanteloup, G., Isambert, N., Seigneuric, R., Fumoleau, P., Garrido, C., & Gobbo, J. (2017). Exosomes in cancer theranostic: Diamonds in the rough. *Cell Adh Migr*, *11*(2), 151-163. https://doi.org/10.1080/19336918.2016.1250999

Dara, M., Dianatpour, M., Azarpira, N., Tanideh, N., & Tanideh, R. (2024). Integrating CRISPR technology with exosomes: Revolutionizing gene delivery systems. *Biochem Biophys Res Commun*, *740*, 151002. https://doi.org/10.1016/j.bbrc.2024.151002

De Haan, P., Van Diemen, F. R., & Toscano, M. G. (2021). Viral gene delivery vectors: the next generation medicines for immune-related diseases. *Hum Vaccin Immunother*, *17*(1), 14-21. https://doi.org/10.1080/21645515.2020.1757989

Dehghani, S., Ocakci, O., Hatipoglu, P. T., Ozalp, V. C., & Tevlek, A. (2025). Exosomes as Biomarkers and Therapeutic Agents in Neurodegenerative Diseases: Current Insights and Future Directions. *Mol Neurobiol*, *62*(7), 9190-9215. https://doi.org/10.1007/s12035-025-04825-5

Dilsiz, N. (2024). A comprehensive review on recent advances in exosome isolation and characterization: Toward clinical applications. *Translational Oncology*, *50*, 102121. https://doi.org/https://doi.org/10.1016/j.tranon.2024.102121

Do, J., Verma, G., Maurice, Y., Abdumanobova, M., Deng, Z., Kalin, T. V., & Kalinichenko, V. V. (2025). Protocol for minicircle production for gene therapy without subsequent cleanup steps. *STAR Protoc*, *6*(3), 103982. https://doi.org/10.1016/j.xpro.2025.103982

Donoso-Quezada, J., Ayala-Mar, S., & González-Valdez, J. (2021). The role of lipids in exosome biology and intercellular communication: Function, analytics and applications. *Traffic (Copenhagen, Denmark)*, *22*. https://doi.org/10.1111/tra.12803

Doyle, L. M., & Wang, M. Z. (2019). Overview of Extracellular Vesicles, Their Origin, Composition, Purpose, and Methods for Exosome Isolation and Analysis. *Cells*, *8*(7). https://doi.org/10.3390/cells8070727

Du, Z., Rizzo, S. A., Sarrafian, T. L., Bagwell, M. S., Mahlberg, R. C., Amontree, A., Schiebel, P., Tauferner, D. M., LeBrasseur, Z. S., Witt, T. A., Nagel, M., Boyd, K. A., De Vitto, H., Hillestad, M. L., Stalboerger, P. G., Houdek, M. T., Sierra, R. J., & Behfar, A. (2025). Engineered BMP2/BMP7 extracellular vesicles induce autocrine BMP release driving SMAD phosphorylation to promote bone formation. *NPJ Regen Med*, *10*(1), 26. https://doi.org/10.1038/s41536-025-00405-2

Elsherbini, A., & Bieberich, E. (2018). Ceramide and Exosomes: A Novel Target in Cancer Biology and Therapy. *Adv Cancer Res*, *140*, 121-154. https://doi.org/10.1016/bs.acr.2018.05.004

Escudero-Cernuda, S., Eiro, N., Fraile, M., Vizoso, F. J., Fernandez-Colomer, B., & Fernandez-Sanchez, M. L. (2025). Limitations and challenges in the characterization of extracellular vesicles from stem cells and serum. *Mikrochim Acta*, *192*(5), 311. https://doi.org/10.1007/s00604-025-07147-4

Fabbiano, F., Corsi, J., Gurrieri, E., Trevisan, C., Notarangelo, M., & D'Agostino, V. G. (2020). RNA packaging into extracellular vesicles: An orchestra of RNA-binding proteins? *J Extracell Vesicles*, *10*(2), e12043. https://doi.org/10.1002/jev2.12043

Fazio, M., Stagno, F., Penna, G., Mirabile, G., & Allegra, A. (2025). Navigating the Landscape of Exosomal microRNAs: Charting Their Pivotal Role as Biomarkers in Hematological Malignancies. *Noncoding RNA*, *11*(5). https://doi.org/10.3390/ncrna11050064

Ferreira, D., Moreira, J. N., & Rodrigues, L. R. (2022). New advances in exosome-based targeted drug delivery systems. *Crit Rev Oncol Hematol*, *172*, 103628. https://doi.org/10.1016/j.critrevonc.2022.103628

Fu, S., Wang, Y., Xia, X., & Zheng, J. C. (2020). Exosome engineering: Current progress in cargo loading and targeted delivery. *NanoImpact*, *20*, 100261. https://doi.org/https://doi.org/10.1016/j.impact.2020.100261

Ghadami, S., & Dellinger, K. (2023). The lipid composition of extracellular vesicles: applications in diagnostics and therapeutic delivery. *Front Mol Biosci*, *10*, 1198044. https://doi.org/10.3389/fmolb.2023.1198044

Gote, V., Bolla, P. K., Kommineni, N., Butreddy, A., Nukala, P. K., Palakurthi, S. S., & Khan, W. (2023). A Comprehensive Review of mRNA Vaccines. *Int J Mol Sci*, *24*(3). https://doi.org/10.3390/ijms24032700

Gregory, C. D., & Rimmer, M. P. (2023). Extracellular vesicles arising from apoptosis: forms, functions, and applications. *J Pathol*, *260*(5), 592-608. https://doi.org/10.1002/path.6138

Haney, M. J., Klyachko, N. L., Zhao, Y., Gupta, R., Plotnikova, E. G., He, Z., Patel, T., Piroyan, A., Sokolsky, M., Kabanov, A. V., & Batrakova, E. V. (2015). Exosomes as drug delivery vehicles for Parkinson's disease therapy. *J Control Release*, *207*, 18-30. https://doi.org/10.1016/j.jconrel.2015.03.033

He, J., Ren, W., Wang, W., Han, W., Jiang, L., Zhang, D., & Guo, M. (2022). Exosomal targeting and its potential clinical application. *Drug Deliv Transl Res*, *12*(10), 2385-2402. https://doi.org/10.1007/s13346-021-01087-1

Henderson, M. L., Zieba, J. K., Li, X., Campbell, D. B., Williams, M. R., Vogt, D. L., Bupp, C. P., Edgerly, Y. M., Rajasekaran, S., Hartog, N. L., Prokop, J. W., & Krueger, J. M. (2024). Gene Therapy for Genetic Syndromes: Understanding the Current State to Guide Future Care. *BioTech (Basel)*, *13*(1). https://doi.org/10.3390/biotech13010001

Hu, B., Zhong, L., Weng, Y., Peng, L., Huang, Y., Zhao, Y., & Liang, X. J. (2020). Therapeutic siRNA: state of the art. *Signal Transduct Target Ther*, *5*(1), 101. https://doi.org/10.1038/s41392-020-0207-x

Huang, L., Wu, E., Liao, J., Wei, Z., Wang, J., & Chen, Z. (2023). Research Advances of Engineered Exosomes as Drug Delivery Carrier. *ACS Omega*, *8*(46), 43374-43387. https://doi.org/10.1021/acsomega.3c04479

Huber, J., Griffin, M. F., Longaker, M. T., & Quarto, N. (2022). Exosomes: A Tool for Bone Tissue Engineering. *Tissue Eng Part B Rev*, *28*(1), 101-113. https://doi.org/10.1089/ten.TEB.2020.0246

Iqbal, Z., Rehman, K., Mahmood, A., Shabbir, M., Liang, Y., Duan, L., & Zeng, H. (2024). Exosome for mRNA delivery: strategies and therapeutic applications. *J Nanobiotechnology*, *22*(1), 395. https://doi.org/10.1186/s12951-024-02634-x

Isaac, R., Reis, F. C. G., Ying, W., & Olefsky, J. M. (2021). Exosomes as mediators of intercellular crosstalk in metabolism. *Cell Metab*, *33*(9), 1744-1762. https://doi.org/10.1016/j.cmet.2021.08.006

Izraely, S., & Witz, I. P. (2021). Site-specific metastasis: A cooperation between cancer cells and the metastatic microenvironment. *Int J Cancer*, *148*(6), 1308-1322. https://doi.org/10.1002/ijc.33247

Janas, T., Janas, M. M., Sapon, K., & Janas, T. (2015). Mechanisms of RNA loading into exosomes. *FEBS Lett*, *589*(13), 1391-1398. https://doi.org/10.1016/j.febslet.2015.04.036

Jankovicova, J., Secova, P., Michalkova, K., & Antalikova, J. (2020). Tetraspanins, More than Markers of Extracellular Vesicles in Reproduction. *Int J Mol Sci*, *21*(20). https://doi.org/10.3390/ijms21207568

Javdani-Mallak, A., Mowla, S. J., & Alibolandi, M. (2025). Tumor-derived exosomes and their application in cancer treatment. *J Transl Med*, *23*(1), 751. https://doi.org/10.1186/s12967-025-06814-7

Kalluri, V. S., Smaglo, B. G., Mahadevan, K. K., Kirtley, M. L., McAndrews, K. M., Mendt, M., Yang, S., Maldonado, A. S., Sugimoto, H., Salvatierra, M. E., Solis Soto, L. M., Haymaker, C., Finch, R., Gagea, M., Fluty, A. C., Ludtke, S. J., Jack Lee, J., Jain, A. K., Varadhachary, G., . . . Kalluri, R. (2025). Engineered exosomes with Kras(G12D) specific siRNA in pancreatic cancer: a phase I study with immunological correlates. *Nat Commun*, *16*(1), 8696. https://doi.org/10.1038/s41467-025-63718-2

Keeler, A. M., Zhan, W., Ram, S., Fitzgerald, K. A., & Gao, G. (2025). The curious case of AAV immunology. *Mol Ther*, *33*(5), 1946-1965. https://doi.org/10.1016/j.ymthe.2025.03.037

Khan, M. (2024). Polymers as Efficient Non-Viral Gene Delivery Vectors: The Role of the Chemical and Physical Architecture of Macromolecules. *Polymers (Basel)*, *16*(18). https://doi.org/10.3390/polym16182629

Khanabdali, R., Mandrekar, M., Grygiel, R., Vo, P. A., Palma, C., Nikseresht, S., Barton, S., Shojaee, M., Bhuiyan, S., Asari, K., Belzer, S., Ansari, K., Coward, J. I., Perrin, L., Hooper, J., Guanzon, D., Lai, A., Salomon, C., Kershner, K., . . . Rice, G. (2024). High-throughput surface epitope immunoaffinity isolation of extracellular vesicles and downstream analysis. *Biol Methods Protoc*, *9*(1), bpae032. https://doi.org/10.1093/biomethods/bpae032

Kim, G., Kim, K.-H., Seo, M., Kim, T., & Chun, H. (2024). High-throughput exosome isolation based on bidirectional flow control through nanoporous membrane. *Sensors and Actuators B: Chemical*, *418*, 136233. https://doi.org/https://doi.org/10.1016/j.snb.2024.136233

Kimiz-Gebologlu, I., & Oncel, S. S. (2022). Exosomes: Large-scale production, isolation, drug loading efficiency, and biodistribution and uptake. *J Control Release*, *347*, 533-543. https://doi.org/10.1016/j.jconrel.2022.05.027

Kolat, D., Hammouz, R., Bednarek, A. K., & Pluciennik, E. (2019). Exosomes as carriers transporting long non-coding RNAs: Molecular characteristics and their function in cancer (Review). *Mol Med Rep*, *20*(2), 851-862. https://doi.org/10.3892/mmr.2019.10340

Komori, T., & Fukuda, M. (2024). Two roads diverged in a cell: insights from differential exosome regulation in polarized cells. *Front Cell Dev Biol*, *12*, 1451988. https://doi.org/10.3389/fcell.2024.1451988

Konoshenko, M. Y., Lekchnov, E. A., Vlassov, A. V., & Laktionov, P. P. (2018). Isolation of Extracellular Vesicles: General Methodologies and Latest Trends. *Biomed Res Int*, *2018*, 8545347. https://doi.org/10.1155/2018/8545347

Krey-Grauert, I., Ferro, I., & Wagner, M. (2025). Antisense oligonucleotide therapies for monogenic disorders. *Med Genet*, *37*(3), 179-187. https://doi.org/10.1515/medgen-2025-2025

Lai, L., Han, X., Tang, Y., Zhou, J., & Cui, W. (2025). Advances in ultrasound-assisted drug delivery and clinical application. *Ultrasonics Sonochemistry*, 107557. https://doi.org/https://doi.org/10.1016/j.ultsonch.2025.107557

Lang, Z., Li, Y., Lin, L., Li, X., Tao, Q., Hu, Y., Bao, M., Zheng, L., Yu, Z., & Zheng, J. (2023). Hepatocyte-derived exosomal miR-146a-5p inhibits hepatic stellate cell EMT process: a crosstalk between hepatocytes and hepatic stellate cells. *Cell Death Discov*, *9*(1), 304. https://doi.org/10.1038/s41420-023-01602-y

Larios, J., Mercier, V., Roux, A., & Gruenberg, J. (2020). ALIX- and ESCRT-III-dependent sorting of tetraspanins to exosomes. *J Cell Biol*, *219*(3). https://doi.org/10.1083/jcb.201904113

Lee, I., Choi, Y., Shin, D. U., Kwon, M., Kim, S., Jung, H., Nam, G. H., & Kwon, M. (2023). Small Extracellular Vesicles as a New Class of Medicines. *Pharmaceutics*, *15*(2). https://doi.org/10.3390/pharmaceutics15020325

Lee, S. T., Im, W., Ban, J. J., Lee, M., Jung, K. H., Lee, S. K., Chu, K., & Kim, M. (2017). Exosome-Based Delivery of miR-124 in a Huntington's Disease Model. *J Mov Disord*, *10*(1), 45-52. https://doi.org/10.14802/jmd.16054

Lee, Y., Kang, S., Thuy, L. T., Son, M., Park, J. Y., Ahn, S. B., Kang, M., Oh, J., Choi, J. S., & Lee, M. (2025). Exosome-membrane and polymer-based hybrid-complex for systemic delivery of plasmid DNA into brains for the treatment of glioblastoma. *Asian J Pharm Sci*, *20*(1), 101006. https://doi.org/10.1016/j.ajps.2024.101006

Lee, Y. J., Shin, K. J., & Chae, Y. C. (2024). Regulation of cargo selection in exosome biogenesis and its biomedical applications in cancer. *Exp Mol Med*, *56*(4), 877-889. https://doi.org/10.1038/s12276-024-01209-y

Li, B., Fang, T., Li, Y., Xue, T., Zhang, Z., Li, L., Meng, F., Wang, J., Hou, L., Liang, X., Zhang, X., & Gu, Z. (2022). Engineered T cell extracellular vesicles displaying PD-1 boost anti-tumor immunity. *Nano Today*, *46*, 101606. https://doi.org/https://doi.org/10.1016/j.nantod.2022.101606

Li, J., Peng, J., Wang, J., & Chen, Z. (2025). The Dual Role of Exosomes in the Tumor Microenvironment: From Pro-Tumorigenic Signaling to Immune Modulation. *Med Research*, *1*(2), 257-284. https://doi.org/https://doi.org/10.1002/mdr2.70022

Li, J., Wang, J., & Chen, Z. (2025). Emerging role of exosomes in cancer therapy: progress and challenges. *Mol Cancer*, *24*(1), 13. https://doi.org/10.1186/s12943-024-02215-4

Li, L., Wang, F., Zhu, D., Hu, S., Cheng, K., & Li, Z. (2025). Engineering exosomes and exosome-like nanovesicles for improving tissue targeting and retention. *Fundam Res*, *5*(2), 851-867. https://doi.org/10.1016/j.fmre.2024.03.025

Li, Q., Wang, H., Peng, H., Huyan, T., & Cacalano, N. A. (2019). Exosomes: Versatile Nano Mediators of Immune Regulation. *Cancers (Basel)*, *11*(10). https://doi.org/10.3390/cancers11101557

Li, T., Yang, Y., Qi, H., Cui, W., Zhang, L., Fu, X., He, X., Liu, M., Li, P. F., & Yu, T. (2023). CRISPR/Cas9 therapeutics: progress and prospects. *Signal Transduct Target Ther*, *8*(1), 36. https://doi.org/10.1038/s41392-023-01309-7

Liu, C., Xia, C., & Xia, C. (2023). Biology and function of exosomes in tumor immunotherapy. *Biomed Pharmacother*, *169*, 115853. https://doi.org/10.1016/j.biopha.2023.115853

Lopes, D., Lopes, J., Pereira-Silva, M., Peixoto, D., Rabiee, N., Veiga, F., Moradi, O., Guo, Z. H., Wang, X. D., Conde, J., Makvandi, P., & Paiva-Santos, A. C. (2023). Bioengineered exosomal-membrane-camouflaged abiotic nanocarriers: neurodegenerative diseases, tissue engineering and regenerative medicine. *Mil Med Res*, *10*(1), 19. https://doi.org/10.1186/s40779-023-00453-z

Luan, X., Sansanaphongpricha, K., Myers, I., Chen, H., Yuan, H., & Sun, D. (2017). Engineering exosomes as refined biological nanoplatforms for drug delivery. *Acta Pharmacol Sin*, *38*(6), 754-763. https://doi.org/10.1038/aps.2017.12

Lyu, C., Sun, H., Sun, Z., Liu, Y., & Wang, Q. (2024). Roles of exosomes in immunotherapy for solid cancers. *Cell Death Dis*, *15*(2), 106. https://doi.org/10.1038/s41419-024-06494-z

Marzouk, R., Gab-Allah, M., & Kim, J. (2025). Polyethylene glycol (PEG)-based precipitation for exosome enrichment: A review on recent developments, current challenges, and future perspectives. *Analytical Science and Technology*, *38*, 42-64. https://doi.org/10.5806/AST.2025.38.2.42

McAndrews, K. M., Xiao, F., Chronopoulos, A., LeBleu, V. S., Kugeratski, F. G., & Kalluri, R. (2021). Exosome-mediated delivery of CRISPR/Cas9 for targeting of oncogenic Kras(G12D) in pancreatic cancer. *Life Sci Alliance*, *4*(9). https://doi.org/10.26508/lsa.202000875

McMullan, E., Joladarashi, D., & Kishore, R. (2025). Unpacking Exosomes: A Therapeutic Frontier for Cardiac Repair. *Curr Cardiol Rep*, *27*(1), 73. https://doi.org/10.1007/s11886-025-02225-8

Mendt, M., Kamerkar, S., Sugimoto, H., McAndrews, K. M., Wu, C. C., Gagea, M., Yang, S., Blanko, E. V. R., Peng, Q., Ma, X., Marszalek, J. R., Maitra, A., Yee, C., Rezvani, K., Shpall, E., LeBleu, V. S., & Kalluri, R. (2018). Generation and testing of clinical-grade exosomes for pancreatic cancer. *JCI Insight*, *3*(8). https://doi.org/10.1172/jci.insight.99263

Miceli, R. T., Chen, T. Y., Nose, Y., Tichkule, S., Brown, B., Fullard, J. F., Saulsbury, M. D., Heyliger, S. O., Gnjatic, S., Kyprianou, N., Cordon-Cardo, C., Sahoo, S., Taioli, E., Roussos, P., Stolovitzky, G., Gonzalez-Kozlova, E., & Dogra, N. (2024). Extracellular vesicles, RNA sequencing, and bioinformatic analyses: Challenges, solutions, and recommendations. *J Extracell Vesicles*, *13*(12), e70005. https://doi.org/10.1002/jev2.70005

Moeinabadi-Bidgoli, K., Rezaee, M., Hossein-Khannazer, N., Babajani, A., Aghdaei, H. A., Arki, M. K., Afaghi, S., Niknejad, H., & Vosough, M. (2023). Exosomes for angiogenesis induction in ischemic disorders. *J Cell Mol Med*, *27*(6), 763-787. https://doi.org/10.1111/jcmm.17689

Mukerjee, N., Maitra, S., Kaur, M., Rekha, M. M., Soothwal, P., Arora, I., Thorat, N. D., Sharma, P. K., & Kaushik, A. (2025). Click chemistry-based modified exosomes: Towards enhancing precision in cancer theranostics. *Chemical Engineering Journal*, *512*, 160915. https://doi.org/https://doi.org/10.1016/j.cej.2025.160915

Nail, H. M., Chiu, C. C., Leung, C. H., Ahmed, M. M. M., & Wang, H. D. (2023). Exosomal miRNA-mediated intercellular communications and immunomodulatory effects in tumor microenvironments. *J Biomed Sci*, *30*(1), 69. https://doi.org/10.1186/s12929-023-00964-w

Nguyen, V. V. T., Witwer, K. W., Verhaar, M. C., Strunk, D., & van Balkom, B. W. M. (2020). Functional assays to assess the therapeutic potential of extracellular vesicles. *J Extracell Vesicles*, *10*(1), e12033. https://doi.org/10.1002/jev2.12033

Nouri, Z., Barfar, A., Perseh, S., Motasadizadeh, H., Maghsoudian, S., Fatahi, Y., Nouri, K., Yektakasmaei, M. P., Dinarvand, R., & Atyabi, F. (2024). Exosomes as therapeutic and drug delivery vehicle for neurodegenerative diseases. *J Nanobiotechnology*, *22*(1), 463. https://doi.org/10.1186/s12951-024-02681-4

Nowak, M., Gorczynska, J., Kolodzinska, K., Rubin, J., & Choromanska, A. (2023). Extracellular Vesicles as Drug Transporters. *Int J Mol Sci*, *24*(12). https://doi.org/10.3390/ijms241210267

O'Brien, J., Hayder, H., Zayed, Y., & Peng, C. (2018). Overview of MicroRNA Biogenesis, Mechanisms of Actions, and Circulation. *Front Endocrinol (Lausanne)*, *9*, 402. https://doi.org/10.3389/fendo.2018.00402

Oppeneer, T., Qi, Y., Henshaw, J., Larimore, K., Melton, A., Puolivali, J., Carter, C., Fant, P., Brennan, S., Wetzel, L. A., Sigg, M. A., Crawford, B. E., Magat, J., Froelich, S., Woloszynek, J. C., & O'Neill, C. A. (2025). Targeting a Novel Site in Exon 51 with Antisense Oligonucleotides Induces Enhanced Exon Skipping in a Mouse Model of Duchenne Muscular Dystrophy. *Nucleic Acid Ther*, *35*(2), 68-80. https://doi.org/10.1089/nat.2024.0049

Palomar-Alonso, N., Lee, M., & Kim, M. (2024). Exosomes: Membrane-associated proteins, challenges and perspectives. *Biochem Biophys Rep*, *37*, 101599. https://doi.org/10.1016/j.bbrep.2023.101599

Pan, L., & Wang, P. (2025). DNA nanotechnology-enabled bioanalysis of extracellular vesicles. *Nanoscale Horiz*. https://doi.org/10.1039/d5nh00557d

Pan, W., Chen, H., Wang, A., Wang, F., & Zhang, X. (2023). Challenges and strategies: Scalable and efficient production of mesenchymal stem cells-derived exosomes for cell-free therapy. *Life Sci*, *319*, 121524. https://doi.org/10.1016/j.lfs.2023.121524

Pofali, P., Mondal, A., & Londhe, V. (2020). Exosome as a Natural Gene Delivery Vector for Cancer Treatment. *Curr Cancer Drug Targets*, *20*(11), 821-830. https://doi.org/10.2174/1568009620666200924154149

Rajput, A., Varshney, A., Bajaj, R., & Pokharkar, V. (2022). Exosomes as New Generation Vehicles for Drug Delivery: Biomedical Applications and Future Perspectives. *Molecules*, *27*(21). https://doi.org/10.3390/molecules27217289

Raju, D., Bathini, S., Badilescu, S., Ghosh, A., & Packirisamy, M. (2022). Microfluidic Platforms for the Isolation and Detection of Exosomes: A Brief Review. *Micromachines (Basel)*, *13*(5). https://doi.org/10.3390/mi13050730

Ramos-Zaldivar, H. M., Polakovicova, I., Salas-Huenuleo, E., Corvalan, A. H., Kogan, M. J., Yefi, C. P., & Andia, M. E. (2022). Extracellular vesicles through the blood-brain barrier: a review. *Fluids Barriers CNS*, *19*(1), 60. https://doi.org/10.1186/s12987-022-00359-3

Ravichandiran, V., Kesharwani, A., Anupriya, Bhaskaran, M., Parihar, V. K., Bakhshi, S., Velayutham, R., & Kumarasamy, M. (2024). Overcoming biological barriers: Precision engineered extracellular vesicles for personalized neuromedicine. *Precision Medicine and Engineering*, *1*(2), 100010. https://doi.org/https://doi.org/10.1016/j.preme.2024.100010

Rodriguez, D. A., & Vader, P. (2022). Extracellular Vesicle-Based Hybrid Systems for Advanced Drug Delivery. *Pharmaceutics*, *14*(2). https://doi.org/10.3390/pharmaceutics14020267

Sadeghi, S., Tehrani, F. R., Tahmasebi, S., Shafiee, A., & Hashemi, S. M. (2023). Exosome engineering in cell therapy and drug delivery. *Inflammopharmacology*, *31*(1), 145-169. https://doi.org/10.1007/s10787-022-01115-7

Saint-Pol, J., & Culot, M. (2025). Minimum information for studies of extracellular vesicles (MISEV) as toolbox for rigorous, reproducible and homogeneous studies on extracellular vesicles. *Toxicology in Vitro*, *106*, 106049. https://doi.org/https://doi.org/10.1016/j.tiv.2025.106049

Salomon, C., Das, S., Erdbrugger, U., Kalluri, R., Kiang Lim, S., Olefsky, J. M., Rice, G. E., Sahoo, S., Andy Tao, W., Vader, P., Wang, Q., & Weaver, A. M. (2022). Extracellular Vesicles and Their Emerging Roles as Cellular Messengers in Endocrinology: An Endocrine Society Scientific Statement. *Endocr Rev*, *43*(3), 441-468. https://doi.org/10.1210/endrev/bnac009

Sanadgol, N., Abedi, M., Hashemzaei, M., Kamran, Z., Khalseh, R., Beyer, C., & Voelz, C. Exosomes as nanocarriers for brain-targeted delivery of therapeutic nucleic acids: advances and challenges. (1477-3155 (Electronic)).

Shahabipour, F., Banach, M., & Sahebkar, A. (2016). Exosomes as nanocarriers for siRNA delivery: paradigms and challenges. *Arch Med Sci*, *12*(6), 1324-1326. https://doi.org/10.5114/aoms.2016.62911

Shamili, F. H., Bayegi, H. R., Salmasi, Z., Sadri, K., Mahmoudi, M., Kalantari, M., Ramezani, M., & Abnous, K. (2018). Exosomes derived from TRAIL-engineered mesenchymal stem cells with effective anti-tumor activity in a mouse melanoma model. *Int J Pharm*, *549*(1-2), 218-229. https://doi.org/10.1016/j.ijpharm.2018.07.067

Shtykalova, S., Deviatkin, D., Freund, S., Egorova, A., & Kiselev, A. (2023). Non-Viral Carriers for Nucleic Acids Delivery: Fundamentals and Current Applications. *Life (Basel)*, *13*(4). https://doi.org/10.3390/life13040903

Skotland, T., Sandvig, K., & Llorente, A. (2017). Lipids in exosomes: Current knowledge and the way forward. *Prog Lipid Res*, *66*, 30-41. https://doi.org/10.1016/j.plipres.2017.03.001

Song, X., Liang, H., Nan, F., Chen, W., Li, J., He, L., Cun, Y., Li, Z., Zhang, W., & Zhang, D. (2025). Autoimmune Diseases: Molecular Pathogenesis and Therapeutic Targets. *MedComm (2020)*, *6*(7), e70262. https://doi.org/10.1002/mco2.70262

Spinelli, S., Tripodi, D., Corti, N., Zocchi, E., Bruschi, M., Leoni, V., & Dominici, R. (2025). Roles, Functions, and Pathological Implications of Exosomes in the Central Nervous System. *Int J Mol Sci*, *26*(3). https://doi.org/10.3390/ijms26031345

Szwedowicz, U., Lapinska, Z., Gajewska-Naryniecka, A., & Choromanska, A. (2022). Exosomes and Other Extracellular Vesicles with High Therapeutic Potential: Their Applications in Oncology, Neurology, and Dermatology. *Molecules*, *27*(4). https://doi.org/10.3390/molecules27041303

Wallen, M., Aqil, F., Spencer, W., & Gupta, R. C. (2023). Exosomes as an Emerging Plasmid Delivery Vehicle for Gene Therapy. *Pharmaceutics*, *15*(7). https://doi.org/10.3390/pharmaceutics15071832

Wang, S., Jin, S., Zhang, J., & Wang, X. (2025). Exosomal miRNAs: Key Regulators of the Tumor Microenvironment and Cancer Stem Cells. *International Journal of Molecular Sciences*, *26*(19).

Wang, S., & Shi, Y. (2022). Exosomes Derived from Immune Cells: The New Role of Tumor Immune Microenvironment and Tumor Therapy. *Int J Nanomedicine*, *17*, 6527-6550. https://doi.org/10.2147/IJN.S388604

Wang, X., Gong, W., Li, R., Li, L., & Wang, J. (2024). Preparation of genetically or chemically engineered exosomes and their therapeutic effects in bone regeneration and anti-inflammation. *Front Bioeng Biotechnol*, *12*, 1329388. https://doi.org/10.3389/fbioe.2024.1329388

Wang, Y., Ma, H., Zhang, X., Xiao, X., & Yang, Z. (2024). The Increasing Diagnostic Role of Exosomes in Inflammatory Diseases to Leverage the Therapeutic Biomarkers. *J Inflamm Res*, *17*, 5005-5024. https://doi.org/10.2147/JIR.S475102

Welsh, J. A., Goberdhan, D. C. I., O'Driscoll, L., Buzas, E. I., Blenkiron, C., Bussolati, B., Cai, H., Di Vizio, D., Driedonks, T. A. P., Erdbrugger, U., Falcon-Perez, J. M., Fu, Q. L., Hill, A. F., Lenassi, M., Lim, S. K., Mahoney, M. G., Mohanty, S., Moller, A., Nieuwland, R., . . . Witwer, K. W. (2024). Minimal information for studies of extracellular vesicles (MISEV2023): From basic to advanced approaches. *J Extracell Vesicles*, *13*(2), e12404. https://doi.org/10.1002/jev2.12404

Wu, S., Zhao, Y., Zhang, Z., Zuo, C., Wu, H., & Liu, Y. (2024). The Advances and Applications of Characterization Technique for Exosomes: From Dynamic Light Scattering to Super-Resolution Imaging Technology. *Photonics*, *11*(2).

Xie, S., Zhang, Q., & Jiang, L. (2022). Current Knowledge on Exosome Biogenesis, Cargo-Sorting Mechanism and Therapeutic Implications. *Membranes (Basel)*, *12*(5). https://doi.org/10.3390/membranes12050498

Xu, M., Ji, J., Jin, D., Wu, Y., Wu, T., Lin, R., Zhu, S., Jiang, F., Ji, Y., Bao, B., Li, M., Xu, W., & Xiao, M. (2023). The biogenesis and secretion of exosomes and multivesicular bodies (MVBs): Intercellular shuttles and implications in human diseases. *Genes Dis*, *10*(5), 1894-1907. https://doi.org/10.1016/j.gendis.2022.03.021

Yakubovich, E. I., Polischouk, A. G., & Evtushenko, V. I. (2022). Principles and Problems of Exosome Isolation from Biological Fluids. *Biochem (Mosc) Suppl Ser A Membr Cell Biol*, *16*(2), 115-126. https://doi.org/10.1134/S1990747822030096

Yang, J., Luo, S., Zhang, J., Yu, T., Fu, Z., Zheng, Y., Xu, X., Liu, C., Fan, M., & Zhang, Z. (2021). Exosome-mediated delivery of antisense oligonucleotides targeting alpha-synuclein ameliorates the pathology in a mouse model of Parkinson's disease. *Neurobiol Dis*, *148*, 105218. https://doi.org/10.1016/j.nbd.2020.105218

Yang, Y. P., Nicol, C. J. B., & Chiang, M. C. (2025). A Review of the Neuroprotective Properties of Exosomes Derived from Stem Cells and Exosome-Coated Nanoparticles for Treating Neurodegenerative Diseases and Stroke. *Int J Mol Sci*, *26*(8). https://doi.org/10.3390/ijms26083915

Yi, Y. F., Fan, Z. Q., Liu, C., Ding, Y. T., Chen, Y., Wen, J., Jian, X. H., & Li, Y. F. (2025). Immunomodulatory effects and clinical application of exosomes derived from mesenchymal stem cells. *World J Stem Cells*, *17*(3), 103560. https://doi.org/10.4252/wjsc.v17.i3.103560

Yudaeva, A., Kostyusheva, A., Kachanov, A., Brezgin, S., Ponomareva, N., Parodi, A., Pokrovsky, V. S., Lukashev, A., Chulanov, V., & Kostyushev, D. (2024). Clinical and Translational Landscape of Viral Gene Therapies. *Cells*, *13*(22). https://doi.org/10.3390/cells13221916

Zeng, H., Guo, S., Ren, X., Wu, Z., Liu, S., & Yao, X. (2023). Current Strategies for Exosome Cargo Loading and Targeting Delivery. *Cells*, *12*(10). https://doi.org/10.3390/cells12101416

Zhang, L., Wu, T., Shan, Y., Li, G., Ni, X., Chen, X., Hu, X., Lin, L., Li, Y., Guan, Y., Gao, J., Chen, D., Zhang, Y., Pei, Z., & Chen, X. (2021). Therapeutic reversal of Huntington's disease by in vivo self-assembled siRNAs. *Brain*, *144*(11), 3421-3435. https://doi.org/10.1093/brain/awab354

Zhang, P., Chen, K., Liu, W., Niu, X., Wang, X., Wang, J., Yao, W., Tang, X., & Tian, W. (2025). Engineered exosomes: a promising design platform for overcoming cancer therapy resistance. *Front Cell Dev Biol*, *13*, 1608480. https://doi.org/10.3389/fcell.2025.1608480

Zhang, S., Shen, J., Li, D., & Cheng, Y. (2021). Strategies in the delivery of Cas9 ribonucleoprotein for CRISPR/Cas9 genome editing. *Theranostics*, *11*(2), 614-648. https://doi.org/10.7150/thno.47007

Zhang, Y., Bi, J., Huang, J., Tang, Y., Du, S., & Li, P. (2020). Exosome: A Review of Its Classification, Isolation Techniques, Storage, Diagnostic and Targeted Therapy Applications. *Int J Nanomedicine*, *15*, 6917-6934. https://doi.org/10.2147/IJN.S264498

Zhang, Y., Lan, M., & Chen, Y. (2024). Minimal Information for Studies of Extracellular Vesicles (MISEV): Ten-Year Evolution (2014-2023). *Pharmaceutics*, *16*(11). https://doi.org/10.3390/pharmaceutics16111394

Zhao, Y., Li, X., Zhang, W., Yu, L., Wang, Y., Deng, Z., Liu, M., Mo, S., Wang, R., Zhao, J., Liu, S., Hao, Y., Wang, X., Ji, T., Zhang, L., & Wang, C. (2021). Trends in the biological functions and medical applications of extracellular vesicles and analogues. *Acta Pharm Sin B*, *11*(8), 2114-2135. https://doi.org/10.1016/j.apsb.2021.03.012

Zhu, X., Gao, M., Yang, Y., Li, W., Bao, J., & Li, Y. (2023). The CRISPR/Cas9 System Delivered by Extracellular Vesicles. *Pharmaceutics*, *15*(3). https://doi.org/10.3390/pharmaceutics15030984

Zou, J., Peng, H., & Liu, Y. (2021). The Roles of Exosomes in Immunoregulation and Autoimmune Thyroid Diseases. *Front Immunol*, *12*, 757674. https://doi.org/10.3389/fimmu.2021.757674

Author Biography

Nihan Oruklu holds a master's degree from the Department of Medical Microbiology at Hacettepe University, and a PhD from the Department of Immunology at Gazi University, Faculty of Medicine, where she currently works as a lecturer. She is a competent researcher who can use many molecular and immunological techniques. Through her publications in peer-reviewed journals, she has demonstrated her expertise across a wide range of topics including monoclonal antibody and vaccine development, infection and mucosal immunology. Dr. Oruklu's motivation to research the topic of exosomes in gene therapy and contribute to this book arises from her enthusiasm for advancing innovative approaches in immunology and translational medicine. She is particularly inspired by the potential of exosomes as natural carriers for gene delivery, viewing them as a transformative tool in the development of next-generation treatments for complex diseases.

CHAPTER 9

PEPTIDE DELIVERY SYSTEMS

DURMUS AYAN

Niğde Ömer Halisdemir University Faculty of Medicine, Niğde, Türkiye

Abstract

Peptide-based therapeutics represent a promising category of pharmaceuticals, characterized by their high specificity, potent biological activity, and reduced off-target effects compared to small-molecule drugs (Fetse et al., 2023). Peptides are integral to various physiological processes and have been investigated for the treatment of diseases such as cancer, metabolic disorders, infectious diseases, and neurological conditions (L. Wang et al., 2022). Despite their therapeutic potential, peptides encounter significant challenges that hinder their clinical application, including rapid enzymatic degradation, poor membrane permeability, low oral bioavailability, and rapid renal clearance (Di, 2014). To overcome these limitations, researchers have developed various peptide delivery systems designed to enhance stability, bioavailability, targeted delivery, and sustained release (Ezike et al., 2023).

This chapter provides an in-depth analysis of the diverse strategies utilized in peptide delivery systems, highlighting their benefits, mechanisms, and contemporary applications. Notably, nanoparticle-based delivery systems have attracted considerable interest due to their ability to shield peptides from enzymatic degradation while facilitating controlled and sustained drug release (Elumalai et al., 2024). Biodegradable nanoparticles, especially those composed of polymers such as poly (lactic-co-glycolic acid) (PLGA) and chitosan, have demonstrated promising outcomes in enhancing peptide stability and bioavailability (Alsaab et al., 2022).

Liposomes and lipid-based carriers represent a highly effective strategy for peptide delivery. Due to their amphiphilic properties, liposomes are capable of encapsulating both hydrophilic and hydrophobic molecules, thereby enhancing peptide transport across biological membranes. Their biocompatibility and potential for functionalization with targeting ligands make them particularly suitable for site-specific peptide delivery (Plaza-Oliver et al., 2021). Similarly, hydrogels, which are three-dimensional water-swollen networks, offer a tunable and sustained-release platform for peptides, rendering them appropriate for localized and long-acting therapies (Thang et al., 2023).

Transdermal peptide delivery has been explored through the use of microneedle-based systems, which present a minimally invasive alternative to conventional injections. Microneedles create microchannels in the skin, facilitating peptide absorption without inducing significant pain or discomfort. This method improves patient compliance, particularly in the management of chronic diseases (T. Liu et al. 2021). Furthermore, chemical modifications, such as PEGylation and lipidation, have been utilized to extend the half-life of peptides by reducing renal clearance and enhancing their stability in circulation. PEGylation involves the conjugation of polyethylene glycol (PEG) molecules to peptides, thereby protecting them from proteolytic degradation, while lipidation enhances membrane permeability and bioavailability (Menacho-Melgar et al. 2019).

Despite these advancements, the delivery of peptides continues to face challenges, including issues related to formulation stability, immunogenicity, and constraints in large-scale manufacturing. Nevertheless, ongoing progress in the fields of nanotechnology, biomaterials, and bioengineering is facilitating the development of next-generation peptide delivery systems that offer enhanced efficacy and improved patient compliance (Xiao et al., 2025).

In conclusion, peptide delivery systems are essential for overcoming the inherent limitations of peptide therapeutics, thereby enabling more effective drug formulations and expanding clinical applications. The continuous advancement of delivery technologies holds significant potential for transforming peptide-based medicine, with implications across various medical fields, including oncology, endocrinology, infectious diseases, and regenerative medicine. Ongoing research and innovation will continue to propel the development of advanced peptide delivery systems, ultimately enhancing patient outcomes and broadening the scope of peptide-based therapies.

Keywords: Peptide therapeutics; Drug delivery systems; Nanoparticles; Liposomes; Hydrogels; Microneedles; PEGylation; Lipidation; Cell-penetrating peptides; Stimuli-responsive delivery; Targeted therapy; Personalized medicine.

Introduction

Peptides have emerged as a crucial category of therapeutic agents due to their inherent biological specificity, potent activity, and reduced side effects compared to conventional small-molecule drugs (Xiao et al., 2025). These short chains of amino acids play essential roles in physiological processes and have been investigated for a wide range of clinical applications, including oncology, endocrinology, infectious diseases, and neurological disorders (L. Wang et al., 2022). However, despite their therapeutic potential, peptides encounter several pharmacokinetic and pharmacodynamic challenges, such as rapid enzymatic degradation, limited membrane permeability, low oral bioavailability, and swift renal clearance (Diao & Meibohm, 2013). This chapter examines the evolving landscape of peptide delivery systems, focusing on technological advancements aimed at overcoming these challenges and enhancing the therapeutic efficacy of peptides.

Challenges in Peptide Drug Delivery

Peptide-based pharmaceuticals exhibit inherent instability within biological systems due to their vulnerability to proteolytic enzymes. Enzymes such as trypsin, chymotrypsin, and elastase, which are prevalent throughout the digestive tract and bloodstream, significantly impede peptide stability. Consequently, therapeutic peptides are rapidly degraded into inactive fragments prior to reaching their intended sites of action. This instability constitutes a primary factor limiting the systemic availability of numerous promising peptide-based therapies (Langguth et al., 1997; De bruyn et al., 2021; Haddadzadegan et al., 2022).

Beyond enzymatic degradation, peptides encounter additional pharmacokinetic obstacles. Their hydrophilic properties and relatively large molecular size hinder their capacity to cross lipid-rich cellular membranes through passive diffusion. This limitation substantially reduces their permeability and cellular uptake, particularly in tissues characterized by tight junctions, such as the intestinal epithelium (Almansour et al., 2018) and the blood-brain barrier (Parrasia et al., 2022). As a result, peptides frequently necessitate alternative delivery methods or carrier systems to effectively reach intracellular or tissue-specific targets (Vasir & Labhasetwar, 2007; Tarvirdipour et al., 2021).

The intestinal epithelium is distinguished by the presence of tight junctions that regulate paracellular permeability, thereby effectively restricting the passage of macromolecules such as peptides (Chelakkot et al., 2018). These tight junctions consist of transmembrane proteins, including claudins and occludin, which form a selective barrier to solutes and ions (Parrasia et al., 2022). Modulating these tight junctions can enhance the paracellular transport of therapeutic peptides. For example, certain membrane-permeant peptides have been demonstrated to transiently reduce intestinal epithelial barrier function, thus facilitating the uptake of poorly absorbed compounds (Yu et al., 2024). The blood-brain barrier (BBB) presents another significant challenge due to its highly selective permeability, which limits the entry of most therapeutic agents, including peptides (D. Wu et al., 2023). To address this issue, strategies such as receptor-mediated transcytosis are under investigation. This approach involves conjugating peptides to ligands that target specific receptors on the BBB, thereby facilitating their transport into the central nervous system. For instance, the use of Angiopep-2, a peptide that targets the low-density lipoprotein receptor-related protein-1 (LRP1), has been explored to enhance the delivery of therapeutic agents across the BBB (Blades et al., 2023).

- To address these challenges, several delivery systems are currently being explored: Cell-Penetrating Peptides (CPPs) are short peptides that enhance the cellular uptake of various molecular cargoes, including therapeutic peptides, by traversing cell membranes(Blades et al., 2023).
- Nanocarriers, including nanoparticles, liposomes, and dendrimers, serve to encapsulate peptides, thereby safeguarding them from degradation and facilitating their transport across biological barriers. These carriers can be engineered to specifically target tissues or cells, thereby enhancing the bioavailability and efficacy of peptide therapeutics (Yusuf et al., 2023).

Another significant limitation is the rapid renal clearance of peptides. Peptides, particularly those with molecular weights below the renal threshold (typically under 50 kDa), are swiftly filtered from the bloodstream by the kidneys and subsequently excreted in the urine. This results in a markedly short plasma half-life, necessitating frequent dosing to sustain therapeutic levels (Czock et al., 2012). Such frequent administration not only imposes a burden on patients but also elevates the risk of side effects and increases healthcare costs.

Oral administration, while advantageous due to its convenience and patient acceptability, presents distinct challenges for peptides. Upon oral intake, peptides encounter the harsh environment of the gastrointestinal (GI) tract, characterized by acidic pH levels in the stomach (pH 1.5–3.5) and digestive enzymes (e.g., pepsin in the stomach, trypsin, and chymotrypsin in the small intestine), which degrade peptide chains prior to absorption. Moreover, even if a portion of the peptide withstands enzymatic hydrolysis, the intestinal epithelium constitutes an additional barrier. Tight junctions between enterocytes restrict paracellular transport, and transcellular uptake mechanisms are largely inefficient for most peptides (Haddadzadegan et al., 2022).

Several peptides exhibit low chemical and conformational stability under physiological conditions. Oxidation, deamidation, and aggregation may occur during storage or post-administration, thereby compromising the therapeutic agent's efficacy and safety. These degradation pathways necessitate meticulous formulation strategies, often involving the use of stabilizing excipients or encapsulation technologies (M. Shi & McHugh, 2023). Intravenous (IV) administration is frequently employed to circumvent these barriers and achieve rapid systemic distribution. However, IV delivery is invasive, may require trained personnel, and is associated with discomfort, risk of infection, and reduced patient adherence, particularly in chronic conditions necessitating long-term treatment. Repeated injections increase the risk of local tissue damage and immunogenic responses (Homayun et al., 2019). Furthermore, immunogenicity remains a concern with peptide therapeutics. Although generally less immunogenic than protein-based biologics, certain peptides can still provoke immune responses, especially if administered repeatedly or if they contain non-natural amino acids or modifications. This can lead to the development of neutralizing antibodies that reduce therapeutic efficacy or cause adverse effects (Achilleos et al., 2025; De Groot et al., 2025).

These cumulative challenges highlight the imperative for innovative delivery strategies that can safeguard peptides from degradation, enhance their permeability and half-life, and facilitate patient-friendly administration routes (Shah et al., 2025). Strategies such as nanoparticle encapsulation, chemical modification, and the utilization of bioresponsive carriers are currently under investigation to address these obstacles and realize the full potential of peptide-based therapeutics (Rawal & Patel, 2021).

Nanoparticle-Based Delivery Systems

Nanotechnology has significantly transformed peptide drug delivery by introducing encapsulation techniques that protect peptides from enzymatic degradation and enable targeted, sustained release. Biodegradable polymeric nanoparticles, such as those composed of poly(lactic-co-glycolic acid) (PLGA) and chitosan, have shown considerable success in enhancing peptide stability and bioavailability (Omidian et al., 2024; Omidian et al., 2025). These nanoparticles not only safeguard the encapsulated peptides but also facilitate controlled drug release, thereby reducing dosing frequency and improving therapeutic outcomes (Omidian et al., 2025).

Poly(lactic-co-glycolic acid) (PLGA)-based nanoparticles have been extensively investigated due to their approval by the FDA, superior biocompatibility, and adjustable degradation rates (Danhier et al., 2012). The copolymer composition, specifically the lactic acid to glycolic acid ratio, along with the molecular weight, can be modified to alter the degradation kinetics, thereby enabling customized release profiles for various therapeutic peptides (J. Zhao et al., 2017). These nanoparticles can be designed to respond to environmental stimuli such as pH or enzymatic activity, facilitating site-specific drug release. For example, pH-sensitive nanoparticles preferentially release their payload in acidic tumor microenvironments or intracellular endosomes, thereby enhancing therapeutic efficacy while minimizing systemic toxicity (Saadat et al., 2021; Bachta et al., 2025).

PLGA nanoparticles demonstrate exceptional compatibility with a variety of administration routes, including oral, nasal, pulmonary, and parenteral pathways. Their diminutive size, typically less than 200 nm, facilitates deep tissue penetration and cellular uptake via endocytosis (Alghareeb et al., 2024; W. Huang & Zhang, 2018). Surface engineering with targeting moieties, such as antibodies, folic acid, or peptides, enables receptor-mediated endocytosis, thereby enhancing site-specific delivery and reducing off-target effects (Suri et al., 2007; Danhier et al., 2010; Kocbek et al., 2007).

Chitosan, a naturally derived polysaccharide sourced from chitin, has garnered significant attention due to its mucoadhesive properties and its capacity to transiently open tight junctions within epithelial layers. This characteristic facilitates the paracellular transport of peptides across mucosal barriers, such as those found in the gastrointestinal and nasal epithelium, thereby rendering chitosan nanoparticles promising candidates for non-invasive delivery strategies (Rosenthal et al., 2012; Mura et al., 2022). Its intrinsic cationic nature enables the formation of electrostatic complexes with negatively charged peptides and nucleic acids, thereby enhancing encapsulation efficiency (M. Ways et al., 2018).

Chitosan nanoparticles can undergo chemical modification to enhance their solubility, stability, and functionality. Derivatives such as trimethyl chitosan and carboxymethyl chitosan have demonstrated improved permeation and reduced aggregation under physiological conditions (Mourya & Inamdar, 2009). Chitosan-based systems are being actively investigated for the intranasal delivery of neuropeptides and vaccine antigens, yielding promising results in both animal and clinical models (Omidian et al., 2024).

Surface modification of nanoparticles through the application of polyethylene glycol (PEG), targeting ligands, or cell-penetrating peptides significantly enhances their stability and specificity towards cells. The process of PEGylation forms a 'stealth' corona around the nanoparticles, which prevents opsonization and subsequent clearance by the mononuclear phagocyte system (MPS), thereby extending their systemic circulation time (Driscoll et al., 2025; Pan et al., 2025). Targeting ligands, such as transferrin, aptamers, or monoclonal antibodies, facilitate the direction of nanoparticles to specific tissues or cell types, thereby improving therapeutic efficacy while minimizing systemic toxicity (Ghosh et al., 2025).

Cell-penetrating peptides (CPPs), such as TAT (trans-activator of transcription) and penetratin, can be conjugated to nanoparticle surfaces to enhance intracellular delivery. These CPPs facilitate endosomal escape and the cytosolic release of peptide cargo, which is particularly advantageous for delivering therapeutic peptides targeting intracellular sites (Grau &Wagner 2024; D. Mai et al., 2024).

Furthermore, nanocarriers can be engineered as multifunctional platforms that integrate imaging agents, targeting ligands, and therapeutic peptides. These theranostic systems facilitate the real-time monitoring of drug distribution and treatment efficacy through modalities such as magnetic resonance imaging (MRI) or fluorescence imaging. This integration of diagnostics and therapy is advancing the development of personalized medicine in peptide-based therapeutics (Azimizonuzi et al., 2025; Al-Thani et al., 2024).

The scalability and reproducibility of nanoparticle production continue to be significant areas of investigation, with methods such as nanoprecipitation, emulsion-solvent evaporation, and microfluidics undergoing optimization for industrial application (Nunziata et al., 2025; Patel & Patel, 2024). In general, nanoparticle-based systems are among the most promising strategies for addressing the inherent limitations of peptide drugs and enhancing their clinical efficacy across a broad range of diseases (Mitchell et al., 2021).

Liposomes and Lipid-Based Carriers

Liposomes, consisting of phospholipid bilayers, present a versatile and biocompatible platform for peptide delivery due to their structural similarity to cellular membranes. Their distinctive amphiphilic properties facilitate the encapsulation of both hydrophilic molecules within the aqueous core and hydrophobic molecules within the lipid bilayer, thereby extending their applicability to a diverse range of therapeutic peptides. These vesicular systems can vary from small unilamellar vesicles (SUVs) to multilamellar vesicles (MLVs), with their size and lamellarity significantly affecting drug loading, release kinetics, and biodistribution(Liu et al., 2022; Pande, 2023).

One of the primary benefits of liposomes is their capacity to improve the pharmacokinetic profile of peptides. Encapsulation serves to protect peptides from enzymatic degradation and premature clearance, thereby facilitating sustained release and extended circulation times. Additionally, surface modifications of liposomes through polyethylene glycol (PEGylation) impart 'stealth' characteristics, allowing them to evade the mononuclear phagocyte system (MPS) and prolong their systemic half-life (Sercombe et al., 2015; Immordino et al., 2006; Allen & Cullis, 2013).

Liposomes can be functionalized with targeting ligands, including monoclonal antibodies, peptides, folic acid, and aptamers, to facilitate site-specific delivery (Driscoll et al., 2025; Cheng et al., 2025). This active targeting approach enhances the accumulation of liposomes in diseased tissues, such as tumors or inflamed areas, through receptor-mediated endocytosis (Driscoll et al., 2025). In the field of oncology, ligand-directed liposomal formulations have demonstrated improved therapeutic indices and reduced off-target effects (Fan et al., 2023).

The clinical efficacy of liposomal formulations in oncological treatment, as exemplified by Doxil® (liposomal doxorubicin), has facilitated their application in peptide drug delivery (Barenholz, 2012; Allen & Cullis, 2013). Liposomal formulations of insulin, calcitonin, and other peptide hormones have shown enhanced stability and increased bioavailability in both preclinical and clinical investigations (H. Wu et al., 2023; H. He et al., 2019; Wibel et al., 2023). These systems are particularly advantageous in addressing the challenges associated with oral peptide delivery by protecting them from the harsh gastrointestinal environment and promoting transcellular transport (Uhl et al., 2023).

Stimuli-responsive liposomes represent an innovative strategy in lipid-based delivery systems. These advanced carriers are designed to release their contents in response to specific physiological or pathological stimuli, such as pH, temperature, enzymes, or redox gradients (Lee & Thompson, 2017). For example, pH-sensitive liposomes maintain stability at physiological pH but destabilize in the acidic tumor microenvironment or endosomes, thereby facilitating the precise release of the peptide payload at the target site (Alrbyawi et al., 2022). Thermosensitive liposomes, which are activated under mild hyperthermic conditions (e.g., 42°C), can be employed in conjunction with localized heating to achieve spatially and temporally controlled drug delivery (Chaudhry et al., 2022).

In addition to traditional liposomes, solid lipid nanoparticles (SLNs) (Ways et al., 2018) and nanostructured lipid carriers (NLCs) have emerged as advanced lipid-based systems (Bukke et al., 2024). SLNs consist of solid lipids and are stabilized by surfactants, offering enhanced physical stability and biocompatibility. They facilitate controlled drug release, improved peptide protection, and the potential for large-scale production through high-pressure homogenization techniques (Bukke et al., 2024).

Nanostructured lipid carriers (NLCs) are characterized by a combination of solid and liquid lipids, which results in an imperfect crystalline structure. This structural feature enhances the drug loading capacity and minimizes drug expulsion during storage. The matrix of NLCs facilitates the incorporation of hydrophobic peptide derivatives or lipid-conjugated peptides, thereby improving solubility and membrane permeation (Shahzadi et al., 2021).

Solid lipid nanoparticles (SLNs) and nanostructured lipid carriers (NLCs) offer significant advantages for the oral, topical, and injectable administration of peptides. Their nanoscale dimensions facilitate the effective traversal of biological barriers and enable accumulation in targeted tissues through the enhanced permeability and retention (EPR) effect. Furthermore, these lipid-based carriers can be surface-modified with mucoadhesive polymers or targeting ligands to enhance delivery precision (Jnaidi et al., 2020).

Recent advancements have facilitated the development of hybrid lipid-polymer nanoparticles, which integrate the structural benefits of polymers with the biocompatibility of lipids. These systems offer customizable release kinetics and multifunctionality, thereby enabling the co-delivery of peptides alongside adjuvants or imaging agents (Mukherjee et al., 2019; Bose et al., 2017).

In summary, liposomes and lipid-based nanocarriers constitute a highly versatile and promising class of delivery systems for peptide therapeutics. Their capacity to protect, transport, and release peptides in a controlled manner, coupled with their compatibility with various administration routes, highlights their increasing significance in the advancement of peptide-based drug development (Zhang et al., 2012; Sercombe et al., 2015).

Hydrogels for Localized and Sustained Delivery

Hydrogels are three-dimensional, hydrophilic polymer networks that possess the capacity to absorb and retain significant quantities of water or biological fluids. These soft, tissue-like materials offer a favorable environment for the encapsulation, protection, and sustained release of peptide therapeutics. Their high water content, structural resemblance to the extracellular matrix (ECM), and excellent biocompatibility render them particularly advantageous for localized treatments and long-term therapeutic interventions across various biomedical applications (Zöller et al., 2025).

Hydrogels can be classified into two primary categories: natural and synthetic. Natural hydrogels, such as alginate, gelatin, hyaluronic acid, chitosan, and collagen, are sourced from biological origins and are characterized by their high biocompatibility and biodegradability (Abou-Okeil et al., 2024). These materials are frequently employed in applications related to wound healing, drug delivery, and tissue regeneration (Abou-Okeil et al., 2024). In contrast, synthetic hydrogels, including polyethylene glycol (PEG), polyacrylamide, and poloxamers, provide adjustable mechanical strength, degradation rates, and chemical functionalities, thereby enabling precise control over drug release kinetics and physical properties (Vigata et al., 2020).

The release dynamics of peptides from hydrogels can be modulated by adjusting the cross-linking density, polymer concentration, and degradation mechanism. Hydrogels may be physically cross-linked, utilizing hydrogen bonding, hydrophobic interactions, or ionic interactions, or chemically cross-linked through covalent bonds, each imparting distinct stability and release characteristics. This adaptability facilitates the design of hydrogels tailored for specific clinical applications, ranging from acute to chronic disease contexts (Tiwari et al., 2023).

Injectable hydrogels constitute a notably promising category of delivery systems. These formulations are liquid at ambient temperature and undergo a sol-to-gel transition upon injection into the body, induced by physiological stimuli such as temperature, pH, or ionic strength. This minimally invasive method facilitates in situ depot formation, allowing for sustained, site-specific release of therapeutic peptides without necessitating surgical implantation. Thermosensitive hydrogels based on polymers such as poly(N-isopropylacrylamide) (PNIPAAm) or poloxamers (Pluronics®) have been extensively investigated for this application (Gradinaru et al., 2025).

Hydrogels present a promising application in the management of chronic wounds and diabetic ulcers, where the sustained release of angiogenic peptides, such as vascular endothelial growth factor (VEGF) and basic fibroblast growth factor (bFGF), can stimulate neovascularization, promote tissue regeneration, and expedite wound closure. Additionally, hydrogel dressings infused with antimicrobial peptides can prevent infection while facilitating tissue repair (Hartmeier et al., 2021; H. Liu & He, 2025).

In the field of neurology, thermosensitive hydrogels have been employed for the intracranial administration of neuropeptides and neurotrophic factors (Zhu et al., 2025). These systems facilitate enhanced peptide retention at the target site, offer protection against enzymatic degradation, and allow for controlled release over prolonged durations, thereby improving therapeutic outcomes in conditions such as Parkinson's disease (Zhu et al., 2025), Alzheimer's disease, and stroke (Fernández-Serra et al., 2019).

Hydrogels have been utilized in cancer therapy for locoregional treatment (P. Lu et al., 2024). Peptide-based cancer vaccines or immunomodulatory peptides can be integrated into injectable hydrogels and administered directly to the tumor site or lymph nodes. This method promotes a sustained immune response while minimizing systemic exposure, thereby reducing adverse effects (C. Liu et al., 2023).

Stimuli-responsive hydrogels have garnered considerable attention in the development of advanced delivery systems. These hydrogels exhibit structural transformations in response to environmental stimuli, including pH, temperature, enzymatic activity, or oxidative stress, thereby facilitating on-demand and site-specific peptide release (El-Husseiny et al., 2022). Enzyme-responsive hydrogels, in particular, degrade selectively in the presence of disease-associated enzymes such as matrix metalloproteinases (MMPs), rendering them especially beneficial in the contexts of cancer and inflammatory diseases (Sobczak, 2022).

Hydrogels are currently being explored in conjunction with other delivery platforms, such as nanoparticles and microneedles, to develop hybrid systems with enhanced functionality (Choi & Kohane, 2024). Nanoparticles encapsulated within hydrogels offer dual protection and enable multidrug loading, while microneedle arrays coated with hydrogel formulations facilitate transdermal peptide delivery with sustained release properties (Alimardani et al., 2021; Cai et al., 2023).

Despite their numerous advantages, hydrogel-based peptide delivery systems face several challenges, including the control of burst release, the achievement of uniform drug distribution, and the maintenance of long-term stability during storage. Addressing these challenges necessitates meticulous formulation design and robust manufacturing processes. Nevertheless, the ongoing development of advanced hydrogel systems holds significant promise for transforming peptide-based therapies, offering customizable, safe, and patient-friendly solutions across a broad spectrum of clinical applications(Li et al., 2025; Pentlavalli et al., 2025).

Microneedle-Based Transdermal Systems

Microneedle technology presents a minimally invasive and patient-friendly alternative to traditional injections for the transdermal delivery of peptides. These micro-projections, typically measuring between 25 and 2000 micrometers in length, are engineered to penetrate the stratum corneum—the outermost layer of the skin—without reaching the deeper, nerve-rich dermis (Nguyen et al., 2023). By creating temporary micropores in the skin, microneedles facilitate the direct entry of peptides into systemic circulation or targeted local tissues, thereby circumventing gastrointestinal degradation and hepatic first-pass metabolism (Zafar et al., 2025).

The principal benefit of microneedle-based systems is their capacity to improve patient adherence, particularly in the management of chronic conditions that necessitate regular dosing, such as diabetes, osteoporosis, and hormonal disorders (Nguyen et al., 2022).

Microneedles can be manufactured from a diverse range of materials, including metals (e.g., stainless steel, titanium), ceramics, silicon, and biocompatible polymers (e.g., hyaluronic acid, polyvinylpyrrolidone, polylactic acid) (Oliveira et al., 2024). Depending on their design and mechanism of action, microneedles are categorized into several types:

- Solid microneedles are employed to create microchannels in the skin, which are subsequently used for the topical application of the drug (Kim et al., 2012).
- Coated microneedles are characterized by a drug layer applied to the needle surface, which dissolves upon insertion into the skin (Ingrole & Gill, 2019).
- Dissolving microneedles, which are composed entirely of biodegradable polymers embedded with a therapeutic agent, dissolve upon skin penetration, thereby releasing the payload (Sartawi et al., 2022).
- Hollow microneedles function analogously to miniature hypodermic needles, facilitating the direct injection of liquid formulations into the skin (Anbazhagan et al., 2025).

Dissolving microneedles are particularly advantageous for peptide delivery due to their favorable safety profile, user-friendliness, and capacity to incorporate a diverse array of bioactive molecules. These microneedles can be customized to regulate the release kinetics of encapsulated peptides by modifying polymer composition, molecular weight, and matrix density (Moawad et al., 2025).

Recent advancements in microneedle technology have facilitated the creation of integrated smart drug delivery platforms. These platforms encompass wearable patches that are equipped with biosensors, microfluidic components, and microprocessors, enabling real-time monitoring and responsive drug administration. For instance, glucose-responsive microneedle systems are capable of continuously monitoring blood glucose levels and administering insulin or GLP-1 analogs in a feedback-controlled manner (Pal et al., 2025; Yang et al., 2022). This methodology not only enhances glycemic control but also significantly improves patient autonomy and quality of life.

Microneedles are currently under investigation for their potential in intradermal vaccine delivery (Kim et al., 2012). Vaccines based on peptides, when administered via microneedles, have been shown to induce strong immune responses with reduced antigen doses compared to traditional intramuscular injections. This dose-sparing effect, coupled with the simplicity of administration, renders microneedles particularly advantageous for large-scale immunization initiatives, especially in settings with limited resources (Nguyen, 2025).

Furthermore, microneedle arrays can be integrated with nanoparticles or liposomes to facilitate dual-layered or sequential delivery strategies, thereby offering synergistic control over drug release and targeting. This hybrid approach enables precise spatiotemporal regulation, allowing for multi-stage therapy or the co-delivery of adjuvants and peptides in immunotherapeutic applications (Q. Lu et al., 2024; S. Huang et al., 2024; Gunawan et al., 2025).

While microneedle systems offer numerous advantages, several challenges must be addressed to fully harness their clinical potential. These challenges include ensuring mechanical robustness during insertion, achieving consistent fabrication at scale, maintaining peptide stability within the matrix, and securing regulatory approval. Nevertheless, ongoing advancements in materials science, device engineering, and biomedical research continue to broaden the applications of microneedle-based delivery, establishing it as a transformative technology for next-generation peptide therapeutics (Bao et al., 2024; Xiao et al., 2025; Adhikari & Pokhrel, 2025).

Chemical Modification Strategies

Chemical modification techniques, such as PEGylation and lipidation, are extensively utilized to enhance the pharmacokinetic profile and therapeutic efficacy of peptide drugs (Zhang et al., 2014; Menacho-Melgar et al., 2019). These strategies effectively address the primary limitations associated with peptide therapeutics, including inadequate metabolic stability, rapid renal clearance, short plasma half-life, and restricted bioavailability. By structurally modifying peptides without significantly diminishing their biological activity, these approaches facilitate improved systemic exposure, dosing convenience, and patient compliance (Baral & Choi, 2025).

PEGylation, a well-established modification technique, entails the covalent attachment of polyethylene glycol (PEG) chains to specific amino acid residues on the peptide molecule. This hydrophilic polymer forms a hydrated shell around the peptide, offering steric hindrance that protects it from proteolytic enzymes and diminishes renal filtration. Additionally, PEGylation enhances solubility in aqueous environments, decreases immunogenicity, and reduces opsonization by the immune system, thereby prolonging circulation time in the bloodstream (Santhanakrishnan et al., 2024; Y. Gao et al., 2023).

Several PEGylated peptide pharmaceuticals have attained regulatory approval and are currently utilized in clinical settings. For instance, peginterferon alfa-2a and alfa-2b represent PEGylated variants of interferon employed in the management of hepatitis B and C (Y.-W. Huang et al., 2022; Lau et al., 2005). These formulations facilitate once-weekly administration as opposed to daily injections, thereby significantly enhancing patient compliance. Pegvisomant, a PEGylated growth hormone receptor antagonist, has been sanctioned for the treatment of acromegaly (Haberbosch & Strasburger, 2023). Nonetheless, emerging evidence suggests that repeated administration of PEGylated drugs may induce the formation of anti-PEG antibodies, potentially diminishing therapeutic efficacy and eliciting hypersensitivity reactions (Kozma et al., 2020). This has led to the investigation of alternative 'stealth' polymers, including polysialic acid, zwitterionic polymers, and hydroxyethyl starch (Q. Zhang et al., 2023; Prasher & Sharma, 2024; Z. Zhang et al., 2024).

Lipidation is a significant technique characterized by the covalent attachment of lipid moieties, such as fatty acids, cholesterol, or aliphatic chains, to peptide backbones (Bech et al., 2018). This modification facilitates non-covalent binding to serum albumin, a long-circulating plasma protein, thereby extending the peptide's half-life by reducing renal clearance and proteolytic degradation (Hijazi, 2021). Additionally, lipidation enhances membrane permeability, increases lipophilicity, and promotes intracellular uptake via endocytosis or membrane fusion (Menacho-Melgar et al., 2019).

Lipid-modified peptides have achieved clinical success in the management of metabolic and endocrine disorders. Liraglutide and semaglutide, which are GLP-1 receptor agonists modified with fatty acid chains, facilitate albumin binding and allow for once-daily or once-weekly subcutaneous administration in the treatment of type 2 diabetes and obesity. These pharmacological agents not only enhance glycemic control but also mitigate cardiovascular risk and promote weight reduction (Tamayo-Trujillo et al., 2024).

Advanced lipidation strategies encompass the utilization of branched lipid structures, dimerization, and dual conjugation techniques to refine pharmacokinetics and enhance receptor interactions (Xiao et al., 2025). Furthermore, prodrug strategies employing reversible lipid conjugation have been devised to facilitate site-specific release of active peptides in response to enzymatic or environmental stimuli (Y. Wang et al., 2017).

In addition to PEGylation and lipidation, several other chemical modification strategies are increasingly being adopted. Techniques such as glycosylation, acetylation, cyclization, and the incorporation of D-amino acids or non-natural amino acids are employed to enhance stability, receptor affinity, and resistance to enzymatic degradation (Ma et al., 2024). Notably, cyclization contributes to increased conformational rigidity and protease resistance, as demonstrated in therapeutic peptides like octreotide and lanreotide (C. Wang et al., 2024).

Furthermore, site-specific conjugation techniques and click chemistry-based methods offer enhanced precision and reproducibility compared to traditional random modification approaches. These technologies facilitate the design of multifunctional peptide conjugates with improved homogeneity, scalability, and potential for clinical translation (Sadiki et al., 2020).

As peptide therapeutics continue to advance, chemical modification strategies remain indispensable in drug design and formulation. By strategically enhancing pharmacological properties while preserving or augmenting biological activity, these modifications facilitate the successful development of next-generation peptide drugs with improved efficacy, safety, and patient adherence (Xiao et al., 2025).

Targeted and Stimuli-Responsive Delivery

Advanced delivery platforms have incorporated targeting mechanisms and environmental responsiveness to facilitate controlled and site-specific peptide release. These intelligent systems are engineered to enhance therapeutic efficacy by delivering peptides directly to diseased tissues, thereby minimizing systemic exposure and off-target effects. This strategic targeting augments drug potency, reduces toxicity, and supports precision medicine approaches across a broad spectrum of diseases (S. Wang et al., 2024; Zhou et al., 2025).

Stimuli-responsive systems, alternatively referred to as "triggered release" systems, utilize either endogenous (internal) or exogenous (external) cues to initiate drug release. Endogenous stimuli encompass alterations in pH, redox potential, enzyme activity, and temperature at the pathological site.

Conversely, exogenous triggers may include the application of light, magnetic fields, ultrasound, or heat to a targeted region (Raza et al., 2019).

pH-responsive carriers are particularly advantageous in cancer therapy, as tumor tissues and intracellular compartments such as endosomes and lysosomes generally exhibit lower pH values compared to normal tissues. Peptide carriers composed of acid-labile materials or pH-sensitive linkers can undergo structural alterations or degradation under acidic conditions, thereby releasing the therapeutic cargo selectively within the tumor microenvironment or upon cellular uptake (X. He et al., 2013; AlSawaftah et al., 2022).

Enzyme-responsive delivery systems exploit the heightened presence of specific enzymes at pathological sites. For example, matrix metalloproteinases (MMPs) are frequently overexpressed in numerous cancerous tissues and inflammatory environments. By integrating MMP-cleavable peptides or linkers into the carrier structure, these systems facilitate precise drug release in response to enzymatic activity, thereby sparing healthy tissues (Zhang et al., 2023; Isaacson et al., 2017). Similarly, delivery vehicles responsive to cathepsins or proteases have been engineered for targeted peptide release within lysosomes or inflammatory lesions (Yadati et al., 2020).

Redox-responsive systems exploit the differential redox potential between extracellular and intracellular environments, particularly the elevated glutathione (GSH) levels found in cancer cells. Linkers containing disulfide bonds undergo cleavage in high GSH concentrations, facilitating peptide release within the cytoplasm. These systems are especially advantageous for peptides that act intracellularly, such as those targeting transcription factors or signaling pathways (Meng et al., 2024; J. Wang et al., 2023).

Exogenous stimuli-responsive platforms facilitate the temporal and spatial regulation of peptide delivery. Light-responsive systems, for instance, employ photosensitive linkers or light-activated carriers to release peptides at the site of irradiation (Xing et al., 2022). Near-infrared (NIR) light is frequently utilized due to its superior tissue penetration and reduced phototoxicity (Tang & Wang, 2021). Magnetic nanoparticles can be directed to specific tissues using an external magnetic field and subsequently heated (magnetothermal therapy) to trigger peptide release from thermosensitive matrices (Graham et al., 2025).

Targeted delivery systems enhance the specificity of peptide therapeutics by incorporating ligands that recognize receptors overexpressed on diseased cells. Common targeting ligands include folic acid (for tumors overexpressing folate receptors), transferrin (for cancers targeted by transferrin receptors), RGD peptides (for integrin-rich vasculature), and monoclonal antibodies (for tumor-associated antigens) (Islam et al., 2025; G. Ji et al., 2024). These ligands are conjugated to the surface of nanoparticles, liposomes, or hydrogels to facilitate receptor-mediated endocytosis (G. Ji et al., 2024).

Aptamer-functionalized systems have emerged as a promising class of targeting platforms due to their high specificity, small size, and ease of synthesis. Aptamers are single-stranded oligonucleotides that bind selectively to target proteins or cells. Nanocarriers decorated with tumor-specific aptamers can achieve precise homing and internalization into cancer cells, delivering peptides directly to intracellular compartments (Fu & Xiang, 2020; Yin et al., 2023).

Multivalent targeting strategies, which involve the utilization of multiple ligands or dual-ligand combinations, significantly enhance cell specificity and uptake efficiency. For example, the combination of folic acid and an antibody fragment on a single nanoparticle can simultaneously exploit multiple receptor pathways, thereby increasing cellular internalization and therapeutic efficacy (YU et al., 2010; Sultana & David, 2023).

Targeted and stimuli-responsive delivery systems are being developed for applications extending beyond oncology. In the context of inflammatory diseases, such as rheumatoid arthritis or inflammatory bowel disease, enzyme-sensitive and ROS-responsive carriers are capable of delivering anti-inflammatory peptides directly to the affected tissues (J. Gao et al., 2024). In neurological disorders, peptide-loaded carriers functionalized with transferrin or lactoferrin can traverse the blood-brain barrier through receptor-mediated transcytosis (B. Ji et al., 2006).

Despite considerable progress, challenges such as ligand stability, immune recognition, and the heterogeneous expression of target receptors persist. Current research endeavors are directed towards optimizing ligand density, enhancing the stealth properties of nanoparticles, and integrating multiplexed targeting strategies (Chehelgerdi et al., 2023).

In summary, targeted and stimuli-responsive delivery platforms constitute a transformative strategy in peptide therapeutics, facilitating precise, efficient, and safe drug administration that is tailored to the physiological and pathological characteristics of individual patients and diseases (Sun & Davis, 2021).

Table 1. Comparison of Peptide-Based Nucleic Acid Delivery Strategies

Delivery Strategy	Mechanism of Action	Key Advantages	Limitations	Applications
Cell-Penetrating Peptides (CPPs)	Direct membrane translocation or endocytosis	Efficient cellular uptake; modifiable sequence	Limited tissue specificity; potential toxicity	siRNA, pDNA, CRISPR-Cas delivery
Nanoparticle Conjugation	Encapsulation or surface binding	Protection from degradation; targeted delivery	Complex formulation; scale-up challenges	siRNA, mRNA, gene therapy
Lipid-Based Carriers (LNPs)	Fusion with lipid membranes	High transfection efficiency; clinical success	Immunogenicity; storage sensitivity	mRNA vaccines, gene editing
Stimuli-Responsive Systems	Release triggered by pH, redox, enzymes	Site-specific release; reduced side effects	Requires precise tuning; heterogeneous responses	Tumor-targeted therapies
Ligand-Targeted Delivery	Receptor-mediated endocytosis	High specificity; low off-target effects	Target heterogeneity; receptor saturation	Tumor, CNS, hepatic targeting
Hybrid Systems (CPP + NP)	Combination of CPPs with NPs or LNPs	Synergistic efficiency; enhanced stability	Complexity of formulation	Combination therapies

Current Limitations and Future Perspectives

Despite notable advancements, peptide delivery technologies continue to encounter several limitations that must be addressed to facilitate their widespread clinical adoption. These challenges encompass various domains, including formulation development, biological compatibility, stability, delivery efficiency, and scalability. The intrinsic instability of peptides, due to their susceptibility to enzymatic degradation and physical or chemical instability during storage, necessitates innovative formulation strategies and robust delivery vehicles (Xiao et al., 2025).

One enduring challenge is achieving a balance between protection and release. Although encapsulation strategies can protect peptides from degradation, attaining precise control over release kinetics without compromising bioactivity remains a technical obstacle (Beach et al., 2024). Furthermore, maintaining the structural integrity and functional conformation of peptides during formulation, storage, and transport necessitates careful optimization of excipients, buffers, and lyophilization techniques (Shi & McHugh, 2023).

Immunogenicity remains a significant concern. While peptides typically exhibit a lower immunogenic potential compared to larger biologics, modifications such as PEGylation or conjugation with carrier systems may provoke immune responses (Suk et al., 2016). The formation of anti-drug antibodies (ADAs) can neutralize therapeutic effects and result in adverse reactions. Advanced techniques in immunoinformatics and in silico modeling are employed to predict and mitigate these risks during drug design (Vaisman-Mentesh et al., 2020).

Large-scale manufacturing and reproducibility present substantial challenges for advanced delivery systems, particularly those involving complex nanocarriers or stimuli-responsive materials. Ensuring batch-to-batch consistency, material purity, and the scale-up of micro- or nano-formulations is not straightforward. Technologies such as microfluidics, continuous manufacturing, and 3D printing are being investigated to enhance scalability and minimize production variability (El-Tanani et al., 2025).

Current research endeavors are focused on the development of effective oral delivery systems, which are considered the "holy grail" of peptide therapeutics. Promising strategies include the utilization of absorption enhancers, such as medium-chain fatty acids, enzyme inhibitors like aprotinin and soybean trypsin inhibitor, and mucoadhesive polymers, for instance, chitosan. Additionally, enteric coatings, nanoparticles, and pH-responsive carriers are under investigation to protect peptides from gastric degradation and enhance their intestinal absorption(Chen et al., 2022; L. Liu et al., 2017).

Microbiome-modulating strategies represent an innovative frontier in scientific research. It is increasingly acknowledged that the gut microbiota plays a pivotal role in drug metabolism and absorption (J. Huang et al., 2023). Emerging concepts, such as modulating the microbiome to enhance peptide stability or utilizing engineered microbial consortia to deliver peptides at mucosal sites, hold significant potential to revolutionize oral and colonic peptide delivery (Taherali et al., 2023).

Regulatory and manufacturing considerations remain essential. It is imperative to streamline compliance with Good Manufacturing Practices (GMP), regulatory approval pathways, and safety assessments to expedite translation. The standardization of evaluation protocols, quality control assays, and regulatory frameworks specifically designed for advanced delivery systems will be critical (P. Lu et al., 2024).

Furthermore, interdisciplinary collaboration is crucial. Integrating expertise from fields such as nanotechnology, materials science, immunology, pharmacokinetics, and clinical medicine can significantly advance the development of next-generation peptide therapeutics (Omidian et al., 2025).

Emerging trends, such as personalized peptide therapy, mRNA-encoded peptide delivery, and gene-editing tools for regulating endogenous peptide production, present promising opportunities (Itoh & Yamada, 2006; Y. Shi et al., 2024). The integration of peptide science with synthetic biology, smart biomaterials, and bioelectronic interfaces holds the potential to develop programmable and responsive peptide therapeutics tailored to the specific needs of individual patients (Parvin et al., 2025; N. Zhao et al., 2023).

In conclusion, although peptide delivery technologies have achieved significant advancements, ongoing efforts are essential to surmount existing challenges and realize their full therapeutic potential. The future of this field resides in the development of intelligent, scalable, and patient-focused delivery platforms that integrate biological understanding with technological innovation, thereby facilitating the provision of safe, effective, and accessible peptide-based treatments to the global population.

Cell-Penetrating Peptides (CPPs) and Nucleic Acid Delivery

In the field of gene therapy, the effective and safe delivery of therapeutic nucleic acids, including plasmid DNA, mRNA, siRNA, miRNA, ASOs, aptamers, and CRISPR components, into target cells represents a significant challenge. These macromolecules often exhibit instability in circulation and encounter various biological barriers, such as enzymatic degradation, limited cellular uptake, and endosomal sequestration upon internalization. Addressing these obstacles necessitates the employment of delivery vectors that are not only efficient but also biocompatible, ensuring the protection of the cargo until it reaches its intracellular target (T. Jiang et al., 2023; Sioson et al., 2021).

Cell-penetrating peptides (CPPs) have emerged as promising tools to address these challenges. Typically consisting of 5–30 amino acids, CPPs possess a net positive charge and/or amphipathic characteristics, enabling interaction with negatively charged cell membranes and facilitating translocation into the cytoplasm. They are capable of delivering a wide range of biological cargos, including nucleic acids, proteins, peptides, and nanoparticles, into various cell types without the need for specific receptors (Du et al., 2025; Said Hassane et al., 2009; Yokoo et al., 2021).

CPPs can be employed in their native form or conjugated with other functional components, such as targeting ligands, endosomal escape enhancers, and shielding molecules like polyethylene glycol (PEG), to enhance delivery efficiency and specificity. Moreover, hybrid nanoformulations incorporating CPPs—such as lipid-based nanoparticles, polymeric micelles, and inorganic scaffolds—have demonstrated improved stability, reduced toxicity, and increased cellular uptake compared to conventional vectors. These characteristics render CPPs particularly promising for clinical translation in gene therapy platforms (Y. Liu et al., 2022; Moreno-Vargas & Prada-Gracia, 2025b).

Structural Classification and Examples

CPPs exhibit structural diversity and can be classified according to their physicochemical properties and mechanisms of interaction with cellular membranes. Such a broad classification facilitates the rational selection and design of CPPs for specific cargo types and target tissues (Ouyang et al., 2022).

Cationic CPPs represent a highly studied class, predominantly composed of arginine and lysine residues. Their substantial positive charge facilitates electrostatic interactions with negatively charged cell membranes, thereby promoting cellular entry (Szabó et al., 2022). Noteworthy examples include TAT (48–60), derived from the HIV-1 transactivator of transcription protein, Penetratin from the Antennapedia homeodomain, and synthetic oligoarginine peptides such as R8 and R9. These CPPs are particularly effective for nucleic acid delivery, although they often require optimization for serum stability and endosomal escape (Shin et al., 2014).

Table 2. Commonly used CPPs and their typical applications

CPP	Type	Nucleic Acid Cargo	Typical Applications	Notes
TAT(48–60)	Cationic	pDNA, siRNA, mRNA, CRISPR RNP	Broad use	High uptake; may require endosomal escape optimization
Penetratin	Cationic	siRNA/ASO	Nuclear targeting studies	NLS-like properties
R8/R9	Cationic	pDNA, siRNA	Simple, modular complexation	Needs modification for serum stability
MPG / Pep-1	Amphipathic	siRNA, mRNA, protein	Co-delivery (protein+NA)	Amphipathic balance is critical
Transportan	Amphipathic	pDNA, siRNA	Strong membrane interaction	Potential cytotoxicity concerns

Amphipathic CPPs are characterized by the presence of both hydrophobic and cationic domains, which facilitate robust interactions with lipid bilayers and promote enhanced membrane translocation. Notable examples include MPG, Pep-1, and Transportan, which can deliver nucleic acids, proteins, or even co-complexes into cells. The amphipathic balance of these peptides is crucial for optimizing delivery efficiency while minimizing cytotoxicity (Khairkhah et al., 2023).

Hydrophobic CPPs, though less prevalent, demonstrate a pronounced affinity for cellular membranes due to their high concentration of nonpolar or aromatic residues (Datta, 2025). These peptides can integrate into membranes and facilitate the delivery of cargo through mechanisms of direct translocation or membrane perturbation. Despite their efficacy, the design of these peptides requires meticulous optimization to mitigate off-target effects and toxicity (Ouyang et al., 2022).

Smart or stimuli-responsive CPPs are designed to react to specific physiological or pathological stimuli, such as variations in pH, redox gradients, or enzyme overexpression. For example, matrix metalloproteinase (MMP)-cleavable peptides facilitate selective activation within tumor microenvironments, whereas redox-sensitive linkers enable cargo release in the reducing intracellular milieu. These designs enhance the control and specificity of CPP-based delivery systems (Perche, 2019).

Ligand-targeted CPPs constitute a versatile class that integrates targeting moieties such as RGD peptides (for integrins), nuclear localization signals (NLS), aptamers, or antibody fragments. These functionalized CPPs facilitate the delivery system's targeting of specific cell types or subcellular compartments, thereby enhancing therapeutic efficacy while minimizing systemic toxicity (Cerrato & Langel, 2022; Longoria-García et al., 2022; Nikitovic et al., 2024).

Cellular Uptake and Endosomal Escape Mechanisms

The intracellular delivery of nucleic acids via CPPs encompasses a multistep process, beginning with initial surface binding and culminating in the localization at the designated subcellular target. A thorough comprehension of each phase is essential for optimizing delivery efficiency and minimizing off-target effects (Guidotti et al., 2017; Ruseska & Zimmer, 2020; Skotland et al., 2015; Teo et al., 2021).

CPPs primarily facilitate cellular uptake through interactions with negatively charged components of the cell membrane. Cationic CPPs, which are abundant in arginine and lysine residues, engage in electrostatic interactions with glycosaminoglycans such as heparan sulfate, as well as with the phosphate groups of membrane phospholipids (R. Zhang et al., 2019). This binding process enhances the concentration of CPP-cargo complexes at the membrane surface, frequently resulting in membrane invagination or direct translocation (Ruseska & Zimmer, 2020).

Several cellular internalization pathways have been identified for CPP-mediated delivery, including clathrin-mediated endocytosis, caveolin-dependent endocytosis, and macropinocytosis (Ruseska & Zimmer, 2020). Each of these mechanisms results in the encapsulation of CPPs and their associated cargo within endosomal compartments (Guidotti et al., 2017). At elevated peptide concentrations or in the presence of specific structural characteristics, such as amphipathic balance, CPPs may circumvent endocytosis altogether, directly translocating across the lipid bilayer through transient pore formation or membrane destabilization (Herce et al., 2009).

Upon internalization via endocytosis, CPP-cargo complexes must successfully escape from endosomal vesicles to prevent degradation and ensure delivery to the cytosol or nucleus. Various mechanisms have been employed to facilitate endosomal escape. The "proton sponge effect," frequently utilized by incorporating histidine residues or co-formulating with polycations, inducing osmotic swelling and rupture of the endosome. Membrane-active peptide segments derived from fusogenic viruses or toxins can also promote escape by destabilizing the endosomal membrane. Furthermore, pH-sensitive lipid and peptide designs enable environment-triggered destabilization, while enzymatically cleavable linkers responsive to intracellular enzymes such as phospholipases or MMPs further enhance release into the cytoplasm (Erazo-Oliveras et al., 2012; Sahni et al., 2020).

For gene delivery strategies necessitating nuclear access, such as plasmid DNA or specific CRISPR constructs, the nuclear envelope represents the ultimate barrier (Alhakamy et al., 2013; Ni et al., 2019). NLS can be integrated into CPPs or conjugates to facilitate active transport through nuclear pores (Ni et al., 2019). Alternatively, leveraging the mitotic window—during which the nuclear membrane temporarily disassembles in the course of cell division—can enhance the passive nuclear entry of larger cargos (Remaut et al., 2014).

Nucleic Acid Complexation and Formulation Strategies

Effective formulation strategies are essential for ensuring stability, bioavailability, and functional delivery of nucleic acids via CPPs. Various methodologies have been developed to enhance the physicochemical compatibility between CPPs and nucleic acid cargos (Porosk & Langel, 2022).

One prevalent technique is non-covalent electrostatic complexation, wherein positively charged CPPs condense negatively charged nucleic acids through ionic interactions (Alhakamy et al., 2013). The efficacy of this process is contingent upon the nitrogen-to-phosphate (N/P) ratio, which requires optimization to achieve a balance between complex stability, particle size, and transfection efficiency (Alhakamy et al., 2013). Optimal formulations generally yield nanoparticles within the 50–200 nm size range, exhibiting moderately positive zeta potentials to enhance cellular uptake while minimizing cytotoxicity (W. Chen et al., 2017).

In addition to non-covalent interactions, covalent conjugation techniques have been utilized to develop more stable CPP–nucleic acid constructs. These techniques include thiol–maleimide coupling, click chemistry (azide–alkyne cycloaddition), and disulfide linkage formation (Behzadipour & Hemmati, 2024; Malinowska et al., 2024). Covalent bonds offer significant advantages when precise control over stoichiometry and site-specific attachment is necessary, particularly in applications that require intracellular stability and controlled release (J. Walsh et al., 2021; Malinowska et al., 2024).

Hybrid delivery systems that integrate CPPs with other carrier platforms confer additional advantages (Dowaidar, 2024). For instance, lipid-based nanoparticles (LNPs) can be functionalized with CPPs through surface adsorption or covalent anchoring using lipid-PEG–CPP conjugates (Aschmann et al., 2024). Similarly, polymeric vectors, such as PEGylated polyethylenimines (PEIs) or poly(β-amino esters), can be co-formulated with CPPs to enhance transfection efficiency and mitigate toxicity (Karlsson et al., 2020). Inorganic cores, such as gold or silica nanoparticles, can also be surface-modified with CPPs to facilitate dual imaging and therapeutic functions (Kovtareva et al., 2024).

Stabilizing agents are frequently incorporated into formulations to maintain structural integrity and enhance pharmacokinetics (Rahban et al., 2023). PEG is commonly employed to provide steric stabilization, minimize protein adsorption, and extend circulation time (Suk et al., 2016). Cholesterol and other sterols may be included to facilitate membrane fusion and delivery, particularly for mRNA cargoes (Patel et al., 2022). pH-sensitive lipids are incorporated to enable endosomal escape in response to acidic intracellular environments (Z.-R. Lu & Sun, 2025).

Adherence to Good Manufacturing Practice (GMP) guidelines is crucial during the synthesis and purification of peptides for clinical-grade applications. Techniques such as solid-phase peptide synthesis (SPPS), reversed-phase high-performance liquid chromatography (RP-HPLC), and mass spectrometry are employed to ensure batch consistency, purity, and identity. Proper characterization of critical quality attributes (CQAs), including particle size, polydispersity index, zeta potential, encapsulation efficiency, and enzymatic stability, is essential to ensure the safety and efficacy of the final product.

Targeting Strategies

To improve the specificity and efficiency of CPP-mediated delivery, a range of targeting strategies has been developed. These strategies are intended to direct the delivery system to specific cells, tissues, or even subcellular compartments, thereby reducing off-target effects and enhancing therapeutic efficacy (Moreno-Vargas & Prada-Gracia, 2025).

Ligand-mediated targeting entails the integration of specific recognition motifs into the CPP sequence or onto the delivery complex. Frequently employed ligands include RGD peptides, which bind to integrin receptors that are overexpressed in numerous tumors, and NLS, which facilitate the nuclear entry of nucleic acid cargos (Martín et al., 2010). Furthermore, mitochondrial targeting sequences can be incorporated to deliver therapeutics aimed at modulating mitochondrial function or signaling (Hong et al., 2024).

Stimuli-responsive systems enhance the environmental control of delivery mechanisms (Rahim et al., 2021). These CPP formulations are designed to activate or disassemble in response to specific physiological or pathological conditions, such as acidic pH, elevated levels of enzymes like MMPs, hypoxic environments, or intracellular redox gradients (Y. Liu t al., 2022). For instance, redox-sensitive linkers facilitate cargo release in the cytoplasm, where glutathione concentrations are high, while pH-sensitive elements enable cargo escape from acidic endosomes (Phillips & Gibson, 2014; H. Zhang et al., 2024).

An essential approach to enhancing CPP-based delivery involves the development of systems capable of traversing biological barriers. These barriers, including mucosal linings, the blood–brain barrier (BBB), and the intestinal epithelium, pose significant challenges to systemic delivery (Ghorai et al., 2023; Kristensen et al., 2016; Wu et al., 2024). To address these challenges, CPPs can be conjugated with moieties that promote transcytosis or mucosal penetration. For instance, transferrin receptor-binding peptides can be employed for BBB traversal, while mucoadhesive modifications can be utilized for intranasal and oral formulations (Ghorai et al., 2023).

By incorporating principles of targeting and stimuli-responsive design, CPPs can be transformed from generic delivery agents into highly selective and controllable vectors, thereby enhancing their suitability for precision gene therapy.

Application Examples and Evidence Level

CPP-based delivery systems have been effectively utilized in a range of gene therapy applications, as evidenced by both in vitro and in vivo studies (Shin et al., 2014). A particularly well-researched application is the delivery of small interfering RNA (siRNA) and antisense oligonucleotides (ASOs), wherein CPPs enhance cellular uptake and facilitate gene silencing through RNA interference or antisense mechanisms (Estupiñán et al., 2025; Mendonça et al., 2021). These methodologies have shown promising outcomes in silencing oncogenes and modulating disease-related pathways in cancer and genetic disorders (Alexander-Bryant et al., 2015; de Morais et al., 2024; Juliano et al., 2008; M. Zhou et al., 2022).

Messenger RNA (mRNA) delivery represents a promising domain in which CPPs have demonstrated significant potential. Given the necessity for rapid and transient expression of therapeutic proteins, mRNA-based therapies benefit from the capacity of CPPs to facilitate swift and efficient payload delivery. The co-formulation with stabilizing components and endosomal escape enhancers further augments mRNA translation efficiency and protein yield (Afzal et al., 2025; Kowalski et al., 2019; Yokoo et al., 2021).

Plasmid DNA (pDNA) delivery via CPPs has been extensively investigated, particularly in strategies necessitating sustained gene expression or genome integration. The incorporation of NLS into CPPs enhances the nuclear delivery of pDNA, which is crucial for transcriptional activity (Nebogatova et al., 2023). These methodologies are pertinent in the fields of vaccine development, regenerative medicine, and long-term gene therapy (Farag et al., 2025; Jiang et al., 2025; Nebogatova et al., 2023; Uchida, 2022).

CRISPR-based genome editing constitutes a pioneering application domain for CPP-mediated delivery (Allemailem et al., 2022). Both ribonucleoprotein (RNP) complexes and plasmid-encoded CRISPR components can be administered using CPPs. RNP delivery offers the benefit of rapid, transient activity with diminished off-target effects, whereas plasmid-based systems facilitate prolonged expression of CRISPR components (Zhang et al., 2021). CPPs enhance the intracellular trafficking and editing efficiency of these tools, particularly when integrated with endosomal escape strategies (Soni et al., 2025).

Furthermore, combination strategies that integrate CPPs with tumor-targeting ligands, such as RGD peptides, and pH-sensitive lipids have demonstrated synergistic effects. These approaches result in enhanced selectivity, improved uptake in pathological tissues, and superior therapeutic outcomes. Such strategies exemplify the versatility and modularity of CPP-based platforms, establishing them as valuable components in next-generation nucleic acid therapeutics (Jadhav et al., 2025; Omidianet al., 2025).

Conclusion

Peptide delivery systems constitute a significant advancement in addressing the inherent limitations associated with peptide-based therapeutics. Although peptides are characterized by high specificity and biological potency, they encounter challenges such as enzymatic degradation, limited membrane permeability, and rapid systemic clearance. The strategic development and implementation of advanced delivery technologies have effectively mitigated many of these obstacles, thereby substantially enhancing the therapeutic index of peptide drugs and expanding their clinical applicability.

Researchers have achieved substantial improvements in peptide stability, bioavailability, and targeted delivery through the use of innovative platforms such as nanoparticles, liposomes, hydrogels, microneedles, and chemical modifications. These systems effectively protect peptides from premature degradation, regulate release rates, and ensure that the active agent reaches its site of action in a biologically effective form. The incorporation of targeting ligands and stimuli-responsive materials has further refined delivery strategies, facilitating site-specific and condition-responsive drug release. Such advancements are crucial for diseases that necessitate localized action or controlled dosing, including cancer, autoimmune diseases, metabolic disorders, and neurodegenerative conditions.

The integration of peptide therapeutics with advanced technologies—such as artificial intelligence, smart biomaterials, wearable delivery devices, and nanotheranostics—signals the advent of a new era in personalized medicine. Patient-specific delivery systems, which can adapt to individual physiological conditions or disease states, are transitioning from a distant aspiration to an emerging reality. These methodologies hold significant potential for tailoring therapies to patient-specific genetic, epigenetic, and environmental factors, thereby enhancing efficacy and reducing adverse effects.

Significantly, these advancements are augmented by enhancements in computational modeling, high-throughput screening, and biosensing technologies, which facilitate the rational design of peptides and their delivery systems. The integration of in silico tools and machine learning expedites the development process by predicting peptide behavior, optimizing formulation parameters, and identifying optimal delivery strategies. As digital health tools continue to progress, their synergy with peptide therapeutics will enable clinicians to make more informed, data-driven treatment decisions.

Looking toward the future, sustained interdisciplinary collaboration will be crucial for overcoming current limitations and translating laboratory-scale innovations into viable clinical solutions. Engagement of stakeholders across academia, biotechnology companies, regulatory authorities, and patient advocacy groups will be essential to ensure that peptide delivery technologies are safe, accessible, and equitably distributed.

In conclusion, peptide delivery systems represent a pivotal advancement in pharmaceutical innovation. Their capacity to convert peptides from delicate molecules into potent, targeted therapeutics highlights their importance in contemporary medicine. As technological capabilities expand and our comprehension of disease mechanisms advances, these delivery platforms will continue to develop, facilitating not only more effective treatments but also transforming the healthcare landscape towards a more personalized, efficient, and compassionate model of care.

References

Abou-Okeil, A., Refaei, R., Moustafa, S. E., & Ibrahim, H. M. (2024). Magnetic hydrogel scaffold based on hyaluronic acid/chitosan and gelatin natural polymers. *Scientific Reports*, *14*(1). https://doi.org/10.1038/s41598-024-78696-6

Achilleos, K., Petrou, C., Nicolaidou, V., & Sarigiannis, Y. (2025). Beyond Efficacy: Ensuring Safety in Peptide Therapeutics through Immunogenicity Assessment. *Journal of Peptide Science*, *31*(6). https://doi.org/10.1002/psc.70016

Adhikari, D., & Pokhrel, S. (2025). Microneedle delivery of protein and peptides: Advances in drug delivery. *Journal of Drug Delivery and Therapeutics*, *15*(2), 86–94. https://doi.org/10.22270/jddt.v15i2.6995

Afzal, A., Abbasi, M. H., Ahmad, S., Sheikh, N., & Khawar, M. B. (2025). Current trends in mRNA technology for cancer therapeutics. *Biomaterials Research*. https://doi.org/10.34133/bmr.0178

Al-Thani, A. N., Jan, A. G., Abbas, M., Geetha, M., & Sadasivuni, K. K. (2024). Nanoparticles in cancer theragnostic and drug delivery: A comprehensive review. *Life Sciences*, *352*, 122899. https://doi.org/10.1016/j.lfs.2024.122899

Alexander-Bryant, A. A., Dumitriu, A., Attaway, C. C., Yu, H., & Jakymiw, A. (2015). Fusogenic-oligoarginine peptide-mediated silencing of the CIP2A oncogene suppresses oral cancer tumor growth in vivo. *Journal of Controlled Release*, *218*, 72–81. https://doi.org/10.1016/j.jconrel.2015.09.026

Alghareeb, S., Asare-Addo, K., Conway, B. R., & Adebisi, A. O. (2024). PLGA nanoparticles for nasal drug delivery. *Journal of Drug Delivery Science and Technology*, *95*, 105564. https://doi.org/10.1016/j.jddst.2024.105564

Alhakamy, N. A., Nigatu, A. S., Berkland, C. J., & Ramsey, J. D. (2013). Noncovalently Associated cell-penetrating Peptides for Gene Delivery Applications. *Therapeutic Delivery*, *4*(6), 741–757. https://doi.org/10.4155/tde.13.44

Alimardani, V., Abolmaali, S. S., Yousefi, G., Rahiminezhad, Z., Abedi, M., Tamaddon, A., & Ahadian, S. (2021). Microneedle Arrays Combined with Nanomedicine Approaches for Transdermal Delivery of Therapeutics. *Journal of Clinical Medicine*, *10*(2), 181. https://doi.org/10.3390/jcm10020181

Allemailem, K. S., Alsahli, M. A., Almatroudi, A., Alrumaihi, F., Alkhaleefah, F. K., Rahmani, A. H., & Khan, A. A. (2022). Current updates of CRISPR/Cas9-mediated genome editing and targeting within tumor cells: an innovative strategy of cancer management. *Cancer Communications*, *42*(12), 1257–1287. https://doi.org/10.1002/cac2.12366

Allen, T. M., & Cullis, P. R. (2012). Liposomal drug delivery systems: From concept to clinical applications. *Advanced Drug Delivery Reviews*, *65*(1), 36–48. https://doi.org/10.1016/j.addr.2012.09.037

Almansour, K., Taverner, A., Turner, J. R., Eggleston, I. M., & Mrsny, R. J. (2018). An intestinal paracellular pathway biased toward positively-charged macromolecules. *Journal of Controlled Release*, *288*, 111–125. https://doi.org/10.1016/j.jconrel.2018.09.003

Alrbyawi, H., Poudel, I., Annaji, M., Boddu, S. H. S., Arnold, R. D., Tiwari, A. K., & Babu, R. J. (2022). PH-Sensitive liposomes for enhanced cellular uptake and cytotoxicity of daunorubicin in melanoma (B16-BL6) cell lines. *Pharmaceutics*, *14*(6), 1128. https://doi.org/10.3390/pharmaceutics14061128

Alsaab, H. O., Alharbi, F. D., Alhibs, A. S., Alanazi, N. B., Alshehri, B. Y., Saleh, M. A., Alshehri, F. S., Algarni, M. A., Almugaiteeb, T., Uddin, M. N., & Alzhrani, R. M. (2022). PLGA-Based Nanomedicine: History of advancement and development in clinical applications of multiple diseases. *Pharmaceutics*, *14*(12), 2728. https://doi.org/10.3390/pharmaceutics14122728

AlSawaftah, N. M., Awad, N. S., Pitt, W. G., & Husseini, G. A. (2022). PH-Responsive Nanocarriers in Cancer Therapy. *Polymers*, *14*(5), 936. https://doi.org/10.3390/polym14050936

Anbazhagan, G., Suseela, S. B., & Sankararajan, R. (2025). Hollow microneedles: from materials to market—a comprehensive review. *Microsystem Technologies*. https://doi.org/10.1007/s00542-025-05854-9

Aschmann, D., Knol, R. A., & Kros, A. (2024). Lipid-Based Nanoparticle Functionalization with Coiled-Coil Peptides for In Vitro and In Vivo Drug Delivery. *Accounts of Chemical Research*, *57*(8), 1098–1110. https://doi.org/10.1021/acs.accounts.3c00769

Azimizonuzi, H., Ghayourvahdat, A., Ahmed, M. H., Kareem, R. A., Zrzor, A. J., Mansoor, A. S., Athab, Z. H., & Kalavi, S. (2025). A state-of-the-art review of the recent advances of theranostic liposome hybrid nanoparticles in cancer treatment and diagnosis. *Cancer Cell International*, *25*(1). https://doi.org/10.1186/s12935-024-03610-z

Bachta, P., Jakhmola, V., Nainwal, N., Joshi, P., Bahuguna, R., Chaudhary, M., Kumar, K., Singh, A., & Kumar, P. (2025b). A comprehensive study on pH-sensitive nanoparticles for the efficient delivery of drugs. *Journal of Advanced Biotechnology and Experimental Therapeutics*, *8*(2), 200. https://doi.org/10.5455/jabet.2025.17

Bao, Q., Zhang, X., Hao, Z., Li, Q., Wu, F., Wang, K., Li, Y., Li, W., & Gao, H. (2024). Advances in Polysaccharide-Based Microneedle systems for the treatment of ocular diseases. *Nano-Micro Letters*, *16*(1). https://doi.org/10.1007/s40820-024-01477-3

Baral, K. C., & Choi, K. Y. (2025). Barriers and Strategies for oral peptide and protein therapeutics delivery: Update on Clinical advances. *Pharmaceutics*, *17*(4), 397. https://doi.org/10.3390/pharmaceutics17040397

Barenholz, Y. (2012). Doxil® — The first FDA-approved nano-drug: Lessons learned. *Journal of Controlled Release*, *160*(2), 117–134. https://doi.org/10.1016/j.jconrel.2012.03.020

Beach, M. A., Nayanathara, U., Gao, Y., Zhang, C., Xiong, Y., Wang, Y., & Such, G. K. (2024). Polymeric nanoparticles for drug delivery. *Chemical Reviews*, *124*(9), 5505–5616.

https://doi.org/10.1021/acs.chemrev.3c00705

Bech, E. M., Pedersen, S. L., & Jensen, K. J. (2018). Chemical Strategies for Half-Life Extension of Biopharmaceuticals: Lipidation and its Alternatives. *ACS Medicinal Chemistry Letters*, *9*(7), 577–580. https://doi.org/10.1021/acsmedchemlett.8b00226

Behzadipour, Y., & Hemmati, S. (2024). Covalent conjugation and non-covalent complexation strategies for intracellular delivery of proteins using cell-penetrating peptides. *Biomedicine & Pharmacotherapy*, *176*, 116910. https://doi.org/10.1016/j.biopha.2024.116910

Blades, R., Ittner, L. M., & Tietz, O. (2023). Peptides for trans-blood–brain barrier delivery. *Journal of Labelled Compounds and Radiopharmaceuticals*, *66*(9), 237–248. https://doi.org/10.1002/jlcr.4023

Bose, R. J., Ravikumar, R., Karuppagounder, V., Bennet, D., Rangasamy, S., & Thandavarayan, R. A. (2017). Lipid–polymer hybrid nanoparticle-mediated therapeutics delivery: advances and challenges. *Drug Discovery Today*, *22*(8), 1258–1265. https://doi.org/10.1016/j.drudis.2017.05.015

Bukke, S. P. N., Venkatesh, C., Rajanna, S. B., Saraswathi, T. S., Kusuma, P. K., Goruntla, N., Balasuramanyam, N., & Munishamireddy, S. (2024). Solid lipid nanocarriers for drug delivery: design innovations and characterization strategies—a comprehensive review. *Deleted Journal*, *6*(6). https://doi.org/10.1007/s42452-024-05897-z

Cai, Y., Fu, X., Zhou, Y., Lei, L., Wang, J., Zeng, W., & Yang, Z. (2023). A hydrogel system for drug loading toward the synergistic application of reductive/heat-sensitive drugs. *Journal of Controlled Release*, *362*, 409–424. https://doi.org/10.1016/j.jconrel.2023.09.004

Cerrato, C. P., & Langel, Ü. (2022). An update on cell-penetrating peptides with intracellular organelle targeting. *Expert Opinion on Drug Delivery*, *19*(2), 133–146. https://doi.org/10.1080/17425247.2022.2034784

Chaudhry, M., Lyon, P., Coussios, C., & Carlisle, R. (2022). Thermosensitive liposomes: a promising step toward localised chemotherapy. *Expert Opinion on Drug Delivery*, *19*(8), 899–912. https://doi.org/10.1080/17425247.2022.2099834

Chehelgerdi, M., Chehelgerdi, M., Allela, O. Q. B., Pecho, R. D. C., Jayasankar, N., Rao, D. P., Thamaraikani, T., Vasanthan, M., Viktor, P., Lakshmaiya, N., Saadh, M. J., Amajd, A., Abo-Zaid, M. A., Castillo-Acobo, R. Y., Ismail, A. H., Amin, A. H., & Akhavan-Sigari, R. (2023). Progressing nanotechnology to improve targeted cancer treatment: overcoming hurdles in its clinical implementation. *Molecular Cancer*, *22*(1). https://doi.org/10.1186/s12943-023-01865-0

Chelakkot, C., Ghim, J., & Ryu, S. H. (2018). Mechanisms regulating intestinal barrier integrity and its pathological implications. *Experimental & Molecular Medicine*, *50*(8), 1–9. https://doi.org/10.1038/s12276-018-0126-x

Chen, G., Kang, W., Li, W., Chen, S., & Gao, Y. (2022). Oral delivery of protein and peptide drugs: from non-specific formulation approaches to intestinal cell targeting strategies. *Theranostics*, *12*(3), 1419–1439. https://doi.org/10.7150/thno.61747

Chen, W., Li, F., Tang, Y., Yang, S., Li, J., Yuan, Z., Liu, Y., Zhou, X., Liu, C., & Zhang, X. (2017). Stepwise pH-responsive nanoparticles for enhanced cellular uptake and on-demand intracellular release of doxorubicin. *International Journal of Nanomedicine*, *Volume 12*, 4241–4256. https://doi.org/10.2147/ijn.s129748

Cheng, Z., Huang, H., Yin, M., & Liu, H. (2025). Applications of liposomes and lipid nanoparticles in cancer therapy: current advances and prospects. *Experimental Hematology and Oncology*, *14*(1). https://doi.org/10.1186/s40164-025-00602-1

Choi, W., & Kohane, D. S. (2024). Hybrid Nanoparticle–Hydrogel systems for drug delivery depots and other biomedical applications. *ACS Nano*, *18*(34), 22780–22792. https://doi.org/10.1021/acsnano.4c06888

Czock, D., Keller, F., & Seidling, H. M. (2012). Pharmacokinetic predictions for patients with renal impairment: focus on peptides and protein drugs. *British Journal of Clinical Pharmacology*, *74*(1), 66–74. https://doi.org/10.1111/j.1365-2125.2012.04172.x

Mai, L. D., Wimberley, S. C., & Champion, J. A. (2024). Intracellular delivery strategies using membrane-interacting peptides and proteins. *Nanoscale*, *16*(33), 15465–15480. https://doi.org/10.1039/d4nr02093f

Danhier, F., Ansorena, E., Silva, J. M., Coco, R., Breton, A. L., & Préat, V. (2012). PLGA-based nanoparticles: An overview of biomedical applications. *Journal of Controlled Release*, *161*(2), 505–522. https://doi.org/10.1016/j.jconrel.2012.01.043

Danhier, F., Feron, O., & Préat, V. (2010). To exploit the tumor microenvironment: Passive and active tumor targeting of nanocarriers for anti-cancer drug delivery. *Journal of Controlled Release*, *148*(2), 135–146. https://doi.org/10.1016/j.jconrel.2010.08.027

Datta, N. (2025). A review on the Cell-Penetrating peptides. *Cell Engineering Connect.*, *1*(1), 1. https://doi.org/10.69709/cellengc.2025.145023

De Bruyn, M., Ceuleers, H., Hanning, N., Berg, M., De Man, J. G., Hulpiau, P., Hermans, C., Stenman, U., Koistinen, H., Lambeir, A., De Winter, B. Y., & De Meester, I. (2021). Proteolytic cleavage of bioactive peptides and Protease-Activated receptors in acute and Post-Colitis. *International Journal of Molecular Sciences*, *22*(19), 10711. https://doi.org/10.3390/ijms221910711

De Groot, A. S., Mattei, A., Gabriel, B., Calderini, J., Roberts, B. J., Lelias, S., McAllister, M., Boyle, C., Martin, W., & Richard, G. (2025). Immunogenicity of generic peptide impurities: current orthogonal approaches. *Pharmaceutical Research*. https://doi.org/10.1007/s11095-025-03843-1

Di, L. (2014). Strategic Approaches to Optimizing Peptide ADME Properties. *The AAPS Journal*, *17*(1), 134–143. https://doi.org/10.1208/s12248-014-9687-3

Diao, L., & Meibohm, B. (2013). Pharmacokinetics and Pharmacokinetic–Pharmacodynamic correlations of therapeutic peptides. *Clinical Pharmacokinetics*, *52*(10), 855–868. https://doi.org/10.1007/s40262-013-0079-0

Dowaidar, M. (2024). Cell-penetrating peptides with nanoparticles hybrid delivery vectors and their uptake pathways. *Mitochondrion*, *78*, 101906. https://doi.org/10.1016/j.mito.2024.101906

Driscoll, J., Gondaliya, P., Zinn, D. A., Jain, R., Yan, I. K., Dong, H., & Patel, T. (2025). Using aptamers for targeted delivery of RNA therapies. *Molecular Therapy*. https://doi.org/10.1016/j.ymthe.2025.02.047

Du, J., Zhang, R., Jiang, S., Xiao, S., Liu, Y., Niu, Y., Zhao, W., Wang, D., & Ma, X. (2025). Applications of cell penetrating peptide-based drug delivery system in immunotherapy. *Frontiers in Immunology*, *16*. https://doi.org/10.3389/fimmu.2025.1540192

El-Husseiny, H. M., Mady, E. A., Hamabe, L., Abugomaa, A., Shimada, K., Yoshida, T., Tanaka, T., Yokoi, A., Elbadawy, M., & Tanaka, R. (2021). Smart/stimuli-responsive hydrogels: Cutting-edge platforms for tissue engineering and other biomedical applications. *Materials Today Bio*, *13*, 100186. https://doi.org/10.1016/j.mtbio.2021.100186

El-Tanani, M., Satyam, S. M., Rabbani, S. A., El-Tanani, Y., Aljabali, A. a. A., Faouri, I. A., & Rehman, A. (2025). Revolutionizing Drug delivery: The impact of advanced materials science and technology on precision medicine. *Pharmaceutics*, *17*(3), 375. https://doi.org/10.3390/pharmaceutics17030375

Elumalai, K., Srinivasan, S., & Shanmugam, A. (2023). Review of the efficacy of nanoparticle-based drug delivery systems for cancer treatment. *Biomedical Technology*, *5*, 109–122. https://doi.org/10.1016/j.bmt.2023.09.001

Erazo-Oliveras, Alfredo, Nandhini Muthukrishnan, Ryan Baker, Ting-Yi Wang, and Jean-Philippe Pellois. 2012. "Improving the Endosomal

Escape of Cell-Penetrating Peptides and Their Cargos: Strategies and Challenges". Pharmaceuticals (Basel, Switzerland) 5 (11): 1177-209. https://doi.org/10.3390/ph5111177.

Estupiñán, H. Y., Baladi, T., Roudi, S., Munson, M. J., Bost, J., Gustafsson, O., Velásquez-Ramírez, D., Bhatt, D. K., Hagey, D., Hekman, D., Andersson, S., Andaloussi, S. E., & Dahlén, A. (2025). Design and screening of novel endosomal escape compounds that enhance functional delivery of oligonucleotide in vitro. *Molecular Therapy — Nucleic Acids*, 102522. https://doi.org/10.1016/j.omtn.2025.102522

Ezike, T. C., Okpala, U. S., Onoja, U. L., Nwike, C. P., Ezeako, E. C., Okpara, O. J., Okoroafor, C. C., Eze, S. C., Kalu, O. L., Odoh, E. C., Nwadike, U. G., Ogbodo, J. O., Umeh, B. U., Ossai, E. C., & Nwanguma, B. C. (2023). Advances in drug delivery systems, challenges and future directions. *Heliyon*, *9*(6), e17488. https://doi.org/10.1016/j.heliyon.2023.e17488

Fan, D., Cao, Y., Cao, M., Wang, Y., Cao, Y., & Gong, T. (2023). Nanomedicine in cancer therapy. *Signal Transduction and Targeted Therapy*, *8*(1). https://doi.org/10.1038/s41392-023-01536-y

Farag, V. E., Devey, E. A., & Leong, K. W. (2024). The Interface of Gene Editing with Regenerative Medicine. *Engineering*. https://doi.org/10.1016/j.eng.2024.10.019

González-Nieto, D., Fernandez-Serra, R., Gallego, R., & Lozano, P. (2019). Hydrogels for neuroprotection and functional rewiring: a new era for brain engineering. *Neural Regeneration Research*, *15*(5), 783. https://doi.org/10.4103/1673-5374.268891

Fetse, J., Kandel, S., Mamani, U., & Cheng, K. (2023). Recent advances in the development of therapeutic peptides. *Trends in Pharmacological Sciences*, *44*(7), 425–441. https://doi.org/10.1016/j.tips.2023.04.003

Fu, Z., & Xiang, J. (2020). Aptamer-Functionalized nanoparticles in targeted delivery and cancer therapy. *International Journal of Molecular Sciences*, *21*(23), 9123. https://doi.org/10.3390/ijms21239123

Gao, J., Li, J., Luo, Z., Wang, H., & Ma, Z. (2024). Nanoparticle-Based Drug delivery systems for inflammatory bowel disease treatment. *Drug Design Development and Therapy*, *Volume 18*, 2921–2949. https://doi.org/10.2147/dddt.s461977

Gao, Y., Joshi, M., Zhao, Z., & Mitragotri, S. (2023). PEGylated therapeutics in the clinic. *Bioengineering & Translational Medicine*, *9*(1). https://doi.org/10.1002/btm2.10600

Ghorai, S. M., Deep, A., Magoo, D., Gupta, C., & Gupta, N. (2023). Cell-Penetrating and Targeted Peptides Delivery Systems as Potential

Pharmaceutical Carriers for Enhanced Delivery across the Blood–Brain Barrier (BBB). *Pharmaceutics*, *15*(7), 1999. https://doi.org/10.3390/pharmaceutics15071999

Ghosh, R., Kumar, M., Kumar, S., Komal, K., Sharma, R., & Kurmi, B. D. (2025). Small molecule therapeutics for receptor-mediated targeting through liposomes in breast cancer treatment: A comprehensive review. *Bioorganic Chemistry*, 108442. https://doi.org/10.1016/j.bioorg.2025.108442

Gradinaru, V. R., Bercea, M., Gradinaru, L. M., Puiu, A., Lupu, A., & Petre, B. A. (2025). Targeting injectable hydrogels: The role of diphenylalanine peptide derivative in the gelation dynamics of Pluronic® F127. *Polymers*, *17*(7), 930. https://doi.org/10.3390/polym17070930

Graham, W., Torbett-Dougherty, M., Islam, A., Soleimani, S., Bruce-Tagoe, T. A., & Johnson, J. A. (2025). Magnetic Nanoparticles and Drug Delivery Systems for Anti-Cancer Applications: A review. *Nanomaterials*, *15*(4), 285. https://doi.org/10.3390/nano15040285

Grau, M., & Wagner, E. (2024). Strategies and mechanisms for endosomal escape of therapeutic nucleic acids. *Current Opinion in Chemical Biology*, *81*, 102506. https://doi.org/10.1016/j.cbpa.2024.102506

Guidotti, G., Brambilla, L., & Rossi, D. (2017). Cell-Penetrating peptides: From basic research to clinics. *Trends in Pharmacological Sciences*, *38*(4), 406–424. https://doi.org/10.1016/j.tips.2017.01.003

Gunawan, M., Bestari, A. N., Ramadon, D., Efendi, A., & Boonkanokwong, V. (2025). Combination of lipid-based nanoparticles with microneedles as a promising strategy for enhanced transdermal delivery systems: A comprehensive review. *Journal of Drug Delivery Science and Technology*, 106807. https://doi.org/10.1016/j.jddst.2025.106807

Haberbosch, L., & Strasburger, C. J. (2023). Efficacy and safety of Pegvisomant in the treatment of acromegaly. *Archives of Medical Research*, *54*(8), 102884. https://doi.org/10.1016/j.arcmed.2023.102884

Haddadzadegan, S., Dorkoosh, F., & Bernkop-Schnürch, A. (2022). Oral delivery of therapeutic peptides and proteins: Technology landscape of lipid-based nanocarriers. *Advanced Drug Delivery Reviews*, *182*, 114097. https://doi.org/10.1016/j.addr.2021.114097

Hartmeier, P. R., Pham, N. B., Velankar, K. Y., Issa, F., Giannoukakis, N., & Meng, W. S. (2020). *Hydrogel Dressings for Chronic wound Healing in Diabetes: Beyond Hydration*. https://pmc.ncbi.nlm.nih.gov/articles/PMC9473423/

He, H., Lu, Y., Qi, J., Zhu, Q., Chen, Z., & Wu, W. (2018). Adapting liposomes for oral drug delivery. *Acta Pharmaceutica Sinica B*, *9*(1), 36–48. https://doi.org/10.1016/j.apsb.2018.06.005

He, X., Li, J., An, S., & Jiang, C. (2013). pH-sensitive drug-delivery Systems for Tumor Targeting. *Therapeutic Delivery*, *4*(12), 1499–1510. https://doi.org/10.4155/tde.13.120

Herce, H., Garcia, A., Litt, J., Kane, R., Martin, P., Enrique, N., Rebolledo, A., & Milesi, V. (2009). Arginine-Rich Peptides Destabilize the Plasma Membrane, Consistent with a Pore Formation Translocation Mechanism of Cell-Penetrating Peptides. *Biophysical Journal*, *97*(7), 1917–1925. https://doi.org/10.1016/j.bpj.2009.05.066

Hijazi, Y. (2021). Prediction of Half-Life Extension of peptides via serum albumin binding: current challenges. *European Journal of Drug Metabolism and Pharmacokinetics*, *46*(2), 163–172. https://doi.org/10.1007/s13318-020-00664-y

Homayun, B., Lin, X., & Choi, H. (2019). Challenges and recent progress in oral drug delivery systems for biopharmaceuticals. *Pharmaceutics*, *11*(3), 129. https://doi.org/10.3390/pharmaceutics11030129

Hong, W., Huang, H., Zeng, X., & Duan, C. (2024). Targeting mitochondrial quality control: new therapeutic strategies for major diseases. *Military Medical Research*, *11*(1). https://doi.org/10.1186/s40779-024-00556-1

Huang, J., Gong, C., & Zhou, A. (2023). Modulation of gut microbiota: a novel approach to enhancing the effects of immune checkpoint inhibitors. *Therapeutic Advances in Medical Oncology*, *15*. https://doi.org/10.1177/17588359231204854

Huang, S., Wen, T., Wang, J., Wei, H., Xiao, Z., Li, B., & Shuai, X. (2024). Nanoparticle-integrated dissolving microneedles for the co-delivery of R848/aPD-1 to synergistically reverse the immunosuppressive microenvironment of triple-negative breast cancer. *Acta Biomaterialia*, *176*, 344–355. https://doi.org/10.1016/j.actbio.2024.01.009

Huang, W., & Zhang, C. (2017). Tuning the Size of Poly(lactic-co-glycolic Acid) (PLGA) Nanoparticles Fabricated by Nanoprecipitation. *Biotechnology Journal*, *13*(1). https://doi.org/10.1002/biot.201700203

Huang, Y., Qin, A., Tsai, C., & Chen, P. (2022). Novel pegylated interferon for the treatment of chronic viral hepatitis. *Viruses*, *14*(6), 1128. https://doi.org/10.3390/v14061128

Immordino, M. L., Dosio, F., & Cattel, L. (2006). *Stealth liposomes: review of the basic science, rationale, and clinical applications, existing and potential*. https://pmc.ncbi.nlm.nih.gov/articles/PMC2426795/

Ingrole, R. S., & Gill, H. S. (2019). Microneedle Coating Methods: A Review with a Perspective. *Journal of Pharmacology and Experimental Therapeutics*, *370*(3), 555–569. https://doi.org/10.1124/jpet.119.258707

Isaacson, K. J., Jensen, M. M., Subrahmanyam, N. B., & Ghandehari, H. (2017). Matrix-metalloproteinases as targets for controlled delivery in cancer: An analysis of upregulation and expression. *Journal of Controlled Release*, *259*, 62–75. https://doi.org/10.1016/j.jconrel.2017.01.034

Islam, S., Ahmed, M. M. S., Islam, M. A., Hossain, N., & Chowdhury, M. A. (2025). Advances in nanoparticles in targeted drug delivery- a review. *Results in Surfaces and Interfaces*, 100529. https://doi.org/10.1016/j.rsurfi.2025.100529

Itoh, K., & Yamada, A. (2006). Personalized peptide vaccines: A new therapeutic modality for cancer. *Cancer Science*, *97*(10), 970–976. https://doi.org/10.1111/j.1349-7006.2006.00272.x

Walsh, S. J., Bargh, J. D., Dannheim, F. M., Hanby, A. R., Seki, H., Counsell, A. J., Ou, X., Fowler, E., Ashman, N., Takada, Y., Isidro-Llobet, A., Parker, J. S., Carroll, J. S., & Spring, D. R. (2020). Site-selective modification strategies in antibody–drug conjugates. *Chemical Society Reviews*, *50*(2), 1305–1353. https://doi.org/10.1039/d0cs00310g

Jadhav, K., Abhang, A., Kole, E. B., Gadade, D., Dusane, A., Iyer, A., Sharma, A., Rout, S. K., Gholap, A. D., Naik, J., Verma, R. K., & Rojekar, S. (2025). Peptide–Drug Conjugates as Next-Generation Therapeutics: Exploring the potential and Clinical progress. *Bioengineering*, *12*(5), 481. https://doi.org/10.3390/bioengineering12050481

Ji, B., Maeda, J., Higuchi, M., Inoue, K., Akita, H., Harashima, H., & Suhara, T. (2005). Pharmacokinetics and brain uptake of lactoferrin in rats. *Life Sciences*, *78*(8), 851–855. https://doi.org/10.1016/j.lfs.2005.05.085

Ji, G., Li, Y., Zhang, Z., Li, H., & Sun, P. (2024). Recent advances of novel targeted drug delivery systems based on natural medicine monomers against hepatocellular carcinoma. *Heliyon*, *10*(2), e24667. https://doi.org/10.1016/j.heliyon.2024.e24667

Jiang, S., Zu, C., Wang, B., & Zhong, Y. (2025). Enhancing DNA vaccine delivery through Stearyl-Modified Cell-Penetrating peptides: improved antigen expression and immune response in vitro and in vivo. *Vaccines*, *13*(1), 94. https://doi.org/10.3390/vaccines13010094

Jiang, T., Gonzalez, K. M., Cordova, L. E., & Lu, J. (2023). Nanotechnology-enabled gene delivery for cancer and other genetic diseases. *Expert Opinion on Drug Delivery*, *20*(4), 523–540. https://doi.org/10.1080/17425247.2023.2200246

Jnaidi, R., Almeida, A. J., & Gonçalves, L. M. (2020). Solid lipid nanoparticles and nanostructured lipid carriers as smart drug delivery systems in the treatment of glioblastoma multiforme. *Pharmaceutics*, *12*(9), 860. https://doi.org/10.3390/pharmaceutics12090860

Juliano, R., Alam, M. R., Dixit, V., & Kang, H. (2008). Mechanisms and strategies for effective delivery of antisense and siRNA oligonucleotides. *Nucleic Acids Research*, *36*(12), 4158–4171. https://doi.org/10.1093/nar/gkn342

Karlsson, J., Rhodes, K. R., Green, J. J., & Tzeng, S. Y. (2020). Poly(beta-amino ester)s as gene delivery vehicles: challenges and opportunities. *Expert Opinion on Drug Delivery*, *17*(10), 1395–1410. https://doi.org/10.1080/17425247.2020.1796628

Khairkhah, N., Namvar, A., & Bolhassani, A. (2023). Application of cell penetrating peptides as a promising drug carrier to combat viral infections. *Molecular Biotechnology*, *65*(9), 1387–1402. https://doi.org/10.1007/s12033-023-00679-1

Kim, Y., Park, J., & Prausnitz, M. R. (2012). Microneedles for drug and vaccine delivery. *Advanced Drug Delivery Reviews*, *64*(14), 1547–1568. https://doi.org/10.1016/j.addr.2012.04.005

Kocbek, P., Obermajer, N., Cegnar, M., Kos, J., & Kristl, J. (2007). Targeting cancer cells using PLGA nanoparticles surface modified with monoclonal antibody. *Journal of Controlled Release*, *120*(1–2), 18–26. https://doi.org/10.1016/j.jconrel.2007.03.012

Kovtareva, S., Kusepova, L., Tazhkenova, G., Mashan, T., Bazarbaeva, K., & Kopishev, E. (2024). Surface modification of mesoporous silica nanoparticles for application in targeted delivery systems of antitumour drugs. *Polymers*, *16*(8), 1105. https://doi.org/10.3390/polym16081105

Kowalski, P. S., Rudra, A., Miao, L., & Anderson, D. G. (2019). Delivering the Messenger: Advances in technologies for therapeutic mRNA delivery. *Molecular Therapy*, *27*(4), 710–728. https://doi.org/10.1016/j.ymthe.2019.02.012

Kozma, G. T., Shimizu, T., Ishida, T., & Szebeni, J. (2020). Anti-PEG antibodies: Properties, formation, testing and role in adverse immune reactions to PEGylated nano-biopharmaceuticals. *Advanced Drug Delivery Reviews*, *154–155*, 163–175. https://doi.org/10.1016/j.addr.2020.07.024

Kristensen, M., Birch, D., & Nielsen, H. M. (2016). Applications and challenges for use of Cell-Penetrating Peptides as delivery vectors for peptide and protein cargos. *International Journal of Molecular Sciences*, *17*(2), 185. https://doi.org/10.3390/ijms17020185

Langguth, P., Bohner, V., Heizmann, J., Merkle, H., Wolffram, S., Amidon, G., & Yamashita, S. (1997). The challenge of proteolytic enzymes in intestinal peptide delivery. *Journal of Controlled Release*, *46*(1–2), 39–57. https://doi.org/10.1016/s0168-3659(96)01586-6

Lau, G. K., Piratvisuth, T., Luo, K. X., Marcellin, P., Thongsawat, S., Cooksley, G., Gane, E., Fried, M. W., Chow, W. C., Paik, S. W., Chang, W. Y., Berg, T., Flisiak, R., McCloud, P., & Pluck, N. (2005). Peginterferon Alfa-2A, lamivudine, and the combination for HBEAG-Positive chronic hepatitis B. *New England Journal of Medicine*, *352*(26), 2682–2695. https://doi.org/10.1056/nejmoa043470

Lee, Y., & Thompson, D. (2017). Stimuli-responsive liposomes for drug delivery. *Wiley Interdisciplinary Reviews Nanomedicine and Nanobiotechnology*, *9*(5). https://doi.org/10.1002/wnan.1450

Li, H., Vora, L. K., Anjani, Q., Abraham, A. M., Cong, Y., Moreno-Castellanos, N., Ballana, E., Muñoz, E. R., Nevot, M., & Donnelly, R. F. (2025). Quality by Design-Guided development of Hydrogel-Forming microneedles for transdermal delivery of enfuvirtide. *ACS Applied Materials & Interfaces*. https://doi.org/10.1021/acsami.5c00499

Liu, C., Liao, Y., Liu, L., Xie, L., Liu, J., Zhang, Y., & Li, Y. (2023). Application of injectable hydrogels in cancer immunotherapy. *Frontiers in Bioengineering and Biotechnology*, *11*. https://doi.org/10.3389/fbioe.2023.1121887

Liu, H., & He, L. (2025). Intelligent hydrogel-based dressings for treatment of chronic diabetic wounds. *World Journal of Diabetes*, *16*(5). https://doi.org/10.4239/wjd.v16.i5.104937

Liu, L., Yao, W., Rao, Y., Lu, X., & Gao, J. (2017). pH-Responsive carriers for oral drug delivery: challenges and opportunities of current platforms. *Drug Delivery*, *24*(1), 569–581. https://doi.org/10.1080/10717544.2017.1279238

Liu, P., Chen, G., & Zhang, J. (2022). A review of liposomes as a drug delivery system: current status of approved products, regulatory environments, and future perspectives. *Molecules*, *27*(4), 1372. https://doi.org/10.3390/molecules27041372

Liu, T., Chen, M., Fu, J., Sun, Y., Lu, C., Quan, G., Pan, X., & Wu, C. (2021). Recent advances in microneedles-mediated transdermal delivery of protein and peptide drugs. *Acta Pharmaceutica Sinica B*, *11*(8), 2326–2343. https://doi.org/10.1016/j.apsb.2021.03.003

Liu, Y., Zhao, Z., & Li, M. (2022). Overcoming the cellular barriers and beyond: Recent progress on cell penetrating peptide modified nanomedicine in combating physiological and pathological barriers. *Asian Journal of Pharmaceutical Sciences*, *17*(4), 523–543. https://doi.org/10.1016/j.ajps.2022.05.002

Longoria-García, S., Sánchez-Domínguez, C. N., & Gallardo-Blanco, H. (2022). Recent applications of cell-penetrating peptide guidance of nanosystems in breast and prostate cancer (Review). *Oncology Letters*, *23*(3). https://doi.org/10.3892/ol.2022.13223

Lu, P., Ruan, D., Huang, M., Tian, M., Zhu, K., Gan, Z., & Xiao, Z. (2024). Harnessing the potential of hydrogels for advanced therapeutic applications: current achievements and future directions. *Signal Transduction and Targeted Therapy*, *9*(1). https://doi.org/10.1038/s41392-024-01852-x

Lu, Q., Kou, D., Lou, S., Ashrafizadeh, M., Aref, A. R., Canadas, I., Tian, Y., Niu, X., Wang, Y., Torabian, P., Wang, L., Sethi, G., Tergaonkar, V., Tay, F., Yuan, Z., & Han, P. (2024). Nanoparticles in tumor microenvironment remodeling and cancer immunotherapy. *Journal of Hematology & Oncology*, *17*(1). https://doi.org/10.1186/s13045-024-01535-8

Lu, Z., & Sun, D. (2025). Mechanism of pH-sensitive amphiphilic endosomal escape of ionizable lipid nanoparticles for cytosolic nucleic acid delivery. *Pharmaceutical Research*. https://doi.org/10.1007/s11095-025-03890-8

Navaneetha, K. M., Sangeetha, S., Sree, R. P., & Narayanasamy, D. (2024). The Science of Solid Lipid Nanoparticles: From Fundamentals to Applications. *Cureus,* 16 (9): e68807. https://doi.org/10.7759/cureus.68807.

Ma, J., Yan, L., Yang, J., He, Y., & Wu, L. (2023). Effect of modification strategies on the biological activity of Peptides/Proteins. *ChemBioChem*, *25*(3). https://doi.org/10.1002/cbic.202300481

Malinowska, A. L., Huynh, H. L., & Bose, S. (2024). Peptide–Oligonucleotide conjugation: Chemistry and therapeutic applications. *Current Issues in Molecular Biology*, *46*(10), 11031–11047. https://doi.org/10.3390/cimb46100655

Martín, I., Teixidó, M., & Giralt, E. (2010). Building Cell Selectivity into CPP-Mediated Strategies. *Pharmaceuticals*, *3*(5), 1456–1490. https://doi.org/10.3390/ph3051456

Menacho-Melgar, R., Decker, J. S., Hennigan, J. N., & Lynch, M. D. (2018). A review of lipidation in the development of advanced protein and peptide therapeutics. *Journal of Controlled Release*, *295*, 1–12. https://doi.org/10.1016/j.jconrel.2018.12.032

Mendonça, M. C. P., Kont, A., Aburto, M. R., Cryan, J. F., & O'Driscoll, C. M. (2021). Advances in the design of (Nano)Formulations for delivery of antisense oligonucleotides and small interfering RNA: focus on the central nervous system. *Molecular Pharmaceutics*, *18*(4), 1491–1506. https://doi.org/10.1021/acs.molpharmaceut.0c01238

Meng, X., Shen, Y., Zhao, H., Lu, X., Wang, Z., & Zhao, Y. (2024). Redox-manipulating nanocarriers for anticancer drug delivery: a systematic review. *Journal of Nanobiotechnology*, *22*(1). https://doi.org/10.1186/s12951-024-02859-w

Mitchell, M. J., Billingsley, M. M., Haley, R. M., Wechsler, M. E., Peppas, N. A., & Langer, R. (2020). Engineering precision nanoparticles for drug delivery. *Nature Reviews Drug Discovery*, *20*(2), 101–124. https://doi.org/10.1038/s41573-020-0090-8

Moawad, F., Pouliot, R., & Brambilla, D. (2025). Dissolving microneedles in transdermal drug delivery: A critical analysis of limitations and translation challenges. *Journal of Controlled Release*, 113794. https://doi.org/10.1016/j.jconrel.2025.113794

Lira, C., Correia, E. M., Bonamino, M., & Vasconcelos, Z. F. M. (2024). Cell-Penetrating peptides and CRISPR-CAS9: a combined strategy for human genetic disease therapy. *Human Gene Therapy*. https://doi.org/10.1089/hum.2024.020

Mourya, V. K., & Inamdar, N. N. (2008). Trimethyl chitosan and its applications in drug delivery. *Journal of Materials Science Materials in Medicine*, *20*(5), 1057–1079. https://doi.org/10.1007/s10856-008-3659-z

Mukherjee, A., Waters, A. K., Kalyan, P., Achrol, A. S., Kesari, S., & Yenugonda, V. M. (2019). Lipid-Polymer Hybrid Nanoparticles as a next-Generation Drug Delivery Platform: State of the Art, Emerging Technologies, and Perspectives. *International Journal of Nanomedicine,* 14:1937-52. https://doi.org/10.2147/IJN.S198353.

Mura, P., Maestrelli, F., Cirri, M., & Mennini, N. (2022). Multiple roles of Chitosan in mucosal drug delivery: an updated review. *Marine Drugs*, *20*(5), 335. https://doi.org/10.3390/md20050335

Nebogatova, J., Härk, H. H., Puskar, A., Porosk, L., Guazzi, P., Dowaidar, M., Langel, Ü., & Kurrikoff, K. (2023). A Method for Using Cell-Penetrating Peptides for Loading Plasmid DNA into Secreted Extracellular Vesicles. *Biomolecules*, *13*(12), 1751. https://doi.org/10.3390/biom13121751

Nguyen, H. X. (2025). Beyond the needle: innovative Microneedle-Based transdermal vaccination. *Medicines*, *12*(1), 4. https://doi.org/10.3390/medicines12010004

Nguyen, H. X., & Nguyen, C. N. (2023). Microneedle-Mediated transdermal delivery of biopharmaceuticals. *Pharmaceutics*, *15*(1), 277. https://doi.org/10.3390/pharmaceutics15010277

Nguyen, T. T., Nguyen, T. T. D., Tran, N., & Van Vo, G. (2021). Advances of microneedles in hormone delivery. *Biomedicine & Pharmacotherapy*, *145*, 112393. https://doi.org/10.1016/j.biopha.2021.112393

Ni, R., Feng, R., & Chau, Y. (2019). Synthetic approaches for nucleic acid delivery: Choosing the right carriers. *Life*, *9*(3), 59. https://doi.org/10.3390/life9030059

Nikitovic, D., Kukovyakina, E., Berdiaki, A., Tzanakakis, A., Luss, A., Vlaskina, E., Yagolovich, A., Tsatsakis, A., & Kuskov, A. (2024). Enhancing tumor targeted therapy: The role of IRGD peptide in advanced drug delivery systems. *Cancers*, *16*(22), 3768. https://doi.org/10.3390/cancers16223768

Nunziata, G., Borroni, A., & Rossi, F. (2025). Advanced microfluidic strategies for core-shell nanoparticles: the next-generation of polymeric and lipid-based drug nanocarriers. *Chemical Engineering Journal Advances*, 100759. https://doi.org/10.1016/j.ceja.2025.100759

Oliveira, C., Teixeira, J. A., Oliveira, N., Ferreira, S., & Botelho, C. M. (2024). Microneedles' device: design, fabrication, and applications. *Macromol—A Journal of Macromolecular Research*, *4*(2), 320–355. https://doi.org/10.3390/macromol4020019

Omidian, H., Cubeddu, L. X., & Wilson, R. L. (2025). Peptide-Functionalized nanomedicine: advancements in drug delivery, diagnostics, and biomedical applications. *Molecules*, *30*(7), 1572. https://doi.org/10.3390/molecules30071572

Omidian, H., Gill, E. J., Chowdhury, S. D., & Cubeddu, L. X. (2024). Chitosan nanoparticles for intranasal drug delivery. *Pharmaceutics*, *16*(6), 746. https://doi.org/10.3390/pharmaceutics16060746

Omidian, H., Wilson, R. L., & Castejon, A. M. (2025). Recent advances in Peptide-Loaded PLGA nanocarriers for drug delivery and regenerative medicine. *Pharmaceuticals*, *18*(1), 127. https://doi.org/10.3390/ph18010127

Ouyang, J., Sheng, Y., & Wang, W. (2022). Recent advances of studies on Cell-Penetrating peptides based on molecular dynamics simulations. *Cells*, *11*(24), 4016. https://doi.org/10.3390/cells11244016

Pal, S., Rakshit, T., Saha, S., & Jinagal, D. (2025). Glucose-Responsive materials for smart insulin delivery: From Protein-Based to Protein-Free design. *ACS Materials Au*, *5*(2), 239–252. https://doi.org/10.1021/acsmaterialsau.4c00138

Pan, J., Wang, Y., Chen, Y., Zhang, C., Deng, H., Lu, J., & Chen, W. (2025). Emerging strategies against accelerated blood clearance phenomenon of nanocarrier drug delivery systems. *Journal of Nanobiotechnology*, *23*(1). https://doi.org/10.1186/s12951-025-03209-0

Pande, S. (2023). Liposomes for drug delivery: review of vesicular composition, factors affecting drug release and drug loading in liposomes. *Artificial Cells Nanomedicine and Biotechnology*, *51*(1), 428–440. https://doi.org/10.1080/21691401.2023.2247036

Parrasia, S., Szabò, I., Zoratti, M., & Biasutto, L. (2022). Peptides as pharmacological carriers to the brain: promises, shortcomings and challenges. *Molecular Pharmaceutics*, *19*(11), 3700–3729. https://doi.org/10.1021/acs.molpharmaceut.2c00523

Parvin, N., Joo, S. W., Jung, J. H., & Mandal, T. K. (2025). Innovative Micro- and Nano-Architectures in Biomedical engineering for therapeutic and diagnostic applications. *Micromachines*, *16*(4), 419. https://doi.org/10.3390/mi16040419

Patel, N. A., & Patel, N. R. (2024). Nano formulations for peptide drug delivery: Overcoming bioavailability and stability challenges. *World Journal of Advanced Research and Reviews*, *22*(1), 2032–2044. https://doi.org/10.30574/wjarr.2024.22.1.0971

Patel, S. K., Billingsley, M. M., Frazee, C., Han, X., Swingle, K. L., Qin, J., Alameh, M., Wang, K., Weissman, D., & Mitchell, M. J. (2022). Hydroxycholesterol substitution in ionizable lipid nanoparticles for mRNA delivery to T cells. *Journal of Controlled Release*, *347*, 521–532. https://doi.org/10.1016/j.jconrel.2022.05.020

Pentlavalli, S., Coulter, S. M., An, Y., Cross, E. R., Sun, H., Moore, J. V., Sabri, A. B., Greer, B., Vora, L., McCarthy, H. O., & Laverty, G. (2025). D-peptide hydrogels as a long-acting multipurpose drug delivery platform for combined contraception and HIV prevention. *Journal of Controlled Release*, *379*, 30–44. https://doi.org/10.1016/j.jconrel.2024.12.052

Perche, F. (2019). Stimuli-Sensitive cell penetrating Peptide-Modified nanocarriers. *Processes*, *7*(10), 727. https://doi.org/10.3390/pr7100727

Phillips, D. J., & Gibson, M. I. (2013). Redox-Sensitive materials for drug delivery: targeting the correct intracellular environment, tuning release rates, and appropriate predictive systems. *Antioxidants and Redox Signaling*, *21*(5), 786–803. https://doi.org/10.1089/ars.2013.5728

Plaza-Oliver, M., Santander-Ortega, M. J., & Lozano, M. V. (2021). Current approaches in lipid-based nanocarriers for oral drug delivery. *Drug Delivery and Translational Research*, *11*(2), 471–497. https://doi.org/10.1007/s13346-021-00908-7

Porosk, L., & Langel, Ü. (2022). Approaches for evaluation of novel CPP-based cargo delivery systems. *Frontiers in Pharmacology*, *13*. https://doi.org/10.3389/fphar.2022.1056467

Prasher, P., & Sharma, M. (2024). ProHES: hydroxyethyl starch's transformative role in anticancer drug delivery. *Future Medicinal Chemistry*, *16*(9), 811–816. https://doi.org/10.4155/fmc-2024-0052

Rahban, M., Ahmad, F., Piatyszek, M. A., Haertlé, T., Saso, L., & Saboury, A. A. (2023). Stabilization challenges and aggregation in protein-based therapeutics in the pharmaceutical industry. *RSC Advances*, *13*(51), 35947–35963. https://doi.org/10.1039/d3ra06476j

Rahim, M. A., Jan, N., Khan, S., Shah, H., Madni, A., Khan, A., Jabar, A., Khan, S., Elhissi, A., Hussain, Z., Aziz, H. C., Sohail, M., Khan, M., & Thu, H. E. (2021). Recent advancements in stimuli responsive drug delivery platforms for active and passive cancer targeting. *Cancers*, *13*(4), 670. https://doi.org/10.3390/cancers13040670

Rawal, S., & Patel, M. (2021). Bio-Nanocarriers for Lung Cancer Management: Befriending the Barriers. *Nano-Micro Letters*, *13*(1). https://doi.org/10.1007/s40820-021-00630-6

Raza, A., Rasheed, T., Nabeel, F., Hayat, U., Bilal, M., & Iqbal, H. M. N. (2019). Endogenous and exogenous Stimuli-Responsive Drug Delivery Systems for Programmed Site-Specific release. *Molecules*, *24*(6), 1117. https://doi.org/10.3390/molecules24061117

Remaut, K., Symens, N., Lucas, B., Demeester, J., & De Smedt, S. (2014). Cell division responsive peptides for optimized plasmid DNA delivery: The mitotic window of opportunity? *Journal of Controlled Release*, *179*, 1–9. https://doi.org/10.1016/j.jconrel.2014.01.013

Rosenthal, R., Günzel, D., Finger, C., Krug, S. M., Richter, J. F., Schulzke, J., Fromm, M., & Amasheh, S. (2012). The effect of chitosan on transcellular and paracellular mechanisms in the intestinal epithelial barrier. *Biomaterials*, *33*(9), 2791–2800. https://doi.org/10.1016/j.biomaterials.2011.12.034

Ruseska, I., & Zimmer, A. (2020). Internalization mechanisms of cell-penetrating peptides. *Beilstein Journal of Nanotechnology*, *11*, 101–123. https://doi.org/10.3762/bjnano.11.10

Saadat, M., Mostafaei, F., Mahdinloo, S., Abdi, M., Zahednezhad, F., Zakeri-Milani, P., & Valizadeh, H. (2021). Drug delivery of pH-Sensitive nanoparticles into the liver cancer cells. *Journal of Drug Delivery Science and Technology*, *63*, 102557. https://doi.org/10.1016/j.jddst.2021.102557

Sadiki, A., Vaidya, S. R., Abdollahi, M., Bhardwaj, G., Dolan, M. E., Turna, H., Arora, V., Sanjeev, A., Robinson, T. D., Koid, A., Amin, A., & Zhou, Z. S. (2020). Site-specific conjugation of native antibody. *Antibody Therapeutics*, *3*(4), 271–284. https://doi.org/10.1093/abt/tbaa027

Sahni, A., Qian, Z., & Pei, D. (2020). Cell-Penetrating peptides escape the endosome by inducing vesicle budding and collapse. *ACS Chemical Biology*, *15*(9), 2485–2492. https://doi.org/10.1021/acschembio.0c00478

Hassane, F. S., Saleh, A. F., Abes, R., Gait, M. J., & Lebleu, B. (2009). Cell penetrating peptides: overview and applications to the delivery of oligonucleotides. *Cellular and Molecular Life Sciences*, *67*(5), 715–726. https://doi.org/10.1007/s00018-009-0186-0

Santhanakrishnan, K. R., Koilpillai, J., & Narayanasamy, D. (2024). PEGylation in Pharmaceutical Development: Current status and emerging trends in macromolecular and immunotherapeutic drugs. *Cureus*. https://doi.org/10.7759/cureus.66669

Sartawi, Z., Blackshields, C., & Faisal, W. (2022). Dissolving microneedles: Applications and growing therapeutic potential. *Journal of Controlled Release*, *348*, 186–205. https://doi.org/10.1016/j.jconrel.2022.05.045

Sercombe, L., Veerati, T., Moheimani, F., Wu, S. Y., Sood, A. K., & Hua, S. (2015). Advances and challenges of liposome Assisted Drug Delivery. *Frontiers in Pharmacology*, *6*. https://doi.org/10.3389/fphar.2015.00286

Shah, S. W. A., Li, X., Yuan, H., Shen, H., Quan, S., Pan, G., Ishfaq, M., Shah, A. U., Xie, H., & Shao, J. (2025). Innovative transdermal drug delivery systems: Benefits, challenges, and emerging application. *BMEMat*. https://doi.org/10.1002/bmm2.70001

Shahzadi, I., Fürst, A., Knoll, P., & Bernkop-Schnürch, A. (2021). Nanostructured lipid carriers (NLCs) for oral peptide drug delivery: About the impact of surface decoration. *Pharmaceutics*, *13*(8), 1312. https://doi.org/10.3390/pharmaceutics13081312

Shi, M., & McHugh, K. J. (2023). Strategies for overcoming protein and peptide instability in biodegradable drug delivery systems. *Advanced Drug Delivery Reviews*, *199*, 114904. https://doi.org/10.1016/j.addr.2023.114904

Shi, Y., Shi, M., Wang, Y., & You, J. (2024). Progress and prospects of mRNA-based drugs in pre-clinical and clinical applications. *Signal Transduction and Targeted Therapy*, *9*(1). https://doi.org/10.1038/s41392-024-02002-z

Shin, M. C., Zhang, J., Min, K. A., Lee, K., Byun, Y., David, A. E., He, H., & Yang, V. C. (2013). Cell-penetrating peptides: Achievements and challenges in application for cancer treatment. *Journal of Biomedical Materials Research Part A*, *102*(2), 575–587. https://doi.org/10.1002/jbm.a.34859

Sioson, V. A., Kim, M., & Joo, J. (2021). Challenges in delivery systems for CRISPR-based genome editing and opportunities of nanomedicine. *Biomedical Engineering Letters*, *11*(3), 217–233. https://doi.org/10.1007/s13534-021-00199-4

Skotland, T., Iversen, T., Torgersen, M., & Sandvig, K. (2015). Cell-Penetrating Peptides: Possibilities and challenges for drug delivery in vitro and in vivo. *Molecules*, *20*(7), 13313–13323. https://doi.org/10.3390/molecules200713313

Sobczak, M. (2022). Enzyme-Responsive Hydrogels as Potential Drug Delivery Systems—State of Knowledge and Future Prospects. *International Journal of Molecular Sciences*, *23*(8), 4421. https://doi.org/10.3390/ijms23084421

Soni, S., Kori, S. K., Nema, P., Iyer, A. K., Soni, V., & Kashaw, S. K. (2024). Cell-Penetrating peptides as keys to endosomal escape and intracellular trafficking in nanomedicine delivery. *Current Medicinal Chemistry*, *32*(7), 1288–1312. https://doi.org/10.2174/0109298673278936240107121907

Suk, J. S., Xu, Q., Kim, N., Hanes, J., & Ensign, L. M. (2015). PEGylation as a strategy for improving nanoparticle-based drug and gene delivery. *Advanced Drug Delivery Reviews*, *99*, 28–51. https://doi.org/10.1016/j.addr.2015.09.012

Suk, J. S., Xu, Q., Kim, N., Hanes, J., & Ensign, L. M. (2015b). PEGylation as a strategy for improving nanoparticle-based drug and gene delivery. *Advanced Drug Delivery Reviews*, *99*, 28–51. https://doi.org/10.1016/j.addr.2015.09.012

Sultana, N., & David, A. E. (2023). Improving Cancer targeting: A study on the effect of Dual-Ligand density on targeting of cells having differential expression of target biomarkers. *International Journal of Molecular Sciences*, *24*(17), 13048. https://doi.org/10.3390/ijms241713048

Sun, Y., & Davis, E. (2021). Nanoplatforms for Targeted Stimuli-Responsive Drug delivery: A review of platform materials and Stimuli-

Responsive release and targeting mechanisms. *Nanomaterials*, *11*(3), 746. https://doi.org/10.3390/nano11030746

Suri, S. S., Fenniri, H., & Singh, B. (2007). Nanotechnology-based drug delivery systems. *Journal of Occupational Medicine and Toxicology*, *2*(1). https://doi.org/10.1186/1745-6673-2-16

Szabó, I., Yousef, M., Soltész, D., Bató, C., Mező, G., & Bánóczi, Z. (2022). Redesigning of Cell-Penetrating peptides to improve their efficacy as a drug delivery system. *Pharmaceutics*, *14*(5), 907. https://doi.org/10.3390/pharmaceutics14050907

Taherali, F., Chouhan, N., Wang, F., Lavielle, S., Baran, M., McCoubrey, L. E., Basit, A. W., & Yadav, V. (2023). Impact of peptide structure on colonic stability and tissue permeability. *Pharmaceutics*, *15*(7), 1956. https://doi.org/10.3390/pharmaceutics15071956

Tamayo-Trujillo, R., Ruiz-Pozo, V. A., Cadena-Ullauri, S., Guevara-Ramírez, P., Paz-Cruz, E., Zambrano-Villacres, R., Simancas-Racines, D., & Zambrano, A. K. (2024). Molecular mechanisms of semaglutide and liraglutide as a therapeutic option for obesity. *Frontiers in Nutrition*, *11*. https://doi.org/10.3389/fnut.2024.1398059

Tang, Y., & Wang, G. (2021). NIR light-responsive nanocarriers for controlled release. *Journal of Photochemistry and Photobiology C Photochemistry Reviews*, *47*, 100420. https://doi.org/10.1016/j.jphotochemrev.2021.100420

Tarvirdipour, S., Skowicki, M., Schoenenberger, C., & Palivan, C. G. (2021). Peptide-Assisted nucleic acid delivery systems on the rise. *International Journal of Molecular Sciences*, *22*(16), 9092. https://doi.org/10.3390/ijms22169092

Teo, S. L. Y., Rennick, J. J., Yuen, D., Al-Wassiti, H., Johnston, A. P. R., & Pouton, C. W. (2021). Unravelling cytosolic delivery of cell penetrating peptides with a quantitative endosomal escape assay. *Nature Communications*, *12*(1). https://doi.org/10.1038/s41467-021-23997-x

Thang, N. H., Chien, T. B., & Cuong, D. X. (2023). Polymer-Based Hydrogels Applied in Drug Delivery: An Overview. *Gels*, *9*(7), 523. https://doi.org/10.3390/gels9070523

Tiwari, O. S., Rencus-Lazar, S., & Gazit, E. (2023). Peptide- and Metabolite-Based Hydrogels: Minimalistic approach for the identification and characterization of gelating building blocks. *International Journal of Molecular Sciences*, *24*(12), 10330. https://doi.org/10.3390/ijms241210330

Uchida, S. (2022). Delivery systems of plasmid DNA and messenger RNA for advanced therapies. *Pharmaceutics*, *14*(4), 810. https://doi.org/10.3390/pharmaceutics14040810

Uhl, P., Bajraktari-Sylejmani, G., Witzigmann, D., Bay, C., Zimmermann, S., Burhenne, J., Weiss, J., Haefeli, W. E., & Sauter, M. (2023). A nanocarrier approach for oral peptide delivery: Evaluation of Cell-Penetrating-Peptide-Modified liposomal formulations in dogs. *Advanced Therapeutics*, *6*(10). https://doi.org/10.1002/adtp.202300021

Vaisman-Mentesh, A., Gutierrez-Gonzalez, M., DeKosky, B. J., & Wine, Y. (2020). The molecular mechanisms that underlie the immune biology of anti-drug antibody formation following treatment with monoclonal antibodies. *Frontiers in Immunology*, *11*. https://doi.org/10.3389/fimmu.2020.01951

Vasir, J., & Labhasetwar, V. (2007). Biodegradable nanoparticles for cytosolic delivery of therapeutics☆. *Advanced Drug Delivery Reviews*, *59*(8), 718–728. https://doi.org/10.1016/j.addr.2007.06.003

Vigata, M., Meinert, C., Hutmacher, D. W., & Bock, N. (2020). Hydrogels as Drug Delivery Systems: A review of Current characterization and Evaluation techniques. *Pharmaceutics*, *12*(12), 1188. https://doi.org/10.3390/pharmaceutics12121188

Wang, C., Shen, Z., Chen, Y., Wang, Y., Zhou, X., Chen, X., Li, Y., Zhang, P., & Zhang, Q. (2024). Research progress on Cyclic-Peptide functionalized nanoparticles for Tumor-Penetrating Delivery. *International Journal of Nanomedicine*, *Volume 19*, 12633–12652. https://doi.org/10.2147/ijn.s487303

Wang, Jiahua, Manzar Abbas, Yu Huang, Junyou Wang, andYuehua Li. 2023. "Redox-Responsive Peptide-Based Complex Coacervates as Delivery Vehicles with Controlled Release of Proteinous Drugs". Communications Chemistry 6 (1): 1-8. https://doi.org/10.1038/s42004-023-01044-8.

Wang, L., Wang, N., Zhang, W., Cheng, X., Yan, Z., Shao, G., Wang, X., Wang, R., & Fu, C. (2022). Therapeutic peptides: current applications and future directions. *Signal Transduction and Targeted Therapy*, *7*(1). https://doi.org/10.1038/s41392-022-00904-4

Wang, S., Wang, X., Luo, Y., & Liang, Y. (2024). A comprehensive review of conventional and stimuli-responsive delivery systems for bioactive peptides: from food to biomedical applications. *Advanced Composites and Hybrid Materials*, *8*(1). https://doi.org/10.1007/s42114-024-01053-8

Wang, Y., Cheetham, A. G., Angacian, G., Su, H., Xie, L., & Cui, H. (2016). Peptide–drug conjugates as effective prodrug strategies for targeted delivery. *Advanced Drug Delivery Reviews*, *110–111*, 112–126. https://doi.org/10.1016/j.addr.2016.06.015

Ways, T. M., Lau, W., & Khutoryanskiy, V. (2018). Chitosan and its derivatives for application in mucoadhesive drug delivery systems. *Polymers*, *10*(3), 267. https://doi.org/10.3390/polym10030267

Wibel, R., Jörgensen, A. M., Laffleur, F., Spleis, H., Claus, V., & Bernkop-Schnürch, A. (2022). Oral delivery of calcitonin-ion pairs: In vivo proof of concept for a highly lipophilic counterion. *International Journal of Pharmaceutics*, *631*, 122476. https://doi.org/10.1016/j.ijpharm.2022.122476

Wu, D., Chen, Q., Chen, X., Han, F., Chen, Z., & Wang, Y. (2023). The blood–brain barrier: Structure, regulation and drug delivery. *Signal Transduction and Targeted Therapy*, *8*(1). https://doi.org/10.1038/s41392-023-01481-w

Wu, H., Nan, J., Yang, L., Park, H. J., & Li, J. (2022). Insulin-loaded liposomes packaged in alginate hydrogels promote the oral bioavailability of insulin. *Journal of Controlled Release*, *353*, 51–62. https://doi.org/10.1016/j.jconrel.2022.11.032

Wu, J., Roesger, S., Jones, N., Hu, C. J., & Li, S. (2024). Cell-penetrating peptides for transmucosal delivery of proteins. *Journal of Controlled Release*, *366*, 864–878. https://doi.org/10.1016/j.jconrel.2024.01.038

Xiao, W., Jiang, W., Chen, Z., Huang, Y., Mao, J., Zheng, W., Hu, Y., & Shi, J. (2025). Advance in peptide-based drug development: delivery platforms, therapeutics and vaccines. *Signal Transduction and Targeted Therapy*, *10*(1). https://doi.org/10.1038/s41392-024-02107-5

Xing, Y., Zeng, B., & Yang, W. (2022). Light responsive hydrogels for controlled drug delivery. *Frontiers in Bioengineering and Biotechnology*, *10*. https://doi.org/10.3389/fbioe.2022.1075670

Yadati, T., Houben, T., Bitorina, A., & Shiri-Sverdlov, R. (2020). The Ins and Outs of Cathepsins: Physiological function and role in Disease Management. *Cells*, *9*(7), 1679. https://doi.org/10.3390/cells9071679

Yang, C., Sheng, T., Hou, W., Zhang, J., Cheng, L., Wang, H., Liu, W., Wang, S., Yu, X., Zhang, Y., Yu, J., & Gu, Z. (2022). Glucose-responsive microneedle patch for closed-loop dual-hormone delivery in mice and pigs. *Science Advances*, *8*(48). https://doi.org/10.1126/sciadv.add3197

Yin, X., He, Z., Ge, W., & Zhao, Z. (2023). Application of aptamer functionalized nanomaterials in targeting therapeutics of typical tumors. *Frontiers in Bioengineering and Biotechnology*, *11*. https://doi.org/10.3389/fbioe.2023.1092901

Yokoo, H., Oba, M., & Uchida, S. (2021). Cell-Penetrating Peptides: Emerging tools for mRNA delivery. *Pharmaceutics*, *14*(1), 78. https://doi.org/10.3390/pharmaceutics14010078

Yu, B., Tai, H. C., Xue, W., Lee, L. J., & Lee, R. J. (2010). Receptor-targeted nanocarriers for therapeutic delivery to cancer. *Molecular Membrane Biology*, *27*(7), 286–298. https://doi.org/10.3109/09687688.2010.521200

Yu, Z., Liu, D., Wu, C., & Zhao, W. (2024). Intestinal absorption of bioactive oligopeptides: paracellular transport and tight junction modulation. *Food & Function*, *15*(12), 6274–6288. https://doi.org/10.1039/d4fo00529e

Yusuf, A., Almotairy, A. R. Z., Henidi, H., Alshehri, O. Y., & Aldughaim, M. S. (2023). Nanoparticles as Drug delivery systems: A review of the implication of nanoparticles' physicochemical properties on responses in biological systems. *Polymers*, *15*(7), 1596. https://doi.org/10.3390/polym15071596

Zafar, S., Rana, S. J., Hamza, M., Hussain, A., Abbas, N., Ghori, M. U., & Arshad, M. S. (2025). Advancements in transdermal drug delivery using microneedles: technological and material perspective. *Discover Pharmaceutical Sciences*, *1*(1). https://doi.org/10.1007/s44395-025-00005-5

Zhang, C., Jiang, G., & Gao, X. (2023). Matrix Metalloproteinase-Responsive Drug Delivery Systems. *Bioconjugate Chemistry*, *34*(8), 1349–1365. https://doi.org/10.1021/acs.bioconjchem.3c00266

Zhang, Q., Li, S., He, L., & Feng, X. (2023). A brief review of polysialic acid-based drug delivery systems. *International Journal of Biological Macromolecules*, *230*, 123151. https://doi.org/10.1016/j.ijbiomac.2023.123151

Zhang, S., Zhi, D., & Huang, L. (2012). Lipid-based vectors for siRNA delivery. *Journal of Drug Targeting*, *20*(9), 724–735. https://doi.org/10.3109/1061186x.2012.719232

Zhang, X., Wang, H., Ma, Z., & Wu, B. (2014). Effects of pharmaceutical PEGylation on drug metabolism and its clinical concerns. *Expert Opinion on Drug Metabolism & Toxicology*, *10*(12), 1691–1702. https://doi.org/10.1517/17425255.2014.967679

Zhang, Z., Sun, H., Giannino, J., Wu, Y., & Cheng, C. (2024). Biodegradable zwitterionic polymers as PEG alternatives for drug delivery. *Journal of Polymer Science*, *62*(10), 2231–2250. https://doi.org/10.1002/pol.20230916

Zhang, H., Li, L., Li, W., Yin, H., Wang, H., & Ke, X. (2024). Endosomal PH, Redox Dual-Sensitive prodrug Micelles based on hyaluronic acid for intracellular camptothecin delivery and active tumor targeting in cancer therapy. *Pharmaceutics*, *16*(10), 1327. https://doi.org/10.3390/pharmaceutics16101327

Zhang, R., Qin, X., Kong, F., Chen, P., & Pan, G. (2019). Improving cellular uptake of therapeutic entities through interaction with components of cell membrane. *Drug Delivery*, *26*(1), 328–342. https://doi.org/10.1080/10717544.2019.1582730

Zhang, S., Shen, J., Li, D., & Cheng, Y. (2020). Strategies in the delivery of Cas9 ribonucleoprotein for CRISPR/Cas9 genome editing. *Theranostics*, *11*(2), 614–648. https://doi.org/10.7150/thno.47007

Zhao, J., Yang, H., Li, J., Wang, Y., & Wang, X. (2017b). Fabrication of pH-responsive PLGA(UCNPs/DOX) nanocapsules with upconversion luminescence for drug delivery. *Scientific Reports*, *7*(1). https://doi.org/10.1038/s41598-017-16948-4

Zhao, N., Song, Y., Xie, X., Zhu, Z., Duan, C., Nong, C., Wang, H., & Bao, R. (2023). Synthetic biology-inspired cell engineering in diagnosis, treatment, and drug development. *Signal Transduction and Targeted Therapy*, *8*(1). https://doi.org/10.1038/s41392-023-01375-x

Zhou, L., Zhang, T., Zhang, L., Deng, Q., Xia, Z., Chen, S., Cheng, D., Qiao, Z., & Wang, H. (2025). Stimuli-Responsive peptide-based nanodrug delivery systems for tumor therapy. *Chemical Communications*. https://doi.org/10.1039/d5cc00950b

Zhou, M., Zou, X., Cheng, K., Zhong, S., Su, Y., Wu, T., Tao, Y., Cong, L., Yan, B., & Jiang, Y. (2022). The role of cell-penetrating peptides in potential anti-cancer therapy. *Clinical and Translational Medicine*, *12*(5). https://doi.org/10.1002/ctm2.822

Zhu, P., Zhao, Z., & Gao, Y. (2025). Advances in hydrogel for diagnosis and treatment for Parkinson's disease. *Frontiers in Pharmacology*, *16*. https://doi.org/10.3389/fphar.2025.1552586

Zöller, K., To, D., & Bernkop-Schnürch, A. (2024). Biomedical applications of functional hydrogels: Innovative developments, relevant clinical trials and advanced products. *Biomaterials*, *312*, 122718. https://doi.org/10.1016/j.biomaterials.2024.122718

Author Biography

I am an Associate Professor of Medical Biochemistry at Niğde Ömer Halisdemir University Faculty of Medicine, board-certified in Medical Biochemistry, with a career dedicated to evidence-based diagnostics, academic excellence, and interdisciplinary research. My expertise spans clinical biochemistry, focusing on the interpretation of liver, kidney, cardiac, endocrine, and metabolic panels, as well as molecular biochemistry and bioinformatics, including gene and microRNA expression, protein–ligand docking, and biomarker discovery in breast and liver cancers.

I actively contribute to quality assurance of laboratory systems, medical education, mentorship, and scientific publishing as both author and reviewer. My goal is to bridge bench and bedside by ensuring laboratory results are analytically precise, clinically meaningful, and actionable in-patient care.

I welcome national and international collaborations in molecular diagnostics, cancer biology, and translational research, and I am open to joint projects, co-authorships, and grant development to advance laboratory medicine.

CHAPTER 10

LIPOSOMES

SANEM GÖKÇEN

Gazi University Faculty of Medicine, Department of Adult Hematology, Ankara, Türkiye.

Abstract

Liposomes are spherical vesicles composed of phospholipid bilayers enclosing an aqueous core. Their size, number of layers, lipid composition, surface modifications, and inclusion of helper lipids such as cholesterol or fusogenic lipids determine both their physical properties and biological behavior. Cationic liposomes can form complexes with nucleic acids, called lipoplexes, which protect DNA or RNA from degradation and promote cellular uptake. Their positive charge facilitates interaction with negatively charged cell membranes, while pH-sensitive or fusogenic lipids aid in escaping from endosomes. Liposomes can be functionalized with ligands, antibodies, or aptamers to achieve targeted delivery to specific cell types. Advantages include biocompatibility, the ability to carry both hydrophilic and hydrophobic molecules, reduced toxicity compared with many viral vectors, prolonged circulation when stealth coatings are applied, controlled release, and design flexibility. However, challenges remain, such as rapid clearance by the immune system, PEG-related immunogenicity, limited transfection efficiency in some tissues, instability during storage, and difficulties in large-scale reproducible manufacturing. Advances in liposome design, including stimuli-responsive systems and lipid–polymer hybrids, are enhancing their utility in non-viral gene therapy for cancer, rare genetic diseases, and immunotherapy. Ongoing research focuses on improving endosomal escape, avoiding immune detection, enhancing tissue-specific targeting, and ensuring scalability and stability. Integration with genome editing tools like CRISPR/Cas and RNA-based therapies such as siRNA or miRNA could further expand their therapeutic potential.

Keywords: Liposomes, Phospholipids, Lipid nanoparticulate, Targeted drug delivery

Introduction

Gene therapy holds significant therapeutic promise; however, the success of this approach depends significantly on the development of safe and efficient gene delivery systems. Among the various vectors explored, liposomes, as nanocarriers for drug and gene delivery, offer several advantages, including improved intracellular accumulation, targeted delivery capabilities, and excellent biocompatibility (Yildiz et al., 2024). Liposomes were first discovered by Dr. Alec D. Bangham and collaborators at the Babraham Institute, University of Cambridge in the 1960s (Bangham & Horne, 1964). The term “Liposome” is derived from the Greek words: “Lipos” meaning fat and “Soma” meaning body (Daraee et al., 2016). The liposomes are convenient, safe and the most commonly used nanocarriers with characteristic phospholipid bilayers which closely resembles the structure of cell membranes. Because of their high biocompatibility, biodegradability, non-immunogenic and non-toxic properties, they are very useful gene carriers today (Akbarzadeh et al., 2013; Gregoriadis, 2016). The mechanisms of liposomes uptake into the cell are adsorption, endocytosis, fusion and lipid exchange (Akbarzadeh et al., 2013). In the biological, biochemical, agricultural and food fields, liposomes have also been found to be ideal systems for the encapsulation of many different active agents. Enzymes, antimicrobial agents and antioxidants are some of the encapsulated substances (Benech et al., 2003; Chai et al., 2013; Gibbs et al., 1999; Torchilin, 2005; Wechtersbach et al., 2012). Importantly, they can protect nucleic acids from enzymatic degradation while improving their intracellular reuptake and altering the pharmacokinetics of the entrapped molecule (Cardador et al., 2023). Owing to these advantages, the use of liposomal formulations in cancer therapy has expanded considerably in recent years. The first examples of preparations that appear in the form of liposomal formulations are Doxil® approved by FDA (Food and Drug Administration) and AmBisome® approved by EMA (European Medicines Agency). Since then, multiple liposomal systems—such as liposomal doxorubicin (PLD) coated with polyethyleneglycol (PEG), uncoated liposomal doxorubicin (NPLD), liposomal daunorubicin (DNX), platinum compounds encapsulated in liposomes, immunoliposomes (antibody-mediated transport) have been developed to create a more effective method in the treatment of cancer (Hofheinz et al., 2005; Stone et al., 2016). Onpattro, the first FDA-approved lipid nanoparticle (LNP)-based nucleic acid therapeutic (siRNA), represents a landmark in the field (Akinc et al., 2019). Pfizer/BioNTech's Comirnaty (BNT162b2) and Moderna's Spikevax (mRNA-1273) vaccines against COVID-19 represent a novel immunization approach using mRNA encapsulated in lipid nanoparticles (mRNA-LNPs). The mRNA encodes the viral spike protein, which triggers an adaptive immune response. This strategy leverages lipid nanoparticle technologies initially developed for gene therapy and drug delivery, incorporating ionizable cationic lipids, PEGylated lipids, phospholipids, and cholesterol (Szebeni et al., 2023).

The use of liposomes is also of particular importance in the treatment of dermatological diseases. Oils, vitamins and ions required for skin health can be encapsulated into liposomes and administered directly to the skin. The biggest advantage of the use of liposomes in the field of dermatology is the long-term and controlled release of active substances. These substances carried by liposomes are accepted by skin tissues. However, it is not possible to say this for preservatives. Due to these substances, allergic reactions may develop (Ahmadi Ashtiani et al., 2016; Castañeda-Reyes et al., 2020; Eroğlu et al., 2016). Beyond IgE-mediated allergy, complement activation-related pseudoallergy (CARPA) has re-emerged as a clinically relevant safety phenotype for liposomal drugs, with new human data in 2024–2025 strengthening the link between infusion reactions and complement activation (Thompson et al., 2025). Extensive reviews on CARPA describe mitigation strategies such as premedication, surface modifications to limit complement activation, and advances in diagnostics, all of which are progressively integrated into modern liposome development strategies (Saxena et al., 2025). A recent area of advancement involves targeted delivery and genetic therapeutics: clinical-stage in vivo CRISPR programs utilizing lipid nanoparticles (LNPs) have demonstrated the feasibility of systemic hepatic delivery and stimulated renewed efforts to translate ligand-directed and stimulus-responsive approaches to liposomal platforms for extrahepatic applications (Kazemian et al., 2022). Taken together, the last 3–5 years have reinforced the therapeutic significance of liposomes and incorporated lessons from LNP vaccinology and gene editing, especially regarding immune modulation, microfluidic manufacturability, and thermo-stable distribution, thus enabling safer and more precise liposomal medicines (Lamichhane et al., 2018; Mukai et al., 2022).

Structure of Liposome

The sizes of the liposomes can range from 20 nm to 20 µm in diameter (Taylor & Morris, 1995). As seen in Figure 1, the three-dimensional ball-like liposomes contain both hydrophilic polar and hydrophobic apolar spaces (Laouini et al., 2012). Generally, liposomes are composed of different types of non-toxic phospholipids, such as phosphatidylcholine, phosphatidylserine and phosphatidylglycerol, and cholesterol (Al Badri et al., 2023). These phospholipids can be of natural origin, semi-synthetic or fully synthetic. Modified phospholipids from natural sources or phospholipids with natural head groups are also commonly used in liposomal formulations. Dilauryl phosphotidyl choline (DLPC), Dimyristoyl phosphotidyl choline (DMPC), Dipalmitoyl phosphotidyl choline (DPPC), Distearoyl phosphotidyl choline (DSPC), Dioleolyl phosphotidyl choline (DOPC), Dilauryl phosphotidylethanolamine (DLPE), Dimyristoyl phosphotidyl ethanolamine (DMPE), Distearoyl phosphotidyl ethanolamine (DSPE), Dioleoyl phosphotidyl ethanolamine (DOPE), Dilauryl phosphotidyl glycerol (DLPG), Distearoyl phosphotidyl serine (DSPS) are among the most commonly used phospholipids in liposome preparation (Samad et al., 2007; Shah et al., 2017). The chemical properties of the phospholipids used in the preparation of liposomes also significantly affect the properties of the liposome. The biodistribution, permeability, release, clearance and surface charge of liposomal formulations are perpetually subject to the chemical nature of the phospholipids (Lombardo & Kiselev, 2022). Accordingly, toxicity, stability and the encapsulation efficiency of liposomes are also influenced by phospholipid types used in their preparation. The hydrophilic-lipophilic balance has been a useful indicator for the prediction of the liposomal vesicle forming ability of an amphiphile. The composition and surface charge of phospholipids also determine the tissue distribution and total kinetics (clearance) of drug-loaded liposome (Andra et al., 2022). When phospholipids are placed to water, their hydrophilic regions tend to move towards the water, while their hydrophobic regions escape interaction with the water and form vesicles. Interactions between phospholipid and water molecules together with Van der Waals interactions between hydrophobic interactions and phospholipid molecules lead to the formation of bilayer membranes (liposomal structure) (Nakhaei et al., 2021; Wang, 2016) (Figure 1). Gangliosides are a class of sphingolipids. They sometimes included in liposome formulations and made available a layer of surface-charged groups to prolong the lifetime of circulating liposomes in the blood stream (E. Sanarova, 2019).

Figure 1: Structure of Liposome

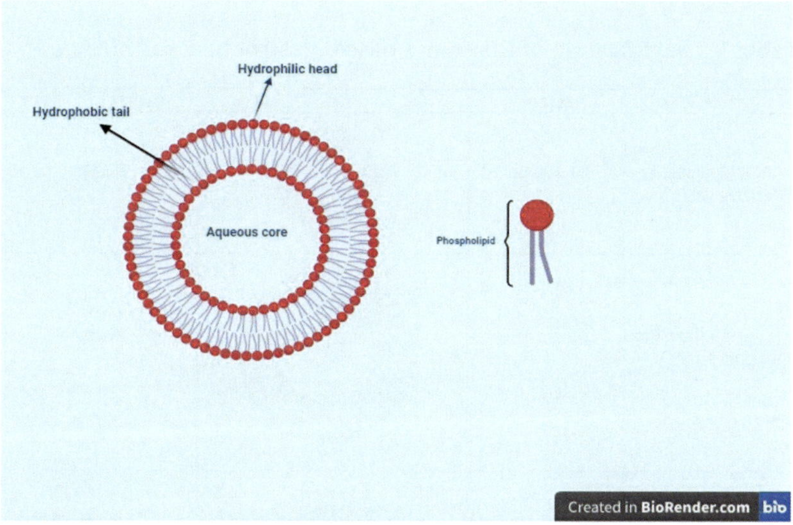

Liposomes are classified according to the number of layers and their size as unilamellar (Small Unilamellar Vesicle=SUV, Large Unilamellar Vesicle=LUV, Giant Unilamellar Vesicles=GUV), multilamellar (Multi Lamellar Vesicle=MLV), oligolamellar (Oligo Lamellar Vesicles=OLV) and multi vesicular vesicles (MVV) (Panday et al., 2016; Sforzi et al., 2020) (Table 1). SUV and MLV are basically used for drug delivery technologies, while GUV are used usually for cell-based models (Tenchov et al., 2021). According to their composition, liposomes are are classified as conventional, pH-sensitive, cationic, fusogenic, immune liposomes and long-circulating liposomes (Barba et al., 2019). Vesicle size is an important parameter to determine the circulation half-life of liposomes. Interaction between liposomes and cell membranes is described by several theories as endocytosis, phagocytosis, adhesion, and absorption into the cell membrane (Nsairat et al., 2022). The propensity of liposomes to evade or be sequestered by the mononuclear phagocyte system correlates with particle size, such that particles above certain size thresholds are more rapidly opsonized and cleared from the bloodstream (Kelly et al., 2011). Tumor accumulation and intratumoral penetration of liposomal formulations are strongly size-dependent: intermediate-to-small nanoscale liposomes penetrate tumor interstitium more effectively than larger vesicles, although optimal dimensions vary with tumor type and microenvironmental pressure (Goins et al., 2016). Cellular uptake mechanisms of liposomes shift with size, since small liposomes are more readily internalized via clathrin- and caveolin-mediated endocytosis, whereas larger vesicles show reduced

Table 1. Classification of liposomes based on structure and size

Vesicle Type	Image	Size	Number of Layers
Small Unilamellar Vesicles (SUV)	20-100 nm	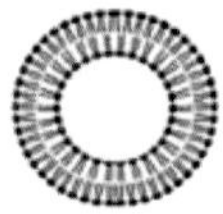	Single
Large Unilamellar Vesicles (SUV)	100 nm-1μm	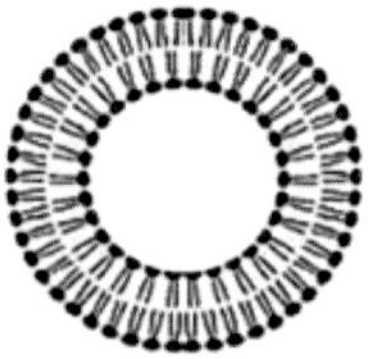	Single
Multivesicular Vesicles (MLV)	> 500 nm	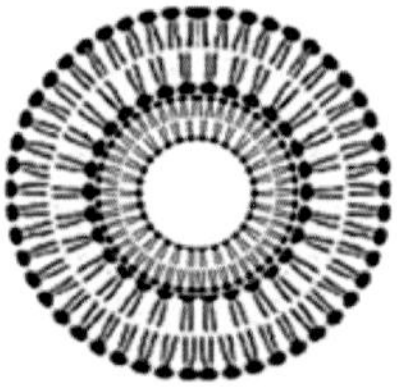	Multiple
Oligo Lamellar Vesicles (OLV)	100 nm-1μm	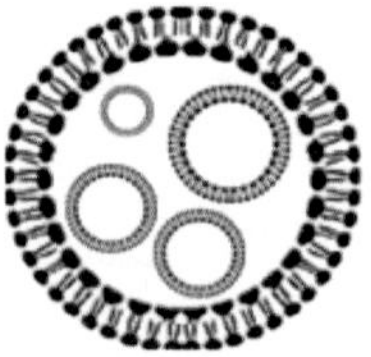	Multiple
Giant Unilamellar Vesicles (GUV)	> 1μm	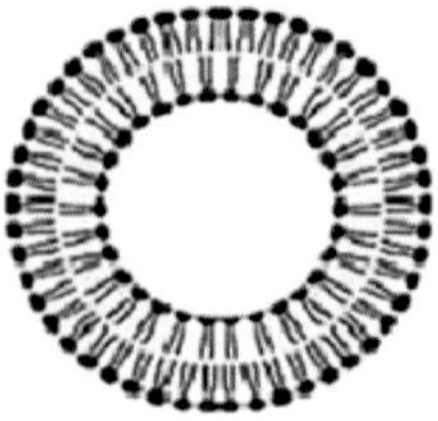	Single

internalization or engage alternative uptake routes (Andar et al., 2013) The efficiency and mechanism of receptor-mediated targeting are modulated by liposome size because ligand accessibility and the membrane curvature of the carrier influence binding avidity and subsequent endocytic internalization (Ashby et al., 2023). Complement activation and infusion-related hypersensitivity reactions (CARPA) have been associated with certain liposome sizes and surface properties, highlighting the interplay between particle dimension and innate immune recognition (Szebeni et al., 2011; Thompson et al., 2025).

The Type of Liposomes

The liposomes can be classified into different types according to their composition and application, including conventional liposomes, charged liposomes, stealth (long circulating) liposomes, actively targeted liposomes (immunoliposomes), stimuli-responsive liposomes and bubble liposomes (Nsairat et al., 2022).

Methods of Preparing The Liposomes

Since the preparation methods will affect the number of layers and the size distribution of the liposomes to be formed, the goal-directed method should be chosen (Kobayashi et al., 2005). The methods for preparations of liposomes include conventional methods as thin film hydration, ether/ethanol injection, reverse phase evaporation, detergent depletion, microfluidic channel method, heating, membrane extrusion, high shear homogenization, sonication methods, and novel methods as freeze drying, dual asymmetric centrifugation, supercritical fluid methods (Andra et al., 2022). The methods used to prepare liposomes generally involve 3 basic steps: Drying of lipids dissolved in organic solvent, formation of liposomes in aqueous media, and analysis of the resulting liposomes (Das; Kobayashi et al., 2005; Wang, 2016). Lipid membranes must first be prepared to study the interactions between membranes and polyphenols (Šturm & Poklar Ulrih, 2021).

a. Bangham Method (Thin-Film Hydration)

MVLs are the most widely used form of liposome. The thin-film and proliposomal methods are most commonly used methods for MLVs preparation (Šturm & Poklar Ulrih, 2021). In the thin-film hydration method, the lipid ingredients are prepared by dissolving it in chloroform or a mixture of chloroform/methanol as an organic solvent. The organic solvent is removed from the lipid film by vacuum drying. Then liquid buffer is added onto the lipid and the lipids swell abruptly, and heterogeneous liposomes are formed. One of the biggest advantages of the thin film hydration method is that it provides high encapsulation efficiency. Repeated freezing and thawing increase the encapsulation efficiency and decrease the lamellarity of MLVs (Ahmed et al., 2019; Zhang, 2017). However, this method has disadvantages such as the use of organic solvents, the long duration of the process, the presence of solvent residue and the low encapsulation rate of water-soluble compounds (Maja et al., 2020) (Figure 2).

Figure 2. Liposome Preparation via Thin Film Hydration

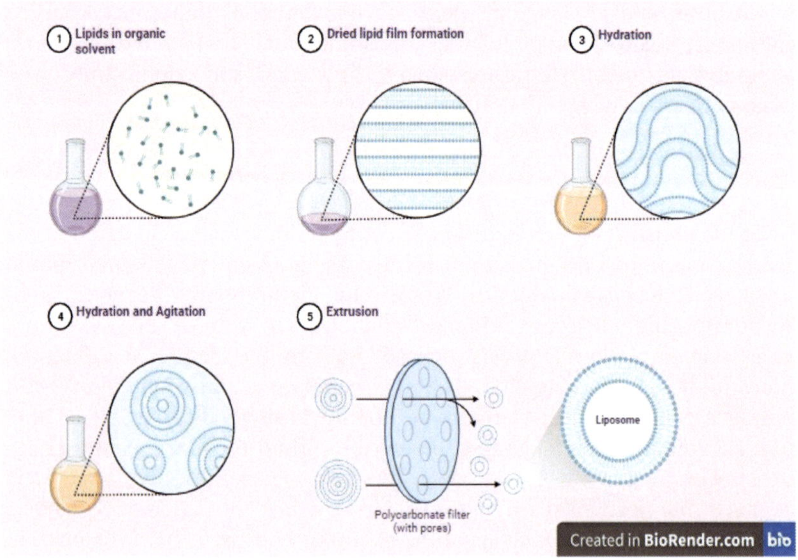

b. Detergent Dialysis Method

Monolayer liposomes were also prepared by the detergent separation technique. Mixed micelles of phospholipids with a detergent such as sodium cholate are prepared, and liposomes are formed as a result of the separation of detergent molecules from these micelles by gel filtration or dialysis (Laouini et al., 2012; Schubert, 2003). During the dialysis process, small-sized surfactant molecules flow out of the dialysis membrane and the phospholipids in the micelles converge to form bilayer liposomes, avoiding exposure to the aqueous phase. Phospholipids form homogeneous single-lamellar vesicles and provide effective encapsulation. Small unilamellar vesicles with high homogeneity can be obtained by dialysis method. The dimensions of liposome structures can be regulated by adjusting the lipid:detergent ratio used during the method (Andra et al., 2022; Zumbuehl & Weder, 1981). Dialysis method requires higher duration (>20 hours) for the formation of liposome structure compared to other methods. Components to be encapsulated may be exposed to detergents and are therefore not considered suitable for encapsulation of detergent sensitive components. In addition, interactions between detergents and encapsulated agents should be carefully considered to prevent loss of bioactive ingredient (Zhao, 2017). The major disadvantages are the need for many steps to achieve size homogenization and the high energy requirement for mass production of liposomes (Laouini et al., 2012).

c. Solvent (Ether or Ethanol) Injection Method

Ethanol or ether injection is a method in which the liposome structure is formed by injecting the lipid material dissolved in the organic phase into the aqueous medium (Meure et al., 2008). In the injection method, the lipid-based component such as phosphatidylcholine, which is targeted, is dissolved in ethanol and then injected into water to form a liposome. Effective removal of toxic solvent such as chloroform, which is used as a solvent during liposome formation, is one of its most important advantages. Solvent and injection method facilitate the scaling of liposomes. The use of ethanol as a safe (GRAS) solvent in the injection method increases the suitability of the method for liposome formation (Ajeeshkumar et al., 2021; Wagner et al., 2006). The biggest disadvantage of this method is organic solvent residue, nozzle clogging in the ether system and the necessity of sterilization (Maja et al., 2020).

d. Reverse Phase Evaporation (REV) Method

This method, based on liposome formation from inverted micelles developed by Szoka and Papahadjopoulos (1978), involves the formation of a water-in-oil emulsion by mixing a small amount of water into the lipid organic solution. A lipid-based film is formed by evaporation of the organic lipid solvent under reduced pressure. The lipid-based structures are then re-dissolved in a second organic phase, usually consisting of diethyl ether and/or isopropyl ether, after the system has been purged with nitrogen.

When buffer solution is added to the dissolved mixture, large monolamellar and oligolamellar structures are formed. After removal of the organic solvent, the system is constantly kept under nitrogen. Vesicles obtained by the reverse phase evaporation method have liquid volume/lipid ratios that are 30 times higher than sonicated vesicles and 4 times higher than multilayered vesicles. A significant part of the liquid phase can remain inside the vesicles and even large macromolecule groups can be kept in the liposome structure with high encapsulation efficiency (Laouini et al., 2012; Maherani et al., 2011; Szoka & Papahadjopoulos, 1978).

e. Extrusion Method

Extrusion method is based on the reduction of multilayered vesicles into small single-layered vesicles by the extrusion process applied through a mini extruder apparatus. The applied high pressure helps the extrusion of vesicles through defined pore sized polycarbonate filters. Properties such as mean diameter and polydispersity of the extruded liposome are affected by the applied pressure, the number of cycles, and the pore size of the filter used. In this method, large vesicles are divided into smaller sizes as they pass through the pores due to the applied pressure. This method is simple, fast, reproducible and shows relatively homogeneous size distributions (Olson et al., 1979; Ong et al., 2016; Schneider et al., 1995). The main factors limiting the application of this method include clogging of pores, product loss and unsuitability for large-scale production (Costa & Santos, 2017).

f. Spray-drying Method

Simple and industrially applicable, spray drying can be used to directly spray dry a mixture of lipids and drugs in the preparation of liposomes (Skalko-Basnet et al., 2000). Spray drying is accepted as a rapid one-step procedure that produces nano-sized particles (Laouini et al., 2012). As a result of liposome aggregation, an increase in particle size distribution during storage and leakage of charged active material are the major issues in spray drying liposomes. To limit this aggregation, biopolymers with opposite charges such as proteins and carbohydrates are used as preservatives by spray drying to improve the kinetics and mechanical stability of liposomes (Yu et al., 2021).

g. Microfluidic Method

Microfluidic system is a high pressure conveying equipment that transforms high fluid pressures into intense shear forces. Liposome production is carried out by suspension of aqueous phase liposomal components in the special chamber of the microplasticizer (Yu et al., 2009). Microfluidizer® technology is considered an applicable technique for large scale pharmaceutical industry productions due to its flexibility for control of globule size and the ability to produce fine particles (Jafari et al., 2007). Microfluidic technology creates large unilamellar vesicles of homogeneous structure and desired size. Also, reproducibility and reduction of post-production processing steps are recognized as another advantage (Al-Amin et al., 2020).

h. Heating Method

The heating method was developed by Mozafari to produce liposomes. In this method, which is based on the hydration of phospholipids, the mixture is heated in the presence of a hydrating agent (propylene glyc ol, glycerol or sorbitol). Gycerol is used as a hydrating agent since it is a water soluble and physiologically accepted chemical. It acts as an isotonizing agent and increase the stability of lipid vesicles by avoiding particle coagulation and sedimentation (Mozafari, 2005). Among all the conventional methods, liposome preparation by heating method stands out because it is simple and fast with less organic solvent residue (Christian Isalomboto et al., 2019). It is stated that since the liposomes prepared by heating method are exposed to high temperature (60-120°C), deterioration may occur in the bioactive components, albeit a little (Ajeeshkumar et al., 2021).

i. Freeze-drying Method

Freeze-drying technique (also called lyophilization) is one of the most widely used methods for liposome preparation. By means of this method, the long-term stability of liposomes is increased and the degradation of sensitive substances encapsulated in the structure of liposomes is hindered (Yu et al., 2021). Overall, the freeze drying process is made up of three stages: (1) freezing, (2) primary drying, and (3) secondary drying (van Winden, 2003). This process may lead to physical changes of the liposomes, such as alterations in the vesicle size, a loss of the encapsulated agent and a loss of membrane integrity (Mozafari, 2005; Yu et al., 2021). The freeze-drying method can be applied to the preparation of sterile and pyrogen-free submicron small size liposomes (Li & Deng, 2004).

j. The Crossflow Injection Method

Crossflow injection method is a new scalable liposome preparation technique for pharmaceutical application. It is specified as a crossflow system consisting of two pipes and an injection hole at the connection point (Wagner et al., 2006; A. Wagner et al., 2002). Lipid concentration, injection whole diameter, injection pressure, buffer flow rate and system performance are stated as important parameters (Andreas Wagner et al., 2002). A minimum buffer flow rate with increased injection pressure has a significant effect on the homogeneity of the liposomes. When high lipid concentrations are injected in environments where injection rates remain constant and pressure exceeds the upper limit of the linear range, the vesicle aggregates show a narrow range of size distribution (Laouini et al., 2012; A. Wagner et al., 2002).

k. Ultrasonication Method

Similar sized and single-compartment liposomes are much more suitable for research and applications compared to MLVs due to better knowledge of their physicochemical properties like permeability, stability, elasticity, toughness etc. (Rideau et al., 2018). The French press, sonication, homogenization and membrane extrusion techniques are often used for conversion of MLVs into SUVs and LUVs (Lombardo & Kiselev, 2022). The idea of using ultrasonic energy for the preparation of SUVs was first put forward by Huang (Huang, 1969). The advantages of liposomes synthesized by sonication are respectively; ease of preparation, no use of potentially toxic organic solvents, advantageous in terms of biodegradation (Dua et al., 2012). Sonication allows large quantities of liposomes to be produced continuously or reproducibly without the use of detergents and toxic chemicals. Disadvantages of the method include degradation of lipids and compounds, and limited internal volume (Ajeeshkumar et al., 2021). The process can be carried out using either an ultrasonic probe or an ultrasonic bath. If the probe type is used, it uses more energy and results in a shorter time, but the titanium particles detached from the probe tip need to be cleaned by ultrafiltration or centrifugation afterwards (Mendez & Banerjee, 2017; New, 1990). Sonication should be done at a temperature just above the phase transition temperature. Otherwise, defective parts are formed in the structures of liposomes (Rieth & Lozano, 2020). The sonication time is also important. More than 5% of the lipids can be deesterified on sonication for up to 1 hour (Andra et al., 2022).

l. Supercritical CO_2 Reverse Phase Evaporation [SCRPE] Method

Supercritical fluid extraction technology is a green technology that uses supercritical fluids such as supercritical carbon dioxide ($ScCO_2$) in its processing methods (Ibáñez et al., 2016). It is referred that the use of ScCO2 as a non-toxic material that can replace organic solvents is one of the promising applications in the pharmaceutical industries for micro- and nano-encapsulation of drugs (Soh & Lee, 2019). GRAS solvents such as ethanol can be used to modify the system, thereby increasing process efficiency (Tsai & Rizvi, 2016). Less solvent usage compared to traditional evaporation methods is one of the remarkable features of supercritical fluid methods. However, some disadvantages of these techniques are mentioned, especially the high cost and the use of complex design (Nkanga et al., 2019). There are two main types of supercritical liquid technologies for the preparation of liposomes, the supercritical antisolvent (SAS) method and the supercritical reverse phase evaporation (SRPE) method (Huang et al., 2014). SCRPE is a one-step method developed for the preparation of liposomes using supercritical carbon dioxide (Otake et al., 2001). This method allows to obtain aqueous dispersions of liposomes through emulsion formation by adding a certain amount of water to a homogeneous mixture of supercritical carbon dioxide. The encapsulation efficiency of these liposomes shows higher values for water-soluble components compared to multilayered vesicles prepared by the Bangham method. The encapsulation efficiency for cholesterol, which is a fat-soluble substance, is expressed as approximately 63%, and SCRPE is stated to be a technique that allows one-step preparation of large monolayer liposomes exhibiting a high encapsulation efficiency for both water-soluble and fat-soluble compounds (Imura et al., 2003; Otake et al., 2006).

m. Supercritical Antisolvent (SAS) Method

In the supercritical antisolvent method, CO_2 acts as an antisolvent and the organic solvent containing the phospholipids is continuously sprayed in the supercritical CO_2 (Trucillo et al., 2020). Dissolution of supercritical CO2 in the liquid phase followed by extraction of organic solvent leads to precipitation of lipid particles. A humidification step of the supercritical liquid phase under pressure is performed to produce liposome structures by precipitation (Shashidhar et al., 2016; Trucillo et al., 2020). The SAS method starts by creating a uniform lipid substance that simulates that done in the conventional method (thin film dispersion), but ScCO2 is used to help dry the phospholipids by removing excess organic solvent. The particles are hydrated in an aqueous buffer to attain liposomes at the nano or micro level, depending on the type of application required. Liposome structures can be more spherical and encapsulation efficiency can be at an optimum level. In addition, the particle size distribution in the SAS method can be more controlled and reproducible (Trucillo et al., 2020). Process conditions of the method are specified as 8-25 MPa for pressure and 35-50°C for temperature. The resulting liposomes are relatively smaller in size, multilamellar vesicles and spherical with a smoother surface, and are more stable physically and chemically (Ajeeshkumar et al., 2021; Karn et al., 2013).

Liposomes for Use in Gene Delivery

Beyond oncology, liposomes have also gained prominence in gene therapy, which we can briefly define as the correction of the genetic structure by replacing the defective gene that causes the disease with healthy copies. Because nucleic acids are negatively charged, cationic liposomes come to the fore as the most suitable vectors to transport genes to the target site (Immordino et al., 2006). Typically, gene delivery platforms are developed to transport nucleic acids (NAs), including plasmid DNA (pDNA) and messenger RNA (mRNA), as well as regulatory small RNAs such as siRNA, miRNA, shRNA, and antisense oligonucleotides (ASOs) (Federica Ponti et al., 2021). For example, previous studies have demonstrated that plasmid DNA (pDNA) encapsulated within neutral stealth liposomes, modified with a targeting peptide, can achieve highly efficient and selective gene delivery to cancer cells in both in vitro and in vivo settings (Levine et al., 2013). In targeted applications, Trojan Horse liposomes—PEGylated liposomes conjugated with monoclonal antibodies—enable receptor-mediated transcytosis of plasmid DNA across biological barriers like the blood–brain barrier, achieving delivery to the brain while avoiding viral vectors (Pardridge, 2020).

Small interfering RNA (siRNA) and messenger RNA (mRNA) therapeutics also require robust delivery systems to navigate extracellular degradation, renal clearance, and cellular barriers, and lipid-based carriers remain among the most extensively studied platforms for this purpose. Because RNA molecules are inherently unstable, numerous carrier platforms, such as lipid nanoparticles (LNPs), have been created to enable RNA therapeutics. The initial demonstration of mRNA delivery with liposomes dates back to 1978

(Jung et al., 2022). Liposomes and modern lipid nanoparticles (LNPs) encapsulate nucleic acids to shield them from extracellular ribonucleases and to facilitate cellular uptake and cytosolic delivery (Tenchov et al., 2021). As summarized in Table 2, LNPs are generally composed of four distinct components, each fulfilling a specific function. These are ionizable cationic lipids (ICLs), helper lipids, cholesterol, and polyethylene glycol (PEG) lipids (Jung et al., 2022; Liu et al., 2024).

Table 2. Components and function of lipids in LNPs for mRNA delivery (Jung et al., 2022).

LNP LIPID COMPONENTS	
1) Ionizable Cationic Lipids	
Functions	Nucleic acids complexation and membrane fusion
Examples	ALC-0315 (Pfizer/BioNTech), SM-102 (Moderna)
2) Phospholipid	
Functions	Complex support. Saturated lipids provide structural stability, while unsaturated lipids promote endosomal destabilization.
Examples	DSPC, DPPC (saturated lipid)-DOPE (unsaturated lipid)
3) Cholesterol	
Functions	Integrity and endosomal release
Examples	Cholesterol
4) PEGylated lipid	
Functions	Hydrophilic surface, steric hindrance, "Stealth" effect
Examples	ALC-0159 (Pfizer/BioNTech), PEG-DMG (Moderna)

Historically, cationic and pH-sensitive liposomes were developed to complex and deliver siRNA in vitro and in vivo, and these early liposomal formulations established key principles for nucleic-acid encapsulation and delivery (Yonezawa et al., 2020). In recent years, conventional cationic liposomes have been successfully modified into Liposome/Protamine/Hyaluronic acid (LPH) NPs and Lipid-Calcium-Phosphate (LCP) NPs, aiming to enhance gene silencing efficiency in vivo while simultaneously minimizing toxicity (Liu & Huang, 2021).

Various engineering approaches have been employed to enhance the stability and translational efficiency of mRNA therapeutics, such as optimizing untranslated regions (UTRs), adding a poly-A tail, capping, and chemically modifying nucleosides (Jung et al., 2022). Liposome-mediated transfection efficiency is significantly influenced by the weight ratio of liposome to plasmid DNA (pDNA), the characteristics of the lipid components, and the effectiveness of pDNA entrapment (Ghanbari Safari & Hosseinkhani, 2013). The chemical nature of the lipid headgroup, particularly whether it is permanently cationic or ionizable, modulates nucleic acid binding strength, endosomal escape, and cytotoxicity (F. Ponti et al., 2021). Cationic lipids are commonly employed in gene delivery, and the incorporation of dioleoylphosphatidylethanolamine (DOPE) as a helper lipid within cationic lipid–DNA complexes has been shown to frequently enhance transfection efficiency (Zuhorn et al., 2005). Formulations of LNPs with DOPE and/or cholesterol are associated with improved transfection performance, primarily through enhanced membrane fusion and facilitated endosomal escape (Sun & Lu, 2023). The charge ratio between lipids and nucleic acids, often expressed as the N/P ratio, is another critical determinant, as it affects particle size, surface charge, and uptake efficiency (Brgles et al., 2012).

An essential but challenging aspect of nanomedicine formulation is the adjustment of zeta potential. The zeta potential (ZP), which reflects colloidal stability, is influenced by surface charge and is typically derived from electrophoretic mobility analysis in suspension (Wang & Keller, 2009). Formulations exhibiting at least ±30 mV are generally recognized as stable (Németh et al., 2022). Particle size and polydispersity index also play crucial roles since nanoscale dimensions maximize cellular internalization and proper intracellular trafficking (Danaei et al., 2018). Surface PEGylation extends circulation time; however, it may diminish cellular uptake unless combined with cleavable linkers or targeting strategies (Suk et al., 2016).

Liposomes and Safety Profile Assessment

Liposomes exhibit notable therapeutic potential; however, their formulation, development, and manufacturing processes are difficult to standardize. In nano-formulations, this difficulty is further intensified by nanoscale physics and chemistry, which introduce numerous parameters that must be thoroughly understood and optimized (Porfire et al., 2019). The development of liposomal formulations through a risk assessment-based Quality by Design (QbD) approach involves systematically identifying and controlling critical factors to ensure product quality and consistency. Key components of a Quality by Design (QbD) strategy include the definition of the Quality Target Product Profile (QTPP), selection of Critical Quality Attributes (CQAs) and Critical Process Parameters (CPPs), Risk Assessment (RA), application of Design of Experiments (DoE), establishment of a Design Space (DS) with control measures, and lifecycle management guided by continuous improvement (Dobó et al., 2022; Németh et al., 2020).

Tools for risk assessment, including Failure Modes and Effects Analysis (FMEA) and Ishikawa diagrams, are utilized to analyze how these factors influence CQAs (Yang et al., 2025). Subsequently, experimental designs like Plackett-Burman and Central Composite Designs are utilized to optimize formulation variables and processing conditions. The approach has been successfully applied in various studies, demonstrating its efficacy in developing stable, reproducible, and high-quality liposomal products (Jain et al., 2019).

Liposomes and Immune System Interactions

Immune system is a multicomponent complex in which many mediators, receptors and cells are interrelated. Liposomal formulations are in strict relationship with immune system. These interactions need to be taken into account to achieve more effective results. Innate immune system is primarily subjected to liposomes in biodistribution. Mononuclear phagocytic system (MPS) and complement system are important parts of important part of the innate immune system. The associated cells are usually macrophages, monocytes, dendritic cells (DCs), and neutrophils (Zahednezhad et al., 2019). In recent years, it was reported that the usage of nanoparticle-based vaccinations has drawn considerable interest to refine vaccine efficacy, immunization strategies, and targeted delivery to obtain coveted immune responses at the cellular level (Diaz-Arévalo & Zeng). In general, nanoparticles (NPs) have the ability to stimulate cytokine and antibody responses. In vaccine development, important delivery systems are liposomes and and liposome-derived nanovesicles such as archaeosomes and virosomes. Liposomes are ideal carriers for antigens and adjuvants (Schwendener, 2014). Almost all liposomes have the capacity to induce varying degrees of complement system activation when exposed to plasma for a sufficient period of time under certain conditions. These reactions can also lead a state of hypersensitivity reaction called c-activation-related pseudo-allergy (CARPA) (Zahednezhad et al., 2019).

The most important problem encountered in the use of liposomes in the medical field has been the clearance of liposomes by the phagocytic system. To solve this problem, scientists have attempted to coat the liposome surface with molecules that do not activate the immune system (Gao et al., 2013). Upon realizing that intravenously administered liposomes are digested by phagocytic cells in the body, these liposomes have become the most suitable drug delivery systems for directing drug molecules to macrophages (Immordino et al., 2006). The use of such liposomes in the treatment of diseases caused by parasites located in the cells of the mononuclear phagocytic system has been a popular topic among researchers. The most common diseases caused by these parasites are leishmaniniasis and fungal infections. Leishmaniniasis is a lethal intramacrophage parasitic disease found in more than 100 million people, usually in tropical regions. The drugs used to treat this disease are extremely toxic. The body is protected from its toxic effects by encapsulating these types of drugs in liposomes and accumulating only in the target area (Basu & Lala, 2004; Tuon et al., 2022).

In order for the liposomes to be directed to a specific target, ligands that can recognize specific units are attached to the appropriate regions of the liposomes. Antibodies covalently bound to the surface of liposomes are targeted to safely deliver drugs to specific surface antigens. Promising results have been obtained in studies with in vivo and in vitro animal models (Xing et al., 2013). Although the use of such formulations is currently limited to animal studies, human trials using antiparasitic liposome formulations have also been initiated in recent years. The most successful in these studies has been the liposome formulations containing Amphotericin B used in human antifungal therapy (Perez et al., 2016). Badiee and et al. utilized the the role of liposomes with different sizes containing the recombinant surface glycoprotein of Leishmania (rgp63) in BALB/c mice, and they evaluated the rate of protection and the type of immune response generated against leishmaniasis. The results indicated that immunization with small size liposomes induces a Th2 response, whereas immunization with large size liposomes induces a Th1 response, and higher interferon γ (IFNγ) levels and immunoglobulin IgG2a/IgG1 ratios (Badiee et al., 2012). Although the use of such formulations is currently limited to studies on animals, studies on humans using antiparasitic liposome formulations have also been initiated in recent years. The most successful of these studies has been the liposome formulations containing Amphoteracin B used in human antifungal therapy (Faustino & Pinheiro, 2020). Drugs used in patients whose immune system does not function correctly are neurotoxic and nephrotoxic. These toxic substances are either cleared by bonding with other drugs or these drugs are encapsulated with liposomes to greatly reduce their toxic effects (Inglut et al., 2020). Similar approaches have been applied in antiviral and antibacterial treatments (Nisini et al., 2018). Antiviral siRNA or retroviral drugs encapsulated with liposome NPs or dendrimers have been found to be better presented to CD4+ T cells by antigen presenting cells (APCs) (Pati et al., 2018).

Conclusion and Future Directions

Liposomes hold great potential as a safe and effective delivery system for drug and gene therapy. Their biocompatibility, targeted delivery capabilities, and ability to encapsulate various active substances have led to their successful use in cancer, infectious disease, and dermatological treatments. In conclusion, the potential of liposomes as drug delivery systems and investigating of immune related interactions of the liposome will provide a basis for future studies to discover the full clinical potential of cancer nanomedicines.

References

Ahmadi Ashtiani, H. R., Bishe, P., Lashgari, N., Nilforoushzadeh, M. A., & Zare, S. (2016). Liposomes in Cosmetics [Review Article]. J Skin Stem Cell, 3(3), e65815. https://doi.org/10.5812/jssc.65815

Ahmed, K. S., Hussein, S. A., Ali, A. H., Korma, S. A., Lipeng, Q., & Jinghua, C. (2019). Liposome: composition, characterisation, preparation, and recent innovation in clinical applications. J Drug Target, 27(7), 742-761. https://doi.org/10.1080/1061186x.2018.1527337

Ajeeshkumar, K. K., Aneesh, P. A., Raju, N., Suseela, M., Ravishankar, C. N., & Benjakul, S. (2021). Advancements in liposome technology: Preparation techniques and applications in food, functional foods, and bioactive delivery: A review. Compr Rev Food Sci Food Saf, 20(2), 1280-1306. https://doi.org/10.1111/1541-4337.12725

Akbarzadeh, A., Rezaei-Sadabady, R., Davaran, S., Joo, S. W., Zarghami, N., Hanifehpour, Y.,…Nejati-Koshki, K. (2013). Liposome: classification, preparation, and applications. Nanoscale Res Lett, 8(1), 102. https://doi.org/10.1186/1556-276x-8-102

Akinc, A., Maier, M. A., Manoharan, M., Fitzgerald, K., Jayaraman, M., Barros, S.,…Cullis, P. R. (2019). The Onpattro story and the clinical translation of nanomedicines containing nucleic acid-based drugs. Nat Nanotechnol, 14(12), 1084-1087. https://doi.org/10.1038/s41565-019-0591-y

Al-Amin, M., Bellato, F., Mastrotto, F., Garofalo, M., Malfanti, A., Salmaso, S., & Caliceti, P. (2020). Dexamethasone Loaded Liposomes by Thin-Film Hydration and Microfluidic Procedures: Formulation Challenges. International Journal of Molecular Sciences, 21(5), 1611. https://www.mdpi.com/1422-0067/21/5/1611

Al Badri, Y. N., Chaw, C. S., & Elkordy, A. A. (2023). Insights into Asymmetric Liposomes as a Potential Intervention for Drug Delivery Including Pulmonary Nanotherapeutics. Pharmaceutics, 15(1). https://mdpi-res.com/d_attachment/pharmaceutics/pharmaceutics-15-00294/article_deploy/pharmaceutics-15-00294-v2.pdf?version=1673836913

Andar, A., Hood, R., Vreeland, W., DeVoe, D., & Swaan, P. (2013). Microfluidic Preparation of Liposomes to Determine Particle Size Influence on Cellular Uptake Mechanisms. Pharmaceutical research, 31. https://doi.org/10.1007/s11095-013-1171-8

Andra, V. V. S. N. L., Pammi, S. V. N., Bhatraju, L. V. K. P., & Ruddaraju, L. K. (2022). A Comprehensive Review on Novel Liposomal Methodologies, Commercial Formulations, Clinical Trials and Patents. BioNanoScience, 12(1), 274-291. https://doi.org/10.1007/s12668-022-00941-x

Ashby, G., Keng, K. E., Hayden, C. C., Gollapudi, S., Houser, J. R., Jamal, S., & Stachowiak, J. C. (2023). Selective endocytic uptake of targeted liposomes occurs within a narrow range of liposome diameter. bioRxiv. https://doi.org/10.1101/2023.07.06.548000

Badiee, A., Khamesipour, A., Samiei, A., Soroush, D., Shargh, V. H., Kheiri, M. T.,…Jaafari, M. R. (2012). The role of liposome size on the type of immune response induced in BALB/c mice against leishmaniasis: rgp63 as a model antigen. Exp Parasitol, 132(4), 403-409. https://doi.org/10.1016/j.exppara.2012.09.001

Bangham, A. D., & Horne, R. W. (1964). Negative Staining of Phospholipids and Their Structural Modification by Surface-Active Agents as Observed in the Electron Microscope. J Mol Biol, 8, 660-668. https://doi.org/10.1016/s0022-2836(64)80115-7

Barba, A. A., Bochicchio, S., Dalmoro, A., & Lamberti, G. (2019). Lipid Delivery Systems for Nucleic-Acid-Based-Drugs: From Production to Clinical Applications. Pharmaceutics, 11(8). https://doi.org/10.3390/pharmaceutics11080360

Basu, M. K., & Lala, S. (2004). Macrophage specific drug delivery in experimental leishmaniasis. Curr Mol Med, 4(6), 681-689. https://doi.org/10.2174/1566524043360186

Benech, R. O., Kheadr, E. E., Lacroix, C., & Fliss, I. (2003). Impact of nisin producing culture and liposome-encapsulated nisin on ripening of Lactobacillus added-Cheddar cheese. J Dairy Sci, 86(6), 1895-1909. https://doi.org/10.3168/jds.S0022-0302(03)73776-X

Brgles, M., Šantak, M., Halassy, B., Forcic, D., & Tomašić, J. (2012). Influence of charge ratio of liposome/DNA complexes on their size after extrusion and transfection efficiency. Int J Nanomedicine, 7, 393-401. https://doi.org/10.2147/ijn.S27471

Cardador, C. M., Muehlmann, L. A., Coelho, C. M., Silva, L. P., Garay, A. V., Carvalho, A.,…Longo, J. P. F. (2023). Nucleotides Entrapped in Liposome Nanovesicles as Tools for Therapeutic and Diagnostic Use in Biomedical Applications. Pharmaceutics, 15(3). https://doi.org/10.3390/pharmaceutics15030873

Castañeda-Reyes, E. D., Perea-Flores, M. J., Davila-Ortiz, G., Lee, Y., & Gonzalez de Mejia, E. (2020). Development, Characterization and Use of Liposomes as Amphipathic Transporters of Bioactive Compounds for Melanoma Treatment and Reduction of Skin Inflammation: A Review. Int J Nanomedicine, 15, 7627-7650. https://doi.org/10.2147/ijn.S263516

Chai, R., Zhang, G., Sun, Q., Zhang, M., Zhao, S., & Qiu, L. (2013). Liposome-mediated mycelial transformation of filamentous fungi. Fungal Biol, 117(9), 577-583. https://doi.org/10.1016/j.funbio.2013.06.008

Christian Isalomboto, N., Alain Murhimalika, B., Nnamdi Ikemefuna, O., & Rui Werner Maçedo, K. (2019). General Perception of Liposomes: Formation, Manufacturing and Applications. In C. Angel (Ed.), Liposomes (pp. Ch. 3). IntechOpen. https://doi.org/10.5772/intechopen.84255

Costa, R., & Santos, L. (2017). Delivery systems for cosmetics - From manufacturing to the skin of natural antioxidants. Powder Technology, 322, 402-416. https://doi.org/https://doi.org/10.1016/j.powtec.2017.07.086

Danaei, M., Dehghankhold, M., Ataei, S., Hasanzadeh Davarani, F., Javanmard, R., Dokhani, A.,…Mozafari, M. R. (2018). Impact of Particle Size and Polydispersity Index on the Clinical Applications of Lipidic Nanocarrier Systems. Pharmaceutics, 10(2). https://doi.org/10.3390/pharmaceutics10020057

Daraee, H., Etemadi, A., Kouhi, M., Alimirzalu, S., & Akbarzadeh, A. (2016). Application of liposomes in medicine and drug delivery. Artif Cells Nanomed Biotechnol, 44(1), 381-391. https://doi.org/10.3109/21691401.2014.953633

Das, S. K. Drug Delivery: Principles and Applications. Am J Pharm Educ. 2006 Aug 15;70(4):94.

Diaz-Arévalo, D., & Zeng, M. Nanoparticle-based vaccines: opportunities and limitations. Nanopharmaceuticals. 2020:135-50. doi: 10.1016/B978-0-12-817778-5.00007-5. Epub 2020 Jan 17.

Dobó, D. G., Németh, Z., Sipos, B., Cseh, M., Pallagi, E., Berkesi, D.,…Csóka, I. (2022). Pharmaceutical Development and Design of Thermosensitive Liposomes Based on the QbD Approach. Molecules, 27(5). https://doi.org/10.3390/molecules27051536

E. Sanarova, A. L., N. Oborotova, O. Orlova, A. Polozkova, M. Dmitrieva, N. Nikolaeva. (2019). Liposome Drug Delivery. Journal of Pharmaceutical Sciences and Research, 11(3), 1148-1155.

Eroğlu, İ., Azizoğlu, E., Özyazıcı, M., Nenni, M., Gürer Orhan, H., Özbal, S.,…Özer, Ö. (2016). Effective topical delivery systems for corticosteroids: dermatological and histological evaluations. Drug Deliv, 23(5), 1502-1513. https://doi.org/10.3109/10717544.2014.960981

Faustino, C., & Pinheiro, L. (2020). Lipid Systems for the Delivery of Amphotericin B in Antifungal Therapy. Pharmaceutics, 12(1). https://doi.org/10.3390/pharmaceutics12010029

Gao, W., Hu, C. M., Fang, R. H., & Zhang, L. (2013). Liposome-like Nanostructures for Drug Delivery. J Mater Chem B, 1(48). https://doi.org/10.1039/c3tb21238f

Ghanbari Safari, M., & Hosseinkhani, S. (2013). Lipid composition of cationic nanoliposomes implicate on transfection efficiency. J Liposome Res, 23(3), 174-186. https://doi.org/10.3109/08982104.2013.779703

Gibbs, B. F., Kermasha, S., Alli, I., & Mulligan, C. N. (1999). Encapsulation in the food industry: a review. Int J Food Sci Nutr, 50(3), 213-224. https://doi.org/10.1080/096374899101256

Goins, B., Phillips, W. T., & Bao, A. (2016). Strategies for improving the intratumoral distribution of liposomal drugs in cancer therapy. Expert Opin Drug Deliv, 13(6), 873-889. https://doi.org/10.1517/17425247.2016.1167035

Gregoriadis, G. (2016). Liposomes in Drug Delivery: How It All Happened. Pharmaceutics, 8(2). https://doi.org/10.3390/pharmaceutics8020019

Hofheinz, R.-D., Gnad-Vogt, S. U., Beyer, U., & Hochhaus, A. (2005). Liposomal encapsulated anti-cancer drugs. Anti-Cancer Drugs, 16(7), 691-707. https://doi.org/10.1097/01.cad.0000167902.53039.5a

Huang, C. (1969). Studies on phosphatidylcholine vesicles. Formation and physical characteristics. Biochemistry, 8(1), 344-352. https://doi.org/10.1021/bi00829a048

Huang, Z., Li, X., Zhang, T., Song, Y., She, Z., Li, J., & Deng, Y. (2014). Progress involving new techniques for liposome preparation. Asian Journal of Pharmaceutical Sciences, 9(4), 176-182. https://doi.org/https://doi.org/10.1016/j.ajps.2014.06.001

Ibáñez, E., Mendiola, J. A., & Castro-Puyana, M. (2016). Supercritical Fluid Extraction. In B. Caballero, P. M. Finglas, & F. Toldrá (Eds.), Encyclopedia of Food and Health (pp. 227-233). Academic Press. https://doi.org/https://doi.org/10.1016/B978-0-12-384947-2.00675-9

Immordino, M. L., Dosio, F., & Cattel, L. (2006). Stealth liposomes: review of the basic science, rationale, and clinical applications, existing and potential. Int J Nanomedicine, 1(3), 297-315.

Imura, T., Otake, K., Hashimoto, S., Gotoh, T., Yuasa, M., Yokoyama, S.,…Abe, M. (2003). Preparation and physicochemical properties of various soybean lecithin liposomes using supercritical reverse phase evaporation method. Colloids and Surfaces B: Biointerfaces, 27(2), 133-140. https://doi.org/https://doi.org/10.1016/S0927-7765(02)00048-6

Inglut, C. T., Sorrin, A. J., Kuruppu, T., Vig, S., Cicalo, J., Ahmad, H., & Huang, H. C. (2020). Immunological and Toxicological Considerations for the Design of Liposomes. Nanomaterials (Basel), 10(2). https://doi.org/10.3390/nano10020190

Jafari, S. M., He, Y., & Bhandari, B. (2007). Production of sub-micron emulsions by ultrasound and microfluidization techniques. Journal of Food Engineering, 82(4), 478-488. https://doi.org/https://doi.org/10.1016/j.jfoodeng.2007.03.007

Jain, A., Hurkat, P., & Jain, S. K. (2019). Development of liposomes using formulation by design: Basics to recent advances. Chemistry and Physics of Lipids, 224, 104764. https://doi.org/https://doi.org/10.1016/j.chemphyslip.2019.03.017

Jung, H. N., Lee, S. Y., Lee, S., Youn, H., & Im, H. J. (2022). Lipid nanoparticles for delivery of RNA therapeutics: Current status and the role of in vivo imaging. Theranostics, 12(17), 7509-7531. https://doi.org/10.7150/thno.77259

Karn, P. R., Cho, W., Park, H. J., Park, J. S., & Hwang, S. J. (2013). Characterization and stability studies of a novel liposomal cyclosporin A prepared using the supercritical fluid method: comparison with the modified conventional Bangham method. Int J Nanomedicine, 8, 365-377. https://doi.org/10.2147/ijn.S39025

Kazemian, P., Yu, S. Y., Thomson, S. B., Birkenshaw, A., Leavitt, B. R., & Ross, C. J. D. (2022). Lipid-Nanoparticle-Based Delivery of CRISPR/Cas9 Genome-Editing Components. Mol Pharm, 19(6), 1669-1686. https://doi.org/10.1021/acs.molpharmaceut.1c00916

Kelly, C., Jefferies, C., & Cryan, S.-A. (2011). Targeted liposomal drug delivery to monocytes and macrophages. Journal of drug delivery, 2011, 727241. https://doi.org/10.1155/2011/727241

Kobayashi, N., Nishikawa, M., & Takakura, Y. (2005). Gene Therapy and Gene Delivery. In Drug Delivery (pp. 305-319). https://doi.org/https://doi.org/10.1002/0471475734.ch14

Lamichhane, N., Udayakumar, T. S., D'Souza, W. D., Simone, C. B., 2nd, Raghavan, S. R., Polf, J., & Mahmood, J. (2018). Liposomes: Clinical Applications and Potential for Image-Guided Drug Delivery. Molecules, 23(2). https://doi.org/10.3390/molecules23020288

Laouini, A., Jaafar-Maalej, C., Blouza, I., Sfar, S., Charcosset, C., & Fessi, H. (2012). Preparation, Characterization and Applications of Liposomes: State of the Art. Journal of Colloid Science and Biotechnology, 1, 147-168. https://doi.org/10.1166/jcsb.2012.1020

Levine, R. M., Pearce, T. R., Adil, M., & Kokkoli, E. (2013). Preparation and characterization of liposome-encapsulated plasmid DNA for gene delivery. Langmuir, 29(29), 9208-9215. https://doi.org/10.1021/la400859e

Li, C., & Deng, Y. (2004). A novel method for the preparation of liposomes: freeze drying of monophase solutions. J Pharm Sci, 93(6), 1403-1414. https://doi.org/10.1002/jps.20055

Liu, Y., & Huang, L. (2021). Preparation and Characterization of siRNA-Loaded Liposomes. In H. J. Ditzel, M. Tuttolomondo, & S. Kauppinen (Eds.), Design and Delivery of SiRNA Therapeutics (pp. 159-169). Springer US. https://doi.org/10.1007/978-1-0716-1298-9_10

Liu, Y., Huang, Y., He, G., Guo, C., Dong, J., & Wu, L. (2024). Development of mRNA Lipid Nanoparticles: Targeting and Therapeutic Aspects. Int J Mol Sci, 25(18). https://doi.org/10.3390/ijms251810166

Lombardo, D., & Kiselev, M. A. (2022). Methods of Liposomes Preparation: Formation and Control Factors of Versatile Nanocarriers for Biomedical and Nanomedicine Application. Pharmaceutics, 14(3). https://doi.org/10.3390/pharmaceutics14030543

Maherani, B., Arab-Tehrany, E., Mozafari, M., Gaiani, C., & M, L. (2011). Liposomes: A Review of Manufacturing Techniques and Targeting Strategies. Current Nanoscience, 7, 436-452. https://doi.org/10.2174/157341311795542453

Maja, L., Željko, K., & Mateja, P. (2020). Sustainable technologies for liposome preparation. The Journal of Supercritical Fluids, 165, 104984. https://doi.org/https://doi.org/10.1016/j.supflu.2020.104984

Mendez, R., & Banerjee, S. (2017). Sonication-Based Basic Protocol for Liposome Synthesis. Methods Mol Biol, 1609, 255-260. https://doi.org/10.1007/978-1-4939-6996-8_21

Meure, L. A., Foster, N. R., & Dehghani, F. (2008). Conventional and Dense Gas Techniques for the Production of Liposomes: A Review.

AAPS PharmSciTech, 9(3), 798-809. https://doi.org/10.1208/s12249-008-9097-x

Mozafari, M. R. (2005). Liposomes: an overview of manufacturing techniques. Cell Mol Biol Lett, 10(4), 711-719.

Mukai, H., Ogawa, K., Kato, N., & Kawakami, S. (2022). Recent advances in lipid nanoparticles for delivery of nucleic acid, mRNA, and gene editing-based therapeutics. Drug Metab Pharmacokinet, 44, 100450. https://doi.org/10.1016/j.dmpk.2022.100450

Nakhaei, P., Margiana, R., Bokov, D. O., Abdelbasset, W. K., Jadidi Kouhbanani, M. A., Varma, R. S.,…Beheshtkhoo, N. (2021). Liposomes: Structure, Biomedical Applications, and Stability Parameters With Emphasis on Cholesterol. Front Bioeng Biotechnol, 9, 705886. https://doi.org/10.3389/fbioe.2021.705886

Németh, Z., Csóka, I., Semnani Jazani, R., Sipos, B., Haspel, H., Kozma, G.,…Dobó, D. G. (2022). Quality by Design-Driven Zeta Potential Optimisation Study of Liposomes with Charge Imparting Membrane Additives. Pharmaceutics, 14(9). https://doi.org/10.3390/pharmaceutics14091798

Németh, Z., Pallagi, E., Dobó, D. G., & Csóka, I. (2020). A Proposed Methodology for a Risk Assessment-Based Liposome Development Process. Pharmaceutics, 12(12). https://doi.org/10.3390/pharmaceutics12121164

New, R. R. C. (1990). Liposomes : a practical approach.

Nisini, R., Poerio, N., Mariotti, S., De Santis, F., & Fraziano, M. (2018). The Multirole of Liposomes in Therapy and Prevention of Infectious Diseases. Front Immunol, 9, 155. https://doi.org/10.3389/fimmu.2018.00155

Nkanga, C., Bapolisi, A., Okafor, N. I., & Krause, R. (2019). General Perception of Liposomes: Formation, Manufacturing and Applications. In.

Nsairat, H., Khater, D., Sayed, U., Odeh, F., Al Bawab, A., & Alshaer, W. (2022). Liposomes: structure, composition, types, and clinical applications. Heliyon, 8(5), e09394. https://doi.org/10.1016/j.heliyon.2022.e09394

Olson, F., Hunt, C. A., Szoka, F. C., Vail, W. J., & Papahadjopoulos, D. (1979). Preparation of liposomes of defined size distribution by extrusion through polycarbonate membranes. Biochim Biophys Acta, 557(1), 9-23. https://doi.org/10.1016/0005-2736(79)90085-3

Ong, S. G., Chitneni, M., Lee, K. S., Ming, L. C., & Yuen, K. H. (2016). Evaluation of Extrusion Technique for Nanosizing Liposomes. Pharmaceutics, 8(4). https://doi.org/10.3390/pharmaceutics8040036

Otake, K., Imura, T., Sakai, H., & Abe, M. (2001). Development of a New Preparation Method of Liposomes Using Supercritical Carbon Dioxide. Langmuir, 17(13), 3898-3901. https://doi.org/10.1021/la010122k

Otake, K., Shimomura, T., Goto, T., Imura, T., Furuya, T., Yoda, S.,…Abe, M. (2006). Preparation of liposomes using an improved supercritical reverse phase evaporation method. Langmuir, 22(6), 2543-2550. https://doi.org/10.1021/la051654u

Panday, H., Rani, R., & Agarwal, V. (2016). Liposome and Their Applications in Cancer Therapy. Brazilian Archives of Biology and Technology, 59. https://doi.org/10.1590/1678-4324-2016150477

Pardridge, W. M. (2020). Brain Delivery of Nanomedicines: Trojan Horse Liposomes for Plasmid DNA Gene Therapy of the Brain. Front Med Technol, 2, 602236. https://doi.org/10.3389/fmedt.2020.602236 Pati, R., Shevtsov, M., & Sonawane, A. (2018). Nanoparticle Vaccines Against Infectious Diseases. Front Immunol, 9, 2224. https://doi.org/10.3389/fimmu.2018.02224

Perez, A. P., Altube, M. J., Schilrreff, P., Apezteguia, G., Celes, F. S., Zacchino, S.,…Morilla, M. J. (2016). Topical amphotericin B in ultradeformable liposomes: Formulation, skin penetration study, antifungal and antileishmanial activity in vitro. Colloids Surf B Biointerfaces, 139, 190-198. https://doi.org/10.1016/j.colsurfb.2015.12.003

Ponti, F., Campolungo, M., Melchiori, C., Bono, N., & Candiani, G. (2021). Cationic lipids for gene delivery: many players, one goal. Chem Phys Lipids, 235, 105032. https://doi.org/10.1016/j.chemphyslip.2020.105032

Ponti, F., Campolungo, M., Melchiori, C., Bono, N., & Candiani, G. (2021). Cationic lipids for gene delivery: many players, one goal. Chemistry and Physics of Lipids, 235, 105032. https://doi.org/https://doi.org/10.1016/j.chemphyslip.2020.105032

Porfire, A., Achim, M., Barbalata, C., Rus, I., Tomuţă, I., & Cristea, C. (2019). Pharmaceutical Development of Liposomes Using the QbD Approach. In (pp. https://www.intechopen.com/online-first/pharmaceutical). https://doi.org/10.5772/intechopen.85374

Rideau, E., Dimova, R., Schwille, P., Wurm, F., & Landfester, K. (2018). Liposomes and polymersomes: a comparative review towards cell mimicking. Chemical Society Reviews, 47. https://doi.org/10.1039/C8CS00162F

Rieth, M. D., & Lozano, A. (2020). Preparation of DPPC liposomes using probe-tip sonication: Investigating intrinsic factors affecting temperature phase transitions. Biochem Biophys Rep, 22, 100764. https://doi.org/10.1016/j.bbrep.2020.100764

Samad, A., Sultana, Y., & Aqil, M. (2007). Liposomal Drug Delivery Systems: An Update Review. Current drug delivery, 4, 297-305. https://doi.org/10.2174/156720107782151269

Saxena, S., Sharma, S., Kumar, G., & Thakur, S. (2025). Unravelling the complexity of CARPA: a review of emerging advancements in therapeutic strategies. Arch Dermatol Res, 317(1), 439. https://doi.org/10.1007/s00403-025-03971-z

Schneider, T., Sachse, A., Rößling, G., & Brandl, M. (1995). Generation of contrast-carrying liposomes of defined size with a new continuous high pressure extrusion method. International Journal of Pharmaceutics, 117(1), 1-12. https://doi.org/https://doi.org/10.1016/0378-5173(94)00245-Z

Schubert, R. (2003). Liposome Preparation by Detergent Removal. Methods in enzymology, 367, 46-70. https://doi.org/10.1016/S0076-6879(03)67005-9

Schwendener, R. A. (2014). Liposomes as vaccine delivery systems: a review of the recent advances. Therapeutic Advances in Vaccines, 2(6), 159-182. https://doi.org/10.1177/2051013614541440

Sforzi, J., Palagi, L., & Aime, S. (2020). Liposome-Based Bioassays. Biology (Basel), 9(8). https://doi.org/10.3390/biology9080202

Shah, M. R., Imran, M., & Ullah, S. (2017). Lipid-Based Nanocarriers for Drug Delivery and Diagnosis.

Shashidhar, G. M., Pravin, G. V., & Manohar, B. (2016). Nano-engineering of liposomes using a supercritical CO2 mediated gas anti-solvent method [10.1039/C6RA09530E]. RSC Advances, 6(62), 57739-57750. https://doi.org/10.1039/C6RA09530E

Skalko-Basnet, N., Pavelic, Z., & Becirevic-Lacan, M. (2000). Liposomes containing drug and cyclodextrin prepared by the one-step spray-drying method. Drug Dev Ind Pharm, 26(12), 1279-1284. https://doi.org/10.1081/ddc-100102309

Soh, S. H., & Lee, L. Y. (2019). Microencapsulation and Nanoencapsulation Using Supercritical Fluid (SCF) Techniques. Pharmaceutics, 11(1), 21. https://www.mdpi.com/1999-4923/11/1/21

Stone, N. R., Bicanic, T., Salim, R., & Hope, W. (2016). Liposomal Amphotericin B (AmBisome(®)): A Review of the Pharmacokinetics, Pharmacodynamics, Clinical Experience and Future Directions. Drugs, 76(4), 485-500. https://doi.org/10.1007/s40265-016-0538-7

Šturm, L., & Poklar Ulrih, N. (2021). Basic Methods for Preparation of Liposomes and Studying Their Interactions with Different Compounds, with the Emphasis on Polyphenols. Int J Mol Sci, 22(12). https://doi.org/10.3390/ijms22126547

Suk, J. S., Xu, Q., Kim, N., Hanes, J., & Ensign, L. M. (2016). PEGylation as a strategy for improving nanoparticle-based drug and gene delivery. Adv Drug Deliv Rev, 99(Pt A), 28-51. https://doi.org/10.1016/j.addr.2015.09.012

Sun, D., & Lu, Z. R. (2023). Structure and Function of Cationic and Ionizable Lipids for Nucleic Acid Delivery. Pharm Res, 40(1), 27-46. https://doi.org/10.1007/s11095-022-03460-2

Szebeni, J., Kiss, B., Bozó, T., Turjeman, K., Levi-Kalisman, Y., Barenholz, Y., & Kellermayer, M. (2023). Insights into the Structure of Comirnaty Covid-19 Vaccine: A Theory on Soft, Partially Bilayer-Covered Nanoparticles with Hydrogen Bond-Stabilized mRNA-Lipid Complexes. ACS Nano, 17(14), 13147-13157. https://doi.org/10.1021/acsnano.2c11904

Szebeni, J., Muggia, F., Gabizon, A., & Barenholz, Y. (2011). Activation of complement by therapeutic liposomes and other lipid excipient-based therapeutic products: prediction and prevention. Adv Drug Deliv Rev, 63(12), 1020-1030. https://doi.org/10.1016/j.addr.2011.06.017

Szoka, F., Jr., & Papahadjopoulos, D. (1978). Procedure for preparation of liposomes with large internal aqueous space and high capture by reverse-phase evaporation. Proc Natl Acad Sci U S A, 75(9), 4194-4198. https://doi.org/10.1073/pnas.75.9.4194

Taylor, K. M. G., & Morris, R. M. (1995). Thermal analysis of phase transition behaviour in liposomes. Thermochimica Acta, 248, 289-301. https://doi.org/https://doi.org/10.1016/0040-6031(94)01884-J

Tenchov, R., Bird, R., Curtze, A. E., & Zhou, Q. (2021). Lipid Nanoparticles─From Liposomes to mRNA Vaccine Delivery, a Landscape of Research Diversity and Advancement. ACS Nano, 15(11), 16982-17015. https://doi.org/10.1021/acsnano.1c04996

Thompson, G. R., 3rd, Sani, G. M., Donnelley, M. A., Figueroa, J. K., Ciuffetelli, R., Trigg, K.,…Dandekar, S. (2025). Liposomal amphotericin B and complement activation-related pseudoallergy (CARPA). Antimicrob Agents Chemother, 69(3), e0169224. https://doi.org/10.1128/aac.01692-24

Torchilin, V. P. (2005). Recent advances with liposomes as pharmaceutical carriers. Nat Rev Drug Discov, 4(2), 145-160. https://doi.org/10.1038/nrd1632

Trucillo, P., Campardelli, R., & Reverchon, E. (2020). Liposomes: From Bangham to Supercritical Fluids. Processes, 8(9), 1022. https://www.mdpi.com/2227-9717/8/9/1022

Tsai, W.-C., & Rizvi, S. S. H. (2016). Liposomal microencapsulation using the conventional methods and novel supercritical fluid processes. Trends in Food Science & Technology, 55, 61-71. https://doi.org/https://doi.org/10.1016/j.tifs.2016.06.012

Tuon, F. F., Dantas, L. R., de Souza, R. M., Ribeiro, V. S. T., & Amato, V. S. (2022). Liposomal drug delivery systems for the treatment of leishmaniasis. Parasitol Res, 121(11), 3073-3082. https://doi.org/10.1007/s00436-022-07659-5

van Winden, E. C. (2003). Freeze-drying of liposomes: theory and practice. Methods Enzymol, 367, 99-110. https://doi.org/10.1016/s0076-6879(03)67008-4

Wagner, A., Platzgummer, M., Kreismayr, G., Quendler, H., Stiegler, G., Ferko, B.,…Katinger, H. (2006). GMP production of liposomes--a new industrial approach. J Liposome Res, 16(3), 311-319. https://doi.org/10.1080/08982100600851086

Wagner, A., Vorauer-Uhl, K., & Katinger, H. (2002). Liposomes produced in a pilot scale: production, purification and efficiency aspects. Eur J Pharm Biopharm, 54(2), 213-219. https://doi.org/10.1016/s0939-6411(02)00062-0

Wagner, A., Vorauer-Uhl, K., Kreismayr, G., & Katinger, H. (2002). The Crossflow Injection Technique: An Improvement of The Ethanol Injection Method. Journal of Liposome Research, 12(3), 259-270. https://doi.org/10.1081/LPR-120014761

Wang, G. (2016). Liposomes as Drug Delivery Vehicles. In Drug Delivery (pp. 272-298). https://doi.org/https://doi.org/10.1002/9781118833322.ch13

Wang, P., & Keller, A. (2009). Natural and Engineered Nano and Colloidal Transport: Role of Zeta Potential in Prediction of Particle Deposition. Langmuir : the ACS journal of surfaces and colloids, 25, 6856-6862. https://doi.org/10.1021/la900134f

Wechtersbach, L., Ulrih, N., & Cigic, B. (2012). Liposomal stabilization of ascorbic acid in model systems and in food matrices. LWT - Food Science and Technology, 45, 43–49. https://doi.org/10.1016/j.lwt.2011.07.025

Xing, H., Tang, L., Yang, X., Hwang, K., Wang, W., Yin, Q.,…Lu, Y. (2013). Selective Delivery of an Anticancer Drug with Aptamer-Functionalized Liposomes to Breast Cancer Cells in Vitro and in Vivo. J Mater Chem B, 1(39), 5288-5297. https://doi.org/10.1039/c3tb20412j

Yang, S., Hu, X., Zhu, J., Zheng, B., Bi, W., Wang, X.,…Wu, Y. (2025). Aspects and Implementation of Pharmaceutical Quality by Design from Conceptual Frameworks to Industrial Applications. Pharmaceutics, 17(5). https://doi.org/10.3390/pharmaceutics17050623

Yildiz, S. N., Entezari, M., Paskeh, M. D. A., Mirzaei, S., Kalbasi, A., Zabolian, A.,…Ertas, Y. N. (2024). Nanoliposomes as nonviral vectors in cancer gene therapy. MedComm, 5(7), e583. https://doi.org/https://doi.org/10.1002/mco2.583

Yonezawa, S., Koide, H., & Asai, T. (2020). Recent advances in siRNA delivery mediated by lipid-based nanoparticles. Adv Drug Deliv Rev, 154-155, 64-78. https://doi.org/10.1016/j.addr.2020.07.022

Yu, B., Lee, R. J., & Lee, L. J. (2009). Microfluidic methods for production of liposomes. Methods Enzymol, 465, 129-141. https://doi.org/10.1016/s0076-6879(09)65007-2

Yu, J., Chuesiang, P., Shin, G., & Park, H. (2021). Post-Processing Techniques for the Improvement of Liposome Stability. Pharmaceutics, 13, 1023. https://doi.org/10.3390/pharmaceutics13071023

Zahednezhad, F., Saadat, M., Valizadeh, H., Zakeri-Milani, P., & Baradaran, B. (2019). Liposome and immune system interplay: Challenges and potentials. Journal of Controlled Release, 305, 194-209. https://doi.org/https://doi.org/10.1016/j.jconrel.2019.05.030

Zhang, H. (2017). Thin-Film Hydration Followed by Extrusion Method for Liposome Preparation. Methods Mol Biol, 1522, 17-22. https://doi.org/10.1007/978-1-4939-6591-5_2

Zhao, L. (2017). Preparation of liposomes and Encapsulation of Bioactives Using Supercritical Carbon Dioxide [Doctoral Thesis, Department of Agricultural, Food and Nutritional

Science University of Alberta, Canada].

Zuhorn, I. S., Bakowsky, U., Polushkin, E., Visser, W. H., Stuart, M. C., Engberts, J. B., & Hoekstra, D. (2005). Nonbilayer phase of lipoplex-membrane mixture determines endosomal escape of genetic cargo and transfection efficiency. Mol Ther, 11(5), 801-810. https://doi.org/10.1016/j.ymthe.2004.12.018

Zumbuehl, O., & Weder, H. G. (1981). Liposomes of controllable size in the range of 40 to 180 nm by defined dialysis of lipid/detergent mixed micelles. Biochim Biophys Acta, 640(1), 252-262. https://doi.org/10.1016/0005-2736(81)90550-2

Author Biography

Sanem Gökçen was born on 1980, April 18th in Ankara, TURKIYE. She graduated from the Medical Biological Sciences Department of Istanbul University, Cerrahpasa Medical Faculty in 2002. She received MSc in 2005 at Medical Biology Department of Istanbul University, Cerrahpasa Medical Faculty and she received Ph.D. degree in 2019 at Immunology Department of Gazi University Medical Faculty. She has been working as an expert from 2009 to present in Molecular Hematology Laboratory at Gazi University Medical Faculty which plays a key role in the diagnosis and management of various malignant and non-malignant disorders, and also provides critical information regarding the clinical management of bone marrow transplant patients. She has been studying on the molecular analysis of a variety of haematological disorders for 12 years.

CHAPTER 11

POLYMER-BASED DELIVERY SYSTEMS FOR NUCLEIC ACID THERAPEUTICS: ADVANCES AND APPLICATIONS

NURCAN GÜMÜŞ,[1,2] UMUT CAN ÖZ[3]

[1] Department of Medical Biology, Faculty of Medicine, Izmir Bakircay University, Izmir, Türkiye
[2] Department of Medical Pharmacology, Faculty of Medicine, Izmir Bakircay University, Izmir, Türkiye
[3] Department of Pharmaceutical Technology, Faculty of Pharmacy, Ankara University, Ankara, Türkiye

Abstract

Gene therapy holds great potential for treating inherited and acquired diseases, including genetic disorders, cancer, neurological disorders, and diabetes mellitus, by delivering nucleic acid therapeutics (DNA or RNA) into specific cells or tissues, facilitating the modulation of gene expression. The success of COVID-19 mRNA vaccines has further highlighted the potential of nucleic acid therapeutics for precise and effective disease management. This success has emphasised that gene therapeutics are an indispensable part of modern medicine. However, the delivery of nucleic acid therapeutics presents significant challenges for their clinical application. These challenges include a short half-life in circulation, poor membrane penetration, difficulties in escaping from endosomes, and insufficient release into the cytosol. In this case, viral vectors and non-viral polymer-carriers have become more attractive as gene delivery vehicles. Even though viral vectors have high transfection efficacies, their clinical implementations have still been limited owing to their inherent immunogenicity and insertional mutagenesis. Non-viral carriers have emerged as a promising option to overcome these obstacles and effectively transport nucleic acid therapeutics to targeted cells or organs.

Polymer-based gene carriers have gained significant interest as effective non-viral carriers attributed to their biocompatibility, biodegradability, versatility in design, and easy surface modification to target specific cells or organs, further enhancing their therapeutic potential. A range of polymers, both natural and synthetic, has been studied for their potential use in gene delivery systems. Polymeric delivery systems, including matrix-type nanoparticles, polymersomes, polyplexes, dendrimers, mesoporous nanoparticles, polymer-lipid hybrid nanoparticles, polyion complexes, and hydrogels, serve as efficient platforms to enable controlled and sustained gene release and facilitate intracellular gene delivery, surmounting biological barriers.

This chapter provides a brief outlook on polymeric nucleic acid carriers with their advantages/disadvantages while emphasising the importance of surface modifications for targeted delivery approaches. Furthermore, it highlights their potential in modern medicine, focusing on current applications in preclinical and clinical studies based on cancer therapy, genetic disorders, and regenerative medicine. In conclusion, this chapter aims to offer a comprehensive understanding of polymeric delivery systems and to exhibit their application potential in modern medicine.

Keywords: Nucleic Acid Therapeutics, Gene Therapy, Gene Delivery, Non-viral carriers, Polymer-Based Delivery Systems

1. Introduction

Gene therapy has emerged as a groundbreaking advancement in molecular medicine, offering the potential to treat diseases at a genetic level. The first human gene therapy studies were perform in the 1990s, (Blaese et al., 1995; Ferrari et al., 1991) since then nucleic acid therapeutics have been used for various inherited or acquired disorders treatment, such as genetic disorders (duchenne muscular dystrophy (Mendell et al., 2020), cystic fibrosis (Reyne et al., 2021), inherited retinal disease (Darrow, 2019) and inherited deafnesse (Qi et al., 2024), cancer (Golan et al., 2015; Mennati et al., 2025), cardiovascular diseases (Cao et al., 2021; Reynolds et al., 2012), neurological disorders (like parkinson (Christine et al., 2022), tay-sachs disease (Flotte et al., 2022) e.g.), and diabetes mellitus (Recino et al., 2019), AIDS (Herskovitz et al., 2021) by directly modifying genetic material to restore or regulate cellular functions. This therapeutic approach enables the correction of disease-associated genetic defects through the insertion, knocking out, or replacement of genetic material, thereby altering gene expression to influence cellular and tissue behaviour (Manohar et al., 2023). Such interventions are achieved through various methodologies, including gene replacement using DNA (Alazzo et al., 2018), saRNA (Dastgerdi et al., 2024) or mRNA (Meo et al., 2021; Polack et al., 2020) gene silencing via siRNA (Alazzo et al., 2022; Golan et al., 2015) or miRNA, and precise genome editing facilitated by CRISPR-Cas9 (Herskovitz et al., 2021) technology. The significance of gene-based interventions has been further emphasised by the rapid development of COVID-19 mRNA vaccines, which demonstrated the efficacy of nucleic acid therapeutics in addressing global health challenges (Meo et al., 2021; Polack et al., 2020; Widge et al., 2020). These advancements highlight the vast potential of gene therapy in transforming modern medicine and providing innovative treatments for previously untreatable conditions.

Efficient gene therapy depends on the intracellular transfer of nucleic acid therapeutics across multiple biological barriers before reaching the target cells or organ, a process referred to as gene delivery (Clima et al., 2021). However, naked nucleic acids (like DNA or RNA) have shown limited effects *in vitro* or *in vivo* studies. Because unmodified DNA or RNA introduced into the bloodstream is susceptible to nuclease degradation, resulting in a short half-life of between a few minutes and one hour (Subhan & Torchilin, 2019). Studies have demonstrated that intravenously administered genetic material is quickly eliminated from circulation (Malhotra et al., 2015). Its negative charge owing to phosphate groups on the molecular backbone, high molecular weight and hydrophilic properties hinder its penetration into cells (Huh et al., 2010). Additionally, nucleic acids can trigger immune responses, show a lack of tissue specificity, experience difficulties in escaping from endosomes, and insufficient release into the cytosol, all of which restrict their therapeutic efficacy (Clima et al., 2021; Subhan & Torchilin, 2019).

To maximise the therapeutic efficacy of nucleic acid therapies, research is being conducted on delivery systems capable of surmounting various extracellular and intracellular barriers to reach the therapeutic sites of action (Malhotra et al., 2015). In this case, viral vectors and non-viral carriers have become more attractive as gene-delivery vehicles. Even though viral vectors have high transfection efficacies, their clinical implementations have still been limited owing to their inherent immunogenicity, insertional mutagenesis, low loading capacity, and difficulties in scale-up and mass-manufacturing (Kumar et al., 2021; Manohar et al., 2023). Non-viral carriers are regarded as a powerful technique for delivering nucleic acid therapeutics to specific cells or organs, owing to their numerous advantages, including low toxicity, capacity for targeted distribution, long-term stability, lack of immunogenicity, and comparatively inexpensive production costs (Clima et al., 2021; Z. Yang et al., 2021). Non-viral carriers can be synthesised utilising a variety of materials such as lipids (e.g., liposomes, solid lipid nanoparticles, and micelles), polymers (e.g., chitosan, polyethyleneimine (PEI), and polylactic-co-glycolic acid), and inorganic materials (e.g., quantum dots, and gold NPs) (Dastgerdi et al., 2024; Kumar et al., 2021; Malhotra et al., 2015).

Polymer-based gene carriers, synthesized from natural (chitosan, dextran, and hyaluronic acid) or synthetic polymers (PEI, poly(*L*-Lysine) (PLL), and poly(β-amino ester) (PBAE)), have emerged as promising alternatives to viral vectors (Alazzo et al., 2022; Thomas et al., 2019). Their key advantages, including biocompatibility, biodegradability, and structural flexibility, enable controlled and sustained gene release while enhancing intracellular delivery by overcoming physiological barriers. This chapter presents a systematic review of polymer-based vectors for nucleic acid delivery, critically evaluating their advantages and drawbacks and emphasising their emerging applications in contemporary medicine. By elucidating the underlying design principles and performance metrics of these polymeric systems, it seeks to furnish a comprehensive framework for understanding their mechanisms of action and to underscore their transformative potential in the development of next-generation therapeutic modalities.

2. Polymeric Nanoparticles as a Delivery System

Polymeric nanoparticles have emerged as promising non-viral vectors for gene delivery, offering a combination of biocompatibility, biodegradability, and structural versatility. These nanoparticles play a critical role in protecting nucleic acids from degradation, facilitating cellular uptake, and promoting efficient intracellular trafficking, thereby improving the overall success of gene delivery strategies (Kumar et al., 2021). Beyond their delivery capabilities, nanoparticles facilitate controlled and sustained release, reduce immunogenicity, and allow for surface functionalization to achieve targeted gene transfer (Yang et al., 2021). These properties make them highly studied biomaterials in both biomedical and biotechnological applications. The key advantages and major drawbacks of polymeric nanoparticles in gene delivery applications will be discussed in the following section.

2.1 Advantages of Polymeric Delivery Systems for Gene Therapy

Polymeric nanoparticles exhibit numerous advantages for gene delivery; however, their most prominent benefits can be categorized as follows: (i) protection of genetic material from enzymatic degradation, (ii) the ability to cross biological barriers, (iii) lower immunogenicity compared to viral vectors, (iv) biocompatibility and biodegradability, (v) facilitation of endosomal escape, (vi) controlled and sustained release profiles, and (vii) versatility in surface functionalization for targeted delivery.

Building on these core advantages, a wide range of polymers is available for the development of polymeric nanocarriers in gene delivery systems, providing significant flexibility to tailor nanoparticle properties for specific therapeutic needs. Owing to their versatile nature, polymers enable precise control over nanoparticle shape, size, composition, and surface charge (Kaczmarek et al., 2018; Ou et al., 2008; Thomas et al., 2019). These physicochemical characteristics are critical determinants of transfection efficiency, as they directly affect biodistribution, cellular uptake, and the accumulation of nanoparticles in tumour tissues. *Vander et al.* demonstrated that the size and condensation capacity of nanoparticles can be tuned by varying the monomer composition within the polymer backbone. In their study, increasing the proportion of ethylenediamine (EDA) led to the formation of more compact nanoparticles and a higher positive charge density of the resulting polymer (Vader et al., 2011). Another study demonstrated that the molecular weight of the polymer significantly influences transfection efficiency, with nanoparticles smaller than 200 nm showing efficient accumulation in HEK cells (Blakney et al., 2020). Moreover, polymeric nanocarriers extend the circulation half-life of nucleic acids by protecting them from nuclease degradation, thereby enhancing their accumulation in tumour regions (Zhang et al., 2018). For instance, *Mahanta et al.* investigated the transfection efficiency of poly(*D*,*L*-lactide-*co*-glycolide) (PLGA) based DNA nanoparticles in comparison to naked DNA using primary astrocytes and primary neuronal cells as *in vitro* models. Their findings demonstrated that the PLGA-DNA nanoparticles achieved a transfection efficiency approximately four times higher than that of naked DNA, highlighting the enhanced gene delivery capability of the nanoparticle-based system in neural cell types (Mahanta et al., 2024).

In addition to physicochemical customisation, another key advantage is the ability of polymeric nanoparticles to overcome biological barriers previously considered insurmountable. Both pre-clinical and clinical studies have suggested that polymeric nanoparticles can pass through barriers such as the blood-brain barrier (BBB) (Malhotra et al., 2015; Zou et al., 2020). For example, *Karlsson et al.* reported that R646 and R647 polymers developed from a PBAE structure functionalised with disulphide bonds displayed high penetration across the BBB and promoted siRNA delivery in both *in vivo* and *in vitro* (Karlsson et al., 2019). To overcome biological barriers and enhance therapeutic accumulation at target sites, nanoparticle surfaces can be functionalized with targeting ligands such as antibodies, peptides, aptamers, transferrin, or angiopeptides (Gajbhiye et al., 2023). These modifications improve tissue penetration, promote cellular internalisation, and help reduce systemic cytotoxicity by increasing therapeutic concentrations at the target region. A different trial illustrated that Angiopep2–modified siRNA nanocapsules (Ang-NCss (siRNA)) exhibited prolonged circulation, successfully penetrated the BBB and accumulated effectively in tumours (Zou et al., 2020). Another approach using a three-layer biomimetic nanocomplex, which utilises red blood cell membrane (RBCm), with poly(*L*-lysine) (PLL-CA), and PEI, and eventually functionalised with the Ang (Angiopep2) peptide, achieved similar results. Being non-immunogenic and biocompatible, the Ang-RBCm-CA/siRNA nano-complex demonstrated prolonged plasma circulation, high BBB transcytosis, and high accumulation in glioblastoma cells (Liu et al., 2020).

Complementing barrier-crossing capabilities, polymer-based nanocarriers can be engineered to be biodegradable and exhibit minimal cellular toxicity. These biodegradable nanoparticles are fabricated from either natural or synthetic polymers (Singh et al., 2019; Thomas et al., 2019). Common natural polymers include structural proteins and polysaccharides such as chitosan, dextran, pullulan, hyaluronic acid, and modified cationic collagen (Duan et al., 2023; Nguyen et al., 2013; Wu et al., 2024). These materials have been widely applied in the delivery of nucleic acids, including siRNA, DNA and miRNA, across various therapeutic fields, with notable applications in cancer therapy and regenerative medicine. Frequently used synthetic polymers include polycaprolactone (PCL), poly(lactic acid) (PLA), poly(*D*,*L*-glycolide) (PLG), poly(ethylene glycol) (PEG), poly(*D*,*L*-lactide-*co*-glycolide) (PLGA), and polycyanoacrylate (PCA), many of which are FDA-approved and have been extensively investigated in biomedical applications, particularly in drug and nucleic acid delivery (Duan et al., 2023; Elsherbeny et al., 2025; Ge et al., 2014; Oyama et al.,

1987). These biodegradable synthetic polymers are composed of low-molecular-weight monomers linked through cleavable bonds such as esters or disulfides that degrade under physiological conditions (Nguyen et al., 2013; Singh et al., 2019). This degradation typically occurs via bulk hydrolysis, enabling a controlled and sustained release of genetic material. For instance, PEG-PCL-PEG hydrogel, synthesised from biodegradable and biocompatible PCL and PEG monomers, facilitates the sustained release of folate-poly(ester amine) (FA-PEA)/DNA complexes through passive hydrolysis and enzymatic cleavage of ester linkages (Yang et al., 2016). Another example is PLA, which degrades through acid-catalysed hydrolysis of its carboxylic acid groups to produce lactic acid. This is further metabolised into glucose, serving as an energy source in cellular pathways (Siparsky et al., 1998). Due to their biocompatibility, tunable degradation rates, and minimal risk of accumulation upon repeated use, biodegradable polymers are increasingly favoured in biomedical research and therapeutic development.

Building on the concept of controlled degradation, polymers can be tailor-designed to fabricate smart nanocarriers that respond to specific stimuli, thereby overcoming limitations of conventional drug and gene delivery systems. By incorporating internal physiological triggers originating from the local environment, including variations in pH, redox conditions, temperature, enzymatic activity and mechanical stress, along with external stimuli such as light, ultrasound, electric fields and magnetic forces, these systems enable precise regulation of drug release (Elsherbeny et al., 2025; Notabi et al., 2023; Wu et al., 2024; Yu et al., 2021). For instance, owing to the pH gradients observed across various tissues, nanocarriers composed of pH-responsive polymers hold great promise for targeted drug delivery (Notabi et al., 2023). While normal tissues maintain a physiological pH of around 7.4, tumours and inflamed tissues typically exhibit a mildly acidic environment (approximately pH 6.8). pH-sensitive delivery systems can exploit this difference to minimise systemic drug exposure and enhance therapeutic agents accumulation at the tumour site, taking advantage of the acidic extracellular environment characteristic of solid tumours (Wells et al., 2019). *Dan et al.* demonstrated that the cellular uptake of pH-responsive miRNA nanocomplexes at pH 6.5 was approximately three times higher than at pH 7.4, showing a significant difference (Yu et al., 2024). Thermo-responsive hydrogels, another commonly used class of stimulus-responsive polymers, undergo a sol–gel phase transition near physiological temperature, enabling their application via injection into target sites (Elsherbeny et al., 2025; Lu et al., 2020). This thermal responsiveness stems from the hydrophilic–hydrophobic balance within their polymeric structure, which alters solubility upon temperature change and induces network gelation (Yu et al., 2024). These smart systems enable sustained drug release and enhanced local therapeutic concentration, improving treatment efficacy (Nguyen et al., 2013).

In addition to their stimulus responsiveness, cationic polymers, a principal category within polymeric nanoparticles, possess the ability to facilitate endosomal escape through the proton sponge mechanism, thereby improving transfection efficiency. After cellular uptake, polyplexes formed through the electrostatic interaction of cationic polymers with negatively charged DNA or RNA become enclosed within endosomes where proton-pumping ATPase channels gradually lower the internal pH. Cationic polymers, such as PEI, can become protonated in response, disrupting endosomal acidification and leading to an influx of chloride ions to balance the charge. This ionic shift leads to water influx, causing osmotic swelling and ultimately rupturing the endosomal membrane, which releases the nanoparticles into the cytoplasm (Akinc et al., 2005). Polymers exhibiting high buffering capacity have demonstrated superior gene transfection efficiency through effective employment of this mechanism.

2.2 Drawbacks of the Polymeric Gene Delivery Vehicles

Although polymeric particles hold great promise as gene delivery systems, the primary obstacle to the clinical application of polymeric nanoparticles remains their cytotoxicity, which affects both cellular and systemic levels. Nanocarriers formed from cationic polymers typically exhibit a high positive surface charge (Lu et al., 2020). This positive charge enhances their interaction with the negatively charged cellular membrane, promoting cellular internalisation (Kumar et al., 2021); however, it also contributes to severe adverse effects by causing cell membrane damage and nonspecific interactions with anionic components in the body, such as plasma proteins and blood cells (Ogris et al., 1999; Vader et al., 2011; Van Der Aa et al., 2011a). To address these limitations, polymers or nanocarriers can be modified with hydrophilic or anionic monomers or polymers, specifically polyethylene glycol (PEG) or polysarcosine (pSar), in order to reduce aggregation, enhance colloidal stability, and mitigate the cytotoxic effects associated with the positive surface charge of polyplexes (Lai et al., 2012; Nomoto et al., 2011; Ogris et al., 1999). Attaching the hydrophilic polymer PEG, a process called PEGylation, is a common strategy to protect nonviral gene vectors from unintended interactions within the bloodstream. This modification also helps evade clearance by the reticuloendothelial system or macrophages, thereby prolonging the circulation time of the vector in the blood (Nomoto et al., 2011; Ogris et al., 1999). As an example of another polymer modification strategy, the incorporation of polysarcosine (pSar) into PBAE polymers has been shown to improve colloidal stability, reduce toxicity, and enhance transfection efficiency. The resulting pSar-modified PBAEs formed sub-200 nm polyplexes with efficient saRNA encapsulation and demonstrated effective gene delivery in colorectal cancer organoids (Bayraktutan et al., 2024). Additionally, co-formulating PBAE/saRNA polyplexes with the non-toxic anionic polymer γ-polyglutamic acid (γ-PGA) partially neutralised the positive surface charge, resulting in significantly enhanced transfection efficiency in HEK293T and A431 cells. This modification led to a notable decrease in zeta potential without altering polyplex size and substantially reduced cytotoxicity in moDC, NIH3T3, and A431 cells. Additionally, γ-PGA improved colloidal stability by minimising the aggregation of the ternary complexes (Dastgerdi et al., 2024). Another strategy would be to use low molecular weight polymers to form nanocarriers because cationic polymers with high molar mass have been demonstrated to have efficient gene transfection, but contribute to increasing toxicity effects, whereas reduced transfection efficiency but lower toxicity has been reported for low molar mass polymers (Sun et al., 2010).

Although the strategies developed so far have significantly improved the transfection efficiency of polymeric nanoparticles and mitigated their cytotoxic effects, further research is essential to ensure their clinical applicability. Comprehensive *in vivo* studies, long-term toxicity assessments, and evaluations of pharmacokinetics and biodistribution are required to better understand the safety profile of these systems. Moreover, the scalability, reproducibility, and regulatory compliance of polymer-based gene delivery platforms must be addressed before they can be translated into routine clinical use.

3. Mechanisms of Gene Delivery Using Polymeric Systems

Nanoparticles are nanocarriers, typically ranging in size from 10 to 1000 nm. The term "nanoparticle" refers to two primary types of polymer-based nanostructures: nanocapsules and nanospheres, which are classified according to their distinct morphological characteristics (Zielinska et al., 2020). Nanocapsules are vesicular systems composed of an inner liquid core, where the therapeutics are typically dissolved and encapsulated, enclosed by a polymeric membrane that governs the release of the active agent. In contrast, nanospheres represent matrix systems in which the therapeutics are uniformly dispersed within a continuous polymeric network or adsorbed onto the surface (Crucho et al., 2017). Depending on the formulation method and polymer type, these nanoparticles can act as reservoir systems (nanocapsules) or matrix systems (nanospheres) (*see* Figure 1). These polymeric nanocarriers are typically formed through non-covalent interactions, including hydrophobic interactions (Hibino et al., 2022), hydrogen bonding (Oyama et al., 1987) and electrostatic interactions (Gurnani et al., 2020). A wide range of hydrophilic and hydrophobic polymer blocks (Elsherbeny et al., 2025), varying in structure, length, and charge, have been utilised to engineer nanoparticles with diverse morphologies, sizes, and stability profiles (Kumar et al., 2021; Rocher et al., 2024; Singh et al., 2019; Yang et al., 2021). This section focuses on the most widely utilised polymeric nanoparticles for gene delivery, including matrix-based systems, polyplexes, dendrimers, polymeric micelles, polymersomes, polyion complexes, lipid–polymer hybrid nanoparticles, hydrogels, and nanogels (*see* Figure 2).

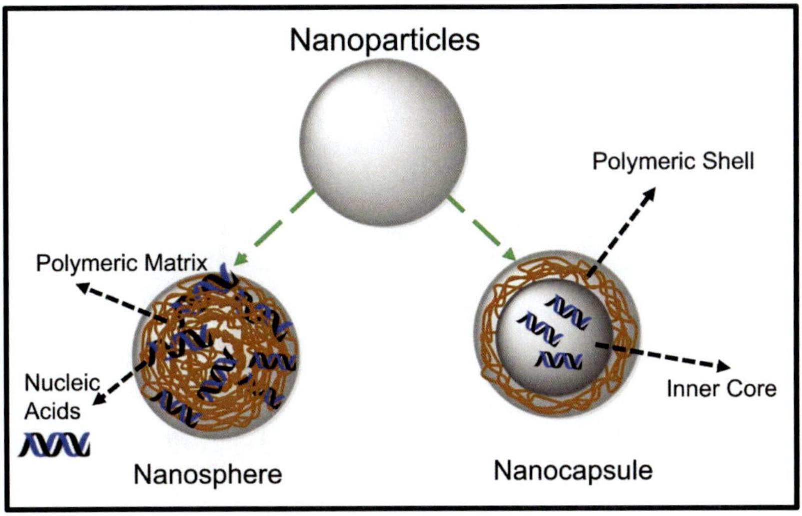

Figure 1: Schematic illustration of polymeric nanoparticles categorised by their morphological structures: nanospheres and nanocapsules.

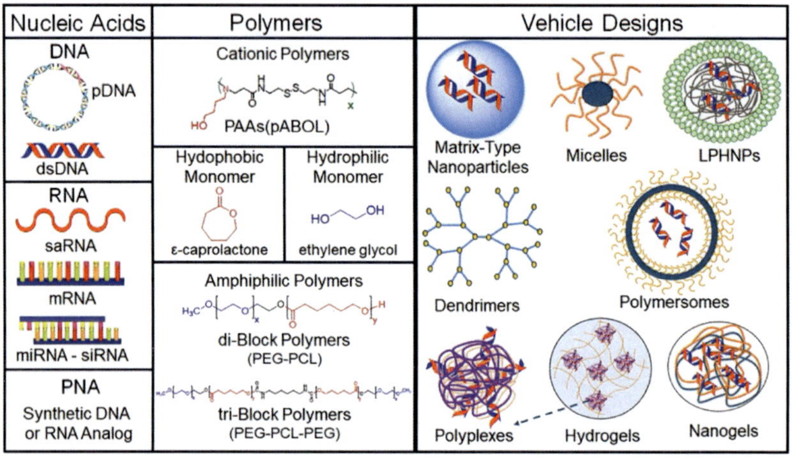

Figure 2: Overview of polymeric nucleic acid delivery vehicle formulations, highlighting representative examples of nucleic acid cargos, polymers, and final vehicle architectures. Common delivery systems include matrix-based nanoparticles, polyplexes, dendrimers, polymeric micelles, polymersomes, lipid–polymer hybrid nanoparticles, hydrogels, and nanogels. Poly(amido amines) (PAAs) are a class of polymers frequently used in gene delivery. One example is pABOL, a PAA synthesised from cystamine bisacrylamide (CBA) and 4-aminobutanol (ABOL) monomers. Additionally, block copolymers are widely employed in nanoparticle design. For instance, PEG-PCL (polyethylene glycol–polycaprolactone) is a di-block copolymer, while PEG-PCL-PEG is a tri-block copolymer. Both are derived from FDA-approved monomers, offering biocompatibility and tunable degradation profiles for therapeutic applications. Peptide Nucleic Acid (PNA). The pDNA, miRNA, siRNA and mRNA icons used in the figures were obtained from bioicons.com and are licensed under CC BY 4.0.

3.1 Matrix-Type Polymeric Nanoparticles

Matrix-type polymeric nanoparticles are comprised of polymers that form a matrix structure, which can encapsulate therapeutic agents such as drugs, proteins, or nucleic acids. These nanoparticles can be fabricated using natural polymers (e.g., chitosan, alginate) or synthetic polymers (e.g., PLGA, PEG, and PCL). One of their key advantages is the ability to provide sustained release of therapeutic compounds. For instance, *Cohen et al.* demonstrated that pDNA-loaded PLGA nanoparticles with a mean size of approximately 600 nm and high encapsulation efficiency (~70%) achieved sustained pDNA release for over a month (Cohen et al., 2000). A separate study reported the development of PLGA nanoparticles coated with mannose-conjugated chitosan for the co-delivery of therapeutic agents and DNA in the treatment of Alzheimer's disease. The mannose moiety enabled targeted interaction with the glucose transporter-1 (GLUT-1) receptor, which is abundantly expressed at the blood-brain barrier, thereby facilitating brain-specific delivery. Meanwhile, the chitosan coating provided a sustained release profile. These PLGA-based nanocarriers were non-toxic, hemocompatible, and demonstrated high transfection efficiency (Mahanta et al., 2024). *Spearman et al.* performed a Phase I clinical trial to evaluate the safety and immunogenicity of a PLGA-based DNA vaccine for HIV treatment. The results demonstrated that the vaccine was generally safe and well-tolerated among participants. Furthermore, the vaccination elicited antigen-specific $CD4^+$ T cell responses, indicating its potential to stimulate cellular immunity (Spearman et al., 2011).

3.2 Polyplexes

Polyplexes, formed due to electrostatic interactions of cationic polymers and nucleic acids, can be taken into cells through endocytosis (C. Lin & Engbersen, 2008) by interacting with the cellular membrane with its positive charges. Thus, polyplexes are able to prolong the half-life of nucleic acids by protecting them from nucleases (Alazzo et al., 2022; Bayraktutan et al., 2024; Dastgerdi et al., 2024; C. Lin & Engbersen, 2008). Cationic polymers such as PEI (Peschel et al., 2023), poly (amido amine) (PAA) (G. Chen et al., 2020; Gurnani et al., 2020), PLL (Alazzo et al., 2022) and PBAE (Bayraktutan et al., 2024) have been heavily investigated as gene delivery systems (Van Der Aa et al., 2011) These polymers are biodegradable, soluble in water (Mateos-Timoneda et al., 2008; Aa et al., 2010), and can be modified easily by adding carboxyl and hydroxyl groups, or targeting ligands and cell-penetrating peptides to enhance transfection efficiency (Lin et al., 2008). For instance, the N-Boc-protected diamines were reported to be able to contribute to improving buffer capacity and transfection efficiency (Ou et al., 2008). Besides the effect of the pendant groups on transfection efficiency, the architectural features of the polymers, notably; linear, dendritic, and branched, have been revealed to have a contribution to improving transfection efficiency by affecting polymer physicochemical properties (Kadlecova et al., 2013; Rocher et al., 2024). Compared to conventional linear cationic polymers, branched polymers can show advantageous physical and chemical properties for nucleic acid condensation due to the variety of amine group environments in their polymer chain, and thus their effective p*K*a (Martello et al., 2012; Sun et al., 2017). For instance, these polymers can exhibit different degrees of protonation, which can affect endosomal escape, and also be synthesised to higher molar mass while retaining structural flexibility (Chen et al., 2009; Kadlecova et al., 2013; Sun et al., 2017). *Martello et al.* reported that hyperbranched CBA-containing PAAs analogues induced higher transfection efficiency as compared to linear polymers (Alazzo et al., 2019).

The aforementioned features not only render cationic polymers a promising class of materials for gene delivery systems but also support their widespread use in the treatment of various diseases. However, as previously mentioned, cationic polymers with high molar weight and increased cation content in the polymer backbone have been associated with elevated toxicity (Sun et al., 2010; Vader et al., 2011). Therefore, achieving an optimal balance between enhanced endocytosis via membrane interaction and minimal membrane damage remains critical when selecting suitable polymers for such applications.

3.3 Dendrimers

Dendrimers are extensively branched polymers exhibiting a three-dimensional structure, characterised by their symmetrical, spherical, and actinomorphic architecture. These polymers consist of a central core with outward-extending, repetitive branches, creating a uniform structure via stepwise covalent assembly (Shen et al., 2010). This distinctive morphology facilitates their efficient utilisation in drug and gene delivery. One of the most researched gene delivery dendrimer topologies is poly(amido amine) (PAMAM), a highly branched cationic polymer developed in the early 1990s (Haensler et al., 1993; Xiong et al., 2019). The dendrimeric structure of PAMAM provides notable advantages for gene delivery, mainly due to its unique architecture containing primary, secondary, and tertiary amine groups. In particular, the high density of primary amines on the surface allows for effective condensation and binding of nucleic acids, leading to the formation of stable complexes with DNA or RNA (Bulkurcuoğlu et al., 2024; Liyanage et al., 2025; Padnya et al., 2024). Researchers have shown that the hyperbranched and dendritic nature of PAMAM facilitates superior gene transfection performance relative to linear counterparts (Khan et al., 2024; Wang et al., 2010). Furthermore, the internal tertiary amine moieties contribute to the "proton sponge effect" during endolysosomal acidification, promoting efficient endosomal escape and enhancing intracellular gene release (Luo et al., 2002; Xiong et al., 2019). The synthesis of PAMAM dendrimers through the number of synthetic growth cycles directly affects their molecular weight, polydispersity, surface charge, and transfection efficacy, so it can be finely tuned through their generation number to optimise delivery performance (Hansen et al., 2024; Khan et al., 2024).

Despite their advantages, including structural uniformity, high loading capacity, a high percentage of amine moieties, low immunogenicity and modifiable surface chemistry (Kadlecova et al., 2013; Sun et al., 2017). PAMAM dendrimers also present challenges such as complicated preparation, inability to be mass produced, poor degradation, rapid clearance from systemic circulation, poor biodegradability and cytotoxicity due to the high positive charge on the surface of PAMAM induced by its terminal amino groups (Luong et al., 2016; Shen et al., 2010). Several strategies have been developed to address these limitations. Due to their high reactivity, the terminal primary amine groups on the surface of PAMAM dendrimers are frequently modified to reduce cytotoxicity, enhance biocompatibility, improve circulation time and enable targeted delivery through conjugation with cell-specific ligands (Ma et al., 2018; Romani et al., 2024). Common approaches include PEGylation, carbohydrate conjugation, acetylation, integration of responsive linkers and the attachment of amino acids or peptides (Bulkurcuoğlu et al., 2024; Hu et al., 2017; Luong et al., 2016). Additionally, incorporating functional groups such as alkyl carboxyl, or cholesteryl chloroformate, helps to balance hydrophobicity and lipophilicity (Lin et al., 2015; Liyanage et al., 2025). For instance, the incorporation of biocompatible PEG branches into PAMAM dendrimers improves their biocompatibility, extends circulation time, decreases clearance, and increases transfection efficiency by up to 20-fold relative to partially degraded dendrimer controls (Luo et al., 2002). The functionalisation of PAMAM dendrimers with linear fluorinated guanidino linkers enhanced DNA condensation and transfection efficiency while maintaining low cytotoxicity (Romani et al., 2024). Beyond terminal functionalisation, structural innovations like the development of various dendrimer topologies (Hansen et al., 2024) or PAMAM-metallic nanoparticle (Z. Xiong et al., 2019) or exosome (Nair et al., 2023) hybrid systems enhance their adaptability and therapeutic potential in biomedical applications.

3.4 Polymeric Micelles and Polymersomes

Amphiphilic block copolymers (di (AB), tri (ABC or ABA)) or graft polymers may self-assemble into various nanostructures in aqueous solution, such as micelles (e.g., spherical, cylindrical), lamellae, and polymersomes (Liaw et al., 2001; Nishiyama & Kataoka, 2006; K. Singh et al., 2022). The resultant architecture of nanostructures is affected by several parameters such as molecular weight, concentration, hydrophilic-lipophilic balance, hydrophilic-to-hydrophobic ratio, chemical structure and block proportions of the polymers as well as external stimuli (the ratio of organic solvent/water composition, ionic strength, pH, and temperature) (Cho et al., 2010; Daubian et al., 2020; Photos et al., 2003). For instance, micelles are typically formed when the hydrophilic section constitutes over 50% of the overall amphiphilic block copolymer, whereas a lower hydrophilic percentage ($35 \pm 10\%$) typically promotes polymersome structures (Discher et al., 1999; Iqbal et al., 2020). *Zhang et al.* showed that the composition of the diblock copolymer of polystyrene-*b*-poly(acrylic acid) (PS-*b*-PAA) plays a crucial role in determining the micelle structure and morphology, which consist of a hydrophobic inner core and a hydrophilic outer shell (Zhang et al., 1996). As the content of the hydrophilic PAA block decreases, the micelles transition through distinct structural forms: from spherical micelles to cylinders, bilayers (vesicles and lamellae), and finally to compound micelles consisting of an assembly of inverted micelles surrounded by a hydrophilic surface (Zhang et al., 1996).

Polymersomes, also referred to as polymeric vesicles, resemble the morphology of liposomes but are composed of amphiphilic block copolymers rather than phospholipids (Cho et al., 2010; Singh et al., 2022). Polymersomes are characterised by hollow structures enclosed by a polymeric bilayer membrane, featuring a hydrophilic inner core and an outer layer formed by a hydrophobic middle section (Ge et al., 2014; Patel et al., 2023; Sinsinbar et al., 2024). Polymersomes are synthesised using high molecular weight amphiphilic block copolymers, and the membrane thickness of polymersomes can be precisely tuned by adjusting the molecular weight of the hydrophobic polymer blocks, which endows them with superior colloidal stability compared to conventional liposomes (Onaca et al., 2009; Photos et al., 2003). *Alibolandi et al.* reported that polymersomes assembled from PEG–PLA diblock copolymers exhibit superior structural stability compared to micelles derived from the same copolymers, which have higher hydrophilic segments (Alibolandi et al., 2015). As a result, polymersomes exhibit strengthened bilayer membranes, making them inherently more robust and durable for drug delivery and biomedical applications.

Both polymeric micelles and polymersomes possess a hydrophobic core and hydrophilic shell, allowing the co-encapsulation of hydrophobic and hydrophilic therapeutics (Laskar et al., 2017). The hydrophobic core serves as a nano-depot for hydrophobic drugs and nucleic acid therapeutics (e.g.,

DNA, oligonucleotides or RNA), while the hydrophilic shell facilitates interaction with the biological environment (Xiong et al., 2011). The tunable nature of copolymer design enables precise control over micelles and polymersome characteristics such as size, morphology, surface functionality, and responsiveness to environmental stimuli (Laskar et al., 2017; Shen et al., 2023; Singh et al., 2022; Wang et al., 2018). Their unique structure makes them highly suitable for delivering a variety of cargo, including anticancer drugs, proteins, DNA, RNA, and vaccines (Afrouz et al., 2023; Wang et al., 2018; Xia et al., 2025). For example, *Shen et al.* developed pH-responsive polymeric micelles based on polycarboxybetaine modified branched PEI for efficient plasmid DNA delivery. These micelles exhibited prolonged blood circulation, enhanced tumour targeting and penetration, and facilitated endosomal escape, ultimately leading to significant tumour growth inhibition in vivo (Shen et al., 2023). Apolipoprotein E (ApoE) peptide functionalised polymersomes, composed of polyethylene glycol, polycarbonate, and spermine segments, were engineered to co-deliver siRNA and chemotherapeutics to the brain. These nanocarriers demonstrated efficient BBB penetration, potent STAT3 gene silencing in glioblastoma cells, and significantly prolonged the median survival of orthotopic GL261 mouse models (Xia et al., 2025).

3.5 Polyion Complexes (PICs)

Forming amphiphilic block copolymers, polymersomes provide high stability, but they suffer from low lateral fluidity and limited permeability to small or hydrophilic molecules. Additionally, organic-solvent-based preparation methods can restrict the encapsulation of fragile biomolecules, such as proteins. Polyion complexes (PICs) have emerged as a promising alternative to overcome the limitations of polymersomes, as PICs can be formed in aqueous media without the need for organic solvents, making the preparation process significantly simpler (Kishimura, 2013). In contrast, PICs are formed via electrostatic interactions, similar to polyplexes, but unlike polyplexes, they can incorporate block copolymers and various polyelectrolytes (Aydinlioglu et al., 2023; Oba et al., 2011; Zhou et al., 2024). *Koide et al.* researchers introduced PIC vesicles known as "PICsomes" synthesised through the electrostatic self-assembly of oppositely charged block copolymers in an aqueous medium (Koide et al., 2006). These block copolymers consist of a hydrophilic nonionic segment, such as PEG, and an ionic segment, either cationic or anionic (Kim et al., 2020; Koide et al., 2006; Zhou et al., 2024). Upon mixing in water, the oppositely charged ionic segments interact to form a polyion complex core, while the hydrophilic

PEG segments extend outward, stabilising the vesicle structure (Aulia et al., 2024a; Aulia et al., 2024b; Oba et al., 2011; Zhou et al., 2024). Recent findings demonstrated that PEGylated polyion complex nanoparticles with mismatched ionic block lengths and vesicle morphology can enhance cellular uptake (Aulia et al., 2024).

PICs can be fabricated using various polymer architectures, including linear, grafted, branched, and dendritic structures (Ando et al., 2024; Aulia et al., 2024b; C. Li et al., 2022). These diverse polymer designs have been utilised to create numerous PIC nanoparticles, which are specifically engineered for the efficient delivery of a wide range of therapeutics. These include genes, small nucleic acids, proteins, and charged macromolecular drugs (Ando et al., 2024; Aydinlioglu et al., 2023; Khan et al., 2024; Kim et al., 2020; Oba et al., 2011; Sueyoshi et al., 2017). For instance, PIC complexes developed by incorporating both electrostatic and hydrophobic interactions between oppositely charged poly(ethylene oxide)-*b*-poly(amino acid) copolymers exhibited minimal cytotoxicity while achieving higher transfection efficiency than standard lipofectamine in HeLa cells (Aydinlioglu et al., 2023). A dual-ligand PIC complex functionalized with rabies virus glycoprotein and Tet1 peptide enabled efficient siRNA delivery to the brain, enhancing BBB penetration and neuronal transfection. This strategy significantly improved the cognitive and spatial memory in alzheimer mice models, demonstrating its potential as a targeted gene delivery carrier for the central nervous system (Jia et al., 2024)

3.6 Lipid–Polymer Hybrid Nanoparticles (LPHNPs)

Lipid–polymer hybrid nanoparticles (LPHNPs) are a class of delivery systems that integrate the advantageous features of both polymeric nanoparticles and lipid-based carriers (Carvalho et al., 2024; Chen et al., 2025; Mennati et al., 2025). These hybrid systems are typically constructed either by co-formulating polymeric components with lipids and therapeutic agents such as mRNA or by embedding polymers directly within traditional lipid nanoparticle (LNP) structures (Di et al., 2022; Kaczmarek et al., 2021). LPHNPs are sophisticated core–shell nanostructures typically composed of two or three integral layers, each contributing distinct functional advantages to the system (Carvalho et al., 2024; Sivadasan et al., 2021). The innermost layer is a polymeric core, which acts as a structural scaffold, offering mechanical strength and a high surface area for efficient therapeutic encapsulation (Sivadasan et al., 2021). This core ensures the structural integrity and storage stability of the nanoparticle and facilitates controlled drug release. Surrounding the polymeric matrix is a lipid monolayer that functions as a biocompatible molecular barrier. This layer plays a critical role in minimising drug leakage from the core and shielding the inner structure from degradation by limiting water diffusion and therefore maintaining the structural integrity and functional stability of the nanoparticle over time (Persano et al., 2021; Zhang et al., 2017). The optional outer lipid–PEG layer forms the third component, serving as a steric stabiliser that prolongs systemic circulation by reducing recognition and clearance by the immune system. This outer shell can also be tailored with targeting ligands (e.g., antibodies, peptides, and aptamers) or stimuli-responsive elements to enable site-specific drug delivery, gene transport, and theranostic applications (Aravind et al., 2012; Chen et al., 2025; Mennati et al., 2025; Zhang et al., 2017). Collectively, the integration of these components allows LPHNPs to combine the strengths of both lipid-based and polymeric systems, offering mechanical stability, tunable release profiles, enhanced biocompatibility, extended circulation time, and efficient therapeutic delivery (Gameiro et al., 2024). LPHNPs can be fabricated using various combinations of natural, synthetic, or semi-synthetic polymers and lipids, each contributing distinct physicochemical properties (Gameiro et al., 2024; Kaczmarek et al., 2021). These properties include diverse particle sizes and morphologies, surface charges, and responsiveness to internal or external stimuli. Such adaptability allows LPHNPs to encapsulate a broad spectrum of bioactive molecules within both their core and outer shell, enhancing their potential for targeted and controlled therapeutic delivery. Commonly used biocompatible polymers for constructing the core of LPHNPs include PLA, PEG, PLGA, PCL, Pluronic F-68, and chitosan (Aravind et al., 2012; Di et al., 2022; González-García et al., 2024; Mennati et al., 2025). Meanwhile, the lipid shell is typically composed of lipids such as myristic acid, phosphatidylcholine (PC), cholesterol, stearic acid, soya phosphatidylcholine (SPC), 1,2-dioleoyl-sn-glycero-3-phosphoethanolamine (DOPE), 1,2-dioleoyl-3-trimethylammonium-propane (DOTAP), 1,2-dipalmitoyl-sn-glycero-3-phosphocholine (DPPC), 1,2-distearoyl-sn-glycero-3-phosphoethanolamine (DSPE), and 1,2-dilauroyl-sn-glycero-3-phosphocholine (DLPC) (Carvalho et al., 2024; González-García et al., 2024; Zhang et al., 2017).

3.7 Hydrogels for Gene Delivery

Hydrogels are structured in a three-dimensional (3D) architecture by crosslinking hydrophilic synthetic or natural polymers in an aqueous environment. The crosslinking allows hydrogels to absorb a substantial volume of water without dissolution, and this high-water content enhances their biocompatibility while also enabling them to match the stiffness of their environment (Peppas et al., 2000). The diversity of polymers used in hydrogel structures allows tuning of several distinct features, such as biocompatibility, biodegradability, and a diverse range of viscoelastic and stiffness properties (Gazaille et al., 2021). Hydrogels have also shown the capability to encapsulate many different therapeutic agents, including DNA, siRNA, hydrophilic/hydrophobic drugs, antibodies, and proteins (Lu et al., 2020; Song et al., 2021; Wanjale et al., 2022; Ye et al., 2023). Being less invasive and injectable, hydrogels enable the sustained local delivery of nucleic acids, which can provide a high local concentration of genetic material while minimising systemic exposure and side effects (Wang et al., 2017). Therefore, hydrogels are gaining significant attention in the treatment of various diseases, including wound healing (Saleh et al., 2019), regenerative medicine applications (Zhang et al., 2021), musculoskeletal diseases (Lolli et al., 2019) and several cancers (Song et al., 2021). The gelation process occurs either in situ or before injection, providing hydrogels with the flexibility to be applied through various means, primarily implantation and injection into the tumour site (Alghamdi et al., 2021). Achieving in situ sol-to-gel transition can be accomplished through chemical or physical stimuli, such as using catalysts or organic solutions, as well as exposure to light or alterations in temperature/pH (Peppas et al., 2000). Due to their in-situ gelation capability, injectable hydrogels have gained significant attention for biomedical applications. This is because the aqueous solution of the hydrogel can fill the irregular edges of the target area and can be easily administered into the target area through injection.

Nucleic acids can be integrated into hydrogels using two distinct strategies. (i) The inclusion of naked RNA relies heavily on physicochemical interactions, including electrostatic or hydrophobic interactions, hydrogen, and covalent bonding between the RNA and the hydrogel structure (Z. Ma et al., 2014; L. L. Wang & Burdick, 2017); and (ii) The loading of encapsulating RNA nanocarriers, such as polyplexes, lipoplexes, or nanoparticles (Song et al., 2021; Wang et al., 2017). Although both methods have been employed for RNAi delivery, nanoparticle-hydrogel composites are widely regarded as the more effective method owing to their manifold benefits. The main benefit is that chemical alteration of RNA or hydrogel polymers is not required. Compared to naked nucleic acid strategies, the nanoparticle-loaded hydrogel approach improves loading capacity, stability, endosomal escape, cellular uptake, and transfection efficiency (Zhong et al., 2023).

For instance, the study conducted by *Song et al.* demonstrated that the intracavitary administration of PLGA-PEG-PLGA hydrogel loaded with shRNA complexes, which target the *CD47* gene, combined with oral TMZ administration, significantly extended the median survival time from 27 days (in the control group) to 73 days (Song et al., 2021). *Lu et al.* demonstrated a 40% reduction in tumour size by employing intratumoral injection of a thermosensitive chitosan-g-poly(N-isopropyl acrylamide) (CPN) hydrogel loaded with GO-CET/CPT11@shRNA, which was described as CPN@GO-CET/CPT11@shRNA. This hydrogel facilitated the co-delivery of shRNA (targeting the stomatin-like protein 2 (*SLP2*) gene) and irinotecan (CPT-11) drug carried with a graphene oxide (GO) nanocarrier conjugated with the CET (cetuximab) antibody (Lu et al., 2020). In another approach, an adhesive hydrogel incorporating hyaluronic acid nanoparticles loaded with a miR-223-5p mimic (miR-223) was developed to promote wound healing (Saleh et al., 2019). Similarly, *Kim et al.* designed a sulfonated chitosan-based hydrogel covalently conjugated with siRNA targeting the noggin gene, aiming to enhance osteogenesis through sustained activation of bone morphogenetic protein (BMP) signalling (Kim et al., 2021). Consequently, the integration of hydrogels with gene delivery systems has the potential to significantly improve therapeutic outcomes.

3.8 Nanogels

Nanogels, also known as hydrogel nanoparticles, are nano-sized colloidal hydrogel particles typically ranging from 10 to 1000 nm, with a common size distribution between 20 and 250 nm, particularly suitable for tissue engineering applications (Li et al., 2025; Mauri et al., 2018). They combine the advantageous properties of both nanomaterials and hydrogels, such as large encapsulation capacity, high swelling ability, and responsiveness to physiological stimuli (e.g., pH, temperature, redox conditions, and/or specific enzymes at the targeted site) (Dong et al., 2020; Notabi et al., 2023). Unlike conventional hydrogels, nanogels are sufficiently small for intravenous administration and are capable of delivering therapeutic agents to specific tissues or cells, thereby enabling targeted treatment at the site of pathological disorders (Mauri et al., 2018). Research has demonstrated that, due to their nanoscale dimensions, nanogels exhibit superior BBB permeability compared to bulk hydrogels (Zhang et al., 2022). Furthermore, their tunable porosity, particle size, surface charge, and hydrophilicity contribute to improved colloidal and dispersion stability, reduced degradation rates, and prolonged retention of loaded therapeutic agents

(Duan et al., 2023). These properties make nanogels promising and versatile platforms for the delivery of drugs and nucleic acids.

Nanogels are nanoscale colloidal hydrogels composed of natural, synthetic, or hybrid polymers, interconnected through physical interactions or chemical cross-linking (Akiyoshi et al., 1993). Natural polymers frequently employed include proteins such as collagen, albumin, and fibrin, as well as polysaccharides like chitosan, hyaluronic acid, alginate, agarose, and heparin (Aslan et al., 2017; Farjadian et al., 2024). On the other hand, synthetic polymers encompass a broader range, including PEG, polyacrylates, PEI, PLA, PCL, polymethacrylates, and dendrimers (Mauri et al., 2018; Notabi et al., 2023; Vinogradov et al., 1999). The functional groups present on these polymers, such as hydroxyl, amide, carboxamide, thiol, and sulfonyl, facilitate three-dimensional network formation and contribute to the hydrophilic nature of nanogels, enabling high water absorption capacity (Farjadian et al., 2024). Although *Akiyoshi et al.* first developed nanogels in 1993 through physical cross-linking of amphiphilic polymers (Akiyoshi et al., 1993), the term "nanogel" was introduced by *Vinogradov et al.* in 1999, referring to a nanosized hydrogel system (~120 nm) synthesised by cross-linking polyethyleneimine and carbonyldiimidazole-activated poly(ethylene glycol) via an emulsification/solvent evaporation method. This system enabled efficient oligonucleotide delivery and demonstrated the ability to overcome drug resistance by enhancing cellular uptake and inhibiting P-glycoprotein expression (Vinogradov et al., 1999).

Since 1999, there has been growing interest in the use of nanogels as delivery systems for nucleic acids. For instance, *Li et al.* synthesised temperature-responsive, low-generation dendrimer-based nanogels via an emulsion-free method. These nanogels demonstrated high yield and purity, tunable particle size, uniform morphology, and excellent colloidal stability (Li et al., 2025). Similarly, *Notabi et al.* developed pH- and redox-responsive smart nanogels for siRNA delivery. These nanogels (DEAEMA-co-HEMA-g-PEGMA) were produced by copolymerising 2-diethylaminoethyl methacrylate (DEAEMA) and 2-hydroxyethyl methacrylate (HEMA), using either tetraethylene glycol dimethacrylate or a disulfide-containing crosslinker, bis(2-methacryloyloxyethyl) disulfide. The resulting nanogels exhibited notable serum stability and effectively delivered siRNA with minimal cytotoxicity. Impressively, they achieved over 90% silencing of e*GFP* in lung cancer cells and successfully induced siRNA-mediated apoptosis by targeting the *POLR2A* gene in squamous carcinoma cells (Notabi et al., 2023). Nanogels have been utilised in various pharmaceutical and medical fields beyond cancer therapy, including vaccine delivery, wound healing, bone regeneration, cardiovascular complications and the treatment of neurological disorders such as multiple sclerosis, parkinson, spinal cord injury (SCI), and alzheimer (Aslan et al., 2017; Farjadian et al., 2024; Fukuyama et al., 2015; Ullah et al., 2022).

4. Conclusion and Future Perspectives

Nucleic acid-based therapy offers a transformative therapeutic strategy for a broad spectrum of diseases, including genetic disorders, viral infections, cardiovascular diseases, neurological disorders, diabetes mellitus, and cancer, by enabling precise modulation and repair of cellular functions. However, the success of these therapies critically depends on the development of efficient and safe delivery systems to overcome the pharmacokinetic limitations of naked nucleic acids. Ideally, an effective gene delivery vector must meet several essential criteria to ensure successful transfection and cellular compatibility. These include (i) possessing a high capacity for nucleic acid encapsulation while enabling efficient cargo release into the cytoplasm, (ii) exhibiting biocompatibility with minimal cytotoxic effects to prevent adverse cellular responses, (iii) maintaining stability in the bloodstream to prevent non-specific interactions with serum proteins and degradation by endonucleases, and (iv) facilitating endosomal escape to ensure the genetic material reaches its intended intracellular target. Beyond these fundamental properties, the physicochemical characteristics of vectors in terms of particle size, morphology and surface modifications critically influence transfection efficiency.

Polymeric gene delivery systems represent a promising class of non-viral vectors, offering advantages including biocompatibility, structural tunability, controlled release, and potential for surface modification. These systems are capable of protecting nucleic acid therapeutics from enzymatic degradation, facilitating cellular uptake, promoting endosomal escape, and enabling efficient cytosolic delivery, thus addressing key challenges in gene therapy. Among these systems, cationic polymers are widely studied for their ability to condense nucleic acids into stable polyplexes, enhancing cellular internalisation. Biodegradable polymers, including PLA, PGA, PLGA, and PEG, are particularly valued for their favourable degradation profiles and safety. Furthermore, other polymeric platforms, including PIC complexes, polymersomes, polymeric micelles, hydrogels and dendrimers, are being actively explored and engineered to improve gene transfection efficiency while minimising associated cytotoxicity. Despite this progress, several challenges still impede the clinical application of polymeric carriers.

Cytotoxicity remains the most critical concern and must be carefully addressed in the design of polymeric gene delivery systems. Achieving an optimal balance between transfection efficiency and cytotoxicity is crucial in polymer selection for gene delivery. This has stimulated increasing interest in biodegradable, stimuli-responsive polymers and hybrid systems that integrate lipids or inorganic components to improve safety while maintaining efficacy.

Future investigation in polymeric gene delivery should emphasise the rational design of next-generation vectors with enhanced targeting specificity, diminished cytotoxicity, and enhanced delivery efficiency. The development of biodegradable and stimuli-responsive systems, along with polymeric implants for sustained and localised delivery, presents considerable potential for advancing therapeutic outcomes. Moreover, the incorporation of advanced bioconjugation techniques, artificial intelligence-driven polymer design, and individualised delivery methodologies may enhance the personalisation of gene therapy applications. To ensure clinical relevance and facilitate regulatory approval, future studies must also address the limitations of current preclinical models by developing standardised disease models that more accurately replicate human physiology. Collectively, these innovations will support the development of safer, more effective, and personalised gene therapies for a wide range of genetic disorders.

References

Afrouz, M., Ahmadi-Nouraldinvand, F., Amani, A., Zahedian, H., Elias, S. G., Arabnejad, F., Yaghoubi, H., Farshad, O., Farazi, N., Jalali, A., & Eskanlou, H. (2023). Preparation and characterization of magnetic PEG-PEI-PLA-PEI-PEG/Fe3O4-PCL/DNA micelles for gene delivery into MCF-7 cells. *Journal of Drug Delivery Science and Technology*, *79*. https://doi.org/10.1016/j.jddst.2022.104016

Akinc, A., Thomas, M., Klibanov, A. M., & Langer, R. (2005). Exploring polyethylenimine-mediated DNA transfection and the proton sponge hypothesis. *Journal of Gene Medicine*, *7*(5), 657–663. https://doi.org/10.1002/jgm.696

Akiyoshi, K., Deguchi, S., Moriguchi, N., Yamaguchi, S., & Sunamoto, J. (1993). Self-Aggregates of Hydrophobized Polysaccharides in Water. Formation and Characteristics of Nanoparticles. In *Macromolecules* (Vol. 26). https://pubs.acs.org/sharingguidelines

Alazzo, A., Al-Natour, M. A., Spriggs, K., Stolnik, S., Ghaemmaghami, A., Kim, D. H., & Alexander, C. (2019). Investigating the intracellular effects of hyperbranched polycation-DNA complexes on lung cancer cells using LC-MS-based metabolite profiling. *Molecular Omics*, *15*(1), 77–87. https://doi.org/10.1039/c8mo00139a

Alazzo, A., Gumus, N., Gurnani, P., Stolnik, S., Rahman, R., Spriggs, K., & Alexander, C. (2022). Investigating histidinylated highly branched poly(lysine) for siRNA delivery. *Journal of Materials Chemistry B*, *10*(2), 236–246. https://doi.org/10.1039/d1tb01793d

Alazzo, A., Lovato, T., Collins, H., Taresco, V., Stolnik, S., Soliman, M., Spriggs, K., & Alexander, C. (2018). Structural variations in hyperbranched polymers prepared via thermal polycondensation of lysine and histidine and their effects on DNA delivery. *Journal of Interdisciplinary Nanomedicine*, *3*(2), 38–54. https://doi.org/10.1002/jin2.36

Alghamdi, M., Gumbleton, M., & Newland, B. (2021). Local delivery to malignant brain tumors: Potential biomaterial-based therapeutic/adjuvant strategies. In *Biomaterials Science* (Vol. 9, Issue 18, pp. 6037–6051). Royal Society of Chemistry. https://doi.org/10.1039/d1bm00896j

Alibolandi, M., Ramezani, M., Abnous, K., Sadeghi, F., & Hadizadeh, F. (2015). Comparative evaluation of polymersome versus micelle structures as vehicles for the controlled release of drugs. *Journal of Nanoparticle Research*, *17*(2). https://doi.org/10.1007/s11051-015-2878-8

Ando, T., Vu, T. N., Nishimura, T., Takahashi, R., & Yusa, S. I. (2024). Synthesis and Characterization of Polyion Complex Micelles with Glycopolymer Shells for Drug Delivery Carriers. *Langmuir*. https://doi.org/10.1021/acs.langmuir.4c03795

Aravind, A., Jeyamohan, P., Nair, R., Veeranarayanan, S., Nagaoka, Y., Yoshida, Y., Maekawa, T., & Sakthi Kumar, D. (2012). ARTICLE AS1411 Aptamer Tagged PLGA-Lecithin-PEG Nanoparticles for Tumor Cell Targeting and Drug Delivery. *Biotechnol. Bioeng*, *109*, 2920–2931. https://doi.org/10.1002/bit.24558/abstract

Aslan, C., Çelebi, N., Değim, I. T., Atak, A., & Özer, Ç. (2017). Development of Interleukin-2 Loaded Chitosan-Based Nanogels Using Artificial Neural Networks and Investigating the Effects on Wound Healing in Rats. *AAPS PharmSciTech*, *18*(4), 1019–1030. https://doi.org/10.1208/s12249-016-0662-4

Aulia, F., & Kishimura, A. (2024). *Recent Progress of Polyion Complex Vesicles (PICsomes) for Biomedical Applications* (pp. 149–183). https://doi.org/10.1007/978-981-97-5288-1_10

Aulia, F., Matsuba, H., Adachi, S., Yamada, T., Nakase, I., Nii, T., Mori, T., Katayama, Y., & Kishimura, A. (2024). Effective design of PEGylated polyion complex (PIC) nanoparticles for enhancing PIC internalisation in cells utilising block copolymer combinations with mismatched ionic chain lengths. *Journal of Materials Chemistry B*, *12*(7), 1826–1836. https://doi.org/10.1039/d3tb02049e

Aydinlioglu, E., Abdelghani, M., Le Fer, G., van Hest, J. C. M., Sandre, O., & Lecommandoux, S. (2023). Robust Polyion Complex Vesicles (PICsomes) Based on PEO-b-poly(amino acid) Copolymers Combining Electrostatic and Hydrophobic Interactions: Formation, siRNA Loading and Intracellular Delivery. *Macromolecular Chemistry and Physics*, *224*(1). https://doi.org/10.1002/macp.202200306

Bayraktutan, H., Kopiasz, R., ElSherbeny, A., Martinez Espuga, M., Gumus, N., Oz, U. C., Polra, K., McKay, P. F., Shattock, R. J., Ordonez Moran, P., Mata, A., Alexander, C., & Gurnani, P. (2024). Polysarcosine functionalised cationic polyesters efficiently deliver self-amplifying mRNA. *Polymer Chemistry*. https://doi.org/10.1039/d4py00064a

Blaese, R. M., Culver, K. W., Miller, A. D., & Carter, C. S. (1995). T lymphocyte-directed gene therapy for ADA- SCID- initial trial results after 4 years. *In Science 1995* Oct 20;270(5235):475-80*. doi: 10.1126 /science.270.5235.475.*

Blakney, A. K., Zhu, Y., McKay, P. F., Bouton, C. R., Yeow, J., Tang, J., Hu, K., Samnuan, K., Grigsby, C. L., Shattock, R. J., & Stevens, M. M. (2020). Big Is Beautiful: Enhanced saRNA Delivery and Immunogenicity by a Higher Molecular Weight, Bioreducible, Cationic Polymer. *ACS Nano*. https://doi.org/10.1021/acsnano.0c00326

Bulkurcuoğlu, B., Gürbüz, M. U., Tyciakova, S., Pavlov, K., Mojzesova, N., Matuskova, M., Tülü, M., & Erçelen, Ş. (2024). Multifunctional PAMAM Dendrimers Carrying SAHA, 5-FU, and a Therapeutic Gene for Targeted Co-Delivery Toward Colorectal Cancer Cells. *Biotechnology Journal*, *19*(11), e202400362. https://doi.org/10.1002/biot.202400362

Cao, G., Xuan, X., Zhang, R., Hu, J., & Dong, H. (2021). Gene Therapy for Cardiovascular Disease: Basic Research and Clinical Prospects. In *Frontiers in Cardiovascular Medicine* (Vol. 8). Frontiers Media SA. https://doi.org/10.3389/fcvm.2021.760140

Carvalho, B. G., Garcia, B. B. M., Godoi, N., Han, S. W., & de la Torre, L. G. (2024). Cationic lipid-coated bPEI/pDNA complexes: Correlation between physicochemical and morphological properties. *Colloids and Surfaces A: Physicochemical and Engineering Aspects*, *700*. https://doi.org/10.1016/j.colsurfa.2024.134795

Chen, G., Wang, Y., Ullah, A., Huai, Y., & Xu, Y. (2020). The effects of fluoroalkyl chain length and density on siRNA delivery of bioreducible poly(amido amine)s. *European Journal of Pharmaceutical Sciences*, *152*. https://doi.org/10.1016/j.ejps.2020.105433

Chen, J., Wu, C., & Oupicky, D. (2009). Bioreducible Hyperbranched Poly (amido amine)s for Gene Delivery. *In Biomacromolecules 2009*, 2921–2927. *doi: 10.1021/bm900724c*

Chen, Y., Li, R., Fu, X., Guo, Y., Yan, S., Tian, L., Zhou, Q., Diao, Y., & Chen, W. (2025). "All in one" lipid-polymer nanodelivery system for gene therapy of ischemic diseases. *Biomaterials*, *313*. https://doi.org/10.1016/j.biomaterials.2024.122799

Cho, H. K., Cheong, I. W., Lee, J. M., & Kim, J. H. (2010). Polymeric nanoparticles, micelles and polymersomes from amphiphilic block copolymer. In *Korean Journal of Chemical Engineering* (Vol. 27, Issue 3, pp. 731–740). https://doi.org/10.1007/s11814-010-0216-5

Christine, C. W., Richardson, R. M., van Laar, A. D., Thompson, M. E., Fine, E. M., Khwaja, O. S., Li, C., Liang, G. S., Meier, A., Roberts, E. W., Pfau, M. L., Rodman, J. R., Bankiewicz, K. S., & Larson, P. S. (2022). Safety of AADC Gene Therapy for Moderately Advanced Parkinson Disease: Three-Year Outcomes from the PD-1101 Trial. *Neurology*, *98*(1), E40–E50. https://doi.org/10.1212/WNL.0000000000012952

Clima, L., Dascalu, A. I., Craciun, B. F., & Pinteala, M. (2021). Polymeric carriers for transporting nucleic acids-contributions to the field. In *New Trends in Macromolecular and Supramolecular Chemistry for Biological Applications* (pp. 133–150). Springer International Publishing. https://doi.org/10.1007/978-3-030-57456-7_7

Cohen, H., Levy, R. J., Gao, J., Fishbein, I., Kousaev, V., Sosnowski, S., Slomkowski, S., & Golomb, G. (2000). Sustained delivery and expression of DNA encapsulated in polymeric nanoparticles. In *Gene Therapy* (Vol. 7). *doi: 10.1038/sj.gt.3301318.*

Crucho, C. I. C., & Barros, M. T. (2017). Polymeric nanoparticles: A study on the preparation variables and characterization methods. In *Materials Science and Engineering C* (Vol. 80, pp. 771–784). Elsevier Ltd. https://doi.org/10.1016/j.msec.2017.06.004

Darrow, J. J. (2019). Luxturna: FDA documents reveal the value of a costly gene therapy. In *Drug Discovery Today* (Vol. 24, Issue 4, pp. 949–954). Elsevier Ltd. https://doi.org/10.1016/j.drudis.2019.01.019

Dastgerdi, N. K., Gumus, N., Bayraktutan, H., Jackson, D., Polra, K., McKay, P. F., Atyabi, F., Dinarvand, R., Shattock, R. J., Martinez-Pomares, L., Gurnani, P., & Alexander, C. (2024). Charge neutralized poly(β-amino ester) polyplex nanoparticles for delivery of self-amplifying RNA. *Nanoscale Advances*, *6*(5), 1409–1422. https://doi.org/10.1039/d3na00794d

Daubian, D., Gaitzsch, J., & Meier, W. (2020). Synthesis and complex self-assembly of amphiphilic block copolymers with a branched hydrophobic poly(2-oxazoline) into multicompartment micelles, pseudo-vesicles and yolk/shell nanoparticles. *Polymer Chemistry*, *11*(6), 1237–1248. https://doi.org/10.1039/c9py01559k

Di, J., Du, Z., Wu, K., Jin, S., Wang, X., Li, T., & Xu, Y. (2022). *Biodistribution and Non-linear Gene Expression of mRNA LNPs Affected by Delivery Route and Particle Size*. https://doi.org/10.1007/s11095-022-03166-5/Published

Discher, B. M., Won, Y. Y., Ege, D. S., Lee, J. C. M., Bates, F. S., Discher, D. E., & Hammer, D. A. (1999). Polymersomes: Tough vesicles made from diblock copolymers. *Science*, *284*(5417), 1143–1146. https://doi.org/10.1126/science.284.5417.1143

Dong, S., Jiang, Y., Qin, G., Liu, L., & Zhao, H. (2020). Methionine-Based pH and Oxidation Dual-Responsive Block Copolymer: Synthesis and Fabrication of Protein Nanogels. *Biomacromolecules*, *21*(10), 4063–4075. https://doi.org/10.1021/acs.biomac.0c00879

Duan, Q. Y., Zhu, Y. X., Jia, H. R., Wang, S. H., & Wu, F. G. (2023). Nanogels: Synthesis, properties, and recent biomedical applications. In *Progress in Materials Science* (Vol. 139). Elsevier Ltd. https://doi.org/10.1016/j.pmatsci.2023.101167

Elsherbeny, A., Bayraktutan, H., Gumus, N., McCrorie, P., Garcia-Sampedro, A., Parmar, S., Ritchie, A. A., Meakin, M., Oz, U. C., Rahman, R., Ashworth, J. C., Grabowska, A. M., Moloney, C., & Alexander, C. (2025). Pentablock thermoresponsive hydrogels for chemotherapeutic delivery in a pancreatic cancer model. *Biomaterials Science*. https://doi.org/10.1039/d4bm01629g

Farjadian, F., Mirkiani, S., Ghasemiyeh, P., Rahbar Kafshboran, H., Mehdi-Alamdarlou, S., Raeisi, A., Esfandiarinejad, R., Soleymani, S., Goshtasbi, G., Firouzabadi, N., Mohammadi-Samani, S., Hossein Morowvat, M., & Doroudian, M. (2024). Smart nanogels as promising platform for delivery of drug, gene, and vaccine; therapeutic applications and active targeting mechanism. In *European Polymer Journal* (Vol. 219). Elsevier Ltd. https://doi.org/10.1016/j.eurpolymj.2024.113400

Ferrari, G., Rossini, S., Giavazzi, R., Maggioni, D., Nobili, N., Soldati, M., Ungers, G., Mavilio, F., Gilboa, E., & Bordignon, C. (1991). An in Vivo Model of Somatic Cell Gene Therapy for Human Severe Combined. In *Source: Science, New Series* (Vol. 251, Issue 4999). *doi: 10.1126/science.1848369.*

Flotte, T. R., Cataltepe, O., Puri, A., Batista, A. R., Moser, R., McKenna-Yasek, D., Douthwright, C., Gernoux, G., Blackwood, M., Mueller, C., Tai, P. W. L., Jiang, X., Bateman, S., Spanakis, S. G., Parzych, J., Keeler, A. M., Abayazeed, A., Rohatgi, S., Gibson, L., … Sena-Esteves, M. (2022). AAV gene therapy for Tay-Sachs disease. *Nature Medicine*, *28*(2), 251–259. https://doi.org/10.1038/s41591-021-01664-4

Fukuyama, Y., Yuki, Y., Katakai, Y., Harada, N., Takahashi, H., Takeda, S., Mejima, M., Joo, S., Kurokawa, S., Sawada, S., Shibata, H., Park, E. J., Fujihashi, K., Briles, D. E., Yasutomi, Y., Tsukada, H., Akiyoshi, K., & Kiyono, H. (2015). Nanogel-based pneumococcal surface protein A nasal vaccine induces microRNA-associated Th17 cell responses with neutralizing antibodies against Streptococcus pneumoniae in macaques. *Mucosal Immunology*, *8*(5), 1144–1153. https://doi.org/10.1038/mi.2015.5

Gajbhiye, K. R., Salve, R., Narwade, M., Sheikh, A., Kesharwani, P., & Gajbhiye, V. (2023). Lipid polymer hybrid nanoparticles: a custom-tailored next-generation approach for cancer therapeutics. In *Molecular Cancer* (Vol. 22, Issue 1). BioMed Central Ltd. https://doi.org/10.1186/s12943-023-01849-0

Gameiro, M., Mano, J. F., & Gaspar, V. M. (2024). Emerging lipid-polymer hybrid nanoparticles for genome editing. In *Polymer Chemistry* (Vol. 15, Issue 34, pp. 3436–3468). Royal Society of Chemistry. https://doi.org/10.1039/d4py00298a

Gazaille, C., Sicot, M., Saulnier, P., Eyer, J., & Bastiat, G. (2021). Local Delivery and Glioblastoma: Why Not Combining Sustained Release and Targeting? In *Frontiers in Medical Technology* (Vol. 3). Frontiers Media S.A. https://doi.org/10.3389/fmedt.2021.791596

Ge, X., Zhang, Q., Cai, Y., Duan, S., Chen, S., Lv, N., Jin, T., Chen, Y., & Yuan, W. (2014). PEG-PCL-DEX polymersome-protamine vector as an efficient gene delivery system via PEG-guided self-assembly. *Nanomedicine*, *9*(8), 1193–1207. https://doi.org/10.2217/nnm.13.83

Golan, T., Khvalevsky, E. Z., Hubert, A., Gabai, R. M., Hen, N., Segal, A., Domb, A., Harari, G., David, B., Raskin, S., Goldes, Y., Goldin, E.,

Eliakim, R., Lahav, M., Kopleman, Y., Dancour, A., Shemi, A., & Galun, E. (2015). RNAi therapy targeting KRAS in combination with chemotherapy for locally advanced pancreatic cancer patients. In *Oncotarget* (Vol. 6, Issue 27 *doi: 10.18632/oncotarget.4183.*

González-García, D., Tapia, O., Évora, C., García-García, P., & Delgado, A. (2024). Conventional and microfluidic methods: Design and optimization of lipid-polymeric hybrid nanoparticles for gene therapy. *Drug Delivery and Translational Research.* https://doi.org/10.1007/s13346-024-01644-4

Gurnani, P., Blakney, A. K., Yeow, J., Bouton, C. R., Shattock, R. J., Stevens, M. M., & Alexander, C. (2020). An improved synthesis of poly(amidoamine)s for complexation with self-amplifying RNA and effective transfection. *Polymer Chemistry*, *11*(36), 5861–5869. https://doi.org/10.1039/d0py00912a

Haensler, J., & Szoka, F. C.'. (1993). Polyamidoamine Cascade Polymers Mediate Efficient Transfection of Cells in Culture+. *Bioconjug Chem.* 1993 Sep-Oct;4(5):372-9. *doi: 10.1021/bc00023a012.*

Hansen, C. B., Janaszewska, A., Dąbrzalska, M., Marcinkowska, M., Klajnert-Maculewicz, B., & Christensen, J. B. (2024). Core-size and geometry versus toxicity in small amino terminated PAMAM dendrimers. *RSC Advances*, *14*(39), 28684–28692. https://doi.org/10.1039/d4ra02020k

Herskovitz, J., Hasan, M., Patel, M., Blomberg, W. R., Cohen, J. D., Machhi, J., Shahjin, F., Mosley, R. L., McMillan, J. E., Kevadiya, B. D., & Gendelman, H. E. (2021). CRISPR-Cas9 Mediated Exonic Disruption for HIV-1 Elimination. *EBioMedicine*, *73.* https://doi.org/10.1016/j.ebiom.2021.103678

Hibino, M., Tanaka, K., Ouchi, M., & Terashima, T. (2022). Amphiphilic Random-Block Copolymer Micelles in Water: Precise and Dynamic Self-Assembly Controlled by Random Copolymer Association. *Macromolecules*, *55*(1), 178–189. https://doi.org/10.1021/acs.macromol.1c02186

Hu, Q., Ding, B., Yan, X., Peng, L., Duan, J., Yang, S., Cheng, L., & Chen, D. (2017). Polyethylene glycol modified PAMAM dendrimer delivery of kartogenin to induce chondrogenic differentiation of mesenchymal stem cells. *Nanomedicine: Nanotechnology, Biology, and Medicine*, *13*(7), 2189–2198. https://doi.org/10.1016/j.nano.2017.05.011

Huh, M. S., Lee, S. Y., Park, S., Lee, S., Chung, H., Lee, S., Choi, Y., Oh, Y. K., Park, J. H., Jeong, S. Y., Choi, K., Kim, K., & Kwon, I. C. (2010). Tumor-homing glycol chitosan/polyethylenimine nanoparticles for the systemic delivery of siRNA in tumor-bearing mice. *Journal of Controlled Release*, *144*(2), 134–143. https://doi.org/10.1016/j.jconrel.2010.02.023

Iqbal, S., Blenner, M., Alexander-Bryant, A., & Larsen, J. (2020). Polymersomes for Therapeutic Delivery of Protein and Nucleic Acid Macromolecules: From Design to Therapeutic Applications. In *Biomacromolecules* (Vol. 21, Issue 4, pp. 1327–1350). American Chemical Society. https://doi.org/10.1021/acs.biomac.9b01754

Jia, T., Wang, H., Chi, W., Zhou, W., Guo, L., Dai, Y., Bian, K., Sun, Z., Ding, X., & Yu, Y. (2024). Knockdown of BACE1 by a multistage brain-targeting polyion complex improved memory and learning behaviors in APP/PS1 transgenic mouse model. *International Journal of Pharmaceutics*, *650*. https://doi.org/10.1016/j.ijpharm.2023.123727

Kaczmarek, J. C., Kauffman, K. J., Fenton, O. S., Sadtler, K., Patel, A. K., Heartlein, M. W., Derosa, F., & Anderson, D. G. (2018). Optimization of a Degradable Polymer-Lipid Nanoparticle for Potent Systemic Delivery of mRNA to the Lung Endothelium and Immune Cells. *Nano Letters*, *18*(10), 6449–6454. https://doi.org/10.1021/acs.nanolett.8b02917

Kaczmarek, J. C., Patel, A. K., Rhym, L. H., Palmiero, U. C., Bhat, B., Heartlein, M. W., DeRosa, F., & Anderson, D. G. (2021). Systemic delivery of mRNA and DNA to the lung using polymer-lipid nanoparticles. *Biomaterials*, *275*. https://doi.org/10.1016/j.biomaterials.2021.120966

Kadlecova, Z., Rajendra, Y., Matasci, M., Baldi, L., Hacker, D. L., Wurm, F. M., & Klok, H. A. (2013). DNA delivery with hyperbranched polylysine: A comparative study with linear and dendritic polylysine. *Journal of Controlled Release*, *169*(3), 276–288. https://doi.org/10.1016/j.jconrel.2013.01.019 https://doi.org/10.1016/j.jconrel.2013.01.019

Karlsson, J., Rui, Y., Kozielski, K. L., Placone, A. L., Choi, O., Tzeng, S. Y., Kim, J., Keyes, J. J., Bogorad, M. I., Gabrielson, K., Guerrero-Cazares, H., Quinõnes-Hinojosa, A., Searson, P. C., & Green, J. J. (2019). Engineered nanoparticles for systemic siRNA delivery to malignant brain tumours. *Nanoscale*, *11*(42), 20045–20057. https://doi.org/10.1039/c9nr04795f

Khan, M. (2024). Polymers as Efficient Non-Viral Gene Delivery Vectors: The Role of the Chemical and Physical Architecture of Macromolecules. In *Polymers* (Vol. 16, Issue 18). Multidisciplinary Digital Publishing Institute (MDPI). https://doi.org/10.3390/polym16182629

Kim, B. S., Naito, M., Chaya, H., Hori, M., Hayashi, K., Min, H. S., Yi, Y., Kim, H. J., Nagata, T., Anraku, Y., Kishimura, A., Kataoka, K., & Miyata, K. (2020). Noncovalent Stabilization of Vesicular Polyion Complexes with Chemically Modified/Single-Stranded Oligonucleotides and PEG-b-guanidinylated Polypeptides for Intracavity Encapsulation of Effector Enzymes Aimed at Cooperative Gene Knockdown. *Biomacromolecules*, *21*(10), 4365–4376. https://doi.org/10.1021/acs.biomac.0c01192

Kim, S., Fan, J., Lee, C. S., Chen, C., & Lee, M. (2021). Sulfonate Hydrogel-siRNA Conjugate Facilitates Osteogenic Differentiation of Mesenchymal Stem Cells by Controlled Gene Silencing and Activation of BMP Signaling. *ACS Applied Bio Materials*, *4*(6), 5189–5200. https://doi.org/10.1021/acsabm.1c00369

Kishimura, A. (2013). Development of polyion complex vesicles (PICsomes) from block copolymers for biomedical applications. In *Polymer Journal* (Vol. 45, Issue 9, pp. 892–897). https://doi.org/10.1038/pj.2013.33

Koide, A., Kishimura, A., Osada, K., Jang, W. D., Yamasaki, Y., & Kataoka, K. (2006). Semipermeable polymer vesicle (PICsome) self-assembled in aqueous medium from a pair of oppositely charged block copolymers: Physiologically stable micro-/nanocontainers of water-soluble macromolecules. *Journal of the American Chemical Society*, *128*(18), 5988–5989. https://doi.org/10.1021/ja057993r

Kumar, R., Santa Chalarca, C. F., Bockman, M. R., Bruggen, C. Van, Grimme, C. J., Dalal, R. J., Hanson, M. G., Hexum, J. K., & Reineke, T. M. (2021). Polymeric Delivery of Therapeutic Nucleic Acids. In *Chemical Reviews* (Vol. 121, Issue 18, pp. 11527–11652). American Chemical Society. https://doi.org/10.1021/acs.chemrev.0c00997

Lai, T. C., Kataoka, K., & Kwon, G. S. (2012). Bioreducible polyether-based pDNA ternary polyplexes: Balancing particle stability and transfection efficiency. *Colloids and Surfaces B: Biointerfaces*, *99*, 27–37. https://doi.org/10.1016/j.colsurfb.2011.09.026

Laskar, P., Dey, J., Banik, P., Mandal, M., & Ghosh, S. K. (2017). In Vitro Drug and Gene Delivery Using Random Cationic Copolymers Forming Stable and pH-Sensitive Polymersomes. *Macromolecular Bioscience*, *17*(4). https://doi.org/10.1002/mabi.201600324

Li, C., Huang, J., Ding, P., Wang, M., Guo, X., Cohen Stuart, M. A., & Wang, J. (2022). Hierarchical polyion complex vesicles from PAMAM dendrimers. *Journal of Colloid and Interface Science*, *606*, 307–316. https://doi.org/10.1016/j.jcis.2021.07.140

Li, X., Ouyang, Z., Hetjens, L., Ni, M., Lin, K., Hu, Y., Shi, X., & Pich, A. (2025). Functional Dendrimer Nanogels for DNA Delivery and Gene Therapy of Tumors. *Angewandte Chemie - International Edition*. https://doi.org/10.1002/anie.202505669

Liaw, J., Chang, S.-F., & Hsiao, F.-C. (2001). In vivo gene delivery into ocular tissues by eye drops of poly(ethylene oxide)-poly(propylene oxide)-poly(ethylene oxide) (PEO-PPO-PEO) polymeric micelles. *Gene Ther.* 2001 Jul;8(13):999-1004. *doi: 10.1038/sj.gt.3301485.*

Lin, C., & Engbersen, J. F. J. (2008). Effect of chemical functionalities in poly(amido amine)s for non-viral gene transfection. *Journal of Controlled Release*, *132*(3), 267–272. https://doi.org/10.1016/j.jconrel.2008.06.022

Lin, J., Hua, W., Zhang, Y., Li, C., Xue, W., Yin, J., Liu, Z., & Qiu, X. (2015). Effect of poly(amidoamine) dendrimers on the structure and activity of immune molecules. *Biochimica et Biophysica Acta - General Subjects*, *1850*(2), 419–425. https://doi.org/10.1016/j.bbagen.2014.11.016

Liu, Y., Zou, Y., Feng, C., Lee, A., Yin, J., Chung, R., Park, J. B., Rizos, H., Tao, W., Zheng, M., Farokhzad, O. C., & Shi, B. (2020). Charge Conversional Biomimetic Nanocomplexes as a Multifunctional Platform for Boosting Orthotopic Glioblastoma RNAi Therapy. *Nano Letters*, *20*(3), 1637–1646. https://doi.org/10.1021/acs.nanolett.9b04683

Liyanage, W., Kannan, G. R., Kannan, S., & Kannan, R. M. (2025). Efficient intracellular delivery of CRISPR-Cas9 ribonucleoproteins using dendrimer nanoparticles for robust genomic editing. *Nano Today*, *61*. https://doi.org/10.1016/j.nantod.2025.102654

Lolli, A., Sivasubramaniyan, K., Vainieri, M. L., Oieni, J., Kops, N., Yayon, A., & van Osch, G. J. V. M. (2019). Hydrogel-based delivery of antimiR-221 enhances cartilage regeneration by endogenous cells. *Journal of Controlled Release*, *309*, 220–230. https://doi.org/10.1016/j.jconrel.2019.07.040

Lu, Y. J., Lan, Y. H., Chuang, C. C., Lu, W. T., Chan, L. Y., Hsu, P. W., & Chen, J. P. (2020). Injectable thermo-sensitive chitosan hydrogel containing CPT-11-loaded EGFR-targeted graphene oxide and SLP2 shRNA for localized drug/gene delivery in glioblastoma therapy. *International Journal of Molecular Sciences*, *21*(19), 1–29. https://doi.org/10.3390/ijms21197111

Luo, D., Haverstick, K., Belcheva, N., Han, E., & Saltzman, W. M. (2002). Poly(ethylene glycol)-conjugated PAMAM dendrimer for biocompatible, high-efficiency DNA delivery. *Macromolecules*, *35*(9), 3456–3462. https://doi.org/10.1021/ma0106346

Luong, D., Kesharwani, P., Deshmukh, R., Mohd Amin, M. C. I., Gupta, U., Greish, K., & Iyer, A. K. (2016). PEGylated PAMAM dendrimers: Enhancing efficacy and mitigating toxicity for effective anticancer drug and gene delivery. In *Acta Biomaterialia* (Vol. 43, pp. 14–29). Elsevier Ltd. https://doi.org/10.1016/j.actbio.2016.07.015

Ma, Y., Sha, M., Cheng, S., Yao, W., Li, Z., & Qi, X. R. (2018). Construction of hyaluronic tetrasaccharide clusters modified polyamidoamine siRNA delivery system. *Nanomaterials*, *8*(6). https://doi.org/10.3390/nano8060433

Ma, Z., Yang, C., Song, W., Wang, Q., Kjems, J., & Gao, S. (2014). Chitosan hydrogel as sirna vector for prolonged gene silencing. *Journal of Nanobiotechnology*, *12*(1). https://doi.org/10.1186/1477-3155-12-23

Mahanta, A. K., Chaulagain, B., Trivedi, R., & Singh, J. (2024). Mannose-Functionalized Chitosan-Coated PLGA Nanoparticles for Brain-Targeted Codelivery of CBD and BDNF for the Treatment of Alzheimer's Disease. *ACS Chemical Neuroscience*. https://doi.org/10.1021/acschemneuro.4c00392

Malhotra, M., Toulouse, A., Godinho, B. M. D. C., Mc Carthy, D. J., Cryan, J. F., & O'Driscoll, C. M. (2015). RNAi therapeutics for brain cancer: Current advancements in RNAi delivery strategies. *Molecular BioSystems*, *11*(10), 2635–2657. https://doi.org/10.1039/c5mb00278h

Manohar, S. K., Gowrav, M. P., & Gangadharappa, H. V. (2023). Materials for Gene Delivery Systems. In *Interaction of Nanomaterials with Living Cells* (pp. 411–437). Springer Nature. https://doi.org/10.1007/978-981-99-2119-5_14

Martello, F., Piest, M., Engbersen, J. F. J., & Ferruti, P. (2012). Effects of branched or linear architecture of bioreducible poly(amido amine)s on their in vitro gene delivery properties. *Journal of Controlled Release*, *164*(3), 372–379. https://doi.org/10.1016/j.jconrel.2012.07.029

Mateos-Timoneda, M. A., Lok, M. C., Hennink, W. E., Feijen, J., & Engbersen, J. F. J. (2008). Poly(amido amine)s as gene delivery vectors: Effects of quaternary nicotinamide moieties in the side chains. *ChemMedChem*, *3*(3), 478–486. https://doi.org/10.1002/cmdc.200700279

Mauri, E., Perale, G., & Rossi, F. (2018). Nanogel Functionalization: A Versatile Approach to Meet the Challenges of Drug and Gene Delivery. In *ACS Applied Nano Materials* (Vol. 1, Issue 12, pp. 6525–6541). American Chemical Society. https://doi.org/10.1021/acsanm.8b01686

Mendell, J. R., Sahenk, Z., Lehman, K., Nease, C., Lowes, L. P., Miller, N. F., Iammarino, M. A., Alfano, L. N., Nicholl, A., Al-Zaidy, S., Lewis, S., Church, K., Shell, R., Cripe, L. H., Potter, R. A., Griffin, D. A., Pozsgai, E., Dugar, A., Hogan, M., & Rodino-Klapac, L. R. (2020). Assessment of Systemic Delivery of rAAVrh74.MHCK7.micro-dystrophin in Children with Duchenne Muscular Dystrophy: A Nonrandomized Controlled Trial. *JAMA Neurology*, *77*(9), 1122–1131. https://doi.org/10.1001/jamaneurol.2020.1484

Mennati, A., Rostamizadeh, K., & Fathi, M. (2025). Dual silencing of integrin αvβ3 receptor and insulin-like growth factor 1 receptor using mPEG-PCL/DDAB hybrid nanoparticle loaded siRNA in breast cancer therapy: An in vitro study on MCF-7 cells. *International Journal of Biological Macromolecules*, *294*. https://doi.org/10.1016/j.ijbiomac.2024.139334

Meo, S. A., bukhari, I. A., & Akram, J. (2021). COVID-19 vaccines: comparison of biological, pharmacological characteristics and adverse effects of Pfizer/BioNTech and Moderna Vaccines. *Eur Rev Med Pharmacol Sci.* 2021Feb;25(3):1663-1669. https://doi.org/10.26355/eurrev_202102_24877

Nair, A., Javius-Jones, K., Bugno, J., Poellmann, M. J., Mamidi, N., Kim, I. S., Kwon, I. C., Hong, H., & Hong, S. (2023). Hybrid Nanoparticle System Integrating Tumor-Derived Exosomes and Poly(amidoamine) Dendrimers: Implications for an Effective Gene Delivery Platform. *Chemistry of Materials*, *35*(8), 3138–3150. https://doi.org/10.1021/acs.chemmater.2c03705

Nguyen, K., Dang, P. N., & Alsberg, E. (2013). Functionalized, biodegradable hydrogels for control over sustained and localized siRNA delivery to incorporated and surrounding cells. *Acta Biomaterialia*, *9*(1), 4487–4495. https://doi.org/10.1016/j.actbio.2012.08.012

Nishiyama, N., & Kataoka, K. (2006). Current state, achievements, and future prospects of polymeric micelles as nanocarriers for drug and gene delivery. In *Pharmacology and Therapeutics* (Vol. 112, Issue 3, pp. 630–648). https://doi.org/10.1016/j.pharmthera.2006.05.006

Nomoto, T., Matsumoto, Y., Miyata, K., Oba, M., Fukushima, S., Nishiyama, N., Yamasoba, T., & Kataoka, K. (2011). In situ quantitative monitoring of polyplexes and polyplex micelles in the blood circulation using intravital real-time confocal laser scanning microscopy. *Journal of Controlled Release*, *151*(2), 104–109. https://doi.org/10.1016/j.jconrel.2011.02.011

Notabi, M. K., Arnspang, E. C., Peppas, N. A., & Andersen, M. (2023). siRNA delivery mediated by pH and redox responsive p(DEAEMA-co-

HEMA-g-PEGMA) nanogels. *Journal of Drug Delivery Science and Technology*, *86*. https://doi.org/10.1016/j.jddst.2023.104510

Oba, M., Miyata, K., Osada, K., Christie, R. J., Sanjoh, M., Li, W., Fukushima, S., Ishii, T., Kano, M. R., Nishiyama, N., Koyama, H., & Kataoka, K. (2011). Polyplex micelles prepared from ω-cholesteryl PEG-polycation block copolymers for systemic gene delivery. *Biomaterials*, *32*(2), 652–663. https://doi.org/10.1016/j.biomaterials.2010.09.022

Ogris, M., Brunner, S., Schü Ller, S., Kircheis, R., & Wagner, E. (1999). PEGylated DNA/transferrin-PEI complexes: reduced interaction with blood components, extended circulation in blood and potential for systemic gene delivery. In *Gene Therapy* (Vol. 6). doi: 10.1038/sj.gt. 3300900.

Onaca, O., Enea, R., Hughes, D. W., & Meier, W. (2009). Stimuli-responsive polymersomes as nanocarriers for drug and gene delivery. In *Macromolecular Bioscience* (Vol. 9, Issue 2, pp. 129–139). https://doi.org/10.1002/mabi.200800248

Ou, M., Wang, X. L., Xu, R., Chang, C. W., Bull, D. A., & Sung, W. K. (2008). Novel biodegradable poly(disulfide amine)s for gene delivery with high efficiency and low cytotoxicity. *Bioconjugate Chemistry*, *19*(3), 626–633. https://doi.org/10.1021/bc700397x

Oyama, H. T., Tang, W. T., & Frank, C. W. (1987). Effect of the Hydrophobic Interaction in the Poly(methacry1ic acid) /Pyrene End-Labeled Poly(ethy1ene glycol) Complex. In *Macromolecules* (Vol. 20). https://doi.org/0024-9297/87/2220-1839

Padnya, P., Shiabiev, I., Pysin, D., Gerasimova, T., Ranishenka, B., Stanavaya, A., Abashkin, V., Shcharbin, D., Shi, X., Shen, M., Nazarova, A., & Stoikov, I. (2024). Non-Viral Systems Based on PAMAM-Calix-Dendrimers for Regulatory siRNA Delivery into Cancer Cells. *International Journal of Molecular Sciences*, *25*(23). https://doi.org/10.3390/ijms252312614

Patel, D., Kuperkar, K., Yusa, S., & Bahadur, P. (2023). Nanoscale Self-Assemblies from Amphiphilic Block Copolymers as Proficient Templates in Drug Delivery. *Drugs and Drug Candidates*, *2*(4), 898–922. https://doi.org/10.3390/ddc2040045

Peppas, N. A., Bures, P., Leobandung, W., & Ichikawa, H. (2000). Hydrogels in pharmaceutical formulations. *European Journal of Pharmaceutics and Biopharmaceutics.* Volume 50, Issue 1, https://doi.org/10.1016/S0939-6411(00)00090-4

Persano, F., Gigli, G., & Leporatti, S. (2021). Lipid-polymer hybrid nanoparticles in cancer therapy: current overview and future directions. In *Nano Express* (Vol. 2, Issue 1). Institute of Physics. https://doi.org/10.1088/2632-959X/abeb4b

Peschel, J. M., Reichel, L. S., Hoffmann, T., Enzensperger, C., Schubert, U. S., Traeger, A., & Gottschaldt, M. (2023). Modification of Branched Poly(ethylene imine) with d-Fructose for Selective Delivery of siRNA into Human Breast Cancer Cells. *Macromolecular Bioscience*, *23*(12). https://doi.org/10.1002/mabi.202300135

Photos, P. J., Bacakova, L., Discher, B., Bates, F. S., & Discher, D. E. (2003). Polymer vesicles in vivo: Correlations with PEG molecular weight. *Journal of Controlled Release*, *90*(3), 323–334. https://doi.org/10.1016/S0168-3659(03)00201-3

Polack, F. P., Thomas, S. J., Kitchin, N., Absalon, J., Gurtman, A., Lockhart, S., Perez, J. L., Pérez Marc, G., Moreira, E. D., Zerbini, C., Bailey, R., Swanson, K. A., Roychoudhury, S., Koury, K., Li, P., Kalina, W. V., Cooper, D., Frenck, R. W., Hammitt, L. L., … Gruber, W. C. (2020). Safety and Efficacy of the BNT162b2 mRNA Covid-19 Vaccine. *New England Journal of Medicine*, *383*(27), 2603–2615. https://doi.org/10.1056/nejmoa2034577

Qi, J., Tan, F., Zhang, L., Lu, L., Zhang, S., Zhai, Y., Lu, Y., Qian, X., Dong, W. X., Zhou, Y., Zhang, Z., Yang, X., Jiang, L., Yu, C., Liu, J., Chen, T., Wu, L., Tan, C., Sun, S., … Chai, R. (2024). AAV-Mediated Gene Therapy Restores Hearing in Patients with DFNB9 Deafness. *Advanced Science*, *11*(11). https://doi.org/10.1002/advs.202306788

Recino, A., Gan, S. U., Sia, K. C., Sawyer, Y., Trendell, J., Kay, R., Gribble, F. M., Reimann, F., Foale, R., Notaridou, M., Holmes, N., Lever, A., Lee, K. O., Nathwani, A., Cooke, A., Calne, R., & Wallberg, M. (2019). Immunosuppression overcomes insulin- and vector-specific immune responses that limit efficacy of AAV2/8-mediated insulin gene therapy in NOD mice. *Gene Therapy*, *26*(1–2), 40–56. https://doi.org/10.1038/s41434-018-0052-5

Reyne, N., Cmielewski, P., McCarron, A., Delhove, J., Parsons, D., & Donnelley, M. (2021). Single-Dose Lentiviral Mediated Gene Therapy Recovers CFTR Function in Cystic Fibrosis Knockout Rats. *Frontiers in Pharmacology*, *12*. https://doi.org/10.3389/fphar.2021.682299

Reynolds, A. M., Holmes, M. D., Danilov, S. M., & Reynolds, P. N. (2012). Targeted gene delivery of BMPR2 attenuates pulmonary hypertension. *European Respiratory Journal*, *39*(2), 329–343. https://doi.org/10.1183/09031936.00187310

Rocher, E. E., Luly, K. M., Tzeng, S. Y., Sunshine, J. C., & Green, J. J. (2024). Efficient Polymeric Nanoparticle Gene Delivery Enabled Via Tri- and Tetrafunctional Branching. *Biomacromolecules*. https://doi.org/10.1021/acs.biomac.4c00954

Romani, C., Gagni, P., Di Pietro, M. E., Sani, M., Sponchioni, M., & Volonterio, A. (2024). Fine-Tuned "Click" Functionalization of PAMAM Dendrimers with a Linear Fluorinated Guanidino Linker: Synthesis, Characterization, and Applications. *Bioconjugate Chemistry*. https://doi.org/10.1021/acs.bioconjchem.4c00434

Saleh, B., Dhaliwal, H. K., Portillo-Lara, R., Shirzaei Sani, E., Abdi, R., Amiji, M. M., & Annabi, N. (2019). Local Immunomodulation Using an Adhesive Hydrogel Loaded with miRNA-Laden Nanoparticles Promotes Wound Healing. *Small*, *15*(36). https://doi.org/10.1002/smll.201902232

Shen, X., Dirisala, A., Toyoda, M., Xiao, Y., Guo, H., Honda, Y., Nomoto, T., Takemoto, H., Miura, Y., & Nishiyama, N. (2023). pH-responsive polyzwitterion covered nanocarriers for DNA delivery. *Journal of Controlled Release*, *360*, 928–939. https://doi.org/10.1016/j.jconrel.2023.07.038

Shen, Y., Zhou, Z., Sui, M., Tang, J., Xu, P., Van Kirk, E. A., Murdoch, W. J., Fan, M., & Radosz, M. (2010). Charge-reversal polyamidoamine dendrimer for cascade nuclear drug delivery. *Nanomedicine*, *5*(8), 1205–1217. https://doi.org/10.2217/nnm.10.86

Singh, A. P., Biswas, A., Shukla, A., & Maiti, P. (2019). Targeted therapy in chronic diseases using nanomaterial-based drug delivery vehicles. *Signal Transduction and Targeted Therapy*, *4*(1). https://doi.org/10.1038/s41392-019-0068-3

Singh, K., Biharee, A., Vyas, A., Thareja, S., & Jain, A. K. (2022). Recent Advancement of Polymersomes as Drug Delivery Carrier. *Current Pharmaceutical Design*, *28*(20), 1621–1631. https://doi.org/10.2174/1381612828666220412103552

Sinsinbar, G., Bindra, A. K., Liu, S., Chia, T. W., Yoong Eng, E. C., Loo, S. Y., Lam, J. H., Schultheis, K., & Nallani, M. (2024). Amphiphilic Block Copolymer Nanostructures as a Tunable Delivery Platform: Perspective and Framework for the Future Drug Product Development. In *Biomacromolecules* (Vol. 25, Issue 2, pp. 541–563). American Chemical Society. https://doi.org/10.1021/acs.biomac.3c00858

Siparsky, G. L., Voorhees, K. J., & Miao3, F. (1998). Hydrolysis of Polylactic Acid (PLA) and Polycaprolactone (PCL) in Aqueous Acetonitrile Solutions: Autocatalysis. In *Journal of Environmental Polymer Degradation* (Vol. 6, Issue 1).

https://doi.org/1064-7546/98/0100-003

Sivadasan, D., Sultan, M. H., Madkhali, O., Almoshari, Y., & Thangavel, N. (2021). Polymeric lipid hybrid nanoparticles (Plns) as emerging drug delivery platform—a comprehensive review of their properties, preparation methods, and therapeutic applications. In *Pharmaceutics* (Vol. 13, Issue 8). MDPI. https://doi.org/10.3390/pharmaceutics13081291

Song, J., Zhang, H., Wang, D., Wang, J., Zhou, J., Zhang, Z., Wang, J., Hu, Y., Xu, Q., Xie, C., Lu, W., & Liu, M. (2021). Hydrogel loading functionalized PAMAM/shRNA complex for postsurgical glioblastoma treatment. *Journal of Controlled Release*, *338*, 583–592. https://doi.org/10.1016/j.jconrel.2021.08.052

Spearman, P., Lally, M. A., Elizaga, M., Montefiori, D., Tomaras, G. D., McElrath, M. J., Hural, J., De Rosa, S. C., Sato, A., Huang, Y., Frey, S. E., Sato, P., Donnelly, J., Barnett, S., & Corey, L. J. (2011). A trimeric, V2-deleted HIV-1 envelope glycoprotein vaccine elicits potent neutralizing antibodies but limited breadth of neutralization in human volunteers. *Journal of Infectious Diseases*, *203*(8), 1165–1173. https://doi.org/10.1093/infdis/jiq175

Subhan, M. A., & Torchilin, V. P. (2019). Efficient nanocarriers of siRNA therapeutics for cancer treatment. *Translational Research*, *214*, 62–91. https://doi.org/10.1016/j.trsl.2019.07.006

Sueyoshi, D., Anraku, Y., Komatsu, T., Urano, Y., & Kataoka, K. (2017). Enzyme-Loaded Polyion Complex Vesicles as in Vivo Nanoreactors Working Sustainably under the Blood Circulation: Characterization and Functional Evaluation. *Biomacromolecules*, *18*(4), 1189–1196. https://doi.org/10.1021/acs.biomac.6b01870

Sun, X., & Zhang, N. (2010). Cationic Polymer Optimization for Efficient Gene Delivery. *Mini-Reviews in Medicinal Chemistry*, *10*(2), 108–125. https://doi.org/10.2174/138955710791185109

Sun, Y., Xian, L., Yu, J., Yang, T., Zhang, J., Yang, Z., Jiang, J., Cai, C., Zhao, X., & Yang, L. (2017). Structure – Function Correlations of Poly (Amido Amine) s for Gene Delivery. *201600297*, 1–16. https://doi.org/10.1002/mabi.201600297

Thomas, T. J., Tajmir-Riahi, H. A., & Pillai, C. K. S. (2019). Biodegradable polymers for gene delivery. In *Molecules* (Vol. 24, Issue 20). MDPI AG. https://doi.org/10.3390/molecules24203744

Ullah, A., & Lim, S. I. (2022). Nanogels: Update on the methods of synthesis and applications for cardiovascular and neurological complications. In *Journal of Drug Delivery Science and Technology* (Vol. 77). Editions de Sante.

https://doi.org/10.1016/j.jddst.2022.103879
Vader, P., Van Der Aa, L. J., Engbersen, J. F. J., Storm, G., & Schiffelers, R. M. (2011). Disulfide-based poly(amido amine)s for siRNA delivery: Effects of structure on siRNA complexation, cellular uptake, gene silencing and toxicity. *Pharmaceutical Research*, *28*(5), 1013–1022. https://doi.org/10.1007/s11095-010-0344-y
van der Aa, L. J., Vader, P., Schiffelers, R. M., & Engbersen, J. F. (2010). Poly(amido amine) copolymers derived from aminobutanol and ethylene diamine are excellent carriers for siRNA delivery. *Journal of Controlled Release: Official Journal of the Controlled Release Society*, *148*(1), e85–e86. https://doi.org/10.1016/j.jconrel.2010.07.061
Van Der Aa, L. J., Vader, P., Storm, G., Schiffelers, R. M., & Engbersen, J. F. J. (2011a). Optimization of poly(amido amine)s as vectors for siRNA delivery. *Journal of Controlled Release*, *150*(2), 177–186. https://doi.org/10.1016/j.jconrel.2010.11.030
Vinogradov, S., Batrakova, E., & Kabanov, A. (1999). Poly(ethylene glycol)-polyethyleneimine NanoGel™ particles: novel drug delivery systems for antisense oligonucleotides. In *Colloids and Surfaces B: Biointerfaces* (Vol. 16). www.elsevier.nl/locate/colsurfb
Wang, F., Gao, J., Xiao, J., & Du, J. (2018). Dually Gated Polymersomes for Gene Delivery. *Nano Letters*, *18*(9), 5562–5568. https://doi.org/10.1021/acs.nanolett.8b01985
Wang, L. L., & Burdick, J. A. (2017). Engineered Hydrogels for Local and Sustained Delivery of RNA-Interference Therapies. *Advanced Healthcare Materials*, *6*(1). https://doi.org/10.1002/adhm.201601041
Wang, X., He, Y., Wu, J., Gao, C., & Xu, Y. (2010). Synthesis and evaluation of phenylalanine-modified hyperbranched poly(amido amine)s as promising gene carriers. *Biomacromolecules*, *11*(1), 245–251. https://doi.org/10.1021/bm901091z
Wanjale, M. V., Jaikumar, V. S., Sivakumar, K. C., Paul, R. A., James, J., & Kumar, G. S. V. (2022). Supramolecular Hydrogel Based Post-Surgical Implant System for Hydrophobic Drug Delivery Against Glioma Recurrence. *International Journal of Nanomedicine*, *17*, 2203–2224. https://doi.org/10.2147/IJN.S348559
Wells, C. M., Harris, M., Choi, L., Murali, V. P., Guerra, F. D., & Jennings, J. A. (2019). Stimuli-responsive drug release from smart polymers. In *Journal of Functional Biomaterials* (Vol. 10, Issue 3). MDPI AG. https://doi.org/10.3390/jfb10030034
Widge, A. T., Rouphael, N. G., Jackson, L. A., & Anderson, E. J. (2020). *Durability of Responses after SARS-CoV-2 mRNA-1273 Vaccination*. https://doi.org/10.1056/NEJMc2032195

Wu, J., Huang, Y., Yu, H., Li, K., Zhang, S., Qiao, G., Liu, X., Duan, H., Huang, Y., So, K. F., Yang, Z., Li, X., & Wang, L. (2024). Chitosan-based thermosensitive hydrogel with long-term release of murine nerve growth factor for neurotrophic keratopathy. *Neural Regeneration Research*, *19*(3), 680–686. https://doi.org/10.4103/1673-5374.380908

Xia, M., Zhao, S., Sun, Z., Shi, Y., Lin, W., Zhong, Z., & Meng, F. (2025). Brain-targeted polymersomes mediating RNAi of STAT3 sensitize glioblastoma to temozolomide and immunotherapy. *Journal of Colloid and Interface Science*, *695*. https://doi.org/10.1016/j.jcis.2025.137751

Xiong, X. B., Falamarzian, A., Garg, S. M., & Lavasanifar, A. (2011). Engineering of amphiphilic block copolymers for polymeric micellar drug and gene delivery. *Journal of Controlled Release*, *155*(2), 248–261. https://doi.org/10.1016/j.jconrel.2011.04.028

Xiong, Z., Alves, C. S., Wang, J., Li, A., Liu, J., Shen, M., Rodrigues, J., Tomás, H., & Shi, X. (2019). Zwitterion-functionalized dendrimer-entrapped gold nanoparticles for serum-enhanced gene delivery to inhibit cancer cell metastasis. *Acta Biomaterialia*, *99*, 320–329. https://doi.org/10.1016/j.actbio.2019.09.005

Yang, Y., Zhao, H., Jia, Y., Guo, Q., Qu, Y., Su, J., Lu, X., Zhao, Y., & Qian, Z. (2016). A novel gene delivery composite system based on biodegradable folate-poly (ester amine) polymer and thermosensitive hydrogel for sustained gene release. *Scientific Reports*, *6*. https://doi.org/10.1038/srep21402

Yang, Z., Guo, Z., Tian, H., & Chen, X. (2021). Enhancers in polymeric nonviral gene delivery systems. In *VIEW* (Vol. 2, Issue 1). John Wiley and Sons Inc. https://doi.org/10.1002/VIW.20200072

Ye, L., Lv, W., He, W., Li, S., Min, Z., Gong, L., Zhang, Q., Teng, C., Sun, S., Lv, L., Guo, Y., & Xin, H. (2023). Reduced malignant glioblastoma recurrence post-resection through the anti-CD47 antibody and Temozolomide co-embedded in-situ hydrogel system. *Journal of Controlled Release*, *359*, 224–233. https://doi.org/10.1016/j.jconrel.2023.05.046

Yu, C., Li, L., Hu, P., Yang, Y., Wei, W., Deng, X., Wang, L., Tay, F. R., & Ma, J. (2021). Recent Advances in Stimulus-Responsive Nanocarriers for Gene Therapy. In *Advanced Science* (Vol. 8, Issue 14). John Wiley and Sons Inc. https://doi.org/10.1002/advs.202100540

Yu, D., Ye, L., Li, B., Mou, F., & Yin, Y. (2024). Preparation and Characterization of pH-Responsive Charge Reversal Nanocomposite for miRNA Delivery. *Journal Wuhan University of Technology, Materials Science Edition*, *39*(4), 1048–1052. https://doi.org/10.1007/s11595-024-2969-4

Zhang, L., & Eisenberg, A. (1996). *Multiple Morphologies and Characteristics of "Crew-Cut" Micelle-like Aggregates of Polystyrene-b-poly(acrylic acid) Diblock Copolymers in Aqueous Solutions*. https://pubs.acs.org/sharingguidelines

Zhang, N., Lin, J., Lin, V. P. H., Milbreta, U., Chin, J. S., Chew, E. G. Y., Lian, M. M., Foo, J. N., Zhang, K., Wu, W., & Chew, S. Y. (2021). A 3D Fiber-Hydrogel Based Non-Viral Gene Delivery Platform Reveals that microRNAs Promote Axon Regeneration and Enhance Functional Recovery Following Spinal Cord Injury. *Advanced Science*, *8*(15). https://doi.org/10.1002/advs.202100805

Zhang, P., An, K., Duan, X., Xu, H., Li, F., & Xu, F. (2018). Recent advances in siRNA delivery for cancer therapy using smart nanocarriers. *Drug Discovery Today*, *23*(4), 900–911. https://doi.org/10.1016/j.drudis.2018.01.042

Zhang, R. X., Ahmed, T., Li, L. Y., Li, J., Abbasi, A. Z., & Wu, X. Y. (2017). Design of nanocarriers for nanoscale drug delivery to enhance cancer treatment using hybrid polymer and lipid building blocks. In *Nanoscale* (Vol. 9, Issue 4, pp. 1334–1355). Royal Society of Chemistry. https://doi.org/10.1039/c6nr08486a

Zhang, Y., Zou, Z., Liu, S., Miao, S., & Liu, H. (2022). Nanogels as Novel Nanocarrier Systems for Efficient Delivery of CNS Therapeutics. In *Frontiers in Bioengineering and Biotechnology* (Vol. 10). Frontiers Media S.A. https://doi.org/10.3389/fbioe.2022.954470

Zhong, R., Talebian, S., Mendes, B. B., Wallace, G., Langer, R., Conde, J., & Shi, J. (2023). Hydrogels for RNA delivery. In *Nature Materials* (Vol. 22, Issue 7, pp. 818–831). Nature Research. https://doi.org/10.1038/s41563-023-01472-w

Zhou, R., Zhou, Y., Yin, M., Ge, C., Yang, Y., Shen, J., & Yin, L. (2024). Inflammation-Responsive Polyion Complex Vesicles for Autoimmune Disease Therapy via Cell-Free DNA Scavenging and Inflammatory Microenvironment Modulation. *ACS Nano*. https://doi.org/10.1021/acsnano.4c10886

Zielinska, A., Carreiró, F., Oliveira, A. M., Neves, A., Pires, B., Nagasamy Venkatesh, D., Durazzo, A., Lucarini, M., Eder, P., Silva, A. M., Santini, A., & Souto, E. B. (2020). Polymeric Nanoparticles: Production, Characterization, Toxicology and Ecotoxicology. In *Molecules* (Vol. 25, Issue 16). MDPI AG. https://doi.org/10.3390/molecules25163731

Zou, Y., Sun, X., Wang, Y., Yan, C., Liu, Y., Li, J., Zhang, D., Zheng, M., Chung, R. S., & Shi, B. (2020). *Single siRNA Nanocapsules for Effective siRNA Brain Delivery and Glioblastoma Treatment. 2000416*, 1–9. https://doi.org/10.1002/adma.202000416

Author Biographies

Nurcan Gumus received her Ph.D. from the School of Pharmacy at the University of Nottingham in 2024 under the supervision of Prof. Cameron Alexander. Since 2024, she has been working in the Department of Medical Biology as an Assistant Professor. Her research focuses on the design and development of biodegradable polymeric nanoparticles and hydrogels for drug and gene delivery, aiming to enhance therapeutic efficacy in systemic and local administration. She utilises polymer chemistry, nanofabrication, and characterisation techniques to optimise carrier properties, including stability, biocompatibility, and controlled release. Dr Gumus evaluates these systems in various in vitro (2D and 3D) and in vivo cancer models, including brain, breast, and pancreatic tumours. Beyond solid tumours, she also explores hematologic malignancies, where her work aims to unravel the biological mechanisms underlying tumour progression, drug response, and the development of multidrug resistance.

Umut Can Oz received his Ph.D. from Ankara University Faculty of Pharmacy in 2017. During his Ph.D., he conducted a part of his thesis research in the Chemistry Department at UCL. He has been working in the Department of Pharmaceutical Technology as an associate professor since 2024, after completing a postdoctoral fellowship with Prof. Cameron Alexander at the University of Nottingham School of Pharmacy. His research interests include developing novel micro- and nano-scale polymeric materials and hydrogel-based biomaterials for drug and nucleic acid delivery.

CHAPTER 12

SYNTHETIC CATIONIC POLYMERS FOR GENE THERAPY

AHMET CESUR,[1,2] UMUT CAN ÖZ[1]

[1]Ankara University, Department of Pharmaceutical Technology, Ankara, Türkiye [2]Ankara University, Institute of Health Sciences, Ankara, Türkiye

Abstract

Synthetic cationic polymers have widespread use to develop non-viral nucleic acid delivery systems. The existence of several positively charged groups on the polymer chain is a typical characteristic of their structures. Both synthetic and natural cationic polymers have been studied for potential therapeutic applications. Synthetic polymers may address the primary challenges associated with lot-to-lot variations of natural polymers. Endosomal escape is a critical bottleneck in gene delivery, presenting a significant challenge for polyplex-based delivery systems. When entrapped in endosomes, these systems often face degradation in lysosomes, which limits the therapeutic efficacy of the polymer-nucleic acid complex after cellular uptake. Strategies such as the proton sponge effect, membrane destabilization, and pH-sensitive polymer designs are employed to facilitate the release of genetic material into the cytoplasm. Among synthetic carriers, polyethylenimine (PEI) has demonstrated high transfection efficiency through its buffering capacity, while poly(β-amino ester)s (PBAEs) offer reduced toxicity despite weaker nucleic acid binding. Recently, research has expanded from traditional plasmid DNA transfer to advanced modalities including mRNA, miRNA, antisense, and siRNA, several of which are now in clinical trials (van den Berg et al., 2021). Despite persistent limitations of toxicity and non-degradability, innovative polymer architectures and delivery platforms continue to improve therapeutic potential. This review highlights advances in synthetic cationic polymers for nucleic acid delivery.

Keywords: Synthetic cationic polymers, Gene therapy, Nucleic acid delivery, Endosomal escape, Non-viral vectors

1. Introduction

Gene therapy aims to modify gene expression or alter the biological properties of living cells for therapeutic purposes. This approach employs a range of nucleic acids including plasmid DNA (pDNA), microRNA (miRNA), small interfering RNA (siRNA), messenger RNA (mRNA), antisense oligonucleotides, and genome editing tools like CRISPR/Cas9. Delivering these therapeutic genes into target cells has gained attention as a promising strategy for the treatment of diverse conditions, including cancer, infectious diseases, and genetic disorders (Gupta et al., 2021; Pan et al., 2021).

While viral vectors have traditionally been investigated for gene delivery, their high immunogenicity, potential oncogenic risks and difficulties in large-scale production have driven the search for safer, more efficient synthetic carriers (Chen et al., 2015). Non-viral vectors, particularly polymer-based systems, offer a versatile and scalable alternative with tuneable properties to enhance gene transfection efficiency while minimizing adverse effects.

Synthetic polymers provide superior structural stability, allowing for controlled gene release and prolonged circulation time. Their chemical flexibility enables precise modifications to optimize strong gene-binding affinity, high buffering capacity, and effective intracellular gene release (Thomas et al., 2016). One of the key advantages of synthetic cationic polymers is their ability to form complexes with anionic nucleic acids through electrostatic interactions. The strength of these interactions can vary depending on the charge density and nitrogen-to-phosphate (N/P) ratio, which influences polyplex stability and transfection efficiency. The cationic nature of these polymers enhances cellular uptake and facilitates endosomal escape, making them highly effective carriers for gene delivery. However, cationic charge can also lead to cytotoxicity, necessitating careful optimization of polymer structure and N/P ratio to balance transfection efficiency and biocompatibility (Lv et al., 2006).

In this chapter, we will discuss the biological and physical challenges encountered in gene delivery caused by synthetic cationic polymers, explore their structural architectures, and analyse well-defined synthetic cationic polymers highlighted in the literature. Additionally, we will examine polymer hybrid systems and recent advancements in the field, including their clinical perspectives.

2. Physical and Biological Challenges in Synthetic Cationic Polymer-Based Gene Delivery

2.1. Physical Challenges

Advancements in material science and synthetic chemistry have enabled the precise design of polymers with controlled topology, size, and transport properties. This progress, alongside sequence-defined polymers and multimodal imaging, facilitates the development of multifunctional polyplexes and cationic polymers as highly efficient and tuneable gene delivery vectors. To address physical challenges in gene delivery, researchers have investigated techniques that adjust charge group composition, alter polymer architecture and molecular weight, and integrate hydrophilic, hydrophobic or stimuli-responsive moieties. Homopolymers and copolymers arranged in statistical, alternating, or block configurations and different topologies including linear, branched, dendritic, or grafted structures have varying degrees of stability and nucleic acid condensation. Furthermore, amphiphilic polymers can self-assemble into micelles or vesicles, which increases their transport capability (Kumar et al., 2021). These advances attempt to balance transfection effectiveness with low cytotoxicity, solving important physical challenges in synthetic cationic polymer-based gene delivery. Some of these key parameters and challenges have been discussed in detail below.

Molecular weight. Low molecular weight (LMW) polymers have poor transfection efficiency but lower toxicity, while high molecular weight (HMW) polymers improve gene delivery but increase toxicity. For example, 22-25 kDa PEI enables effective gene transfer due to facilitated endosomal escape but has high toxicity, whereas LMW PEI is less toxic but ineffective for transfection. PEI F25-LMW (~4-10 kDa) exhibits high DNA/siRNA delivery efficiency with low toxicity and long-term stability. High DNA/siRNA delivery efficiency, minimal toxicity, and long-term stability were demonstrated using a PEI F25-LMW (~4-10 kDa) (Sun and Zhang, 2010). Increased transfection efficacy is due to a narrow molecular weight distribution and smaller complex size, which promotes greater cellular absorption.

Charge density and zeta potential. Charge density indicates the overall charge of a polymer per unit of volume or surface area, whereas zeta potential is a parameter that measures the surface charge and its electrostatic impact in a biological environment. High charge density in cationic polymers improves transfection effectiveness by inducing strong nucleic acid condensation, but it also increases cytotoxicity. This duality illustrates the fundamental delivery dilemma, in which increased efficacy typically compromises safety. Thus, precision-tuning of charge properties remains a cornerstone in optimizing polymer design for clinical translation. For example, PEI having high charge density promotes the development of compact polyplexes, which improves gene transport, but it also impairs cell membrane integrity, resulting in toxicity. Both PEI transfection effectiveness and cytotoxicity are affected by both charge density and molecular weight, emphasizing the need of establishing a balance between these two parameters (Amin et al., 2013). In addition, in order to evaluate the effect of zeta potential, Dosta et al. developed poly(beta-amino ester) (PβAE) polymers integrating various combinations of oligopeptides with negatively and positively charged residues to modulate the zeta potential of the resulting polyplexes. Interestingly, they observed that the measured zeta potential did not correspond to the predicted charge density. Instead, polymer packing and the specific nature of the cationic functional groups exerted a significant influence on surface charge (Dosta et al., 2015). These findings highlight that zeta potential is a multifaceted parameter that cannot be accurately controlled only by adjusting the ratio of charged moieties. While zeta potential remains a valuable tool for assessing formulation properties and structure–activity relationships, it does not always reliably predict cellular uptake or transfection efficiency. This observation emphasizes that physicochemical metrics alone cannot fully account for biological performance. A more holistic approach that includes cellular assays and in vivo models is therefore essential for accurate evaluation.

The nitrogen to phosphorus (N/P) ratio, described as the ratio of nitrogen (N) atoms in cationic head groups of synthetic polymers to phosphorus (P) atoms in the phosphate backbone of nucleic acids in a transfection polyplex and, it is an important metric in improving gene delivery methods. This ratio controls the balance between transfection efficacy and cytotoxicity. The optimal N/P ratio varies across different vector delivery systems, influenced by factors including zeta potential, particle size, and the inherent properties of the cationic polymer. While higher N/P ratios can enhance transfection efficiency by improving DNA binding and stability, they may also increase cytotoxicity, necessitating a careful balance (Ma et al., 2021).

Protein corona formation. Due to the high surface free energy of nanoparticles, which causes the adsorption of different molecules, especially proteins, the protein corona develops (Chakraborty et al., 2020). Electrostatic interactions, Van der Waals forces, hydrophobic interactions, hydrogen bonds, and π-π stacking are some of the interactions that could involve in corona formation.

Nanoparticles are recognized by the reticuloendothelial system primarily through binding to the plasma proteins albumin, lipoproteins and macroglobulins. This immunological identification triggers a series of biological reactions that direct delivered polyplexes to the spleen or liver, blocking them from reaching their target tissue or organs. Furthermore, interactions between nanoparticles and serum proteins can drastically alter their size and zeta potential. Maiolo et al. prepared 25 kDa b-PEI/DNA polyplexes cultured in a medium with Fetal Bovine Serum (FBS) concentrations ranging from 0% to 50% prior to transfection, the study demonstrated a clear dependence of transfection efficiency on FBS levels in HeLa cell cultures, with a marked decrease observed at the highest concentration of 50% FBS (Maiolo et al., 2018). These results highlight the critical influence of biological fluids on the behaviour of polyplexes. It underscores the importance of assessing gene delivery systems under physiologically relevant conditions rather than relying solely on serum-free models. To combat serum instability, various strategies have been used, including phosphonium-containing polymer blocks, carbohydrate moieties, fluorination and PEG based stealth nanoparticle coatings.

2.2. Biological Challenges

While achieving effective nucleic acid delivery, the polyplex must balance two apparently opposing characteristics: it needs to provide protection and maintain stability of itself outside the target cell whereas break down and release undamaged nucleic acid once inside the cell. Polymer-based vectors need to avoid being quickly cleared outside of the cell by the reticuloendothelial system, which removes biologically active substances from the body. These nonviral carriers must overcome distinct physiological barriers associated with different routes of administration: intravenous injection, mucosal injection, topical application and oral delivery. In environments with high salt content, electrolytes can neutralize the electrostatic forces between the cationic polyplexes and the anionic DNA backbone, reducing stability and increasing the likelihood of clustering (Danielsen et al., 2005). Moreover, when administered systemically in living organisms, these carriers encounter additional challenges, which may involve uptake by immune cells, degradation by enzymes such as DNAses, RNAses, or proteases, hydrolytic breakdown, and the potential activation of immune responses through toll-like receptor pathways or cytokine induction.

Cytotoxicity. Nucleic acids must pass through the cell membrane and enter the cytosol in order to become active once they have reached the target cells. Cytocompatibility of gene delivery vector are closely related to toxicity since cell membrane integrity is important for cell survival. Synthetic cationic polymer-based polyplexes, cause considerable cytotoxicity when they interact with anionic membranes and proteins. Incorporation of hydrophilic features, including carbohydrate or PEG moieties, can reduce nuclear permeability and serve as a strategy to mitigate cytotoxicity. Polymer degradation products may also cause toxicity via reactive oxygen species, depending on the polymer structure. Pishavar et al. modified PAMAM dendrimers by introducing alkylcarboxylate-PEG and cholesterol, which elevated gene delivery. Their adjustments increased transfection efficiency and cellular absorption while lowering cytotoxicity. Masking the amine groups on the dendrimer surface improved the hydrophilic-hydrophobic balance of the vector, leading to inhibition of tumour growth in C26 tumour-bearing mice without notable toxicity to major organs (Pishavar et al., 2018).

Immunogenicity. The immune system acts as a considerable extracellular barrier to gene transport, activating non-specific defensive mechanisms immediately upon the introduction of polyplexes (Zhao et al., 2017). While viral vectors elicit stronger innate immune responses, non-viral gene delivery techniques can also stimulate immunological pathways, resulting in inflammatory cytokine release and macrophage-mediated clearance. Poly-L-lysine (PLL), PAMAM dendrimers and PEI, all positively charged polymers, dramatically activate complement cascades; however, this activity is markedly reduced upon association with nucleic acids. Studies have demonstrated that complement activation is polymer-length dependent, with cationic oligomers demonstrating lower immunological responses than longer polymer chains. Cyclodextrin-based cationic oligomer polyplex systems have been shown to effectively inhibit complement activation in vivo. Furthermore, naked nucleic acids can function as immunostimulants, given that toll-like receptors (TLRs) TLR7/8, TLR3, and TLR9 recognize single-stranded RNA, double-stranded RNA, and unmethylated CpG-rich DNA, respectively. These receptors activate strong immunological responses, which, useful for vaccines or cancer immunotherapies but, present a significant obstacle for gene therapy due to excessive cytokine production and inflammation. Höbel et al. revealed that systemic administration of PEI F25-LMW/siRNA polyplexes results in efficient delivery. Immunocompatibility tests Proinflammatory Cytokine Analysis (ELISA) performed and TNF-α and IFN-γ levels were measured to determine whether PEI/siRNA complexes triggered a proinflammatory response. Research revealed no hepatotoxicity, proinflammatory cytokine production, or other negative outcomes linked to PEI F25-LMW/siRNA polyplexes. Furthermore, tumour investigations indicated that siRNA administration resulted in effective vascular endothelial growth factor (VEGF) knockdown, which decreased tumour cell proliferation and angiogenesis (Han-En et al., 2012).

Cellular uptake. Positively charged gene delivery vehicles, exemplified by unmodified PEI, are believed to associate with cell surfaces through non-specific electrostatic interactions with the anionic glycocalyx, a glycosaminoglycan-rich layer composed of proteoglycans and glycolipids. Upon attachment to the plasma membrane, polyplexes become entrapped in membrane-bound vesicles like caveosomes or macropinosomes. Multiple studies have shown that cationic polyplexes are internalized through cells via clathrin-dependent and independent endocytosis, caveolae-mediated endocytosis, and macropinocytosis. While tailored polymeric carriers enhance delivery effectiveness through ligand receptor interactions, specifically the binding of folate to its receptor, they face challenges, including off-target binding and competition from endogenous ligands. Hydrophobic changes to polycations improve their contact with the cell membrane, aiding the uptake process. Researchers found that conjugating palmitic acids with PEI and PLL dramatically improved their binding affinity to bone marrow stromal cells in a degree of substitution-dependent manner. Furthermore, PEI modified with pendant hexyl or dodecyl chains interacted well with phospholipids, however untreated PEI did not interact efficiently (Liu et al., 2010).

Endosomal entrapment plays a essential role in determining the efficiency of gene expression, with the intracellular trafficking pathway of polyplexes particularly the endo-lysosomal route. Following endocytosis, early endosomes are formed, during which a pH drop from neutral to approximately 6.0 occurs. This acidification is driven by the action of membrane-bound vacuolar-type ATPases (V-ATPases), which function as proton pumps. Early endosomes differentiate into sorting endosomes, where their contents can be recycled back into the extracellular environment via exocytosis or other intracellular recycling processes involving the trans-Golgi network. Alternatively, the cargo may be guided to the lysosomal degradation route. In this situation, endosomes mature into late endosomes, where membrane-bound V-ATPases continue to decrease the pH to around 5.5-5.0. Late endosomes can also merge with lysosomes, which maintain a very acidic environment, providing ideal circumstances for lysosomal hydrolases to breakdown cellular components (Bus et al., 2018).

Both exocytosis and the lysosomal degradation pathway play crucial roles in transfection efficiency, but they pose significant challenges that must be overcome through successful escape from these compartments. The fate of polyplexes and their transfection efficiency are largely determined by intracellular trafficking routes, meaning polyplexes need to avoid being trapped in endocytic vesicles early in the endocytosis process to prevent either enzymatic degradation or expulsion of the cargo from the cell. Therefore, strategies that exploit endocytic sorting or manipulate vesicular dynamics may significantly enhance nuclear delivery outcomes. Understanding these routes could also aid in tailoring vectors for specific cell types or tissues. After escaping the endosome, the cargo must be separated from its carrier and directed to its intended location. Plasmid DNA (pDNA) must travel a considerable distance within the cytoplasm before reaching the nucleus. If nucleic acids are released prematurely into the peripheral cytoplasm, they may lose their protective environment, increasing the likelihood of degradation by nucleases. Therefore, releasing pDNA or pDNA-based polyplexes around the nucleus is considered more favourable than in the densely structured regions of the cytoplasm. Endosomal escape remains the primary obstacle for effective intracellular delivery of RNA and DNA (Patel et al., 2020; Varkouhi et al., 2011).

Endosomal escape theories

The "proton sponge" theory

The internalization of protons into endo-lysosomes by vATPase was a key factor in the action of a proton sponge. It is demonstrated that bafilomycin, a particular vATPase inhibitor, prevents the transfection, although chloroquine, which becomes protonated itself, promotes the transfection. Additionally, endosomal escape is facilitated by free PEI that is co-delivered with polyplexes but not linked to particles. Several positively charged polymers including PAMAM and poly dimethyl aminoethyl methacrylate (PDMAEMA) have demonstrated the capacity to act as a "proton sponge" by having strong buffering capabilities over a wide pH range (5.0 to 8.0). However, because of conflicting experimental data, the "proton sponge" theory is still subjected to argument in the research area (Shtykalova et al., 2023). Four main points have been discussed in relation to this hypothesis: the ability of positively charged polymers to buffer endosomes, their potential to avoid lysosomal involvement, preventing acidification within endo-lysosomal compartments, and their ability to cause endo-lysosomes to rupture or lyse completely. The most contentious feature of the "proton sponge" concept is whether it causes total lysis or rupture of the endo-lysosomal membrane. It has been debated whether proton binding by PEI within the endosome may provide a significant osmotic gradient to counteract V-ATPase action. According to studies, a critical PEI concentration is necessary to create sufficient membrane tension to cause rupture. Electron microscopy studies have revealed that PEI aggregates adhere to the lysosomal membrane, generating partial disruptions rather than complete rupture. This suggests that the mechanism of endosomal escape may involve more nuanced membrane perturbations than previously assumed. Such findings could inspire the design of polymers with controlled membrane-interaction profiles to fine-tune intracellular delivery. Similar results have been reported for cyclo-dextran, and poly(methacrylate)-based polyplexes. Live-cell confocal imaging also demonstrated nucleic acid release via temporary local bursts or nanoscale holes, whereas endosomes remained structurally intact. These findings imply that endosomal release arises through localized membrane instability and transitory nanoscale hole creation, rather than total lysis (Bus et al., 2018).

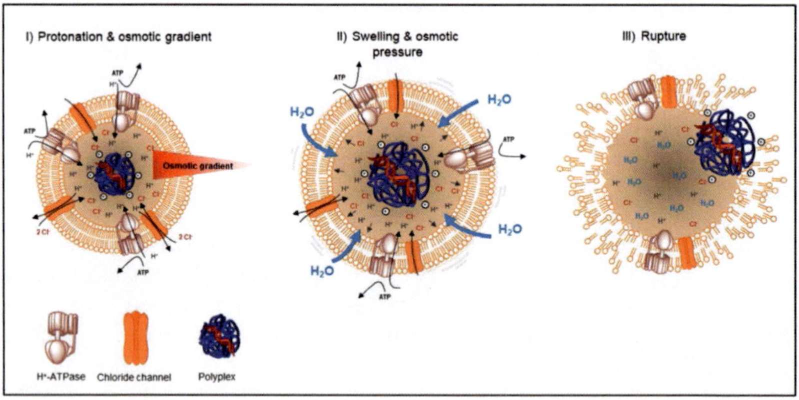

Figure 1. The figure illustrates the "proton sponge" hypothesis in three steps for a cationic polyplex inside an endo-lysosome: I) Protonation & Osmotic Gradient: The polyplex buffers protons in the acidic endo-lysosome, causing H^+ and Cl^- ions to accumulate via V-ATPase and chloride channels, creating an osmotic gradient. II) Swelling & Osmotic Pressure: Water enters the compartment to balance the ion buildup, leading to swelling and increased pressure in the endo-lysosome. III) Rupture: The swollen endo-lysosome bursts due to the pressure, releasing the polyplex and its cargo into the cytoplasm for further cellular action. Reprinted with permission from Ref. (Bus et al., 2018).

The polyplex-mediated membrane disruption

The membrane structure of early endosomes resembles that of the plasma membrane, whose primary constituents are neutral lipids composed of sphingolipids and sterols. The interaction of charged polymers and membrane vesicles is critical in this hypothesis and can be understood by studying the inner leaflet of the endo-lysosomal membrane. Cytotoxicity studies have shown that PEI and other amino-containing polymers can disrupt membranes (Bus et al., 2018). Research combining experimental and computational simulations has demonstrated that the interaction between PEI and anionic lipids enables the polymer to penetrate the hydrophobic region of the membrane bilayer. This mechanism promotes the translocation of anionic lipids across the membrane in a process known as lipid flip-flop and enhances the membrane permeation of charged biomolecules, particularly nucleic acids.

The polymer-mediated membrane disruption

A revised version of the theory above was developed by proposing that unlike the earlier model, free positively charged polymer chains disrupt the endo-lysosomal membrane by directly intercalating into it, leading to membrane damage and facilitating endosomal escape. This model could also account for the cytotoxic effects observed with cationic polymers, particularly PEI, which has been shown to disrupt the integrity of lipid membranes in mitochondria or the endoplasmic reticulum. The presence of excess polymer during polyplex preparation, indicated by high N/P ratios, is considered advantageous for achieving elevated transfection efficiencies. This phenomenon can be attributed to the observation that only a small fraction of PEI participates in complex formation, while the majority (70–80%) remains unbound in solution. The excess free PEI plays a critical role in improving cellular uptake and intracellular transport of polyplexes, a process that is not dependent on the polymer's molecular weight. As pH decreases, the protonation of PEI's amino groups induces electrostatic repulsion, causing the polymer to adopt an extended conformation (Bus et al., 2018). The densely charged cationic segments along the polymer chains establish a polar microenvironment, facilitating the permeation of water molecules across the lipid bilayer. This strong interaction and deep penetration of PEI into the membrane ultimately lead to the generation of transient aqueous channels or nanopores.

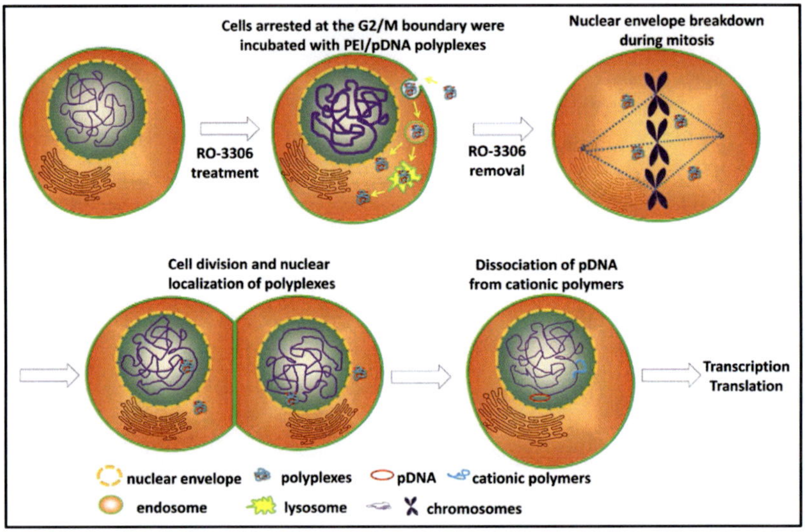

Figure 2. Schematic representation illustrates the intracellular trafficking of PEI/pDNA polyplexes in cancer cells treated with RO-3306. HeLa cells are synchronized at the G2/M boundary of the cell cycle using RO-3306 and incubated with PEI/pDNA polyplexes for 3 hours, during which the polyplexes escape from endosomes or lysosomes. The removal of RO-3306 allows the cells to rapidly and synchronously enter mitosis. The disappearance of the nuclear envelope during metaphase facilitates the localization of polyplexes into the nuclear region, and some polyplexes remain inside the nuclei after the nuclear envelope reforms in the daughter cells. Once inside the nucleus, the pDNA dissociates from PEI, enabling gene transcription followed by translation. Reprinted with permission from Ref. (Zhou et al., 2016).

Nuclear envelope barrier. In polymer-based pDNA delivery, the nuclear envelope which fully encloses genetic material plays a crucial intracellular barrier role. Naturally, nanoparticles larger than 25 nm struggle to pass through nuclear pores. Given that polymer/pDNA polyplexes typically exhibit a particle size of around 100 nm, their entry into the nucleus in an intact form is challenging. Instead, nuclear entry is thought to occur primarily upon the breakdown of the nuclear envelope during mitosis. Zhou et al. employed RO-3306, a selective and reversible CDK1 inhibitor, to stabilize cells at the G2/M phase transition, thereby increasing the population of mitotic cells with a disassembled nuclear envelope during transfection. This pharmacological approach highlights the interplay between cell cycle regulation and gene delivery, suggesting that synchronizing cells may be a valuable auxiliary method to boost nuclear access for large polyplexes. Their findings demonstrate that RO-3306 enhances the transfection efficiency of PEI polyplexes by promoting nuclear localization of both PEI and pDNA. However, this effect was less concern for the charge-reversal polymer poly[(2-acryloyl)ethyl(p-boronic acid benzyl)diethylammonium bromide] (B-PDEAEA), which undergoes stimulus-responsive degradation in the cytoplasm, releasing free pDNA prior to nuclear entry (Zhou et al., 2016). We will discuss charge reversal polymers in the following sections of this chapter.

In another study, Gillard et al. demonstrated that pDNA enters the nucleus primarily through nuclear pores (NPCs) rather than during mitosis (Gillard et al., 2014). Their theory was supported by experiments using wheat germ agglutinin (WGA), which inhibited nuclear pore entry and significantly reduced transfection efficiency to below 10%. Transfection efficiency was determined by the percentage of cells expressing green fluorescence protein (GFP), as measured by flow cytometry. Their findings also showed that polymer/pDNA complexes must dissociate before passing through NPCs, as large complexes (~200 nm) cannot fit through the ~25 nm nuclear pores. Among the tested polymers, their newly synthesized diblock copolymer, poly(DMAEA-b-(ImPAA-co-BA)) (A-C3), delivered more pDNA into the nucleus than PEI Max, likely due to its enhanced endosomal escape and controlled dissociation near the nuclear membrane. Furthermore, by interacting with nuclear pore components, the hydrophobic butyl acrylate segments in A-C3 could have promoted nuclear transport. These findings highlight the significance of polymer design in increasing the success of nucleic acid delivery via nuclear targeting and controlled dissociation. Similarly, Riera et al, also demonstrated that DNA release takes place in the perinuclear area prior to nuclear delivery (Riera et al., 2019). They used PβAE polyplex by mixing 1,4 butanediol diacrylate and hexylamine in a 1:1 ratio. Polyplex effectively condense and protect pDNA during cellular uptake. They monitored polyplex stability in real-time using super-resolution microscopy (dSTORM), which showed that DNA release takes place in the perinuclear area prior to nuclear delivery. They also discovered that unbound PβAE molecules in the cytoplasm are essential for promoting intracellular trafficking and polyplex formation. Since cells with higher nuclear pDNA levels expressed more GFP, their investigation also demonstrated a substantial link between nuclear pDNA levels and gene expression efficiency.

3. Structural Architecture of Synthetic Cationic Polymers

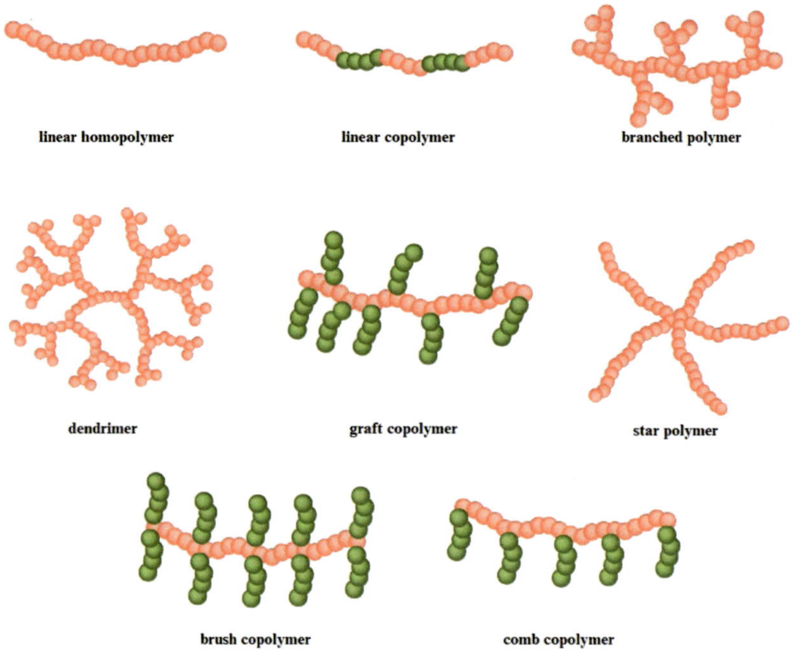

Figure 3. Common polymer architectures are defined by the types of monomers incorporated and their spatial arrangement.

3.1. Linear Polymers

Linear polymers are recognized for their simple structure and ease of modification presenting them an essential group of nanomaterials for non-viral gene delivery.

PLL is a synthetic linear polypeptide made up of repeating L-lysine units. Although it offers easy chemical modification and functionalization potential, PLL has limitations including instability of complexes in serum, poor endosomal escape, and cytotoxicity. In the late 20th century, researchers found that attaching ligands to PLL covalently greatly improved receptor-mediated endocytosis. For instance, asialoorosomucoid (ASOR), a ligand for the sialoglycoprotein receptor on hepatocytes, when linked to PLL, significantly boosted receptor-mediated endocytosis and plasmid uptake. Moreover, PLL modified with transferrin or folic acid was developed, resulting in notable advancements in pDNA transfection into cancer cells (Cai et al., 2023).

Linear PEI (lPEI) is another featured linear arranged cationic polymer made up of secondary amino groups and ethylene units (-NH-CH_2CH_2-). Although PEI has been widely researched and employed as a gene delivery carrier, its primary limitation is its toxicity. Its significant positive charge density originates from the protonated amino groups located on every third atom along its chain. The initial comprehensive analysis of linear PEI was documented by Saegusa et al., who began with the cationic ring-opening polymerization (ROP) of 2-oxazoline, followed by the hydrolysis of poly(2-oxazoline) in an alkaline environment. Since that time, poly(2-oxazoline)s have frequently served as starting materials for producing lPEI through hydrolysis under either alkaline or acidic conditions (Samal et al., 2012).

3.2. Branched and Dendritic Polymers

Branched polymers. Among synthetic branched cationic polymers, poly(β-amino ester)s (PβAEs) are synthesized via a Michael addition reaction combining acrylate derivatives and amine-containing compounds (Liu et al., 2019; Fornaguera et al., 2019). Owing to their intrinsic biodegradability, biocompatibility, and pH-responsive behaviour, PβAEs have gained significant interest as carriers for nucleic acid delivery. The polymer backbone contains ester linkages that undergo hydrolytic cleavage under physiological conditions, generating low-molecular-weight byproducts, namely bis(β-amino acids) and diols, which are generally regarded as non-toxic to mammalian systems. Highly branched variants of PβAEs are typically synthesized through the incorporation of triacrylate monomers and amines bearing dual reactive functionalities. These hyperbranched architectures have demonstrated utility in the delivery of minicircle DNA, particularly in therapeutic strategies targeting neurological pathologies.

In 2018, Fornaguera et al. developed a formulation by conjugating retinol to oligopeptide-modified PβAE, utilizing it as an active targeting agent for the liver (Iqbal et al., 2022). This formulation was subsequently combined with mRNA to create nanoparticles. The resulting modified system exhibited optimized biodistribution, cell-specific transfection, and successful accumulation in the liver as intended. This research highlights the ability to achieve precise and targeted delivery of PβAE using a specific targeting moiety.

In addition to PβAEs, branched forms of other synthetic cationic polymers, among them PEI, oligoethyleneimine (OEI), and PLL, have been developed under specific conditions, and their applications have been examined in a range of studies.

Dendritic polymers. These symmetrical, hyperbranched polymers feature a tree-like structure, with branches of monomer units extending outward from a central core in all directions. Every dendrimer typically consists of a core and multiple branches, the length and number of branches vary depending on the dendrimer's generation. With each generational increase, the number of surface sites on the branches doubles, starting from initial binding points of the core. Dendrimers are distinguished from other macromolecules by the dendritic effect, which is observed in two forms: a divergence in properties relative to their linear counterparts, referred to as the multivalent effect, and variation in the magnitude of specific characteristics, including biocompatibility, binding affinity to cargo molecules, and transfection efficiency, as a function of increasing generation, referred to as the generation effect. Unlike linear or branched polymers, which lack structural uniformity due to random polymerization and thus cannot have their generation defined, dendrimers benefit significantly from the generation effect. This effect is a key factor in their superiority over other polymer types for biological uses, making the selection of the right generation and chemical structure critical for addressing specific research challenges. The dendritic effect's magnitude can be influenced by the core's size and nature, as well as the level of coordination among the terminal functional groups.

Cationic triethanolamine (TEA)-PAMAM G5 has demonstrated potential as a delivery system for Dicer-substrate siRNAs (dsiRNAs), which are siRNA precursors, enabling multitarget suppression of the HIV. Zhou et al. showed that in vitro application in human lymphocytes resulted in over a two-fold reduction in the expression of p24, a critical viral protein. In vivo experiments using HIV-infected humanized mouse models produced even more striking outcomes: administration of TEA-PAMAM G5 complexes combined with a mixture of four dsiRNAs (dsiTAT, dsiREV, dsiCD4, and dsiTNPO3) in mice resulted in undetectable levels of viral particles, alongside a reduction in the total CD4+ lymphocyte population. Typically, a decline in CD4+ T-cell numbers represents a significant medical concern, often necessitating specific isolation measures before and after radiotherapy (Dzmitruk et al., 2018).

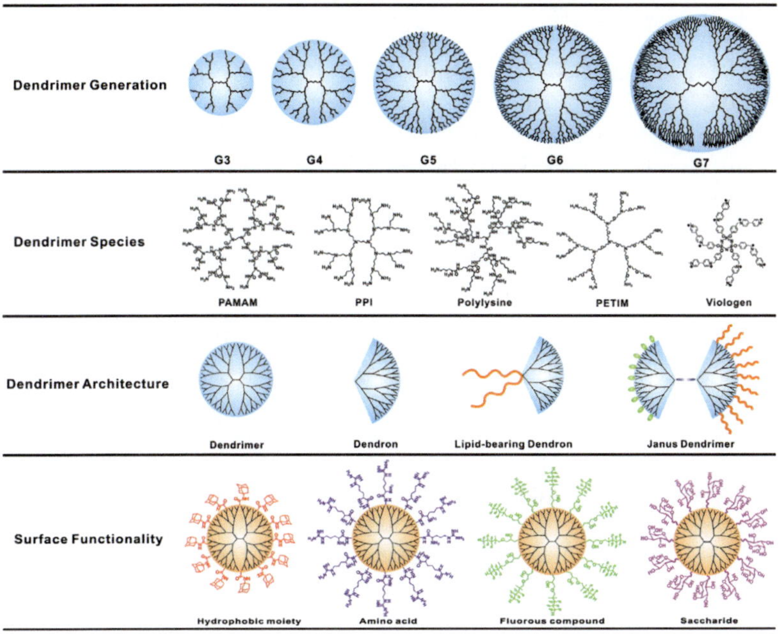

Figure 4. Figure illustrates the major dendrimer generations, species, architectures, and surface functionalities studied in the literature. Reprinted with permission from Ref. (Hu et al., 2016).

3.3. Grafting and Star-shaped polymers

Graft copolymers. Grafting is a technique that involves attaching side chains (grafts) to a polymer backbone to modify its physical, chemical, or biological properties. Polycationic graft copolymers are macromolecules in which multiple cationic polymer chains, often called "combs," are attached to a central polymer backbone. While these short oligocations typically have low transfection efficiency on their own, grafting them onto a backbone increases charge density and enhances gene delivery performance. Various graft polymer-based platforms have been studied for nucleic acid delivery, including those based on PDMAEMA, PEI, oligoamines, and oligopeptide combs. The key factors influencing their effectiveness include the quantity, type, and length of the positively charged grafts. When representing graft polymers, a lowercase "g" is placed between the two monomer names. In this section, only grafting is emphasized, while brush- and comb-like polymers will be discussed in later sections (Porello et al., 2024).

Lu and colleagues synthesized N-maleated chitosan (NMC) grafted PEI (800 Da) copolymers using a Michael addition reaction. The incorporation of LMW PEI enhanced the solubility and buffering capacity of all resulting copolymers. Among them, NMC_{5k}-g-PEI and NMC_{10k}-g-PEI demonstrated transfection efficiencies similar to PEI (25 kDa) but with reduced cytotoxicity in both 293T and HeLa cells, while NMC_{50k}-g-PEI exhibited higher cytotoxicity and lower transfection activity. The higher molecular weight of NMC_{50k}-g-PEI enabled it forming more effective complexes with free DNA via electrostatic interactions which hindered DNA dissociation inside cells, ultimately hindering DNA translation (Lu et al., 2009).

PEGylation (grafting with PEG) with relatively LMW and a low degree of substitution has been demonstrated to enhance the transfection performance of polyplexes. This not only supports the stealth role of PEG in immune evasion but also shows its potential to improve intracellular trafficking. Such dual benefits position PEGylation as a key strategy in designing next-generation vectors. Additionally, it imparts stealth properties to the polyplexes, reducing their visibility to the immune system and enhancing their stability in biological environments. To reduce the cytotoxicity and aggregation associated with PEI, PEI-grafted PEGs (PEI-g-PEG) incorporating PEG chains exceeding 5 kDa were developed, leveraging the charge-shielding effect of PEG to lower the surface charge of the polyplexes. Martin and colleagues synthesized a range of PEI and PEG copolymers, revealing that PEG molecular weight primarily influenced polyplex size by affecting aggregation tendencies. Specifically, grafting with PEG_{5000} enabled both low and HMW PEI-based copolymers to form small polyplexes with minimal aggregation, whereas using PEG_{550} resulted in larger aggregates when complexed with oligonucleotides, regardless of PEI molecular weight.

Star-shaped polymers have gained attention in the delivery of genetic material, largely owing to their high efficiency in facilitating gene expression, precise molecular structure, and flexibility for modification. These polymers are a specific type of branched macromolecule, consisting of linear polymer chains connected to a central core, with a single branching point per molecule. Their simple production, high molecular weights, adaptability, and unique properties have made them increasingly popular for gene delivery applications. Many star polymers with polycationic arms have been developed for gene transfection; however, associated toxicity issues often limit their effectiveness (Hynynen, 2008; Chen et al., 2019). Neoh et al. investigated the synthesis and transfection efficiency of star-shaped copolymers composed of either PDMAEMA homopolymer arms or

PDMAEMA-b-PEG diblock copolymer arms. To construct multifunctional initiators, they functionalized β-cyclodextrin (β-CD) with ATRP-initiator groups, which subsequently enabled the polymerization of PDMAEMA arms that were later elongated with a PEGEEMA block (Kumar et al., 2021). Relative to HMW lPEI and PDMAEMA controls, these star copolymers, particularly those bearing PDMAEMA and PDMAEMA-b-PEG arms at N/P ratios of 20 to 30, achieved approximately five-fold greater transfection efficiency in HEK293 cells.

3.4. Brush polymers

Brush-like polymers are distinct branching structures generated by connecting short side chain molecules to a core backbone chain. Macromonomers are huge molecules that include one or more functional groups and can act as monomers in polymerization operations. Brush-like macromolecules are typically synthesized using three techniques: "grafting-through," which forms the brush-like polymer by polymerizing macromonomers; "grafting-to," which fully attaches the side chains to an existing backbone; and "grafting-from," which builds the brush-like polymer by polymerizing monomers directly from the backbone. Polymerizing macromonomers allows for the successful production of highly defined brush polymers with dense grafting. The study of Reineke and Dalal (US 2023/0414784 A1), patented by the University of Minnesota, explores cationic bottlebrush polymers for gene delivery, synthesized using RAFT polymerization followed by ROMP with 2-(dimethylamino)ethyl methacrylate (DMAEMA) monomers (Heights, 2023). The synthesized polymer demonstrated a 60-fold higher transfection efficiency than linear polymers, achieving up to 60% EGFP+ expression in HEK293 cells. Toxicity studies showed high cell viability (~80–90%) at N/P 5 and 7.5, with increased toxicity at N/P 10. Confocal microscopy confirmed superior nuclear delivery efficiency, highlighting bottlebrush polymers as a scalable and effective non-viral gene delivery platform.

3.5. Comb polymers

Comb polymers represent a unique subclass of macromolecules distinguished by a linear backbone structure (the “shaft”) bearing regularly spaced, functional side chains (the “teeth”) as part of the repeating monomeric units. Owing to their favourable balance between high transfection efficacy and minimal cytotoxicity, these materials have gained recognition as promising vectors for gene delivery applications. Typically, comb polymers are constructed with a hydrophobic main chain and oligolysine-based side chains, facilitating the formation of stable polyplexes through electrostatic interactions with nucleic acids. Experimental evidence indicates that comb polymers frequently outperform several commercially available transfection agents, offering enhanced efficiency while preserving high levels of cellular viability. The hydrophobic nature of the backbone is believed to play a pivotal role in modulating DNA binding affinity, as it reduces nonspecific interactions and lowers the binding free energy, thereby improving transfection efficiency.

Olden and colleagues conducted a comprehensive evaluation of various positively charged polymers for gene transfer in both immortalized and primary human T cells. Their study demonstrated that specifically designed comb- and sunflower-shaped poly(2-hydroxyethyl methacrylate)-graft-poly(dimethylaminoethyl methacrylate) (PHEMA-g-PDMAEMA) structures could achieve transfection efficiencies approaching 50% in Jurkat T cells, while maintaining over 90% cell viability and negligible cytotoxicity. Moreover, they optimized several critical parameters to enhance transfection efficiency in primary T cells: pre-activation duration, cell seeding density, nucleic acid dosage, culture conditions and cytokine supplementation. These efforts culminated in the successful delivery of both mRNA and plasmid DNA into CD4+ and CD8+ primary human T lymphocytes, achieving transfection rates of up to 25% and 18%, respectively, without distressing cell health (Olden et al., 2018).

4. Well-Defined Synthetic Cationic Polymers for Gene Delivery

Research on polymer-based systems dates back to the 1960s, when positively charged proteins, among them histones and protamines, were found to enhance the transfer of genetic material. By the 1970s, pioneering cationic polymers including DEAE-dextran, polyornithine, PLL, and polyarginine were introduced for enhancing cellular uptake and condensing DNA. These initial experiments revealed that gene transport could be promoted through electrostatic attraction between cationic polymers and anionic nucleic acids.

In a 1962 study, Smull and Ludwig demonstrated that single-stranded poliovirus RNA, when isolated with phenol and combined with cationic proteins, could significantly raise infection rates up to 100-fold (Smull and Ludwig, 1962). Similarly, in 1965, Vaheri and Pagano discovered that

DEAE-dextran and similar polymers substantially enhanced viral infectivity (Vaheri and Pagano, 1965). Building on this, McCutchan and Pagano reported in 1968 that the use of DEAE-dextran could amplify the transfer of SV40 DNA by as much as 100,000 times. Vaheri and Pagano hypothesized that the polymer formed a protective layer around the RNA, likely through electrostatic interaction with the cellular membrane, as they observed a notable effect in cells pretreated with DEAE-dextran (Wagner, 2014).

In the 1980s, targeted gene delivery became an important goal and Wu G.Y. and Wu C.H. established receptor-mediated gene transfection utilizing PLL conjugates. This was followed by transferrin-PLL complexes, which increased receptor-specific absorption and gene transfer efficiency. The introduction of PEI in the 1990s marked a significant advance in gene transport due to its proton sponge effect, which enhanced endosomal escape. During this time, PAMAM dendrimers and biodegradable polyesters were investigated as safer options for DNA compaction and intracellular transport. In the 2000s, the focus shifted to developing biodegradable, biocompatible, and multifunctional cationic polymers. Cyclodextrin-based polymers, amphiphilic polymers, and dynamic polyconjugates are among the innovations that have arisen to increase safety and targeting. Micelleplexes, cross-linked micelles, and polymersomes were also studied for their controlled release and improved transfection effectiveness. Studies have shown that altering polymeric nanoparticles with PEGylation, pH-responsive components, and receptor-targeting ligands can enhance circulation time while reducing off-target effects (Otmane et al., 1995; Kataoka et al., 2012; Zhang and Wagner, 2017).

Today, synthetic cationic polymer research is evolving and include nanotechnology, polymer chemistry, and tailored drug delivery systems. These advancements aim to increase biocompatibility, decrease cytotoxicity, and improve gene therapy results, opening the way for safer and more effective non-viral gene delivery methods in clinical settings.

After providing the history in the previous paragraphs, this chapter will now focus on the prominent groups of well-defined synthetic cationic polymers in the following sections.

4.1. Polyethyleneimine (PEI)

Polyethylenimine (PEI), a polyamine polymer, has been widely used in gene transfection since the late 20th century. It is relatively safe compared to viral vectors, straightforward to synthesize and easy to modify. PEI consists of primary, secondary, and tertiary amines, offering a strong buffering capacity facilitating effective endosomal release and contains secondary and tertiary amines with pKa values ranging between physiological and lysosomal pH levels. However, a drawback of PEI is its cytotoxicity, which stems from its high molecular weight and excess positive charges. The gene delivery performance and cellular toxicity of PEI demonstrate a strong molecular weight dependence. While LMW PEIs (1.8 kDa) show favourable biocompatibility, their limited DNA condensation capacity results in suboptimal transfection outcomes. In a comprehensive study by Liu and colleagues (Stanford, 2013), examined how polymer characteristics influence both transfection efficacy and cellular toxicity. LMW-PEI was conjugated with a GFP-encoding plasmid and evaluated in CM7221 cells. Their work demonstrated that while LMW-PEI/DNA complexes could achieve substantial gene expression (~55% in CM7221 cells), this effectiveness diminished with increasing polymer molecular weight. Notably, this reduction in transfection efficiency was accompanied by a corresponding increase in cytotoxic effects, highlighting the critical balance between polymer size and biological performance in gene delivery applications. To address this reduced efficacy, hydrophobic groups can be attached to the polymers, promoting the formation of self-assembled cationic polymer structures that enhance the stability of the complexes formed with nucleic acids and polymers. Non-degradable PEI's limitations have been addressed by developing degradable PEI derivatives incorporating various biodegradable linkages such as ester, disulfide, imine, carbamate, amide, and ketal bonds. Current clinical development of PEI-based gene delivery systems shows promise in oncology applications, with both the jetPEI® platform and linear PEI derivatives advancing through clinical trials for major cancer indications. These synthetic vectors offer substantial advantages in terms of chemical versatility their amine-rich structure permits straightforward functionalization with stabilizing polymers, targeting moieties for tissue-specific delivery, or chemotherapeutic payloads for combination therapies. This multifunctional adaptability presents PEI derivatives as particularly robust platforms for next-generation gene delivery medicine development.

Wang and colleagues developed a novel gene delivery system by modifying PEI with lithocholic acid (LCA) to enhance its stability and reduce cytotoxicity (Kristi et al., 2017). They synthesized LCA-PEI (lp) and further complexed it with hyaluronic acid (HA) to form a complex (DlpH). The researchers optimized the formulation by adjusting the lp/pDNA ratio and evaluated its stability, gene transfection performance, and cellular uptake in both in vitro and tumour-bearing mice models. Their findings revealed that DlpH polyplexes, with a higher lp/pDNA ratio, was more resistant to enzymatic degradation and heparin displacement, leading to improved transfection efficiency in vitro. However, in vivo experiments demonstrated a tumour-size-dependent effect, where DlpH-based polyplexes performed well in smaller tumours (<300 mm³) but was less effective in larger tumours (>500 mm³). Wang et al. attributed this difference to tumour-associated macrophages (TAMs), which preferentially internalized lp/PDNA complexes in advanced tumours, reducing its availability for transfection in tumour cells. Their study highlights the need to consider tumour microenvironment factors when designing gene delivery systems and suggests that standard in vitro screening may not always accurately predict in vivo performance.

PEI, as a synthetic cationic polymer for gene therapy is currently being evaluated in clinical trials. Several PEI-based formulations are under investigation for their potential in cancer and infectious disease therapies. The DTA-H19 formulation, developed by the Hebrew University of Jerusalem, is in a Phase I/II clinical trial for bladder neoplasms through intravesical administration (NCT00393809). Another DTA-H19 formulation by BioCancell Ltd. is being tested in a Phase II clinical trial for superficial bladder cancer (NCT00595088), while BC-819, another PEI-based vector from BioCancell Ltd., is undergoing a Phase I trial for transitional cell carcinoma of the bladder (NCT01878188) (Sharma et al., 2021).

Poly(2-oxazoline)-based polymers, can be described as a class of synthetic cationic polymers that excel in forming polyplexes, offering distinct advantages over traditional polymers. Research has demonstrated that poly(2-oxazolines) (POx) possess beneficial properties, including tuneable hydrophobicity and a simple chemistry that enables precise tailoring of block orientation and lengths. In fact, lPEI can be synthesized through the hydrolysis of poly(2-alkyl-2-oxazoline)s. Two hydrophilic POx monomers, 2-methyl-2-oxazoline (MeOx) and 2-ethyl-2-oxazoline (EtOx), are notable for their biocompatibility, in vivo stability, and diminished production of reactive oxygen species (ROS). Studies have shown that amphiphilic POx block copolymers enhance the delivery of drug combination formulations and effectively solubilize previously insoluble drugs with high efficiency. Additionally, research highlights the use of POx cationic block copolymers in formulating plasmid DNA (pDNA) into polyplexes, which exhibit lower serum binding compared to other polymer-based polyplexes (Yamaleyeva et al., 2023).

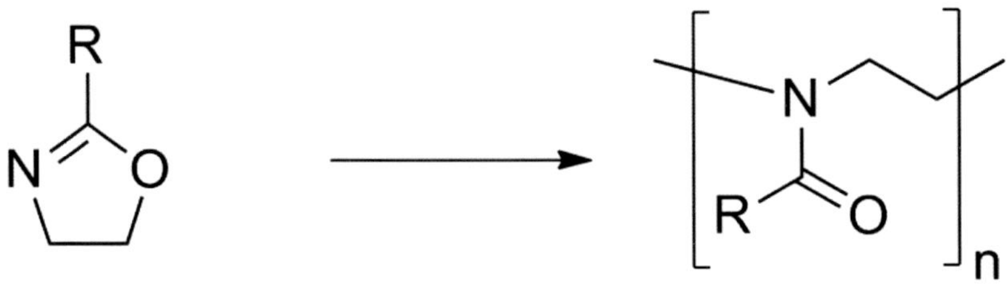

Figure 5. Ring opening polymerization of poly(oxazoline)s.

Bus et al., introduced a new generation of PEI copolymers from partially hydrolysed poly(EtOx-stat-EI) and functionalized using thiol–ene chemistry to introduce primary amines (Bus et al., 2017). These copolymers were synthesized by varying the primary-to-secondary amine ratio; they formed stable complexes with pDNA and siRNA and achieved efficient transfection with lower cytotoxicity than linear PEI. Unlike previous systems, these copolymers displayed minimal protein interactions, preventing aggregation in serum-containing media and enabling efficient cellular uptake. Confocal and electron microscopy studies revealed that polyplexes remained individually localized within endosomes rather than forming clusters, suggesting a membrane interaction-based release mechanism instead of the proton sponge effect. Overall, this polymeric system offers an effective and less toxic alternative for gene delivery, demonstrating high potential for complex transfection applications, including hard-to-transfect cells and in vivo studies.

4.2. Poly(amino acid)s

Poly(amino acid)s have been broadly studied as nucleic acid carriers due to their fundamental ability to interact with genes, forming compact, virus-like structures. These polycations can effectively condense DNA, promoting its delivery into cells. However, formulations based on these polymers can sometimes exhibit toxicity, with lower molecular weight variants generally being more cytotoxic. Among the first poly(amino acid)s utilized for targeted gene transfection was PLL, which was used by incorporating specific ligands that recognize cell surface receptors. Despite their potential, PLL and similar polycations often face limitations, particularly in endosomal escape. At physiological pH, these polycations are fully protonated, which reduces their buffering capacity within endosomes and hinders their ability to promote endosomal escape (Piotrowski-Daspit et al., 2020).

To address these limitations, researchers have devised a range of strategies to enhance the functionality of poly(amino acid)s, with copolymerization being one of the primary approaches. One approach involves integrating low molecular weight polycations with other polymer segments to create copolymers that combine the benefits of both components. A notable example is the work by Fu et al., who examined the development of a tri-block biodegradable, poly(lactic acid)-poly(ethylene glycol)-poly(L-lysine) (PLA-PEG-PLL), as a synthetic vector for gene delivery (Fu et al., 2011). Their study aimed to address the challenges posed by conventional cationic polymers including low transfection efficiency and high cytotoxicity. The results demonstrated that the nanoparticles formed with PLA-PEG-PLL exhibited higher gene transfection efficiency (31.63% in HeLa cells, 21.64% in HepG2 cells) compared to PEI. Furthermore, the addition of PEG increased nanoparticle stability by reducing interactions with serum proteins, thereby improving gene transfection under physiological conditions.

In addition to copolymerization, incorporating biodegradable units into poly(amino acid)s has accepted to be another effective strategy for enhancing gene delivery efficiency. As an example of this is poly[N-[N-(2-aminoethyl)-2-aminoethyl]aspartamide] (P[Asp(DET)]), synthesized by Ithaka et al., which demonstrated exceptional endosomal escape properties due to its pH-responsive membrane destabilization (Itaka et al., 2010). This resulted in highly efficient gene transfection with minimal cytotoxicity. The biodegradability of P[Asp(DET)] plays a crucial role in reducing cumulative toxicity, unlike non-degradable polycations such as N-substituted polyglutamide (P[Glu(DET)]). As P[Asp(DET)] undergoes controlled degradation into non-toxic byproducts, it maintains cellular homeostasis even with repeated administrations. This feature is especially relevant for chronic or multi-dose gene therapies, where cumulative toxicity presents a significant limitation for many traditional polycations. This characteristic ensures sustained gene expression while minimizing long-term cytotoxic effects, making it a promising alternative to traditional polycations like PEI. These findings underscore the potential of biodegradable poly(amino acid)s in gene delivery, offering a safe and efficient solution for next-generation non-viral gene carriers that prioritize both biocompatibility and high transfection efficiency.

Poly-L-ornithine (PLO) is another noteworthy poly(amino acid), which shows many similarities with PLL but has been shown to exhibit a tenfold higher transfection efficiency. Ramsay and Gumbleton determined that PLO condenses pDNA at lower positive/negative charge ratios compared to PLL (Gumbleton, 2002). Furthermore, PLO/pDNA complexes were more resistant to disruption than PLL/pDNA complexes at the same polycation/pDNA mass ratio (Cai et al., 2023). Despite these advantages, like other positively charged poly(amino acid)s, PLO faces limitations in facilitating endosomal escape, which continues to restrict its overall transfection efficiency.

4.3. Polyesters

Poly(beta-amino ester)s (PβAEs) are biodegradable cationic polymers studied for nucleic acid and drug delivery extensively due to their high transfection efficiency, effective endosomal escape, and stimuli-responsive release characteristics (Lynn et al., 2001). PβAE copolymers are typically synthesized through a Michael addition reaction and developed using three main strategies (Iqbal and Zhao, 2022):

1. **Controlled polymerization**, where acrylate or amine-terminated precursors are end-capped with specific agents to form linear PβAEs.
2. **Functionalization**, which involves reacting amine-capped PβAEs with diverse functional molecules to yield copolymers under tailored conditions.
3. **Nanoparticle formation**, stable nanoparticles are formed at optimized copolymer-to-nucleic acid ratios through electrostatic interactions to improve cellular uptake and gene expression.

The first high-throughput PβAE library was introduced by Lynn et al. in 2001, synthesizing 140 variants from 7 diacrylates and 20 amines. Building upon this, Anderson et al. developed a second-generation library in 2005, comprising 486 polymers with 70 distinct structures of polymers varied molecular weights (Cordeiro et al., 2019). These were systematically designed from monomers previously identified as having high transfection efficiency.

Beyond favourable physicochemical properties, structure activity relationship (SAR) studies have become critical in guiding the rational design of PβAEs. Minor modifications to the polymer backbone, side chains, or end-groups can substantially impact key parameters that influence nanoparticle formation, cellular uptake, and intracellular gene release, including molecular weight, hydrophobicity, and charge density. For example, increased hydrophobicity can enhance membrane interaction, while disulfide bonds promote reductive degradation inside cells. Similarly, tertiary amines in the polymer backbone contribute to the "proton sponge" effect, facilitating endosomal escape (Iqbal et al., 2020).

A recent SAR study by Luly et al. evaluated four PβAE polymers with distinct backbone (B), side chain (S), and end-cap (E) combinations (Luly et al., 2022). The copolymer comprising 1,4-butanediol diacrylate (B), 4-amino-1-butanol (S), and 2-(3-aminopropylamino)ethanol (E) demonstrated superior transfection efficiency in HEK 293F and CHO-S cell lines, outperforming 25 kDa PEI. This success arose from optimized nanoparticle characteristics that combined a reduced particle size of 200 to 350 nanometers with an elevated zeta potential and enhanced endosomal escape, all driven by an increased density of protonatable amines. Moreover, despite minor increase in cytotoxicity at higher doses, the polymer maintained a favourable safety-efficacy balance, yielding 4.5- to 8.2-fold higher recombinant protein production across varying scales.

Importantly, end-group modifications have been identified as particularly influential in determining transfection performance. In a pivotal study by Sunshine et al., libraries of linear PβAEs were synthesized with varied backbones, side chains, and end-groups (Elzeny et al., 2017). Despite forming nanoparticles of similar size (~130–150 nm) and surface charge (+21 to +29 mV), gene delivery efficiency was strongly influenced by the end-group structure. Variants terminated with acrylate exhibited negligible uptake and transfection, while amine-capped polymers with 2-(3-aminopropylamino)ethanol achieved between 75 and 94 percent cellular uptake and up to 89% transfection in COS-7 cells. Although PEI exhibited stronger buffering per unit mass, the lower cytotoxicity of PβAEs allowed higher dosing, leading to a greater overall buffering effect and improved gene delivery.

In a recent study, Bayraktutan et al., developed polysarcosine-functionalized cationic poly(β-amino ester)s (pSar-PBAEs) to enhance the delivery of self-amplifying mRNA (saRNA) (Bayraktutan et al., 2024). To address the limitations of existing polyplex systems such as toxicity and PEG-induced reactogenicity, they synthesized triblock copolymers by conjugating polysarcosine to both ends of PBAE chains. Polyplexes containing varying ratios of pSar-modified and unmodified PBAEs (0–100%) were prepared and evaluated for RNA encapsulation efficiency, particle size, and in vitro transfection capacity. The formulations achieved complete RNA encapsulation and <200 nm particle sizes, with the 50% pSar-containing formulation showing the highest reporter gene expression in Caco-2 cells. Further studies in 3D colorectal cancer organoids demonstrated efficient core penetration and high transfection levels. These results underline the significance of pSarylated PBAEs as effective synthetic cationic polymers for improving nucleic acid delivery in gene therapy.

Despite their advantages, PβAEs face challenges including serum instability and potential cytotoxicity, which have prompted strategies like PEGylation and copolymerization to enhance biocompatibility and targeting. These developments position PβAE-based systems as promising non-viral vectors for gene therapy and controlled drug release, with SAR-guided engineering playing a pivotal role in their continued optimization.

PHP (Poly(4-hydroxy-L-proline ester)), a positively charged, biodegradable and water-soluble polyester derived from natural sources like collagen and gelatine, has emerged as a promising nucleic acid vector because of its ability to form stable electrostatic complexes with DNA. Although PHP loses 50% of its molecular weight within two hours under physiological conditions, it ultimately degrades completely into monomeric hydroxyproline over a three-month period (Cai et al., 2023; Stanford, 2013). Li and Huang developed and evaluated a copolymer poly(D,L-lactide-co-4-hydroxy-L-proline) (PLHP) for its potential use as a sustained gene delivery vector (Stanford, 2013). pDNA was encapsulated within PLHP-based microspheres using a solvent evaporation and emulsion method. The release profile of pDNA from these microspheres showed an initial burst release, followed by a sustained and gradual release that extended up to 18 days. In comparison to widely utilized carriers such as PEI and PLL, the PLHP/pDNA formulation exhibited prolonged gene expression activity lasting over one week. These findings suggest that PLHP is a promising candidate for long-term gene delivery applications, owing to its favourable biodegradability and biocompatibility.

Polyphosphoester (PPE) based systems are among the most promising carriers in gene therapy due to their biodegradable structure and biocompatibility. Containing phosphoester bonds in their backbone, PPEs can be readily degraded under physiological conditions through enzymatic or chemical hydrolysis, allowing for controlled release of genetic material. Cationic PPE polymers are particularly effective at forming stable complexes with polyanionic molecules through electrostatic interactions, with siRNA and plasmid DNA being common examples. These complexes can efficiently deliver genetic cargo to target cells and sustain gene expression in the serum media, without the need for another transfection agent (Elzeny et al., 2017; Tambe et al., 2019). Elzeny et al., synthesized cationic PPE nanoparticles and successfully complexed with siRNA to form stable nanocarriers. These PPE-siRNA complexes maintained their structural integrity in physiological conditions and demonstrated efficient in vivo gene delivery in mice through IV injection. Compared to PEI, PPEs exhibited superior safety; animal mortality was observed even at doses more than 130 mg/kg, whereas PEI showed an LD_{50} of approximately 61.7 mg/kg (Elzeny et al., 2017). Similarly, Wen et al. developed a cationic PPE derivative named (poly{[(cholesteryl oxocarbonylamido ethyl) methyl bis(ethylene) ammonium iodide] ethyl phosphate}) (PCEP), which formed 60–80 nm micelles with positive surface charge. These PPE micelles were able to effectively condense plasmid DNA, protect it from degradation, and transfect various cell lines including HEK293, Caco-2, and HeLa cells. Their results demonstrated strong transfection efficiency without triggering significant cytotoxicity, indicating their promise for non-viral gene delivery applications. These findings collectively underline PPEs as highly versatile carriers in gene delivery providing low toxicity, tuneable surface properties, and the capacity for multi-modal therapeutic payloads. Their potential extends beyond siRNA or plasmid DNA delivery to gene–drug combination strategies, opening new avenues in precision medicine and cancer therapeutics (Tambe et al., 2019).

Oligo(carbonate-b-α-amino ester)s. Charge-altering releasable transporters (CART)s, a class of synthetic polymers with cationic properties engineered to package, protect, and deliver mRNA into target cells with high efficiency. Unlike traditional lipid nanoparticles (LNPs), CARTs undergo a dynamic charge-altering degradation process, transitioning from polycationic carriers into neutral byproducts upon cellular entry. This unique feature facilitates endosomal escape and efficient mRNA release while minimizing cytotoxicity, thereby making CARTs a compelling alternative platform for therapeutic applications. Notably, Wilk et al. demonstrated that CARTs can be successfully used to generate cytotoxic primary anti-CD19 chimeric antigen receptor natural killer (CAR NK) cells while maintaining their native phenotype (Wilk et al., 2020). This result marks an important step forward in successfully delivering genetic material into resting primary human NK cells and highlights the promise of CARTs for future clinical applications involving this challenging lymphocyte type.

Building upon this foundation, several specialized CART variants have been developed to enhance cell-type specificity and functionality. For instance, β-amido carbonate-based CARTs (bAC-CARTs), reported by Li et al., incorporate a biodegradable backbone that improves mRNA transfection efficiency in T cells (Li et al., 2023). Oleyl/nonenyl amphiphilic CARTs (ONA-CARTs), developed by Wilk et al., feature hydrophobic lipid blocks that are specifically optimized for delivery to NK cells (Tambe et al., 2019). Among the most innovative designs are difluoroboron diketonate (BDK)-tagged CARTs (BDK-CARTs), described by Haabeth et al., which combine fluorescent tracking capability with potent delivery performance

(Haabeth et al., 2018). These oligo(carbonate-b-α-amino ester) structures self-assemble with mRNA under mildly acidic conditions (pH 5.5) and release their cargo intracellularly through pH-triggered degradation into neutral, biocompatible byproducts. BDK-CARTs have shown exceptional spleen-targeting efficiency (>90% localization) and achieved high transfection rates in immune cells—approximately 50% in dendritic cells and 25% in B cells. Furthermore, when co-delivered with a CpG oligonucleotide adjuvant, they treated 40% of tumour-bearing mice after only three low-dose administrations, demonstrating significant potential in cancer immunotherapy.

Despite their advantages, which include real-time tracking through BDK fluorescence and low toxicity, BDK-CARTs also exhibit certain limitations. These include limited transfection efficiency in hepatocytes (<5%) and the need for acidic formulation, which may complicate clinical translation. Additionally, while the BDK moiety enhances experimental visualization, its potential immunogenicity poses challenges for human use. Nonetheless, BDK-CARTs have outperformed peptide vaccines in preclinical models, particularly in activating tumour-specific T cells without the use of viral vectors or electroporation (Haabeth et al., 2018). These advancements illustrate the versatility and promise of CART-based systems as next-generation delivery platforms for mRNA therapeutics, with broad applications across immunotherapy, gene editing, and cell engineering.

4.4. Poly(amidoamid)s (PAMAM)s

Dendrimers are a unique type of nano biopolymers known as highly promising nanocarriers for targeted drug and nucleic acid delivery. These synthetic macromolecules, named from the Greek word "dendron" meaning tree, feature distinctive multiple branched layers. Dendrimers have the advantage of being monodisperse, meaning each molecule shows identical globular well-defined shape and size after their synthesis, unlike other polymers that result from uncontrolled polymerization (Grund et al., 2011; Tang et al., 1996). A typical dendrimer comprises three key components: a central core, which serves as the starting point of synthesis and is often a multifunctional molecule; branching units that extend outward from the core in repetitive layers known as "generations"; and terminal functional groups on the surface, which vary depending on the synthesis method and the dendrimer's generation (Kalomiraki et al., 2015). This precise architecture indicates their potential in advanced medical applications. Dendrimers with positively charged surfaces effectively bind to negatively charged biological membranes, enhancing their utility for delivering therapeutics inside cells. However, this characteristic can also lead to toxic effects, such as cytotoxicity and haemolysis. To mitigate these issues, the dendrimer surface can be altered with substances like carbohydrates, PEG, or acetate, which help neutralize the positive charge and reduce toxicity. Beyond drug delivery, this versatility also enables the use of dendrimers as gene carriers (Markowicz-Piasecka and Mikiciuk-Olasik, 2016). Cationic dendrimers including PLL, PPI, and PAMAM can interact with polyanionic DNA to form stable polyplexes. Additionally, microRNA and siRNA delivery employ predominantly five cationic dendrimer classes (PLL, PPI, PAMAM, carbosilane [CBS] and phosphorus dendrimers).

Among dendritic polymers, PAMAM dendrimers represent the most extensively studied class due to their synthetic versatility and commercial availability (Nguyen and Szoka, 2012). These highly branched nanostructures are typically constructed around core molecules ranging from simple linear amines (e.g., ethylenediamine or diaminobutane) to more complex branched architectures (e.g., triethanolamine) or synthetic scaffolds like polyphenylene-vinylidenes. The characteristic branching pattern emerges from nitrogen junction points connected by aliphatic aminoamide chains, with terminal primary amines providing critical nucleic acid binding functionality.

Notably, structural modifications influence dendrimer performance. Szoka and colleagues proposed that partially degraded ("fractured") PAMAM dendrimers exhibit remarkable (>50-fold) improvements in transfection efficiency compared to their intact counterparts, attributable to their more flexible, open architectures. This finding sparked considerable interest in engineering PAMAM derivatives that combine advantageous features from both synthetic and biological systems to create optimized nucleic acid carriers (Stanford, 2013).

Core modifications represent another powerful strategy for enhancing gene delivery. Tomalia and colleagues demonstrated this principle through the development of lipid-cored PAMAM dendrimers, which exhibit fundamentally different membrane interaction capabilities compared to traditional ammonia- or ethylenediamine-cored variants. Diaminododecane-cored dendrimers stand out depending on their architecture supports interactions with phospholipids and surfactants on both the surface and within internal cavities, a functionality that conventional dendrimers confined to external binding lack. This dual interaction mode provides superior membrane affinity, positioning these modified dendrimers as particularly promising candidates for advanced gene delivery applications.

However, not every PAMAM is a dendrimer; for example, Gurnani et al. optimized the synthesis of poly(cystamine bisacrylamide-co-4-amino-1-butanol) (pABOL), a PAMAM-based polymer, to improve its efficacy as a delivery vector for self-amplifying RNA (Gurnani et al., 2020a). Conventional PAMAM synthesis methods are frequently time-consuming and inefficient; so, they set a microwave-assisted method that reduced polymerization time from 48 hours to 4 hours while preserving repeatability. The optimized synthesis conditions produced low-viscosity polymer solutions, which facilitated scalability and large-scale production. To assess the biological efficacy of pABOL, transfection studies were performed using the HEK293T cell line and a luciferase-encoding saRNA model. The research showed that pABOL successfully formed polyplexes with saRNA, facilitating effective gene delivery. The data revealed that pABOL polymers with well-defined molecular weights and low dispersity achieved the highest transfection efficiency, while those with wider molecular weight ranges displayed diminished performance. These results underscore potential of pABOL as a robust gene delivery vehicle, positioning it as a valuable candidate for RNA vaccine development and nucleic acid therapeutics.

4.5. Poly(methacrylate)s

Poly(methacrylate)s have gained attention as effective synthetic cationic gene carriers due to their tuneable physicochemical properties, ability to condense nucleic acids, and potential for endosomal escape. These polymers confer ease of synthesis, structural versatility, and reduced immunogenicity relative to viral vectors. This section explores the role of poly(methacrylate)-based polymers in gene therapy, highlighting their mechanisms, advantages, and recent developments in the field (Rungsardthong et al., 2001).

Among polyelectrolytes with low cationic strength, Poly(2-(dimethylamino)ethyl methacrylate) (PDMAEMA) has been extensively studied as a gene delivery vector. Their tertiary amine side groups enable the effective condensation of genetic material into nanoparticles, which aids cellular absorption. PDMAEMA-based polymers provide transfection efficiency equivalent to the "gold standard" branching polyethyleneimine (PEI, 25 kDa) while being less toxic (Góis et al., 2018). Advances in polymerization methods, notably Atom Transfer Radical Polymerization (ATRP), have permitted the synthesis of a wide range of PDMAEMA topologies, including linear copolymers, star-shaped, comb-like, and branching structures. Olden et al. demonstrated that comb polymers grafted with PDMAEMA exhibit impressive cell viability and transfection efficiency in human T-cell transfection experiments. The effectiveness of these comb polymers in nucleic acid delivery has prompted interest in combining them with physical delivery methods including sonoporation, to improve in vivo performance (Khan, 2024).

Poly(2-(diisopropylamino) ethyl methacrylate) (PDPA), another promising methacrylate derivative, displays a pH-dependent transition from hydrophilic to hydrophobic behaviour around a pH of 6.2. This property makes it particularly appealing for biomedical applications. PDPA-based copolymers have been employed in non-viral gene delivery systems, leveraging their ability to form micellar nanoparticles and pH-responsive polymersomes for effective DNA encapsulation. Baptista et al. developed pH-responsive nanoparticles based on POEOMA-b-PDPA block copolymers for RNA encapsulation, protection, and intracellular delivery (Baptista et al., 2023). The PDPA block provided pH sensitivity, enabling RNA complexation under acidic conditions due to the protonation of its tertiary amines, while the POEOMA segment enhanced solubility and stability. The copolymers demonstrated high encapsulation efficiencies (~89–91%) and successfully protected RNA from enzymatic degradation. Moreover, transfection studies in A549 lung cancer cells showed effective RNA delivery and gene silencing. These findings identify POEOMA-b-PDPA as a promising non-viral gene carrier and underscore its suitability for pH-dependent applications in cancer therapy.

While POEOMA-b-PDPA block copolymers provide pH-responsive behaviour for RNA delivery, their charge transition is limited to cationic-to-neutral/hydrophobic conversion at physiological pH. In contrast, acrylate-based polyelectrolytes exhibit true charge reversal, where their surface charge shifts from cationic to anionic depending on the environmental pH. This property is particularly advantageous for gene delivery, as it allows for strong electrostatic interactions during complexation, followed by triggered release under specific physiological conditions. Charge-reversible nanoparticles have gained significant attention in drug delivery and diagnostic applications due to their ability to dynamically alter their surface charge in response to environmental stimuli (Veider et al., 2024). At the end of this section, we will mention about acrylate-based polymers with charge reversal capabilities and their implications for advanced gene delivery systems. This transition offers a key advantage in navigating biological barriers. For example, negatively charged nanoparticles can avoid early clearance and immune detection, while their ability to switch to a cationic state in response to specific stimuli enhances cellular uptake, endosomal escape, and precise drug delivery. This approach effectively resolves the "polycation dilemma", where traditional cationic NPs achieve strong cellular uptake but are hindered by toxicity and quick elimination from the body. Ros et al. developed polycations based on N,N-(dimethylamino)ethyl acrylate (DMAEA) that undergo hydrolysis-driven charge shifting to improve DNA delivery while reducing toxicity (Ros et al., 2020). Initially, these copolymers have a high cationic charge for effective DNA binding and cellular uptake. At physiological pH, hydrolysis transforms the DMAEA side chains into anionic acrylic acid, lowering the cationic charge and forming polyampholytes that lessen the toxicity typical of cationic vectors. Notably, 80 mol% DMAEA achieved ~95% DNA uptake efficiency in HeLa cells, surpassing standard PEI systems with much lower cytotoxicity. This charge-reversal mechanism enabled efficient intracellular DNA release, positioning these copolymers as promising, biocompatible gene delivery carriers. Results highlight the value of charge-shifting strategies in advancing safer, more effective non-viral nucleic acid therapeutics.

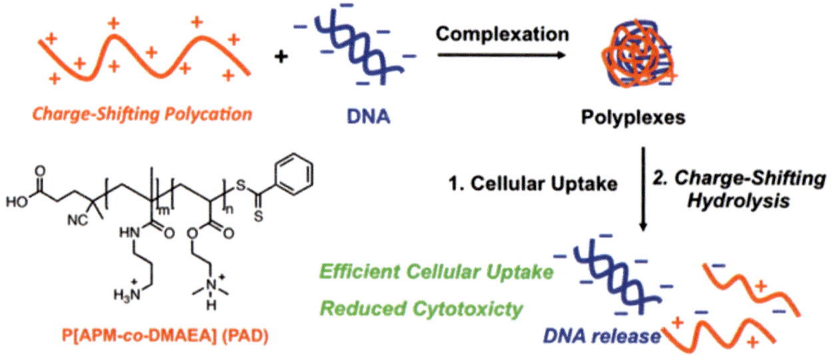

Figure 6. The charge-shifting property of copolymers can enhance intracellular DNA release by weakening electrostatic interactions. Additionally, a decrease in overall cationic charge may help lower cytotoxicity. Reprinted with permission from Ref. (Ros et al., 2020).

In another study, Gurnani et al. synthesized a range of poly(dimethylaminoethyl acrylate) PDMAEA copolymers with varying levels of hydrophobicity and assessed their effectiveness in delivering saRNA (Gurnani et al., 2020b). The charge-reversal mechanism of copolymers, triggered by the hydrolysis of PDMAEA side chains, allowed them to shift from a polycationic to a polyanionic state, promoting efficient RNA release. Copolymers with greater hydrophobicity showed improved polyplex stability and higher transfection efficiency in vitro, while more hydrophilic versions excelled in vivo, achieving better gene expression in mouse models. These results underscore the importance of tuning polymer hydrophobicity in charge-reversible gene carriers, highlighting the necessity of customizing polymer structures to enhance RNA delivery efficiency and biocompatibility across diverse biological media.

Oz et al., reported the polymersome-mediated intracellular delivery of the pro-apoptotic BikDDA gene using two different peptide-copolymer covalent conjugation strategies for prostate cancer targeting (Oz et al., 2020). They used the BikDDA gene as a therapeutic agent on prostate cancer cells and employed poly[oligo(ethyleneglycol) methacrylate]-co-poly[2-(diisopropylamino) ethyl methacrylate] ($P(OEG_{10}MA)_{20}–PDPA_{100}$) copolymersomes as a non-viral gene transfection tool. The targeted delivery of BikDDA into prostate cancer cells (LNCaP) was achieved by conjugating the PSMA-targeting moiety (peptide 563) to the $P(OEG10MA)_{20}–PDPA_{100}$ copolymer using either succinimidyl 4-(N-maleimidomethyl)cyclohexane-1-carboxylate (SMCC) as a bifunctional linker or by attaching a maleimide-modified targeting peptide onto a thiol-terminated $P(OEG_{10}MA)_{20}–PDPA_{100}$ copolymer. The results showed that the peptide 563-conjugated polymersomes exhibited enhanced cellular uptake by LNCaP cells compared to healthy prostate cells, indicating cell-specific delivery and increased Bik mRNA expression and cell death in the cancer cells. The authors conclude that these targeted pH-sensitive polymersomes show promise for developing novel therapies against prostate cancer.

4.6. Polymer Hybrids

Hybrid systems are innovative approaches in gene delivery that combine the advantages of different materials to enhance efficiency. Significant attention has been devoted to integrating synthetic cationic polymers PEI and PLL with the natural polymers chitosan and hyaluronic acid. These combinations enhance stability, cellular uptake, and biocompatibility, while reducing cytotoxicity. Polymer-coated nanoparticles and multilayered delivery platforms are designed to optimize gene transfection, offering controlled release and improved therapeutic outcomes (Jiang et al., 2008).

Pinnapireddy et al. developed PEI-based hybrid gene carriers by integrating linear PEI polyplexes with glycosylated artificial viral envelopes (AVE) that mimic the lipid compositions of HIV and HSV viral envelopes (Pinnapireddy et al., 2019). These hybrid vectors were formulated using anionic liposomes providing enhanced stability and serum resistance.

Physicochemical characterization confirmed that the hybrid vectors maintained a size of ~180–200 nm and a net positive surface charge, facilitating efficient cellular uptake. Transfection studies using a luciferase reporter assay demonstrated that glycosylated hybrid vectors exhibited a more than five-fold increase in transfection efficiency relative to PEI. This improvement was ascribed to dual internalization pathways, including clathrin- and caveolae-mediated endocytosis, as confirmed by uptake inhibition studies. Moreover, cytotoxicity and hemocompatibility assessments revealed minimal toxicity (~85% cell viability) and negligible haemolysis or coagulation issues. These PEI-based glycosylated hybrid vectors exhibited superior gene transfection efficiency and improved biocompatibility, positioning them as promising candidates for non-viral synthetic gene delivery applications.

In the mid-1990s, Dr. Mark Davis from the California Institute of Technology designed synthetic polycations utilizing cyclodextrins, which are cyclic glucose-based oligomers (Heidel, 2011). Cyclodextrins, already widely used as drug solubilizers due to their high-dose tolerability, were chemically modified and incorporated into polymers to create cyclodextrin-containing polycations (CDPs). These CDPs spontaneously interact with nucleic acids in solution, forming CDP–NA complexes that enhance cellular uptake and facilitate gene delivery. Building upon the early developments of cyclodextrin-based polycations for gene delivery, Zuckerman et al. designed polycationic cyclodextrin nanoparticles (CDP-NPs) for siRNA delivery to the glomerular mesangium (Zuckerman et al., 2015). These nanoparticles, composed of CDPs complexed with siRNA, were formulated to enable systemic intravenous administration. The study demonstrated that CDP-NPs effectively localized to the glomerular mesangium with minimal deposition in other kidney regions. Moreover, uptake by mesangial cells was significantly enhanced by surface modification with mannose or transferrin ligands, facilitating receptor-mediated internalization. The CDP-NPs successfully delivered siRNA to mesangial cells, leading to target gene knockdown in a reporter mouse model, highlighting their potential as a targeted synthetic gene delivery system.

Shen et al. have developed traceable nano-biohybrid complexes as CRISPR-Chem vectors, introducing a novel strategy for Alzheimer's disease treatment (Shen et al., 2021). The researchers designed a polymeric carrier system based on DOPA-modified poly-lysine (DOPA-PLys) to deliver both CRISPR/Cas9 for BACE1 gene knockout and Fluvastatin for amyloid-beta (Aβ) clearance. This system was further modified with Rabies virus glycoprotein (RVG) to facilitate blood-brain barrier (BBB) penetration, and superparamagnetic iron oxide nanoparticles (SPIONs) were incorporated for MRI traceability.

The resulting CRISPR/Cas9 plasmids loaded nano-biohybrid (CF-TBIO) complexes, with their high-density positive charge, efficiently formed complexes with anionic CRISPR/Cas9 plasmids, enhancing their gene therapy potential. In vitro experiments demonstrated that CF-TBIO successfully crossed the BBB, targeted neurons, and was internalized via receptor-mediated endocytosis. Due to proton sponge effect, CF-TBIO escaped from endosomes, allowing CRISPR/Cas9 to reach the nucleus efficiently. In Alzheimer mouse models, Shen et al. found that CF-TBIO successfully knocked out the BACE1 gene with 41.1% efficiency, reduced Aβ levels, and significantly improved cognitive function. MRI imaging confirmed that CF-TBIO effectively reached target regions and could be tracked in vivo using SPIONs. These findings highlight the potential of synthetic cationic polymers as effective CRISPR delivery systems.

One of the recent studies conducted by Pang et al. introduced PEG-PBAE-His (PPH) polyplexes as a pH-sensitive siRNA delivery platform for lung cancer treatment (Pang et al., 2025). The polyplex consists of PEG for stability, PBAE, synthesized from 4-amino-1-butanol and adipic acid divinyl ester, facilitates siRNA complexation, and histidine (His) for facilitating endosomal escape. At alkaline pH, PPH remains negatively charged, preventing aggregation, while in acidic environments, protonation induces charge reversal, enhancing cellular uptake and endosomal siRNA release for ALK gene silencing. PEI is widely recognized for its toxicity as a vector, that lead to a survival rate of less than 27% in H3122 cells at concentrations over 1 μM. PPH vehicles showed good cell viability throughout concentrations up to 4 μM, indicating low intrinsic cytotoxicity. The study found that inhaling PPH polyplexes substantially reduced lung tumour burden in an orthotopic NSCLC xenograft mice model, as revealed by a significant reduction in bioluminescence imaging (BLI) signals, lower lung weight, and higher survival rates. The ALK knockdown demonstrated 84.5% tumour growth suppression compared to the control group, with therapeutic benefits lasting about a month. Additionally, systemic administration via intravenous injection also inhibited tumour growth, at a slightly lower rate (74.8%), while maintaining body weight and reducing tumour volume. The findings collectively highlight that PPH polyplexes enable efficient siRNA delivery, robust ALK silencing, and substantial tumour suppression in vivo, regardless of the administration route.

5. Clinical Outlook

In vivo and in vitro investigations continue to demonstrate the potential of synthetic cationic polymers as non-viral vectors for various types of DNA and RNA delivery. Nevertheless, their transition to clinical applications has progressed at a slower rate than that of viral vectors, primarily due to several intrinsic limitations. A key constraint is their reduced transfection efficiency in vivo, where synthetic polymers encounter challenges such as instability in serum, rapid systemic clearance, and suboptimal cellular internalization. Moreover, issues related to toxicity and biocompatibility have hampered their broader acceptance. Many cationic polymers, including PEI, exhibit cytotoxicity stemming from their robust electrostatic interactions with cellular membranes, which can result in membrane destabilization and the induction of oxidative stress. Synthetic gene delivery methods approaching clinical implementation primarily consist of phosphorothioate compounds, unencapsulated plasmid DNA, lipid-based systems, and to a lesser extent, polymeric vectors. Several of these approaches have already received approval or are on track for potential approval for human use. The widespread adoption of naked cargo delivery and liposomal drug carriers can likely be attributed to their simplicity and the extensive experience gained from working with liposomal-based systems (Mintzer and Simanek, 2009; Hou et al., 2021; Pack et al., 2005).

A linear positively charged polymer containing cyclodextrin units is capable of binding siRNA by forming complexes and can be functionalized with targeting and stabilizing components through host–guest supramolecular interactions, especially involving adamantane-based linkers. Originally introduced by Mark Davis, this modular approach has been further refined by incorporating non-polymeric cyclodextrins with LMW PEI side chains, which are stabilized using pH-responsive polyketal poly-adamantanes. Additionally, cyclodextrin polymers have been explored for tumour-targeted combination therapies involving both chemotherapeutic agents and plasmid DNA. However, phase I clinical trials have indicated some toxicity associated with these cyclodextrin-based polymer systems (Lostalé-Seijo and Montenegro, 2018).

Another significant barrier is endosomal escape, a critical step in which synthetic vectors exhibit limited efficiency in releasing their nucleic acid payloads into the cytoplasm, often leading to lysosomal degradation prior to nuclear entry. In contrast to viral vectors, which possess naturally evolved mechanisms to overcome such intracellular obstacles, synthetic systems depend on chemical modifications that remain under optimization.

Additionally, the lack of precise targeting specificity poses a further challenge, as many synthetic carriers rely on passive diffusion or non-specific interactions, limiting their capacity to selectively deliver therapeutic genes to specific diseased cells or tissues (Liu et al., 2019; Park et al., 2010). Despite their advantages in cost-effectiveness and scalability relative to viral vectors, synthetic polymers also face regulatory and manufacturing hurdles. The structural heterogeneity of these polymers can complicate clinical application. However, advancements in polymer chemistry through the development of biodegradable pH-responsive carriers are gradually overcoming these limitations. The increasing variety of non-viral materials designed for effective in vivo cell transfection highlights the remarkable synergy between chemistry and biology. These significant advancements drive innovative gene therapy strategies and offer promising prospects for the future of human health (Muhammad et al., 2020; Yin et al., 2013).

6. Conclusion and Future Perspective

Synthetic positively charged polymers have gained attention as viable alternative for viral vectors in gene therapy, primarily because of their adaptable structures, ease of large-scale production, and lower potential to trigger immune responses. Their capacity to form stable complexes with genetic material, enhance internalization by cells, and support the release of nucleic acids from endosomal compartments has positioned them as central elements in non-viral delivery system research (Chen et al., 2013). However, despite significant progress, cytotoxicity, serum instability and limited in vivo transfection efficiency continue to pose obstacles to widespread clinical use.

One of the key achievements of the synthetic cationic gene delivery research has been the development of diverse polymer architectures, including linear, branched, dendritic, and grafted structures, as well as hybrid systems combining synthetic and natural polymers (Schaffert and Wagner, 2008; Malek et al.,2008). These innovations have enabled tailored solutions for specific therapeutic applications. Additionally, PEGylation, biodegradable design, and charge-shifting mechanisms have enhanced biocompatibility while preserving stability and improving targeting capabilities. Notably, some polymer-based systems, particularly those using PEI and cyclodextrins, have advanced to clinical trials, demonstrating potential in cancer therapy and genetic disorders (Chen et al., 2018).

Future research should prioritize precision engineering in polymer design and stimuli-responsive features to fine-tune therapeutic performance. Incorporating cell-specific ligands and harnessing the capabilities of nanotechnology could significantly enhance targeted delivery while reducing off-target side effects. An exciting frontier lies in combining gene-editing tools like CRISPR-Cas9 with smart delivery systems, offering synergistic approaches to address multifactorial diseases. However, overcoming biological barriers, with particular emphasis on endosomal escape and efficient nuclear transport, remains a critical challenge in attaining strong in vivo efficacy. To support clinical translation and reproducibility, standardized manufacturing processes and regulatory frameworks must also be established.

As synthetic cationic polymers advance, integrating them with emerging technologies, namely AI-guided design and high resolution bioimaging, holds significant promise for the future of gene therapy. Through interdisciplinary collaboration and sustained innovation, these platforms are assured not only to meet recent unmet medical needs but to unlock a new era of personalized, transformative therapeutics.

References

Amin, Z.R, Rahimizadeh, M., Eshghi, H., Dehshahri, A., Ramezani, M. (2013). The effect of cationic charge density change on transfection efficiency of Polyethylenimine. *Iran J Basic Med Sci., 16*(2), 150–6

Baptista, B., Oliveira, A.SR, Mendonça P, Serra, A.C, Coelho, J.FJ, Sousa, F. (2023). pH-responsive nanoparticles based on POEOMA-b-PDPA block copolymers for RNA encapsulation, protection and cell delivery. *Biomater Adv., 145*

Bayraktutan, H., Kopiasz, RJ, Elsherbeny, A., Martinez, E.spuga M, Gumus, N., Oz, U.C, et al (2024). Polysarcosine functionalised cationic polyesters efficiently deliver self-amplifying mRNA. *Polym Chem., 15*(18), 1862–76

Bus, T., Traeger, A., Schubert, U.S (2018). The great escape: How cationic polyplexes overcome the endosomal barrier. *J Mater Chem B., 6*(43), 6904–18

Bus, T., Englert, C., Reifarth, M., Borchers, P., Hartlieb, M., Vollrath, A., et al (2017). 3Rd Generation Poly(Ethylene Imine)S for Gene Delivery. *J Mater Chem B., 5*(6), 1258–74

Cai, X., Dou, R., Guo, C., Tang, J., Li, X., Chen, J., et al (2023). Cationic Polymers as Transfection Reagents for Nucleic Acid Delivery. *Pharmaceutics., 15*(5), 1–24

Chakraborty, D., Ethiraj, K.R, Mukherjee, A. (2020). Understanding the relevance of protein corona in nanoparticle-based therapeutics and diagnostics. *RSC Adv., 10*(45), 27161–72

Chen, X., Tian, H., Guan, X. (2015). Polymeric Gene Carriers. *Wiley Blackwell 6., 9783527334*, 171–202

Chen, W., Hong, Y., Zhang, T., Kong, D., Zhang, M., Zhang, Q., et al (2019). Star-shaped poly(2-aminoethyl methacrylate)s as non-viral gene carriers: Exploring structure-function relationship. *Colloids Surfaces B Biointerfaces., 181*. https://doi.org/10.1016/j.colsurfb.2019.06.029

Chen, C.K, Jones, C.H, Mistriotis, P., Yu, Y., Ma, X., Ravikrishnan, A., et al (2013). Poly(ethylene glycol)-block-cationic polylactide nanocomplexes of differing charge density for gene delivery. *Biomaterials, 34*(37), 9688–99. https://doi.org/10.1016/j.biomaterials.2013.08.063

Chen, J., Wang, K., Wu, J., Tian, H., Chen, X. (2018). Polycations for Gene Delivery: Dilemmas and Solutions. *Bioconjug Chem., 30*(2), 338–49

Cordeiro, RA, Serra, A., Coelho, J.FJ, Faneca, H. (2019). Poly(β-amino ester)-based gene delivery systems: From discovery to therapeutic applications. *J Control Release, 310*. https://doi.org/10.1016/j.jconrel.2019.08.024

Danielsen, S., Maurstad, G., Stokke, B.T (2005). DNA-polycation complexation polyplex stability in the presence of competing polyanions. *Biopolymers., 77*(2), 86–97

Dosta, P., Segovia, N., Cascante, A., Ramos, V., Borrós S (2015). Surface charge tunability as a powerful strategy to control electrostatic interaction for high efficiency silencing, using tailored oligopeptide-modified poly(beta-amino ester)s (PBAEs). *Acta Biomater, 20*, 82–93. https://doi.org/10.1016/j.actbio.2015.03.029

Dzmitruk, V., Apartsin, E., Ihnatsyeu-Kachan, A., Abashkin, V., Shcharbin, D., Bryszewska, M. (2018). Dendrimers show promise for siRNA and microrna therapeutics. *Pharmaceutics., 10*(3), 1–25

Elzeny, H., Zhang, F., Ali, E.N, Fathi, H.A, Zhang, S., Li, R., et al (2017). Polyphosphoester nanoparticles as biodegradable platform for delivery of multiple drugs and siRNA. *Drug Des Devel Ther, 11*, 483–96. https://doi.org/10.2147/DDDT.S128503

Fornaguera, C., Guerra-Rebollo, M., Lázaro MÁ, Cascante, A., Rubio, N., Blanco, J., et al (2019). In Vivo Retargeting of Poly(beta aminoester) (OM-PBAE) Nanoparticles is Influenced by Protein Corona. *Adv Healthc Mater., 8*(19), 1–11

Fu, C., Sun, X., Liu, D., Chen, Z., Lu, Z., Zhang, N. (2011). Biodegradable tri-block copolymer poly(lactic acid)-poly(ethylene glycol)-poly(L-lysine)(PLA-PEG-PLL) as a non-viral vector to enhance gene transfection. *Int J Mol Sci., 12*(2), 1371–88

Gillard, M., Jia, Z., Hou, JJC, Song, M., Gray, P.P, Munro, T.P, et al (2014). Intracellular trafficking pathways for nuclear delivery of plasmid DNA complexed with highly efficient endosome escape polymers. *Biomacromolecules., 15*(10), 3569–76

Grund, S., Bauer, M., Fischer, D. (2011). Polymers in drug delivery-state of the art and future trends. *Adv Eng Mater., 13*(3), 61–87

GUMBLETON ER and M (2002). Polylysine and Polyornithine Gene Transfer Complexes: A Study of Complex Stability and Cellular Uptake as a Basis for their Differential in-vitro Transfection Efficienc. *J Drug Target., 10*(1), 11–21

Gupta, A., Andresen, J.L, Manan, R.S, Langer, R. (2021). Nucleic acid delivery for therapeutic applications. *Adv Drug Deliv Rev, 178*, 113834. https://doi.org/10.1016/j.addr.2021.113834

Gurnani, P., Blakney, A.K, Yeow, J., Bouton, C.R, Shattock, R.J, Stevens, M.M, et al (2020a). An improved synthesis of poly(amidoamine)s for complexation with self-amplifying RNA and effective transfection. *Polym Chem., 11*(36), 5861–9

Gurnani, P., Blakney, A.K, Terracciano, R., Petch, J.E, Blok, A.J, Bouton, C.R, et al (2020b). The in Vitro, Ex Vivo, and in Vivo Effect of Polymer Hydrophobicity on Charge-Reversible Vectors for Self-Amplifying RNA. *Biomacromolecules., 21*(8), 3242–53

Góis JR, Reis, F., Almeida, A.M, Pereira, P., Sousa, F., Serra, A.C, et al (2018). Preparation of well-defined brush-like block copolymers for gene delivery applications under biorelevant reaction conditions. *Colloids Surfaces B Biointerfaces, 169*, 107–17. https://doi.org/10.1016/j.colsurfb.2018.05.004

Haabeth, O.AW, Blake, T.R, McKinlay, C.J, Waymouth, R.M, Wender, P.A, Levy, R. (2018). mRNA vaccination with charge-altering releasable transporters elicits human T cell responses and cures established tumors in mice. *Proc Natl Acad Sci U S A., 115*(39)

HE T, LF L, GJ D, WT W, SC C, ML K, et al (2012). Pro-opiomelanocortin gene delivery suppresses the growth of established Lewis lung carcinoma through a melanocortin-1 receptor-independent pathway. *J Gene Med., 14*(1), 44–53

Heidel, J.D (2011). Cyclodextrin-containing polycations for nucleic acid delivery. *Cold Spring Harb Protoc., 6*(11), 1319–22

Heights, V., Data, R.USA, Classiflcation, P. (2023). (19) United States (U) Patent Application Publication oltIehruse Polymer.

Hou, X., Zaks, T., Langer, R., Dong, Y. (2021). Lipid nanoparticles for mRNA delivery. *Nat Rev Mater, 6*(12), 1078–94. https://doi.org/10.1038/s41578-021-00358-0

Hynynen, K. (2008). Ultrasound for drug and gene delivery to the brain. *Adv Drug Deliv Rev., 60*(10), 1209–17

Iqbal, S., Zhao, Z. (2022). Poly (β amino esters) copolymers: Novel potential vectors for delivery of genes and related therapeutics. *Int J Pharm, 611*. https://doi.org/10.1016/j.ijpharm.2021.121289

Iqbal, S., Qu, Y., Dong, Z., Zhao, J., Rauf, K.han A, Rehman, S., et al (2020). Poly (β-amino esters) based potential drug delivery and targeting polymer; an overview and perspectives (review). *Eur Polym J, 141*. https://doi.org/10.1016/j.eurpolymj.2020.110097

Itaka, K., Ishii, T., Hasegawa, Y., Kataoka, K. (2010). Biodegradable polyamino acid-based polycations as safe and effective gene carrier minimizing cumulative toxicity. *Biomaterials, 31*(13), 3707–14. https://doi.org/10.1016/j.biomaterials.2009.11.072

Jiang, H.L, Kim, T.H, Kim, Y.K, Park, I.Y, Cho, M.H, Cho, C.S (2008). Efficient gene delivery using chitosan-polyethylenimine hybrid systems. *Biomed Mater., 3*(2), 25013

Kalomiraki, M., Thermos, K., Chaniotakis, N.A (2015). Dendrimers as tunable vectors of drug delivery systems and biomedical and ocular applications. *Int J Nanomedicine., 11*, 1–12

Kataoka, K., Harada, A., Nagasaki, Y. (2012). Block copolymer micelles for drug delivery: Design, characterization and biological significance. *Adv Drug Deliv Rev., 64*

Khan, M. (2024). Polymers as Efficient Non-Viral Gene Delivery Vectors: The Role of the Chemical and Physical Architecture of Macromolecules. *Vol. 16, Polymers.,*

Kristi, L. (2017). Stringer, Bulent Turan, Lisa McCormick, Modupeoluwa Durojaiye, Laura Nyblade, Mirjam-Colette Kempf, Bronwen Lichtenstein and JMT. *HHS Public Access. Physiol Behav., 176*(3), 139–48

Kumar, R., Santa, C.halarca CF, Bockman, M.R, Bruggen, C. Van, Grimme, C.J, Dalal, R.J, et al (2021). Polymeric Delivery of Therapeutic Nucleic Acids. *Chem Rev., 121*(18), 11527–652

Li, Z., Amaya, L., Pi, R., Wang, S.K, Ranjan, A., Waymouth, R.M, et al (2023). Charge-altering releasable transporters enhance mRNA delivery in vitro and exhibit in vivo tropism. *Nat Commun., 14*(1)

Liu, Z., Zhang, Z., Zhou, C., Jiao, Y. (2010). Hydrophobic modifications of cationic polymers for gene delivery. *Prog Polym Sci, 35*(9), 1144–62. https://doi.org/10.1016/j.progpolymsci.2010.04.007

Liu, Y., Li, Y., Keskin, D., Shi, L. (2019). Poly(β-Amino Esters): Synthesis, Formulations, and Their Biomedical Applications. *Adv Healthc Mater., 8*(2), 1–24

Liu, Y., Zhao, N., Xu, F.J (2019). PH-Responsive Degradable Dextran-Quantum Dot Nanohybrids for Enhanced Gene Delivery. *ACS Appl Mater Interfaces., 11*(38), 34707–16

Lostalé-Seijo, I., Montenegro, J. (2018). Synthetic materials at the forefront of gene delivery. *Nat Rev Chem., 2*(10), 258–77. https://doi.org/10.1038/s41570-018-0039-1

Lu, B., Wang, C.F, Wu, D.Q, Li, C., Zhang, X.Z, Zhuo, R.X (2009). Chitosan based oligoamine polymers: Synthesis, characterization, and gene delivery. *J Control Release, 137*(1), 54–62. https://doi.org/10.1016/j.jconrel.2009.03.004

Luly, K.M, Yang, H., Lee, S.J, Wang, W., Ludwig, S.D, Tarbox, H.E, et al (2022). Poly(Beta-Amino Ester)s as High-Yield Transfection Reagents for Recombinant Protein Production. *Int J Nanomedicine., 17*

Lv, H., Zhang, S., Wang, B., Cui, S., Yan, J. (2006). Toxicity of cationic lipids and cationic polymers in gene delivery. *J Control Release., 114*(1), 100–9

Lynn, D.M, Anderson, D.G, Putnam, D., Langer, R. (2001). Accelerated discovery of synthetic transfection vectors: Parallel synthesis and screening of a degradable polymer library [20]. *J Am Chem Soc., 123*(33), 8155–6

Ma, K., Mi, C.L, Cao, X.X, Wang, T.Y (2021). Progress of cationic gene delivery reagents for non-viral vector. *Appl Microbiol Biotechnol., 105*(2), 525–38

Maiolo, D., Colombo, J., Beretta, J., Malloggi, C., Candiani, G., Baldelli, B.ombelli F (2018). The polyplex, protein corona, cell interplay: Tips and drawbacks. *Colloids Surfaces B Biointerfaces, 168*, 60–7. https://doi.org/10.1016/j.colsurfb.2018.01.040

Malek, A., Czubayko, F., Aigner, A. (2008). PEG grafting of polyethylenimine (PEI) exerts different effects on DNA transfection and siRNA-induced gene targeting efficacy. *J Drug Target., 16*(2), 124–39

Markowicz-Piasecka, M., Mikiciuk-Olasik, E. (2016). Dendrimers in drug delivery. *Nanobiomaterials in Drug Delivery: Applications of Nanobiomaterials.,*

Mintzer, M.A, Simanek, E.E (2009). Nonviral vectors for gene delivery. *Chem Rev., 109*(2), 259–302

Muhammad, K., Zhao, J., Ullah, I., Guo, J., Ren, X.K, Feng, Y. (2020). Ligand targeting and peptide functionalized polymers as non-viral carriers for gene therapy. *Biomater Sci., 8*(1), 64–83

Nguyen, J., Szoka, F.C (2012). Nucleic acid delivery: The missing pieces of the puzzle? Acc Chem Res. ,

Olden, B.R, Cheng, Y., Yu, J.L, Pun, S.H (2018). Cationic polymers for non-viral gene delivery to human T cells. *J Control Release, 282*. https://doi.org/10.1016/j.jconrel.2018.02.043

OTMANE BOUSSIF*, FRANK LEZOUALC'Ht, MARLA ANTONIETrA ZANTA* MDMergny, DANIEL SCHERMANt, BARBARA DEMENEIXt, A.J-PB (1995). A versatile vector for gene and oligonucleotide transfer into cells in culture and in vivo: Polyethylenimine. *Proc Natl Acad Sci USA Vol 92, pp,* -7301

Oz, U.C, Bolat, Z.B, Poma, A., Guan, L., Telci, D., Sahin, F., et al (2020). Prostate cancer cell-specific BikDDA delivery by targeted polymersomes. *Appl Nanosci, 10*(9), 3389–401. https://doi.org/10.1007/s13204-020-01287-0

Pack, D.W, Hoffman, A.S, Pun, S., Stayton, P.S (2005). Design and development of polymers for gene delivery. *Nat Rev Drug Discov., 4*(7), 581–93

Pan, X., Veroniaina, H., Su, N., Sha, K., Jiang, F., Wu, Z., et al (2021). Applications and developments of gene therapy drug delivery systems for genetic diseases. *Asian J Pharm Sci, 16*(6), 687–703. https://doi.org/10.1016/j.ajps.2021.05.003

Pang, J., Chen, X., Lin, Z., Yao, S., Wang, W., Wu, H. (2025). Inhalable pH-responsive charge-reversal polymer-small interfering RNA polyplexes for directed gene therapy of anaplastic lymphoma kinase fusion-positive lung cancer. *J Control Release, 381*. https://doi.org/10.1016/j.jconrel.2025.113644

Park, I.K, Singha, K., Arote, R.B, Choi, Y.J, Kim, W.J, Cho, C.S (2010). PH-responsive polymers as gene carriers. *Macromol Rapid Commun., 31*(13), 1122–33

Patel, S., Ashwanikumar, N., Robinson, E., Xia, Y., Mihai, C., Griffith, J.P, et al (2020). Naturally-occurring cholesterol analogues in lipid nanoparticles induce polymorphic shape and enhance intracellular delivery of mRNA. *Nat Commun., 11*(1), 1–13

Pinnapireddy, S.R, El, A.ssy MR, Schlote, P., Bakowsky, U. (2019). Glycosylated artificial virus-like hybrid vectors for advanced gene delivery. *Polymers (Basel)., 11*(2), 1–9

Piotrowski-Daspit, A.S, Kauffman, A.C, Bracaglia, L.G, Saltzman, W.M (2020). Polymeric vehicles for nucleic acid delivery. *Adv Drug Deliv Rev., 156*, 119–32

Pishavar, E., Attaranzadeh, A., Alibolandi, M., Ramezani, M., Hashemi, M. (2018). Modified PAMAM vehicles for effective TRAIL gene delivery to colon adenocarcinoma: in vitro and in vivo evaluation. *Artif Cells, Nanomedicine Biotechnol, 46*. https://doi.org/10.1080/21691401.2018.1500372

Porello, I., Bono, N., Candiani, G., Cellesi, F. (2024). Advancing nucleic acid delivery through cationic polymer design: non-cationic building blocks from the toolbox. *Polym Chem., 15*(28), 2800–26

Riera, R., Feiner-Gracia, N., Fornaguera, C., Cascante, A., Borrós S, Albertazzi, L. (2019). Tracking the DNA complexation state of pBAE polyplexes in cells with super resolution microscopy. *Nanoscale., 11*(38), 17869–77

Ros, S., Freitag, J.S, Smith, D.M, Stöver HDH (2020). Charge-Shifting Polycations Based on N, N-(dimethylamino)ethyl Acrylate for Improving Cytocompatibility during DNA Delivery. *ACS Omega., 5*(16), 9114–22

Rungsardthong, U., Deshpande, M., Bailey, L., Vamvakaki, M., Armes, S.P, Garnett, M.C, et al (2001). Copolymers of amine methacrylate with poly(ethylene glycol) as vectors for gene therapy. *J Control Release., 73*

Samal, S.K, Dash, M., Vlierberghe, S. Van, Kaplan, D.L, Chiellini, E., Blitterswijk, C. van, et al (2012). Cationic polymers and their therapeutic potential. *Chem Soc Rev., 41*(21), 7147–94

Schaffert, D., Wagner, E. (2008). Gene therapy progress and prospects: Synthetic polymer-based systems. *Gene Ther., 15*(16), 1131–8

Sharma, D., Arora, S., Singh, J., Layek, B. (2021). A review of the tortuous path of nonviral gene delivery and recent progress. *Int J Biol Macromol, 183*. https://doi.org/10.1016/j.ijbiomac.2021.05.192

Shen, J., Lu, Z., Wang, J., Hao, Q., Ji, W., Wu, Y., et al (2021). Traceable Nano-Biohybrid Complexes by One-Step Synthesis as CRISPR-Chem Vectors for Neurodegenerative Diseases Synergistic Treatment. *Adv Mater., 33*(27), 1–10

Shtykalova, S., Deviatkin, D., Freund, S., Egorova, A., Kiselev, A. (2023). Non-Viral Carriers for Nucleic Acids Delivery: Fundamentals and Current Applications. *Life., 13*(4)

SMULL CE, LUDWIG EH (1962). Enhancement of the plaque-forming capacity of poliovirus ribonucleic acid with basic proteins. *J Bacteriol., 84*, 1035–40

Stanford, P. (2013). Nanotechnology for the Delivery of Therapeutic Nucleic Acids. *Nanotechnology for the Delivery of Therapeutic Nucleic Acids.,*

Sun, X., Zhang, N. (2010). Cationic Polymer Optimization for Efficient Gene Delivery. *Mini-Reviews Med Chem., 10*(2), 108–25

Tambe, P., Sayed, N., Paknikar, K.M, Gajbhiye, V. (2019). Poly(Phospho Ester) and Poly(Phosphazene) Nanoparticles as a Promising Tool for Anticancer Therapeutics. *Polymeric Nanoparticles as a Promising Tool for Anti-cancer Therapeutics. Elsevier Inc,* https://doi.org/10.1016/B978-0-12-816963-6.00007-8

Tang, M.X, Redemann, C.T, Szoka, F.C (1996). Tang-1996-In vitro gene delive.pdf. *Bioconjugate Chem., 7*(6), 703–14

Thomas, T.J, Tajmir-Riahi, H.A, Thomas, T. (2016). Polyamine–DNA interactions and development of gene delivery vehicles. *Amino Acids., 48*(10), 2423–31

Vaheri, A., Pagano, J.S (1965). Infectious poliovirus RNA: a sensitive method of assay. *Virology., 27*(3), 434–6

van den Berg A I. (2021) Polymeric delivery systems for nucleic acid therapeutics: Approaching the clinic. Journal of Controlled Release, 331, 121–141. https://doi.org/10.1016/j.jconrel.2021.01.014

Varkouhi, A.K, Scholte, M., Storm, G., Haisma, H.J (2011). Endosomal escape pathways for delivery of biologicals. *J Control Release, 151*(3), 220–8. https://doi.org/10.1016/j.jconrel.2010.11.004

Veider, F., Sanchez, A.rmengol E, Bernkop-Schnürch A (2024). Charge-Reversible Nanoparticles: Advanced Delivery Systems for Therapy and Diagnosis. *Small., 20*(3), 1–19

Wagner, E. (2014). Polymers for Nucleic Acid Transfer-An Overview. *Vol. 88, Advances in Genetics. Elsevier,* https://doi.org/10.1016/B978-0-12-800148-6.00008-0

Wilk, AJ, Weidenbacher, N.LB, Vergara, R., Haabeth, O.AW, Levy, R., Waymouth, R.M, et al (2020). Charge-altering releasable transporters enable phenotypic manipulation of natural killer cells for cancer immunotherapy. *Blood Adv., 4*(17), 4244–55

Yamaleyeva, D.N, Makita, N., Hwang, D., Haney, M.J, Jordan, R., Kabanov, A. V (2023). Poly(2-oxazoline)-Based Polyplexes as a PEG-Free Plasmid DNA Delivery Platform. *Macromol Biosci., 23*(11), 1–12

Yin, L., Song, Z., Kim, K.H, Zheng, N., Gabrielson, N.P, Cheng, J. (2013). Non-viral gene delivery via membrane-penetrating, mannose-targeting supramolecular self-assembled nanocomplexes. *Adv Mater., 25*(22), 3063–70

Zhang, P., Wagner, E. (2017). History of Polymeric Gene Delivery Systems. *Top Curr Chem., 375*(2), 1–39

Zhao, X., Li, X., Zhao, Y., Cheng, Y., Yang, Y., Fang, Z., et al (2017). Immune activities of polycationic vectors for gene delivery. *Front Pharmacol., 8*

Zhou, X., Liu, X., Zhao, B., Liu, X., Zhu, D., Qiu, N., et al (2016). Jumping the nuclear envelop barrier: Improving polyplex-mediated gene transfection efficiency by a selective CDK1 inhibitor RO-3306. *J Control Release, 234*, 90–7. https://doi.org/10.1016/j.jconrel.2016.05.042

Zuckerman, J.E, Gale, A., Wu, P., Ma, R., Davis, M.E (2015). SiRNA delivery to the glomerular mesangium using polycationic cyclodextrin nanoparticles containing siRNA. *Nucleic Acid Ther., 25*(2), 53–64

Author Biographies

Ahmet Cesur graduated with a Bachelor of Pharmacy degree from Ankara University, Türkiye. Following his undergraduate studies, he was awarded the YLSY scholarship by the Turkish Ministry of National Education. Through this program, he began his PhD studies in Pharmaceutical Sciences at the University of Houston, USA. His research focuses on synthetic cationic polymers, nucleic acid delivery systems. He presented his team's work as a poster at the 14th International Symposium on Pharmaceutical Sciences, the study focused on the design of a novel hydrogel system with thermo-responsive properties to enhance the controlled release and bioavailability of diclofenac sodium. His long-term goal is to establish an independent academic laboratory that fosters scientific innovation and collaboration between universities and industry.

Umut Can Oz received his Ph.D. in Ankara University Faculty of Pharmacy in 2017. During his Ph.D., he conducted a part of his thesis research in the Chemistry Department at UCL. He has been working in the Department of Pharmaceutical Technology as an associate professor since 2024, after completing a postdoctoral fellowship with Prof. Cameron Alexander at the University of Nottingham School of Pharmacy. His research interests include developing novel micro- and nano-scale polymeric materials and hydrogel-based biomaterials for drug and nucleic acid delivery.

CHAPTER 13

INORGANIC NANOPARTICLES

HÜSEYIN IZGORDÜ

Phd, Department of Chemistry, Osmangazi University, Eskişehir, Türkiye

Abstract

Nanoparticles are particles less than 100 nanometers (nm) in size and exhibit different and superior properties compared to bulk materials. Nanotechnology, the field of nanoparticles, can overcome several limitations associated with conventional delivery systems, from large-scale problems such as biodistribution through cell-specific targeting, molecule delivery to specific organelles and other approaches, to smaller-scale obstacles such as intracellular transport. Inorganic nanoparticles (iNPs) consist of an inorganic core that is passivated by an organic ligand shell. Inorganic nanoparticles include metals, semiconductor materials, and metal oxides. INPs have been widely used in the biomedical field as therapeutic drugs for disease treatment because of their controllable size and unique optical, electrical, magnetic, and catalytic properties. With these properties, inorganic nanoparticles have potential applications in improving the quality of human life, improving medical conditions, early detection, diagnosis, treatment, and monitoring of various diseases. For example, various cancer treatment systems based on inorganic nanoparticles have developed extensively over the past two decades, including photodynamic therapy, nanoprobes, hyperthermia, and drug delivery. This makes inorganic nanoparticles a potential target for developing effective multifunctional cancer therapies. Inorganic materials such as gold, iron, and silica have been used to synthesize nanostructured materials for various drug delivery and imaging applications. These iNPs are precisely described and can be designed to have a wide range of sizes, structures, and geometries. The best-studied gold iNPs (AuNPs) are used in various forms such as nanospheres, nanorods, nanostars, nanoshells, and nanocages. Moreover, iNPs have unique physical, electrical, magnetic, and optical properties depending on the properties of the base material itself. Iron oxide is another widely investigated material for iNP synthesis, and iron oxide NPs constitute the majority of FDA-approved inorganic nanomedicines. Magnetic iron oxide NPs composed of magnetite (Fe3O4) or maghemite (Fe2O3) have superparamagnetic properties at certain sizes and have been successfully used as contrast agents, drug delivery vehicles, and thermal-based therapeutics. Other common iNPs are calcium phosphate and silica iNPs, which have been successfully used in gene and drug delivery. Due to their magnetic, radioactive, or plasmonic properties, iNPs are uniquely qualified for use in diagnostics, imaging, and photothermal therapy. The use of iNPs in medicine enables more specialized therapies, such as improved cellular targeting, fewer off-target effects, and multidrug therapies. In conclusion, inorganic nanoparticles play an important role in advances in nanotechnology in the field of healthcare, offering innovative approaches to diagnostics and therapeutics. However, more research and development work is needed to increase their efficacy in clinical applications and to address issues such as potential toxicity.

Keywords: Inorganic nanoparticles, Nanomedicine, Drug delivery, Cancer therapy

1. Introduction

When considering nanotechnology in a broad context, its roots can be traced back to ancient civilizations. For instance, lead sulfide (PbS) nanocrystals have been identified as a key component in hair dye formulations used as early as the Greco-Roman period (Walter et al., 2006). The use of gold nanoparticles also has deep historical roots, particularly in medicine. In 1449, the Flemish glassmaker John Utynam received a patent in England for producing stained glass infused with gold nanoparticles, while the Swiss physician and alchemist Paracelsus (Von Hohenheim) is known to have prepared and administered gold nanoparticles to patients for therapeutic purposes in the early 16th century. Remarkably, carbon nanotubes, another form of nanomaterial, were discovered within the blades of ancient Damascus swords, contributing to their exceptional strength and resilience — a metallurgical achievement that dates back over 400 years (Reibold et al., 2006; Ramsden, 2011). Similarly, silver has a long history as a therapeutic agent. During World War II, J. N. Burst introduced silver-based treatments for burn victims, and silver nanoparticles have since become well-established as powerful antimicrobial agents, effectively treating infections, burns, and diabetic wounds (Bhattacharyya et al., 2011).

Nanotechnology refers to the exploration and control of materials at the nanoscale, typically ranging from 1 to 100 nanometers, where substances exhibit unique size-dependent properties (Leon, 2020). This field serves as a critical bridge between the physical and biological sciences, providing innovative tools for precise disease detection through advanced sensing technologies (Gupta, 2017). Working at the atomic and molecular levels within this size range, nanotechnology has been a major catalyst for breakthroughs in biomedical science, including the design of novel drug delivery systems for chronic conditions such as cancer and diabetes (Haleem, 2023). The exceptionally small size of nanomaterials allows them to overcome many of the challenges faced by conventional therapies, including limited drug bioavailability and non-specific targeting. By enabling controlled drug release and enhancing the speed of drug discovery, nanotechnology significantly improves therapeutic outcomes (Shi, 2010). Additionally, nano-scale drug carriers can pass through the blood vessel walls without harming the vascular endothelium, ensuring that drugs reach their target tissues while minimizing systemic exposure (Patra et al., 2018). This targeted approach not only prevents enzymatic degradation but also maintains higher local drug concentrations, making nanotechnology a highly effective alternative to traditional drug delivery methods. Furthermore, nanomedicines stand out for their precisely defined size, shape, biocompatibility, and biodegradability, which collectively enable effective disease management with fewer side effects (Shapira et al., 2011).

This figure visually summarizes that nanomaterials are divided into four main categories based on their size: zero-dimensional (0D), one-dimensional (1D), two-dimensional (2D) and three-dimensional (3D) nanomaterials. Each category is based on at least one dimension of the material being on the nanometer scale (1-100 nm).

- **Zero-dimensional (0D)** nanomaterials include particles that are nanoscopic in all dimensions. Examples of this group are nanoparticles and fullerenes. These structures are usually spherical and have quantum confinement effects.
- **One-dimensional (1D)** nanomaterials have nanoscopic dimensions in only one dimension. Nanotubes and nanohorns belong to this group. These structures can exhibit exceptional mechanical, electrical and thermal properties thanks to their high length-to-diameter ratio.

- **Two-dimensional (2D)** nanomaterials are sheet-like structures that are nanoscopic in thickness but have two other dimensions of micrometers or larger. These materials, such as nanosheets and nanolayers, have high surface area and surface-dependent properties.
- **Three-dimensional (3D)** nanomaterials are composed of nanostructures organized in all dimensions. Structures such as nanotubes and nanowire arrays allow for versatile applications due to their volumetric organization.

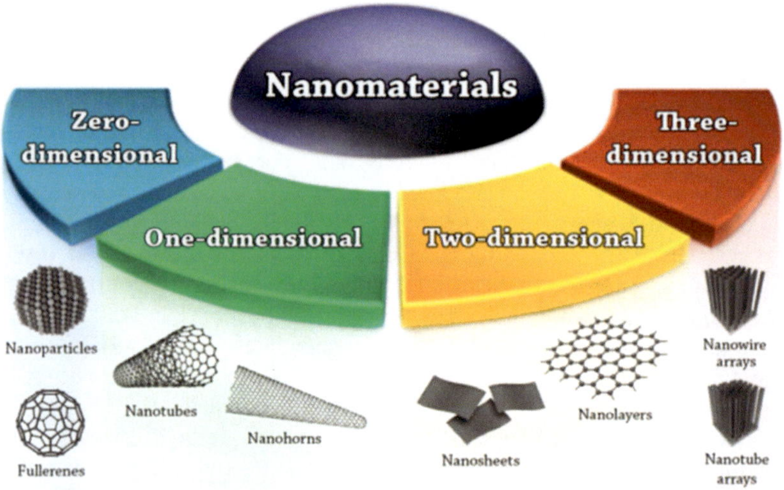

Figure 1. Nanomaterial classification on the basis of dimensionality (Joudeh and Linke, 2022)

This classification serves as a foundational structure for comprehending the physical and chemical characteristics of inorganic nanomaterials and effectively directing them toward suitable applications (Joudeh and Linke, 2022). Nanotechnology offers several key advantages, including:

1. The ability to create materials that exhibit unique combinations of properties not typically found in conventional substances.
2. Nanoscale devices, by their nature, require smaller amounts of material, consume less energy, and benefit from enhanced functionality as their dimensions decrease, providing broader access to innovative technologies.

3. It provides a versatile manufacturing approach, often referred to as a "personal nano-factory," capable of producing a wide range of nanostructures (Ramsden, 2011).

Compared to conventional drug delivery methods, inorganic nanoparticles in particular can offer various benefits by overcoming the pharmacokinetic and pharmacodynamic limitations of potential drug molecules (Kanika et al., 2024). Nanomaterials and nanoparticles have been the basis of nanoscience activities for decades. Inorganic nanoparticles are emerging as a potential drug delivery technology in the current field of materials sciences due to their unique physical properties, which are being developed worldwide (Viswanath et al., 2017). Another important advantage of INPs is that their surface can be easily functionalized, i.e., coated with various ligands, antibodies, peptides, or biomolecules such as DNA/RNA for biological targeting. This makes them not just a passive carrier but a "smart system" that actively contributes to targeted therapy. For example, nanoparticles coated with antibodies that recognize cancer cell-specific proteins can target only tumor cells without affecting healthy cells. Furthermore, by designing drugs that are sensitive to environmental stimuli such as pH, temperature, and magnetic field, etc., drugs can be activated only in the diseased target area. Metallic inorganic nanoparticles with specific physicochemical properties have attracted the attention of scientists for more than a century and are now frequently used in biomedical, engineering, and medical research. These nanomaterials can be synthesized and conjugated with antibodies, ligands, and related drugs because of their ability to be modified with various chemical functional groups and used in biotechnology, magnetic separation, target analyte preconcentration, targeted drug delivery, and vehicle technology (Mody et al., 2010). While nanoparticles exhibit different properties from the bulk samples of the same material, groups of nanoparticles can also have collective properties that are different from those exhibited by individual nanoparticles and bulk samples. The orderly assembly of nanoparticles on surfaces and interfaces is crucial for the realization of multifaceted functions (Altavilla 2016). The structure formed by the assembly of nanoparticles creates new nanostructures with unpredictable collective, intrinsic physical properties. These properties can be used for multipurpose applications in nanoelectronics, spintronics, biosensors, etc. (Nie et al., 2010).

In the last 20 years, nanotechnology has seen remarkable advancements, particularly in the biomedical sciences, where it has become a cornerstone for innovations in targeted drug delivery, biosensing, and medical imaging. At the heart of these applications are nanoparticles, which play a crucial role as carriers for therapeutic compounds and imaging agents, enhancing the precision and effectiveness of diagnostic and therapeutic strategies. Given their direct interaction with biological systems, ensuring biocompatibility remains a critical consideration in the design and synthesis of nanomaterials intended for biomedical use. To facilitate the selective recognition of biomolecules, thereby enhancing targeted delivery and molecular sensing capabilities, it is common to modify the surfaces of these nanomaterials with specific recognition groups (Chun-Pei et al., 2022).

Inorganic nanoparticles, which generally encompass a range of metals, semiconductor compounds, and metal oxides, have garnered significant attention in biomedical research due to their precisely tunable sizes and distinctive physical properties, including optical behavior, electrical conductivity, magnetic attributes, catalytic capabilities, and strong biocompatibility. These characteristics make them promising candidates for applications in early disease detection, diagnosis, treatment, and long-term monitoring, offering potential benefits for improving human health and medical outcomes. For instance, over the past two decades, numerous cancer treatment strategies based on inorganic nanoparticles have been developed, including photodynamic therapy, nanoprobe systems, hyperthermia, and advanced drug delivery platforms, highlighting their potential as versatile and effective tools for cancer therapy (Ma et al., 2023). The success of these nanoparticle-based approaches in oncology has also encouraged their exploration in the field of stem cell biotechnology. Inorganic nanoparticles provide stable microenvironments, influencing the behavior and fate of stem cells over extended periods through their physical and chemical interactions. For example, these nanomaterials can impact stem cell functions by creating specialized nano-environments that regulate cell fate and enable long-term in vivo monitoring. Additionally, their diverse morphologies and structures allow for spatially controlled stem cell differentiation, offering innovative strategies for precisely directing stem cell behaviors. Typically, inorganic nanoparticles interact with stem cells via endocytosis or exocytosis, leading to distinct cellular responses depending on the nanoparticle type and local environment, thus offering unique opportunities for targeted stem cell manipulation (Ma et al., 2023).

2. Structure and Basic Properties of Inorganic Nanoparticles (INP)

2.1. Composition of inorganic nanoparticles

Among inorganic NPs, the most widely used are gold, silver, iron oxide, and magnetic and quantum dots. Gold nanoparticles (AuNPs) are used in the transport and release of pharmaceuticals because they have unique chemical and physical properties. The gold core is essentially inert and its most important property is non-toxic. A second advantage is that they are very easy to synthesize (Huang et al., 2023). AuNPs are synthesized both chemically and biologically (green synthesis). Nowadays, the biological synthesis of AuNPs is more accepted as it does not use hazardous reducing agents. The surfaces of the AuNPs can be easily functionalized with molecules or substances. Thus, the stability and dispersion of AuNPs in organic media have become advantageous. Furthermore, these surface modifiers can be used as targeting moieties to deliver drugs to the target site. The surface modification of AuNPs is quite easy; thus, cancerous tissues can be targeted using passive and active targeting mechanisms with AuNPs (Khan, 2019).

Silver NPs (AgNPs) have potential importance in different applications such as interactions between biomolecules, sensing and imaging (Fathima and Mujeeb, 2021). In addition, AgNPs have anticancer, good antimicrobial, antifungal, anti-inflammatory, antidiabetic and wound healing activities (Sondi and Salopek-Sondi, 2004; Khan, 2019). AgNPs are mainly used in biotechnology, medicine, electronics, engineering, magnetic fields and also in environmental remediation. Due to these excellent properties, AgNPs are used alone or in combination with other pharmacological and diagnostic agents for the treatment or screening of various diseases (Chen and Schluesener, 2008).

Magnetic nanoparticles (NPs) based on iron oxides occur in various forms in nature, including magnetite (Fe_3O_4), maghemite (γ-Fe_2O_3), hematite (α-Fe_2O_3), wüstite (FeO), and several phases of iron (III) oxide (α, β, γ, and ε), as well as bernadine ($Fe(OH)_3$) and lepidocrocite (δ-FeOOH) (Teja and Koh, 2009; Muzibur et al., 2011). The magnetic properties of these materials arise from the strong magnetic moment of the iron atom, which has four unpaired electrons in its 3d orbitals. In addition to their intrinsic magnetic characteristics, such as superparamagnetism, high coercivity, low Curie temperature, and elevated magnetic susceptibility, these nanoparticles also feature a core-shell structure, typically composed of an iron oxide core surrounded by an outer shell of inorganic materials (Wu et al., 2008; Teja and Koh, 2009). Commonly used coatings for iron oxide nanoparticles (FeONPs) include silica, gold, and gadolinium, which not only enhance their stability but also provide functional surfaces for the attachment of various biological ligands, making them highly versatile for biomedical applications (Gupta, 2017). Due to these unique properties, magnetic nanoparticles have found widespread use across multiple fields, including magnetic fluids, data storage, catalysis, medical diagnostics, magnetic resonance imaging (MRI) contrast agents, and targeted cancer therapies (Wu et al., 2008; Teja and Koh, 2009).

Carbon nanoscale NPs play a key role in science and nanotechnology (Saleh and Gupta, 2016). Carbon is the main element in carbon-based NPs (Makhlouf and Barhoum, 2018). Carbon exists in several allotropic forms. Diamond, graphite, and buckminsterfullerene are among the common allotropes (Smith et al., 2019). Carbon-based materials such as hydrocarbons, graphite, graphene, and coal are frequently used in the synthesis of carbon NPs. Coal has been discovered to be one of the low-cost and abundant precursors for the production of carbon nanostructured materials compared to other materials (Raj and Manoj, 2022). Metal NPs (MNPs) have been the center of attention of scientists in recent years due to their great potential in nanotechnology. The possibility of synthesis in different sizes, shapes and with various surface modifications allows MNPs to conjugate with antibodies, target ligands and drugs. Thanks to these properties, they have a wide range of applications (Khan, 2020).

2.2. Controlled Size and Surface Modifications

Nanoparticles (NPs) are often found in nature in non-crystalline or low symmetry forms. The size of these particles and the composition of the aggregates they form are the main determinants of their most stable structural form. This also directly affects the physical and chemical properties of NPs (Vinita et al., 2023). Nowadays, understanding the physicochemical properties of NPs and revealing their structure-function relationships is an important research area for scientists. However, this process is limited by our capacity to study nanoscale structures. Different characterization techniques are based on different physical principles and provide only partial insights into the properties of NPs. Moreover, these characterization methods themselves can directly influence the measured parameters, further complicating the interpretation of the results. To be soluble in aqueous media, NP surfaces must have a certain electrostatic charge. This charge can be achieved by the covalent attachment of biomolecules containing charged functional groups to the surface. This process is often referred to as surface functionalization and involves chemically modifying NPs with biomolecules, metal ions, or polymeric structures (Christian et al., 2008). The type of functional groups plays a dominant role in determining many properties of NPs such as solubility, interactions with cell membranes and other biomacromolecules. In this context, the three-dimensional structure of NPs can be studied using advanced characterization methods such as coherent X-ray diffraction (Moyu et al., 2011). The encounter of NPs with cells in biological environments may result in the adsorption of serum proteins on their surfaces. This facilitates their uptake into cells, usually via receptor-mediated endocytosis (Khan et al., 2007). However, in some applications, it is desirable that NPs do not interact with biological surfaces. Especially in in vivo applications, proteins adsorbed on the surface can lead to agglomeration of NPs and rapid clearance by the reticuloendothelial system. This may reduce the efficiency of the drug and gene delivery systems.

Furthermore, non-specific interactions can cause NPs to bind with the cell membrane or extracellular matrix, which can have negative consequences such as off-target labeling or false detection. To mitigate such effects, NP surfaces can be coated with bioinert, neutral ligands such as poly(ethylene glycol) (PEG). PEG is known as a polymer with high resistance to protein adsorption (Xie et al., 2007). The structure of the nanoparticles can generally be divided into two components, the "core" and the "shell". The shell, which usually has a different chemical composition than the core, is located on the surface and determines the interaction of the particle with the external environment. Core/shell structures are widely used in the development of property-directed and functional NPs. For example, quantum dots with a cadmium selenide (CdSe) core and zinc sulfide (ZnS) shell show quantum yields above 50% (Ding et al., 2017; Malik et al., 2002). The production of such structures is not random; it is the product of controlled synthesis processes. For example, iron nanoparticles (FeNPs) rapidly form iron oxide layers on their surface after synthesis. Although these layers do not envelop the entire particle, the NP is no longer considered a pure iron structure, but a core-shell structure (Santos et al., 2017). In the physical sciences, the core of the NP is often considered the essential component of the structure. Many physicochemical and toxicological properties of NPs are directly related to this core composition. However, focusing only on the core can sometimes be misleading. In some examples, evaluations without considering the composition of the entire NP lead to erroneous results (Wuister et al., 2004). During the synthesis of NPs, the formation of a specific crystalline phase is not always expected.

Inorganic NPs can exist in more than one phase and these phases can co-exist. This can lead to unpredictable changes in the physicochemical properties of the particle (Christian & O'Brien, 2005; Rempel et al., 2006). In this context, controlling and understanding the phase behavior of NPs is of great importance for the design of the targeted properties.

2.3. Electrical, magnetic and optical properties

The stability of nanoparticles (NPs) in manufacturing processes and their efficiency in various applications are directly related to their electrical, magnetic, and optical properties. The properties of NPs such as large surface area, high mechanical strength, pronounced optical responses, and chemical reactivity make them attractive for many technological and biomedical applications. The optical properties of NPs, especially their absorbance capacity, have been analyzed by spectrophotometric methods (Rastar et al., 2012). These properties are mostly related to their electron structure and size-dependent quantum effects. In particular, noble metal NPs exhibit a strong extinction band in the UV-visible region, which is not observed in bulk metals. This feature occurs when the incident photon frequency collectively excites free electrons in the conduction bands, a phenomenon termed "localized surface plasmon resonance" (LSPR) (Eustis & El-Sayed, 2006). LSPR is a mechanism that provides light scattering equivalent to the efficiency of fluorophores and significantly enhances local electromagnetic fields near the NP surface. This results in an extremely high molar excitation coefficient specific to the resonant wavelength. The spectral peak of LSPR varies depending on the size, shape, distance between NPs, their dielectric constants, and the optical properties of the medium (e.g. solvent, substrate or adsorbates) (Trindade et al., 2001). In terms of magnetic properties, NPs exhibit unusual behavior, especially when they are reduced to small sizes. In NPs with a size in the range of about 10-20 nm, magnetic effects are markedly enhanced due to disordered electronic distributions. These superparamagnetic properties make NPs valuable in various applications such as catalysis, biomedicine, magnetic resonance imaging (MRI), data storage, and water purification (Arati et al., 2013; Qi et al., 2016). Research confirms that NPs in this size range perform best. Reiss and Hütten (2005) stated that NPs with a diameter of 10-20 nm are the optimum size in terms of electrical and magnetic performance. In NPs of this scale, magnetic effects suppress other physical effects, which significantly increases their usability in a wide range of applications (Reiss & Hütten, 2005; Priyadarshana et al., 2015; Faivre & Bennet, 2016).

2.4. Biocompatibility and stability

Most inorganic NPs are synthesized in an environmentally friendly way using a bottom-up approach. This characteristic allows INPs to have greater selectivity and biological activity against targeted cells without causing any harm to normal cells. This selectivity and biocompatibility are the most important properties of NPs that enable their future use as drug substitutes in biomedical applications. Among the metal oxide NPs, zinc oxide NPs have many important new physical and chemical properties such as high mechanical and thermal stability, pyro and piezo electric effect, ultraviolet absorbance, biocompatibility, and antimicrobial activity (Balcha et al., 2016). Inorganic AgNPs are non-toxic, excellent bactericidal agents with good biocompatibility, high thermal stability, and chemical reactivity (Kumar et al., 2012). MgONPs possess unique physicochemical properties such as high chemical stability, electrical permeability, photocatalytic efficiency, thermal conductivity, physical and mechanical strength, dielectric resistance, low toxic, and high biocompatibility.

3. Biomedical Applications of Inorganic Nanoparticles

3.1. Diagnostics and Imaging

One of the main goals in medical and biomedical research is to increase the efficacy of therapeutic agents while minimizing adverse effects on healthy cells. In order to achieve this goal, it is of great importance to improve the delivery efficiency of drug delivery systems and to provide specific targeting properties. In this context, biomedical imaging techniques contribute to diagnostic processes by providing valuable information about molecular distribution in both in vitro and in vivo environments. Biomedical applications based on inorganic nanoparticles (NPs) are widely investigated due to their high accessibility and versatile functional properties. In the design of an effective delivery and imaging system, the biological barriers that NPs may encounter inside the body before reaching target tissues should be taken into account. NPs, which usually enter the circulation via injection or oral route, pass through the circulatory system and try to reach the target cells. However, in this process, the risk of being perceived as a foreign body by the organism and destroyed constitutes one of the biggest challenges (Chun-Pei et al., 2022). Therefore, the biocompatibility and surface properties of NPs need to be optimized to ensure targeted delivery and long circulation time. NPs are considered promising tools for numerous biomedical applications such as targeted drug delivery, in vivo therapeutics, molecular imaging and cancer therapy (Garcia et al., 2020). However, the ability of the human immune system to recognize and neutralize foreign materials is a major factor limiting the applicability of NP-based systems (Pratiwi et al., 2019; Malachowski & Hassel, 2020; Papini et al., 2020). Moreover, processes such as protein corona formation reduce the target recognition capacity of ligands on the surface and can negatively affect the functionality of NPs by altering the surface chemistry (Rampado et al., 2020). NPs without adequate surface modification can access solid tumor tissues based solely on enhanced permeability and retention (EPR), which in most cases offers limited efficiency (Subhan et al., 2021). To overcome these problems, various engineering strategies have been developed, such as rearranging the surface chemistry of NPs, coating them with functional ligands and optimizing their geometrical properties. However, although NP research is still active, it is approaching its limits in some aspects. Much of the available data has been obtained under controlled laboratory conditions, where unexpected biological reactions are likely to be encountered in real-life scenarios (Dang and Guan., 2020). Therefore, it is not surprising that many NP-based drug delivery systems have not received clinical approval. On the other hand, recent studies on nanodevices and nanotechnological systems have opened new horizons in the field. For example, microchip systems integrating poly(3,4-ethylenedioxythiophene)-based nanofiber mats can capture and release rare circulating tumor cells in a controlled manner through electrical stimulation (Zhu et al., 2017). Similarly, noninvasive prenatal diagnosis systems (Hou et al., 2017), versatile biosensor platforms (Chou et al., 2019), isolation of cancer cells with microfluidic chips (Zhu et al., 2019) and nanobiotechnological applications for neuron manipulation (Valdembri et al., 2021; Li and Burgess 2020) show that these technologies are increasingly finding their place in clinical and research settings.

3.2. Use in Cancer Treatment

Nanotechnology has emerged as a rapidly growing discipline in science and technology, finding extensive use as a drug delivery platform for a wide range of therapeutic agents, including small molecules, genes, proteins, and peptides (Kim et al., 2010). In contrast to conventional therapies, nanoparticle-based drug delivery systems enable both the diagnosis and treatment of cancer cells simultaneously, offering a more integrated therapeutic approach. With ongoing progress in nanotechnology and medical sciences, a diverse array of nanoparticles and nanomaterials has been developed from various metals, including gold, silver, iron, copper, cobalt, platinum, and cobalt. Among these, gold nanoparticles (AuNPs) have emerged as a particularly popular choice for drug delivery applications, largely due to their exceptional optical characteristics and surface plasmon resonance (SPR) properties, which make them highly suitable for use in biomedical and pharmaceutical research (Dykman and Khlebtsov, 2016).

Due to their distinctive physicochemical and optoelectronic characteristics, inorganic nanomaterials are increasingly being explored as therapeutic agents. One significant application is nanoparticle-mediated hyperthermia, which requires the ability to effectively deliver energy deep into tissues. Recently, core-shell nanomaterials have been developed for hyperthermia treatments using near-infrared (NIR) radiation (Sam et al., 2004). For example, silica-coated gold nanorods exhibit strong NIR scattering, with their optical properties being tunable by adjusting the core and shell thickness, shifting their resonance from the visible to the NIR spectrum. Hirsch et al. demonstrated that silica-gold nanoshells can be used for NIR-induced photothermal therapy to treat human breast cancer cells in both in vitro and in vivo studies. Their in vivo experiments, which involved 4-6 minutes of NIR exposure, generated localized heating to approximately 37.4 ± 6.6 °C, resulting in irreversible tissue damage as confirmed by MRI analysis (Hirsch et al., 2003). Similarly, El-Sayed et al. showed that gold nanorods could serve as contrast agents for both molecular imaging and targeted photothermal therapy when exposed to NIR. They further demonstrated that gold nanorods conjugated with anti-EGFR antibodies can differentiate between normal (HaCaT) and cancerous (HOC-313 and HSC-3) cells, requiring approximately half the energy to damage malignant cells compared to healthy cells when exposed to Ti:sapphire lasers (800 nm, 40-160 W/cm^2) (Huang et al., 2006; Hynes and Lane, 2005). Expanding on these findings, Griffin et al. explored the use of PT-cAu-TNF-α (where PT represents thiol-derived polyethylene glycol) for targeted TNF-α delivery combined with hyperthermia to treat SCK mouse mammary carcinoma. Their approach used contrast-enhanced Doppler ultrasound to assess tumor perfusion, and the combination of PT-cAu-TNF-α with heat was found to significantly reduce cell viability, achieving only 21% survival relative to control groups (Visaria et al., 2006; Billadeau et al., 2005).

In another comparative study, antibody-coated gold-based nanomaterials, including silica-coated Au nanoshells, hollow Au/Ag nanospheres, and Au nanorods, were tested against HeLa (cervical cancer), TCC (bladder cancer), and A549 (lung cancer) cells. This investigation revealed that silica-coated Au nanoshells required the fewest particles to achieve effective photodestruction under NIR irradiation at 808 nm, highlighting their superior efficiency compared to other nanostructures (Cheng et al., 2009; Rai et al., 2009).

Photothermal therapy (PTT) is a localized, minimally invasive treatment approach that utilizes thermal energy to target and destroy cancer cells, making it an appealing option for localized cancer therapy. In PTT, nanoparticles introduced into malignant tissues are exposed to near-infrared (NIR) laser light, leading to localized heating that effectively eradicates cancerous cells. This method relies on longer wavelength light, typically in the 700-1200 nm range, which minimizes damage to surrounding healthy tissues due to its lower energy and deeper tissue penetration. An ideal photothermal agent should exhibit strong NIR absorption, high biocompatibility, minimal toxicity, and a maximum light-to-heat conversion efficiency, characterized by a high absorption cross-section. Among the available photothermal materials, gold-based compounds have become the most widely utilized, given their excellent optical properties. However, concerns about their undefined long-term toxicity remain a significant challenge for clinical applications. Magnetic nanoparticles (MNPs) have emerged as promising alternatives for photothermal therapy due to their ability to integrate with other photothermal agents, potentially enhancing therapeutic effectiveness. Nevertheless, the relatively low molar absorption coefficients of MNPs in the NIR range present a limitation, which can be addressed through controlled nanoparticle clustering to improve their optical performance (Sun et al., 2023).

The medical applications of platinum nanoparticles (PtNPs) are less established compared to their more widely known counterparts, such as cisplatin and its derivatives, which are commonly used as chemotherapeutic agents (Hall et al., 2007). However, recent studies have highlighted the potential of platinum nanoparticles in biomedical applications, particularly when combined with other nanoparticles in core-shell structures. For instance, yolk-shell nanoparticles like FePt@CoS2 have demonstrated significantly higher cytotoxicity against HeLa cells, with an IC_{50} value of 35.5 ± 4.7 ng Pt/ml, compared to cisplatin's IC_{50} of 230 ng Pt/ml, indicating a more potent anticancer effect (Gao et al., 2007). This enhanced efficacy is largely attributed to the structural modifications that reduce overall cytotoxicity while improving therapeutic outcomes. Additionally, platinum nanoparticles have been successfully incorporated with multi-walled carbon nanotubes (MWCNTs) to enhance the sensitivity of electrochemical biosensors and improve their catalytic efficiency. This approach has increased the DNA detection sensitivity to as low as 1.0×10^{-11} mol/L (Wang et al., 2006).

Moreover, recent advancements have shown that face-centered cubic (fcc) FePt nanoparticles conjugated with luteinizing hormone-releasing hormone (LHRH) peptides via phospholipids can inhibit tumor growth in ovarian cancer cells (OVA2780) that overexpress LHRH receptors. This process is pH-dependent, with optimal activity observed in acidic environments (approximately pH 4.8), reflecting the typically acidic microenvironment of tumors (Xu et al., 2009). The antitumor effect is primarily driven by the generation of hydroxyl radicals (HO•) through the catalytic decomposition of hydrogen peroxide (H_2O_2) mediated by Fe^{2+}, offering a promising platform for targeted drug delivery and molecular imaging, including MRI, due to their strong contrast enhancement properties. Cancer progression and metastasis involve multiple steps, including the crucial role of cancer cell adhesion molecules (CCAMs), which facilitate the adhesion and migration of tumor cells within the bloodstream (Okegawa et al., 2004; Bendas and Borsig, 2012). These molecules have specific surface receptors that enable both homotypic (same cell type) and heterotypic (different cell type) interactions, leading to metastatic spread (Sun et al., 2016; Harjunpaa et al., 2019). Additionally, many cancer cells express CD47, a surface protein that helps them evade immune surveillance by transmitting a "don't eat me" signal to macrophages (Lian et al., 2019; Siegler et al., 2020a). Taking advantage of this characteristic, researchers have developed nanoparticle systems coated with cancer cell membranes (CCMs) to enhance their biocompatibility and targeting specificity.

3.2.1. Role of calcium phosphate (CaP) and silica NPs in gene transfer

Gene delivery systems and the auxiliary components used in them are indispensable tools in modern molecular medicine, particularly in cancer treatment and regenerative medicine. In addition to viral vectors, calcium phosphate (CaP) and silica nanoparticles have garnered significant attention due to their high biocompatibility, low toxicity, and effective nucleic acid loading capacity. Compared to viral vectors, these inorganic nanoparticles are considered safer and more stable carrier systems for DNA, RNA, and siRNA delivery. CaP can effectively bind negatively charged nucleic acids through electrostatic interactions and protect them from enzymatic degradation and breakdown. Its pH-sensitive solubility properties facilitate the release of the genetic payload following endocytosis, thereby enhancing transfection efficiency with minimal cytotoxicity (Roy et al., 2003).

Silica nanoparticles are promising gene delivery systems due to their large surface areas, tunable pore sizes, and, most importantly, ease of surface functionalization. Their porous structure allows for the simultaneous loading of nucleic acids and therapeutic agents, enabling applications where gene and drug delivery are carried out in tandem. Functionalized silica nanoparticles can protect nucleic acids from degradation and provide controlled intracellular release under various physiological conditions, which increases their appeal (Slowing et al., 2007).

Overall, calcium phosphate and silica-based nanoparticles represent versatile and efficient non-viral gene delivery systems with strong potential for future biomedical and therapeutic applications.

3.2.2. Mesoporous silica nanoparticles (MSN).

Mesoporous materials, as defined by the International Union of Pure and Applied Chemistry (IUPAC), are characterized by pore sizes ranging from 2 to 50 nanometers (Brühwiler, 2010). The concept of mesoporous silica nanoparticles (MSNs) was introduced nearly four decades ago, and since then, these materials have garnered significant attention due to their highly tunable pore sizes (typically 2-6 nm), adjustable particle sizes (50-300 nm), large surface areas, high pore volumes, and excellent biocompatibility. These features make MSNs ideal candidates for drug delivery systems, as their internal and external surfaces provide abundant space for the attachment of various functional groups, enabling precise drug loading and controlled release. An effective nanocarrier should possess adjustable pore and particle sizes to accommodate different types of pharmaceutical molecules. MSNs are particularly well-suited for this purpose, as their high surface area and porous architecture facilitate the adsorption and release of a wide range of therapeutic agents. Moreover, their biocompatibility and enhanced permeability and retention (EPR) effect enable them to selectively target cancer cells, improving drug delivery efficiency (Tang et al., 2012). MSNs can be broadly classified into two primary categories: conventional mesoporous silica nanoparticles and hollow or rattle-type mesoporous silica nanoparticles (Popat et al., 2012). These structures can be synthesized using both soft and hard templating methods, allowing for precise control over their physical and chemical properties. Importantly, smart MSNs can be engineered to release their therapeutic cargo in response to various external stimuli, such as redox conditions, pH changes, magnetic fields, temperature shifts, enzyme activity, and light exposure, making them highly adaptable for targeted drug delivery applications (Wang et al., 2015; Sun et al., 2023).

Calcium phosphate (CaP) is a naturally occurring inorganic compound found primarily in bones and teeth. It is well-regarded for its exceptional biocompatibility, biodegradability, high capacity for drug loading, and sensitivity to pH changes, making it a promising material for biomedical applications. It has been extensively used in biomedical research since the 16th century. Despite these advantages, CaP-based nanoparticles face a major limitation in vivo, as they are often non-specifically captured by the reticuloendothelial system (RES) macrophages, reducing their overall therapeutic efficacy. This challenge has driven the development of tumor-targeted CaP nanosystems to enhance specificity in cancer treatments. One promising approach involves the use of A54 peptide, a liver cancer-targeting ligand that specifically binds to BEL-7402 liver cancer cells. Nanoparticles modified with A54 peptides have been shown to accumulate more effectively at liver tumor sites, significantly improving cellular uptake and targeting efficiency compared to non-modified counterparts. Previous studies have demonstrated that A54-functionalized nanoparticles exhibit enhanced internalization and specificity for BEL-7402 cells, thereby potentially increasing drug bioavailability at the tumor site while minimizing off-target toxicity to healthy tissues (Zhang et al., 2020).

4. Specific Inorganic Nanoparticle Types and Uses

4.1. Gold Nanoparticles (AuNPs)

Rapid advances in the fields of nanotechnology and medicine have made it possible to use a large number of inorganic nanoparticles produced from various metals such as gold, silver, copper, iron, platinum, and cobalt in biomedical applications. These nanoparticles can be synthesized by both biological (e.g. plant or microbial origin) and physicochemical methods. Among these materials, gold nanoparticles (AuNPs) have attracted attention due to their simple production process, high specific surface area, surface plasmon resonance (SPR) properties, chemical stability, and easy functionalization of their surfaces. These properties have made AuNPs an attractive option for both the diagnosis of malignancies and targeted drug delivery systems (Singh et al., 2018). Gold nanoparticles can selectively infiltrate the tumor site thanks to their non-toxic nature, lack of immunogenic effects, and high permeability/permeability (EPR) effects, which can lead to more effective therapeutic outcomes (Singh et al., 2018). Physical (laser ablation, microwave and UV irradiation), chemical and biological synthesis methods are among the main techniques of AuNP production. However, chemical synthesis processes often involve toxic chemicals, which may have environmental and biological drawbacks. In contrast, biosynthesis methods, especially those using plant extracts or microorganisms, have attracted great interest due to their environmental friendliness (Singh et al., 2016; Sun et al., 2023).

AuNPs have come to the forefront, especially in stem cell research and regenerative medicine, due to their superior biocompatibility and functionalization potential. Various studies have shown that AuNPs can be phagocytosed in mesenchymal stem cells (hMSCs) without being cytotoxic and can affect cellular behaviors (proliferation, differentiation). For example, AuNPs with surfaces modified with amine, carboxyl, or hydroxyl groups showed minimal effect on cellular differentiation while increasing cellular uptake. However, some surface modifications (e.g. AuNP-COOH) can exert suppressive effects on osteogenic differentiation markers (Singh et al., 2018). These results suggest that the surface properties of AuNPs may be decisive on cellular responses and can be made suitable for regenerative medicine applications with customized surface designs. AuNPs also have several uses in cancer diagnosis and treatment thanks to their strong optical and physical properties. Structures with different geometries such as gold nanorods, nanocubes, nanostars, nanocages, and nanospheres are used for both diagnostic and therapeutic purposes thanks to their surface plasmon resonance and near-infrared (NIR) light absorption properties (Aldewachi et al., 2017). Among these structures, Au nanorods in particular are frequently preferred in light-based therapeutic approaches such as photothermal therapy (PTT) and photodynamic therapy (PDT) (Ali et al., 2017). AuNPs can be designed for surface modifications to be used in many fields from biosensors to imaging agents. For example, AuNPs modified with glutamine and lysine can induce the in situ production of photothermal agents by triggering the intra-tumor enzymatic activity (Liu et al., 2023). Furthermore, AuNPs tagged with tumor-targeted peptides containing isoDGR motifs can improve treatment efficacy by enabling the delivery of therapeutic agents to tumor tissues (Gasparri et al., 2019). Such strategies reveal the potential for the multifunctional use of AuNPs as drug carriers, diagnostic platforms, or therapeutic agents (Kong et al., 2017; Sun et al., 2023).

In conclusion, gold nanoparticles are considered as a versatile nano-tool in the biomedical field thanks to their high biocompatibility, chemical functionalization capacity, optical properties, and suitability for surface engineering. Their advantages, especially in areas such as diagnosis, imaging, drug delivery, and photothermal and photodynamic therapy, make them promising for advanced clinical applications.

4.2. *Iron Oxide Nanoparticles (IONP)*

Iron oxide nanoparticles (IONPs) typically have core sizes ranging from 10 to 100 nanometers and consist of synthetic versions of naturally occurring magnetic minerals like magnetite (Fe_3O_4) and maghemite (γ-Fe_2O_3). In addition to these primary forms, IONPs can also be engineered by alloying iron oxides with other transition metals such as copper, cobalt, and nickel, further enhancing their magnetic and functional properties. The phenomenon of superparamagnetism, especially at sizes below 10-20 nm, makes these nanoparticles highly valuable for biomedical applications. Superparamagnetic particles rapidly magnetize when an external magnetic field is applied; however, they show no permanent residual magnetism when the field is removed, making them ideal for safe and controlled biological applications (Palanisamy, 2019). Due to their unique magnetic properties, iron oxide nanoparticles are commonly utilized as contrast agents in medical imaging, particularly in magnetic resonance imaging (MRI). These nanoparticles can be synthesized using a variety of methods, including thermal decomposition, co-precipitation, hydrothermal processes, sonochemical approaches, microemulsion techniques, and microwave-assisted synthesis. Despite this wide range of production methods, chemical synthesis remains the most prevalent approach, owing to its scalability and control over particle size and shape (Cano et al., 2017). Another important application area of iron oxide nanoparticles in the biomedical field is targeted drug delivery. For this purpose, smart carrier systems functionalized with stimulus-sensitive polymer coatings (e.g. pH, temperature) are being developed. These polymers can undergo phase changes, solubility changes, and conformational transformations depending the environmental stimuli. Indeed, in a recent study, polymer-coated IONPs exhibited behavior sensitive to temperature and pH gradients (Dadfar et al., 2022). The ability of an external magnetic field to orient such nanoparticles enhances the therapeutic efficacy by enabling the delivery of therapeutic agents to specific sites. IONPs also play an important role in the transportation of genetic material. Because of the negatively charged phosphate groups of nucleic acids such as DNA and RNA, iron oxide nanoparticles are usually functionalized with cationic lipids or polymers to interact with these molecules. In this respect, IONPs are among the theranostic nano-platforms that can perform diagnosis (diagnostic) and treatment (therapeutic) simultaneously (Santhosh et al., 2013; Sun et al., 2023). One of the most common uses of IONPs in clinical applications is stem cell imaging. Non-invasive monitoring of stem cells in living organisms after transplantation is important to evaluate the success of the treatment process. Superparamagnetic iron oxide nanoparticles (SPIONs) have been used as an effective tool for labeling mesenchymal stem cells (MSCs) along with transfection agents (Palanisamy et al., 2023). Due to their high contrast and biocompatibility in MRI systems, SPIONs are considered to be among the most clinically promising nanoimaging agents for monitoring stem cell therapies. With the rapid development of nanotechnology, metal and metal oxide nanoparticles offer groundbreaking opportunities in biomedical applications. Materials such as gold and iron oxide nanoparticles play critical roles in both diagnosis and treatment processes thanks to their superior physical, chemical, and biological properties. While gold nanoparticles stand out with their surface plasmon resonance, biocompatibility, easy surface functionalization, and effectiveness in photothermal therapy, iron oxide nanoparticles have a wide range of uses, especially in magnetic resonance imaging (MRI) and targeted drug delivery systems thanks to their superparamagnetic properties. Both nanoparticle groups have great potential in areas such as stem cell therapy, cancer diagnosis and treatment, and it is predicted that revolutionary advances in biomedicine will be possible with the development of even more intelligent, safe and target-specific nanocarrier systems in future studies.

4.3. Quantum dots

Quantum dots (QDs) are among the smart nanoparticles that have attracted attention in the biomedical field, especially in applications such as imaging and drug delivery, thanks to their unique photophysical properties. These nanoparticles, usually composed of group II-VI elements, are designed to contain hundreds to thousands of atoms (Zrazhevskiy et al. 2010). Using QDs, both drug delivery to the target site and simultaneous imaging of tumors are possible during treatment (Yan et al. 2020). Commercially available QDs consist of three main components: a core of the semiconductor material, a shell such as ZnS that surrounds this core, and a coating material that provides stability (Bajwa et al. 2016). This two- or three-layer structure increases the stability of the QDs and allows for functional modifications. The diameters of the QDs generally range from 2 to 10 nm, making them well suited for cellular-level monitoring applications. Their small size makes them usable as imaging agents in drug delivery systems. Furthermore, the chemical flexibility of their surfaces makes it possible to modify them with different functional groups. In this respect, QDs can be widely used in applications such as targeted drug release and real-time monitoring of biomolecular interactions (Qi et al. 2008). Quantum dots can be produced by top-down or bottom-up synthesis strategies. Top-down methods include physical techniques such as molecular beam epitaxy, ion implantation, e-beam and X-ray lithography (Bertino, 2007). In contrast, colloidal QDs are usually synthesized by self-assembly after chemical reduction in solution, i.e., bottom-up (Sun et al. 2023). These structure and fabrication advantages make the QDs stand out as multifunctional nanoplatforms. Thanks to their superior photophysical properties and nanometric size, quantum dots stand out as strong candidates for both diagnostic and drug delivery applications. Their core-shell-coating structure allows for high stability and controlled surface modification, while their multifunctional properties, such as real-time imaging and targeted drug release, distinguish them from classical nanoparticles. The combination of tumor targeting, drug delivery, and imaging on the same platform has made quantum dots an indispensable component of smart nanotheranostic systems. In the future, the development of biocompatible, non-toxic, and clinically suitable QDs will pave the way for more sensitive and effective approaches for treating complex diseases such as cancer.

4.4. Carbon nanotubes

Carbon nanotubes (CNTs) are a distinctive type of carbon allotrope, belonging to the fullerene family, known for their diverse range of structures, including hollow spheres, ellipsoids, cylindrical tubes, and other intricate forms. At the molecular level, a CNT is essentially a graphene sheet rolled into a seamless, cylindrical shape. CNTs are typically classified into two primary categories based on their structure: single-walled carbon nanotubes (SWCNTs), which consist of a single graphene layer, and multi-walled carbon nanotubes (MWCNTs), which are composed of multiple concentric graphene cylinders (Liu, 2011). Due to their strong optical absorption in the near-infrared (NIR) spectrum, CNTs are considered promising candidates for photothermal ablation therapies. Additionally, nanoparticles in the 50 to 100 nm size range are known for their efficient cellular uptake, allowing MWCNTs to traverse various intracellular barriers. To further enhance their functionality, SWCNTs can be PEGylated, which allows for precise localization within specific cellular compartments and improves their biocompatibility and solubility. While simple heating of carbon black or graphite in controlled flame environments can produce CNTs, this method lacks control over key parameters like size, structural integrity, and purity. To overcome these limitations, more advanced methods such as electric arc discharge, chemical vapor deposition (CVD), and laser ablation have been developed (Cantoro et al., 2006). SWCNTs are often preferred for drug delivery over MWCNTs due to their more defined walls and lower tendency to form structural defects, enhancing their stability and therapeutic efficacy (Eatemadi et al., 2014). Their remarkable thermodynamic and optical properties make them ideal candidates for cancer detection, bioimaging, and therapeutic applications. Functionalization, either through chemical or physical modification, is a critical step in enhancing CNT performance. For example, PEGylation not only increases their water solubility but also helps them evade the reticuloendothelial system (RES), thereby reducing systemic toxicity (Lay et al., 2011). An interesting example of this is the conjugation of cyclosporine A (CsA) to amine-terminated phospholipid-PEG chains, which were attached to SWCNTs via cleavable ester bonds, demonstrating the potential of PEGylated SWCNTs for drug delivery (Hadidi et al., 2013). Recent findings also suggest that functionalized CNTs can cross the blood-brain barrier, further broadening their therapeutic potential (Wang et al., 2015). Beyond their applications in drug delivery, carbon nanotubes (CNTs) have demonstrated significant potential in the delivery of genetic materials, including plasmid DNA, small interfering RNA (siRNA), antisense oligonucleotides, and aptamers. They have also been explored for use in thermal ablation techniques for targeted tumor destruction (Bao et al., 2018). Additionally, CNTs are gaining attention as powerful diagnostic tools, with promising applications in the early detection of cancer (Chen et al., 2018; Sun et al., 2023).

5. Conclusion

Nanoparticle research has emerged as a highly dynamic and rapidly evolving field, attracting significant scientific interest due to its wide-ranging applications in biomedicine, environmental science, electronics, and advanced materials. In recent years, the volume of published research in this area has grown exponentially, with more than 100,000 scientific papers on nanoparticles appearing in the literature. This substantial body of work represents a critical foundation for future scientific discoveries and technological innovations, highlighting the importance of this field in shaping next-generation technologies. One of the key drivers of this progress is the availability of a diverse array of inorganic nanoparticles, synthesized through a variety of methods, which has paved the way for the development of innovative drug delivery systems and diagnostic tools. However, despite these advancements, significant challenges remain before these nanosystems can be widely adopted in clinical settings. Critical issues such as biocompatibility, toxicity, immune response, and long-term safety must be thoroughly addressed. Additionally, the precise mechanisms of cellular uptake, subcellular trafficking, and biodistribution are still not fully understood, which presents a major hurdle for translating laboratory-scale successes into clinical applications. Given their remarkable physical and chemical properties, including high surface area-to-volume ratios, tunable optical and electronic features, and environmental stability, inorganic nanoparticles hold immense potential for industrial and biomedical applications. These materials are not only promising for targeted drug delivery and precision medicine but also for environmental remediation, energy storage, catalysis, and optoelectronic devices. As such, the development of scalable, cost-effective, and environmentally friendly production methods will be crucial for their widespread adoption. Looking ahead, the future of nanoparticle research will likely focus on addressing these fundamental challenges while simultaneously exploring new frontiers such as theranostics, nanomedicine, and personalized therapies. Moreover, advances in nanoparticle surface engineering, including functionalization with specific ligands and antibodies, will enhance their targeting precision and therapeutic efficacy. This will not only improve the effectiveness of treatments for previously incurable diseases but also reduce off-target effects, thereby enhancing patient outcomes and overall healthcare quality. In conclusion, inorganic nanoparticles are poised to play a transformative role in the next wave of technological and medical breakthroughs. Their integration into clinical practice holds the potential to revolutionize the diagnosis, treatment, and prevention of complex diseases, significantly improving human health. However, achieving this vision will require a deeper understanding of their interactions at the cellular and molecular levels, as well as a concerted effort to overcome the remaining scientific and engineering challenges. Ultimately, these efforts will contribute to global economic growth and pave the way for a new era of precision medicine, benefiting future generations (Bhattacharyya et al., 2010).

References

Aldewachi, H., Chalati, T., Woodroofe, M. N., Bricklebank, N., Sharrack, B., & Gardiner, P. (2017). Gold nanoparticle-based colorimetric biosensors. *Nanoscale, 10*(1), 18–33. https://doi.org/10.1039/C7NR06367A

Ali, M. R., Ibrahim, I. M., Ali, H. R., Selim, S. A., El-Sayed, M. A., & El-Sayed, I. H. (2017). Efficacy, long-term toxicity, and mechanistic studies of gold nanorods photothermal therapy of cancer in xenograft mice. *Proceedings of the National Academy of Sciences of the United States of America, 114*(15), E3110–E3118. https://doi.org/10.1073/pnas.1619302114

Altavilla, C., & Ciliberto, E. (Eds.). (2016). *Inorganic nanoparticles: Synthesis, applications, and perspectives*. CRC Press. https://doi.org/10.1201/b19949

Bajwa, N., Mehra, N. K., Jain, K., & Jain, N. K. (2016). Pharmaceutical and biomedical applications of quantum dots. *Artificial Cells, Nanomedicine, and Biotechnology, 44*(2), 758–768. https://doi.org/10.3109/21691401.2015.1052468

Bao, X., Yuan, Y., Chen, J., Zhang, B., Li, D., Zhou, D., Jing, P., Xu, G., Wang, Y., Holá, K., Shen, D., Wu, C., Song, L., Liu, C., Zbořil, R., & Qu, S. (2018). In vivo theranostics with near-infrared-emitting carbon dots: Highly efficient photothermal therapy based on passive targeting after intravenous administration. *Light: Science & Applications, 7,* 91. https://doi.org/10.1038/s41377-018-0090-1

Bendas, G., & Borsig, L. (2012). Targeting selectins in cancer therapy. *Biochimica et Biophysica Acta (BBA) - General Subjects, 1820*(3), 309–318. https://doi.org/10.1016/j.bbagen.2011.06.012

Bertino, M. F., Sun, Y.-P., Rice, C., & Edelstein, A. S. (2007). Quantum dots by ultraviolet and X-ray lithography. *Nanotechnology, 18*(31), 315603. https://doi.org/10.1088/0957-4484/18/31/315603

Bhattacharyya, S., Bhattacharya, R., Curley, S., McNiven, M. A., & Mukherjee, P. (2010). Nanoconjugation modulates the trafficking and mechanism of antibody-induced receptor endocytosis. *Proceedings of the National Academy of Sciences of the United States of America, 107*(33), 14541–14546. https://doi.org/10.1073/pnas.1006507107

Bhattacharyya, S., Kudgus, R. A., Bhattacharya, R., & Mukherjee, P. (2011). Inorganic nanoparticles in cancer therapy. *Pharmaceutical Research, 28*(2), 237–259. https://doi.org/10.1007/s11095-010-0318-0

Billadeau, M. A., & Morrison, H. (1995). Photoaquation of cis-dichlorobis(1,10-phenanthroline)chromium(III) and the photochemical and thermal reactions of this complex with native calf-thymus DNA. *Journal of Inorganic Biochemistry, 57*(3), 249–270. https://doi.org/10.1016/0162-0134(94)00029-A

Brühwiler, D. (2010). Postsynthetic functionalization of mesoporous silica. *Nanoscale, 2*(6), 887–892. https://doi.org/10.1039/C0NR00039F

Cai, Y., Deng, T., Pan, Y., & Zink, J. I. (2020). Use of ferritin capped mesoporous silica nanoparticles for redox and pH triggered drug release in vitro and in vivo. *Advanced Functional Materials, 30*(23), 2002043. https://doi.org/10.1002/adfm.202002043

Cano, M., Núñez-Lozano, R., Dumont, Y., Larpent, C., & de la Cueva-Méndez, G. (2016). Synthesis and characterization of multifunctional superparamagnetic iron oxide nanoparticles (SPION)/C60 nanocomposites assembled by fullerene–amine click chemistry. *RSC Advances, 6*(74), 70374–70382. https://doi.org/10.1039/C6RA14047E

Cantoro, M., Hofmann, S., Pisana, S., Scardaci, V., Parvez, A., Ducati, C., Ferrari, A. C., & Robertson, J. (2006). Catalytic chemical vapor deposition of single-wall carbon nanotubes at low temperatures. *Nano Letters, 6*(5), 1107–1112. https://doi.org/10.1021/nl060068y

Chang, X., Zhang, Y., Sun, Z., Li, J., Wang, H., Chen, Q., & Liu, Y. (2022). Multifunctional Au-modified Ti_3C_2-MXene for photothermal/enzyme dynamic/immune synergistic therapy. *Nano Letters, 22*(12), 8321–8330. https://doi.org/10.1021/acs.nanolett.2c03260

Cheng, F. Y., Chen, C. T., & Yeh, C. S. (2009). Comparative efficiencies of photothermal destruction of malignant cells using antibody-coated silica@Au nanoshells, hollow Au/Ag nanospheres, and Au nanorods. *Nanotechnology, 20*(42), 425104. https://doi.org/10.1088/0957-4484/20/42/425104

Chou, L.-Y. T., Ming, K., & Chan, W. C. (2019). Engineering nanoparticles to target cancer. *ACS Nano, 13*(6), 6561–6569. https://doi.org/10.1021/nn204165v

Dadfar, S. M., Roemhild, K., Drude, N. I., von Stillfried, S., Knüchel, R., Kiessling, F., & Lammers, T. (2019). Iron oxide nanoparticles: Diagnostic, therapeutic and theranostic applications. *Advanced Drug Delivery Reviews, 138,* 302–325. https://doi.org/10.1016/j.addr.2019.01.005

Dang, Y., & Guan, J. (2020). Nanoparticle-based drug delivery systems for cancer therapy. *Smart Materials in Medicine, 1,* 10–19. https://doi.org/10.1016/j.smaim.2020.04.001

Dykman, L. A., & Khlebtsov, N. G. (2016). Multifunctional gold-based nanocomposites for theranostics. *Biomaterials, 108,* 13–34. https://doi.org/10.1016/j.biomaterials.2016.08.040

Eatemadi, A., Daraee, H., Karimkhanloo, H., Kouhi, M., Zarghami, N., Akbarzadeh, A., Abasi, M., Hanifehpour, Y., & Joo, S. W. (2014). Carbon nanotubes: Properties, synthesis, purification, and medical applications. *Nanoscale Research Letters, 9*(1), 393. https://doi.org/10.1186/1556-276X-9-393

Fathima, T., & Mujeeb, A. (2021). Silver nanoparticles and their interactions with biomolecules. *Materials Science & Engineering C, 119,* 111548. https://doi.org/10.1016/j.msec.2020.111548

Gao, J., Liang, G., Zhang, B., Kuang, Y., Zhang, X., & Xu, B. (2007). FePt yolk-shell nanocrystals as a potent agent to kill HeLa cells. *Journal of the American Chemical Society, 129*(5), 1428–1433. https://doi.org/10.1021/ja067785e

Garcia Ribeiro, R. S., Belderbos, S., Danhier, P., Gallo, J., Manshian, B. B., Gallez, B., Bañobre, M., de Cuyper, M., Soenen, S. J., Gsell, W., & Himmelreich, U. (2019). Targeting tumor cells and neovascularization using RGD-functionalized magnetoliposomes. *International journal of nanomedicine*, *14*, 5911–5924. https://doi.org/10.2147/IJN.S214041

Gasparri, A. M., Colombo, F., Curnis, F., Sacchi, A., & Corti, A. (2019). Boosting interleukin-12 antitumor activity and synergism with immunotherapy by targeted delivery with IsoDGR-tagged nanogold. *Small, 15*(28), 1903462. https://doi.org/10.1002/smll.201903462

Gupta, R. (2017). Diabetes treatment by nanotechnology. *Journal of Biotechnology & Biomaterials, 7*(3), 268. https://doi.org/10.4172/2155-952X.1000268

Hadidi, N., Kobarfard, F., Nafissi-Varcheh, N., & Aboofazeli, R. (2013). PEGylated single-walled carbon nanotubes as nanocarriers for cyclosporin A delivery. *AAPS PharmSciTech, 14*(2), 593–600. https://doi.org/10.1208/s12249-013-9944-2

Haleem, A., Javaid, M., Singh, R. P., Rab, S., & Suman, R. (2023). Applications of nanotechnology in the medical field: A brief review. *Global Health Journal, 7*(2), 70–73. https://doi.org/10.1016/j.glohj.2023.02.008

Hall, M. D., Mellor, H. R., Callaghan, R., & Hambley, T. W. (2007). Basis for design and development of platinum(IV) anticancer complexes. *Journal of Medicinal Chemistry, 50*(15), 3403–3411. https://doi.org/10.1021/jm070280u

Harjunpää, H., Ascierto, P. A., Lipson, E. J., & Grosso, J. F. (2019). Immunoregulatory role of tumor cell-expressed CD47 in cancer. *Frontiers in Immunology, 10,* 1324. https://doi.org/10.3389/fimmu.2021.739048

He, Y., Al-Mureish, A., & Wu, N. (2021). Nanotechnology in the treatment of diabetic complications: A comprehensive narrative review. *Journal of Diabetes Research, 2021,* 1–10. https://doi.org/10.1155/2021/6612063

Hirsch, L. R., Stafford, R. J., Bankson, J. A., Sershen, S. R., Rivera, B., Price, R. E., Hazle, J. D., Halas, N. J., & West, J. L. (2003). Nanoshell-mediated near-infrared thermal therapy of tumors under magnetic resonance guidance. *Proceedings of the National Academy of Sciences of the United States of America, 100*(23), 13549–13554. https://doi.org/10.1073/pnas.2232479100

Hou, K. K., Pan, H., Schlesinger, P. H., & Wickline, S. A. (2017). Integrin-targeted nanoparticles for drug delivery. *ACS Nano, 11*(7), 6739–6747. https://doi.org/10.1021/acsami.3c12776

Huang, H., Liu, R., Yang, J., Dai, J., Fan, S., Pi, J., Wei, Y., & Guo, X. (2023). Gold nanoparticles: Construction for drug delivery and application in cancer immunotherapy. *Pharmaceutics, 15*(7), 1868. https://doi.org/10.3390/pharmaceutics15071868

Huang, X., El-Sayed, I. H., Qian, W., & El-Sayed, M. A. (2006). Cancer cell imaging and photothermal therapy in the near-infrared region by using gold nanorods. *Journal of the American Chemical Society, 128*(6), 2115–2120. https://doi.org/10.1021/ja057254a

Hynes, N. E., & Lane, H. A. (2005). ERBB receptors and cancer: The complexity of targeted inhibitors. *Nature Reviews Cancer, 5*(5), 341–354. https://doi.org/10.1038/nrc1609

Joudeh, N., & Linke, D. (2022). Nanoparticle classification, physicochemical properties, characterization, and applications: A comprehensive review for biologists. *Journal of Nanobiotechnology, 20*(1), 262. https://doi.org/10.1186/s12951-022-01477-8

Khan, I. (2020). Recent advances in metal nanoparticles. *Journal of Materials Chemistry B, 8*(32), 7312–7329. https://doi.org/10.1039/D5TA04223B

Khan, M. A. (2019). Functionalized gold nanoparticles in cancer therapy. *Nano Research, 12*(5), 1083–1093. https://doi.org/10.3390/pharmaceutics15071932

Kim, B. Y., Rutka, J. T., & Chan, W. C. (2010). Nanomedicine. *New England Journal of Medicine, 363*(25), 2434–2443. https://doi.org/10.1056/NEJMra0912273

Kong, F.-Y., Zhang, J.-W., Li, R.-F., Wang, Z.-X., Wang, W.-J., & Wang, W. (2017). Unique roles of gold nanoparticles in drug delivery, targeting and imaging applications. *Molecules, 22*(9), 1445. https://doi.org/10.3390/molecules22091445

Kumar, D., Saini, N., Jain, N., Sareen, R., & Pandit, V. (2013). Gold nanoparticles: An era in bionanotechnology. *Expert Opinion on Drug Delivery, 10*(3), 397–409. https://doi.org/10.1517/17425247.2013.749854

Lay, C. L., Liu, J., & Liu, Y. (2011). Functionalized carbon nanotubes for anticancer drug delivery. *Expert Review of Medical Devices, 8*(5), 561–566. https://doi.org/10.1586/erd.11.34

Leon, L., Chung, E. J., & Rinaldi, C. (2020). A brief history of nanotechnology and introduction to nanoparticles for biomedical applications. In E. J. Chung & C. Rinaldi (Eds.), Nanoparticles for biomedical applications (pp. 1–4). Elsevier. https://doi.org/10.1016/B978-0-12-816662-8.00001-1

Li, C., Wang, J., Wang, Y., Gao, H., Wei, G., Huang, Y., & Zhang, L. (2019). Recent progress in drug delivery. Acta Pharmaceutica Sinica B, 9(6), 1145–1162. https://doi.org/10.1016/j.apsb.2019.08.003

Li, J., & Burgess, D. J. (2020). Nanomedicine-based drug delivery towards tumor biological and immunological microenvironment. *Acta Pharmaceutica Sinica B, 10*(11), 2110–2124. https://doi.org/10.1016/j.apsb.2020.05.008

Li, Z., de Barros, A. L. B., Soares, D. C. F., Moss, S. N., & Alisaraie, L. (2017). Functionalized single-walled carbon nanotubes: Cellular uptake, biodistribution and applications in drug delivery. *International Journal of Pharmaceutics, 524*(1–2), 41–54. https://doi.org/10.1016/j.ijpharm.2017.03.017

Lian, S., Xie, X., Lu, Y., Jia, L., & Liang, Z. (2019). CD47/SIRPα signaling in cancer immune evasion. *Journal of Hematology & Oncology, 12*(1), 34. https://doi.org/10.1016/j.coi.2012.01.010

Liu, T., Li, X., Wang, J., Chen, Y., Zhang, L., & Zhao, H. (2023). Tumor-specific photothermal-therapy-assisted immunomodulation via multiresponsive adjuvant nanoparticles. *Advanced Materials, 35*(1), 2300086. https://doi.org/10.1002/adma.202300086

Liu, Z., Robinson, J. T., Tabakman, S. M., Yang, K., & Dai, H. (2011). Carbon materials for drug delivery & cancer therapy. *Materials Today, 14*(7–8), 316–323. https://doi.org/10.1016/S1369-7021(11)70161-4

Ma, X., Luan, Z., & Li, J. (2023). Inorganic nanoparticles-based systems in biomedical applications of stem cells: Opportunities and challenges. *International Journal of Nanomedicine, 18,* 143–182. https://doi.org/10.2147/IJN.S384343

Makhlouf, A. S. H., & Barhoum, A. (Eds.). (2018). *Handbook of nanoparticles.* Springer. https://doi.org/10.1007/978-3-319-13188-7

Malachowski, K., & Hassel, B. A. (2020). Nanoparticle systems for cancer immunotherapy. *Cancer Immunology, Immunotherapy, 69*(3), 367–378. https://doi.org/10.1007/s00262-020-02530-2

Manral, K., Singh, A., & Singh, Y. (2024). Nanotechnology as a potential treatment for diabetes and its complications: A review. *Diabetes & Metabolic Syndrome: Clinical Research & Reviews, 18*(11–12), 103159. https://doi.org/10.1016/j.dsx.2024.103159

Menon, J. U., Jadeja, P., Tambe, P., Vu, K., Yuan, B., Nguyen, K. T., & Saha, D. (2013). Nanomaterials for photo-based diagnostic and therapeutic applications. *Theranostics, 3*(3), 152–166. https://doi.org/10.7150/thno.5327

Mody, V. V., Siwale, R., Singh, A., & Mody, H. R. (2010). Introduction to metallic nanoparticles. *Journal of Pharmacy and Bioallied Sciences, 2*(4), 282–289. https://doi.org/10.4103/0975-7406.72127

Mody, V., Siwale, R., Singh, A., & Mody, H. (2010). Introduction to metallic nanoparticles. *Journal of Pharmacy and BioAllied Sciences, 2*(4), 282–289. https://doi.org/10.4103/0975-7406.72127

Nasrollahzadeh, M., Sajadi, S. M., Sajjadi, M., & Issaabadi, Z. (2019). An introduction to nanotechnology. In M. Nasrollahzadeh, S. M. Sajadi, M. Sajjadi, Z. Issaabadi, & M. Atarod (Eds.), Interface science and technology (Vol. 28, pp. 1–27). Elsevier. https://doi.org/10.1016/B978-0-12-813586-0.00001-8

Nie, Z., Petukhova, A., & Kumacheva, E. (2010). Properties and self-assembly of inorganic nanoparticles. *Nature Nanotechnology, 5*(1), 15–25. https://doi.org/10.1038/nnano.2009.453

Okegawa, T., Pong, R. C., Li, Y., & Hsieh, J. T. (2004). Integrin-mediated cell adhesion and invasion in cancer. *International Journal of Oncology, 25*(2), 437–444. https://doi.org/10.3892/ijo.25.2.437

Palanisamy, K. L., Vignesh, K., & Karthikeyan, N. (2023). Applications and toxicology of iron oxide nanoparticles. In P. K. Rai (Ed.), *Iron oxide nanoparticles: Advances in science and technology* (pp. 1–20). IntechOpen. https://doi.org/10.5772/intechopen.1001336

Palanisamy, S., & Wang, Y.-M. (2019). Superparamagnetic iron oxide nanoparticulate system: Synthesis, targeting, drug delivery and therapy in cancer. *Dalton Transactions, 48*(31), 9490–9515. https://doi.org/10.1039/C9DT00459A

Papini, E., Silvestri, A., Taddei, C., & Pozzi, D. (2020). Mechanisms of nanoparticle uptake and trafficking in cells. *Advanced Drug Delivery Reviews, 158,* 34–64. https://doi.org/10.1016/j.addr.2020.06.001

Patra, J. K., Das, G., Fraceto, L. F., Campos, E. V., Rodriguez-Torres, M. D., Acosta-Torres, L. S., Diaz-Torres, L. A., Grillo, R., Swamy, M. K., Sharma, S., Habtemariam, S., & Shin, H. S. (2018). Nano based drug delivery systems: Recent developments and future prospects. *Journal of Nanobiotechnology, 16*(1), 1–33. https://doi.org/10.1186/s12951-018-0392-8

Popat, A., Liu, J., Lu, G. Q., & Qiao, S. Z. (2012). A pH-responsive drug delivery system based on chitosan coated mesoporous silica nanoparticles. *Journal of Materials Chemistry, 22*(22), 11173–11178. https://doi.org/10.1039/C2JM30501A

Pratiwi, F. W., Nugraha, R., Wulandari, D. R., Rahmawati, Y., Santoso, S. P., Iman, R. N., & Sari, I. P. (2019). Nanoparticle delivery systems in cancer therapy. *Pharmaceutics, 11*(8), 401.

https://doi.org/10.3390/pharmaceutics11080401

Qi, L., & Gao, X. (2008). Emerging application of quantum dots for drug delivery and therapy. *Expert Opinion on Drug Delivery, 5*(3), 263–267. https://doi.org/10.1517/17425247.5.3.263

Rai, M., Yadav, A., & Gade, A. (2009). Silver nanoparticles as a new generation of antimicrobials. *Biotechnology advances*, *27*(1), 76–83. https://doi.org/10.1016/j.biotechadv.2008.09.002

Raj, M., & Manoj, S. V. (2022). Coal-based carbon nanomaterials. *Materials Today: Proceedings, 56,* 115–120. https://doi.org/10.1016/j.matpr.2022.03.082

Ramsden, J. (2011). *Nanotechnology: An introduction* (2nd ed.). William Andrew.

Reibold, M., Paufler, P., Levin, A. A., Kochmann, W., Pätzke, N., & Meyer, D. C. (2006). Carbon nanotubes in an ancient Damascus sabre. *Nature, 444*(7117), 286. https://doi.org/10.1038/444286a

Reibold, M., Paufler, P., Levin, A. A., Kochmann, W., Pätzke, N., & Meyer, D. C. (2006). Carbon nanotubes in an ancient Damascus saber. *Nature, 444*(7117), 286. https://doi.org/10.1038/444286a

Roy, I., Mitra, S., Maitra, A., & Mozumdar, S. (2003). Calcium phosphate nanoparticles as novel non-viral vectors for targeted gene delivery. *International journal of pharmaceutics*, *250*(1), 25–33. https://doi.org/10.1016/s0378-5173(02)00452-0

Saleh, T. A., & Gupta, V. K. (2016). Functionalization of carbon-based nanomaterials. *Environmental Nanotechnology, 5*(3), 183–192. https://doi.org/10.1016/B978-0-323-95931-5.00014-2

Sam, M., Hwang, J., Chanfreau, G., & Abu-Omar, M. M. (2004). Hydroxyl radical is the active species in photochemical DNA strand scission by bis(peroxo)vanadium(V) phenanthroline. *Inorganic Chemistry, 43*(26), 8447–8455. https://doi.org/10.1021/ic0486419

Santhosh, P. B., & Ulrih, N. P. (2013). Multifunctional superparamagnetic iron oxide nanoparticles: Promising tools in cancer theranostics. *Cancer Letters, 336*(1), 8–17. https://doi.org/10.1016/j.canlet.2013.04.032

Shapira, A., Livney, Y. D., Broxterman, H. J., & Assaraf, Y. G. (2011). Nanomedicine for targeted cancer therapy: Towards the overcoming of drug resistance. *Drug Resistance Updates, 14*(3), 150–163. https://doi.org/10.1016/j.drup.2011.01.003

Shi, J., Votruba, A. R., Farokhzad, O. C., & Langer, R. (2010). Nanotechnology in drug delivery and tissue engineering: From discovery to applications. *Nano Letters, 10*(9), 3223–3230. https://doi.org/10.1021/nl102184c

Siegler, E. L., Kim, Y. J., & Wang, P. (2016). Nanomedicine targeting the tumor microenvironment: Therapeutic strategies to inhibit angiogenesis, remodel matrix, and modulate immune responses. *Journal of Cellular Immunotherapy, 2*(2), 69–78. https://doi.org/10.1016/j.jocit.2016.08.002

Singh, P., Kim, Y. J., Zhang, D., & Yang, D. C. (2016). Biogenic silver and gold nanoparticles synthesized using red ginseng root extract, and their applications. *Artificial Cells, Nanomedicine, and Biotechnology, 44*(2), 811–816. https://doi.org/10.3109/21691401.2015.1008514

Singh, P., Kim, Y. J., Zhang, D., & Yang, D. C. (2018). In vitro anti-inflammatory activity of spherical silver nanoparticles and monodisperse hexagonal gold nanoparticles by fruit extract of *Prunus serrulata*: A green synthetic approach. *Artificial Cells, Nanomedicine, and Biotechnology, 46*(8), 2022–2032. https://doi.org/10.1080/21691401.2017.1408117

Singh, P., Pandit, S., Beshay, M., Mokkapati, V. R. S. S., & Mijakovic, I. (2018). Gold nanoparticles in diagnostics and therapeutics for human cancer. *International Journal of Molecular Sciences, 19*(6), 1979. https://doi.org/10.3390/ijms19071979

Slowing, I. I., Trewyn, B. G., & Lin, V. S. (2007). Mesoporous silica nanoparticles for intracellular delivery of membrane-impermeable proteins. *Journal of the American Chemical Society*, *129*(28), 8845–8849. https://doi.org/10.1021/ja0719780

Smith, R. J., Brown, T., Clark, P., & Wilson, M. (2019). Carbon allotropes in nanomedicine. *Nanomedicine, 14*(8), 971–989. https://doi.org/10.3390/ma11020295

Sondi, I., & Salopek-Sondi, B. (2004). Silver nanoparticles as antimicrobial agent: A case study on *E. coli* as a model for Gram-negative bacteria. *Journal of Colloid and Interface Science, 275*(1), 177–182. https://doi.org/10.1016/j.jcis.2004.02.012

Subhan, M. A., Yousaf, M., Faiyaz, M., Nisar, M. F., Khan, M. I., & Siddique, R. (2021). Tumor targeting strategies for nanomedicine. *Pharmaceutics, 13*(4), 478. https://doi.org/10.3390/pharmaceutics13040478

Sun, L., Liu, H., Ye, Y., Zhang, Y., Zhang, Z., Wang, H., Chen, X., & Zhao, Y. (2023). Smart nanoparticles for cancer therapy. *Signal Transduction and Targeted Therapy, 8,* 418. https://doi.org/10.1038/s41392-023-01642-x

Sun, Y., Chen, Y., Shen, J., Yao, Y., Xu, F., Chen, H., Jin, H., & Wang, J. (2016). Multifunctional nanoparticles for tumor targeting and cancer therapy. *Theranostics, 6*(10), 1520–1531.

https://doi.org/10.7150/thno.16018
Tang, F., Li, L., & Chen, D. (2012). Mesoporous silica nanoparticles: Synthesis, biocompatibility and drug delivery. *Advanced Materials, 24*(12), 1504–1534. https://doi.org/10.1002/adma.201104763
Valdembri, D., & Serini, G. (2021). The roles of integrins in cancer. *Faculty Reviews, 10,* 45. https://doi.org/10.12703/r/10-45
Visaria, R. K., Griffin, R. J., Williams, B. W., Ebbini, E. S., Paciotti, G. F., Song, C. W., Colvin, O. M., & Bischof, J. C. (2006). Enhancement of tumor thermal therapy using gold nanoparticle-assisted tumor necrosis factor-α delivery. *Molecular Cancer Therapeutics, 5*(4), 1014–1020. https://doi.org/10.1158/1535-7163.MCT-05-0381
Viswanath, B., & Kim, S. (2017). Influence of nanotoxicity on human health and environment: The alternative strategies. In D. M. Whitacre (Ed.), *Reviews of environmental contamination and toxicology* (Vol. 242, pp. 61–104). Springer. https://doi.org/10.1007/398_2016_12
Walter, J., Brown, S. D. M., & Turner, A. P. L. (2006). Hair dyes in ancient times. *Journal of Archaeological Science, 33*(7), 1022–1029. https://doi.org/10.1016/j.jas.2006.01.014
Walter, P., Welcomme, E., Hallegot, P., Verger, I., Bréniaux, R., Lefebvre, M. A., Gallet, X., Veyssière, P., Fort, A., & Mille, B. (2006). Early use of PbS nanotechnology for an ancient hair dying formula. *Nano Letters, 6*(10), 2215–2219. https://doi.org/10.1021/nl061493u
Wang, J. T.-W., & Al-Jamal, K. T. (2015). Functionalized carbon nanotubes: Revolution in brain delivery. *Nanomedicine, 10*(17), 2639–2642. https://doi.org/10.2217/nnm.15.114
Wang, X., Liu, F., Andavan, G. T. S., Jing, X., Singh, K., Yazdanpanah, V. R., Koratkar, N., Kang, Y., Chen, P., & Ajayan, P. M. (2006). Carbon nanotube-DNA nanoarchitectures and electronic functionality. *Small, 2*(11), 1356–1365. https://doi.org/10.1002/smll.200600056
Wang, Y., Zhao, Q., Han, N., Bai, L., Li, J., Liu, J., Che, E., Hu, L., Zhang, Q., Jiang, T., & Wang, S. (2015). Mesoporous silica nanoparticles in drug delivery and biomedical applications. *Nanomedicine: Nanotechnology, Biology and Medicine, 11*(2), 313–327. https://doi.org/10.1016/j.nano.2014.09.014
Wu, C.-P., Zhang, J., Chen, L., Li, Q., & Zhou, W. (2022). Nanomedicine strategies to target cancer stem cells. *Journal of Nanobiotechnology, 20*(1), 12. https://doi.org/10.37349/etat.2023.0015
Xu, C., Yuan, Z., Kohler, N., Kim, J., Chung, M. A., & Sun, S. (2009). FePt yonanoparticles as an Fe reservoir for controlled Fe release and tumor inhibition. *Journal of the American Chemical Society, 131*(42), 15346–15351. https://doi.org/10.1021/ja905938a

Yan, X., Ma, J., Yu, K., Li, J., Yang, L., Liu, J., Wang, J., & Cai, L. (2020). Highly green fluorescent Nb_2C MXene quantum dots for Cu^{2+} ion sensing and cell imaging. *Chinese Chemical Letters, 31*(12), 3173–3177. https://doi.org/10.1016/j.cclet.2020.05.020

Yang, R., Yang, X., Zhang, Z., Zhang, Y., Wang, S., Cai, Z., Jia, Y., Ma, Y., Zheng, C., Lu, Y., Roden, R., & Chen, Y. (2006). Single-walled carbon nanotubes-mediated in vivo and in vitro delivery of siRNA into antigen-presenting cells. *Gene Therapy, 13*(24), 1714–1723. https://doi.org/10.1038/sj.gt.3302808

Yang, S., Zhang, R., Su, Y., Zhou, L., & Dong, C.-M. (2019). Tumor-targeted biodegradable multifunctional nanoparticles for cancer theranostics. *Chemical Engineering Journal, 378,* 122171. https://doi.org/10.1016/j.cej.2019.122171

Yang, S., Zhou, L., Su, Y., Zhang, R., & Dong, C.-M. (2019). One-pot photoreduction to prepare NIR-absorbing plasmonic gold nanoparticles tethered by amphiphilic polypeptide copolymer for synergistic photothermal-chemotherapy. *Chinese Chemical Letters, 30*(2), 187–191. https://doi.org/10.1016/j.cclet.2018.02.015

Zhang, N., Lu, C., Shu, G., Li, J., Chen, M., Chen, C., Lv, X., Xu, X., Weng, W., Weng, Q., Tang, B., Du, Y., & Ji, J. (2020). Gadolinium-loaded calcium phosphate nanoparticles for magnetic resonance imaging of orthotopic hepatocarcinoma and primary hepatocellular carcinoma. *Biomaterials Science, 8*(7), 1961–1972. https://doi.org/10.1039/c9bm01544b

Zhao, Z., Zhou, Z., Bao, J., Wang, Z., Hu, J., Chi, X., Ni, K., Wang, R., Chen, X., & Gao, J. (2022). Recent advances in engineering iron oxide nanoparticles for effective magnetic resonance imaging. *Bioactive Materials, 12,* 214–245. https://doi.org/10.1016/j.bioactmat.2021.10.014

Zhu, Y., Feijen, J., & Zhong, Z. (2018). Dual-targeted nanomedicines for enhanced tumor treatment. *Nano Today, 18,* 65–85. https://doi.org/10.1016/j.nantod.2017.12.007

Zrazhevskiy, P., Sena, M., & Gao, X. (2010). Designing multifunctional quantum dots for bioimaging, detection, and drug delivery. *Chemical Society Reviews, 39*(11), 4326–4354. https://doi.org/10.1039/b915139g

Author Biography

Hüseyin İzgördü completed his bachelor's and master's degrees in biology at Kütahya Dumlupınar University and successfully completed his doctorate in molecular biology at Eskişehir Technical University. Specializing in cancer research and nanotechnology-based drug development, İzgördü is currently pursuing his postdoctoral research at Eskişehir Osmangazi University. His work, supported by various national and international scholarships, focuses on topics such as cancer biology, cell death mechanisms, and sphingolipid metabolism. He has participated in numerous scientific research projects, including TÜBİTAK projects, as a director and researcher. His academic achievements include articles published in high-impact journals and presentations at international scientific congresses. Hüseyin İzgördü has participated in numerous training and workshops that have contributed to his professional development and has also won awards aimed at inspiring young researchers. İzgördü aims to make a difference in the health sciences by presenting innovative approaches to cancer biology and has also contributed to biology education through his teaching experience.

CHAPTER 14

TRANSPOSON-BASED DELIVERY SYSTEMS AS A STRATEGIC PIONEER IN GENE THERAPY: A COMPREHENSIVE OVERVIEW

YASEMIN KARTAL, PHD

Department of Physiology, Kırklareli University, Kırklareli, Türkiye

Abstract

Gene therapy, an advanced medical approach employed to treat or prevent certain diseases by manipulating gene expression and reprogramming cellular biological properties, has exhibited considerable advancements in recent years. The widespread application of gene therapy in medicine necessitates the capacity to achieve stable integration of genetic information via gene delivery systems in a manner that ensures efficiency, safety, as well as cost-effectiveness. Since the early stages of gene therapy, viral vector systems have been presented as the majority and attractive vehicles to transfer specific genetic materyal to particular target cells. However, transposons, defined as mobile genetic elements, have recently emerged as promising vectors for gene therapy, offering the potential to overcome some of limitations of commonly employed viral vectors. Transposons or transposable elements (TEs) have the potential to evolve into powerful tools to modify the architecture of genomes and as such, transposon-based technologies can play a game-changer role in the both physiological and pathological processes. TEs exist within the genomes of bacteria, plants and mammals, and are categorized into two major classes depending on the transposition processes. Class I TEs, or retrotransposons, act via reverse-transcribed RNA intermediates and propagate within the genome via a "copy-and-paste" mechanism. In contrast, Class II TEs, or DNA transposons, mobilize via a DNA intermediate and transpose in the genome in a "cut-and-paste" fashion. Sleeping Beauty (SB), PiggyBac (PB), as well as Tol2 are the most widely studied transposon systems in basic research and preclinical applications. The straightforward and encouraging results obtained in preclinical studies indicated that SB and PB-based gene therapy applications are highly promising approaches for clinical investigations. However, Tol2 transposon gene therapy remains relatively limited compared to SB and PB transposons. The first-in-human clinical trial (Phase-I/IIA; EudraCT: 2019-001264-30) with virus-free chimeric antigen receptor (CAR) gene transfer utilizing the cutting-edge SB-based technology to treat multiple myeloma. Despite the promising outcomes obtained from Phase I/II clinical trials, the effectiveness and safety of transposons must be rigorously assessed on an individualized basis, considering critical factors such as cell type, specific target of disease as well as transfection methods.

Keywords: Gene therapy, non-viral vectors, piggyBac, Sleeping Beauty, Tol2, transposon.

1. Introduction

Gene therapy is defined as a therapeutic strategy that incorporates groundbreaking biotechnological interventions with the potential to revolutionize modern medicine (Tamura & Toda, 2020; Bhagat et al., 2024). This technology is applied to transfer of genetic material into the target cells to replace or modify a nonfunctional or defective gene with *in- vivo* and *ex-vivo* strategies (Tang & Xu, 2020). The first successful gene transfer in human was conducted in 1989 and was approved by National Institutes of Health, representing a landmark in the field (O'Reilly et al., 2012). Gene delivery systems are fundamental tools of gene therapy, broadly classified into viral and non-viral vectors each offering distinct advantages (specificity and efficiency) and limitations (off-target effects, immunogenic and inflammatory responses) (Sayed et al., 2022; Bhagat et al., 2024). Viral vectors which have been genetically modified to eliminate their pathogenic potential are widely utilized in gene delivery due to their high transduction efficiency and stable gene expression, however, certain challenges remain such as immunotoxicity and safety concerns (Li et al., 2023; Yudaeva et al., 2024). Viral vector-based gene therapy application relies on three principal vector platforms: adeno-associated viruses (AAVs), adenoviruses, as well as lentiviruses (Li et al., 2023). In addition, viral vector-based delivery systems have been employed in both preclinical and clinical trials (Lundstrom, 2023). Nevertheless, gene delivery systems based on non-viral vector platforms have attracted significant attention in clinical applications offering several advantages including lower toxicity, reduced cytotoxicity, lack of immunogenicity as well as diminished biosafety challenges compared to viral vector mediated gene delivery systems (Begum et al., 2019; Zu & Gao, 2021; Ginn et al., 2024). Furthermore, non-viral vectors exhibit a higher genetic payload capacity and offer easier production than viral vectors (Yin et al., 2014).

Transposons, stated as mobile genetic elements, have demonstrated significant progress in both preclinical and clinical research related to gene therapy in recent years, owing to the aforementioned advantages of non-viral vectors ([a]Tipanee et al., 2017; [b]Tipanee et al., 2017). Transposons, or transposable elements (TEs), first described by Barbara McClintock in the maize genome in 1950, have emerged as pivotal regulators of both physiological and pathological processes across all domains of life, including prokaryotic and eukaryotic organisms (Colonna Romano & Fanti, 2022; Schmitz & Querques, 2024). Although transposons were initially regarded as "genomic parasites", labeled as "junk DNA" or referred to as "jumping genes" due to their ability to move from one genomic location to another, accumulating evidence over the past decades has revealed their potential to serve as powerful modulators of gene expression, drivers of genomic diversity, and pivotal contributors to genome evolution (Colonna Romano & Fanti, 2022; Tang & Liang, 2024). Additionality, TEs have the capacity to remodel or alter the host genome through diverse mechanisms, including insertional mutagenesis, deletions, duplications as well as translocations (Ayarpadikannan & Kim, 2014).

Transposons can be broadly categorized into two well-defined classes based on the type of the transposition intermediates and propagation strategies: Class I TEs (or retrotransposons) and Class II TEs (or DNA transposons) (Schmitz & Querques, 2024). Class I TEs, mobilize within the genome via a "copy-and-paste" mechanism that relies on reverse-transcribed RNA intermediates. Their transposition process entails transcription of the element, followed by reverse transcription, and ultimately integration into the target DNA (Ayarpadikannan & Kim, 2014). In contrast, Class II TEs transpose within the genome via a "cut-and-paste" mechanism that does not involve reverse-transcribed RNA intermediates; instead, it relies solely on DNA molecules as the transposition substrate. This process involves the generation of DNA double-strand breaks (DSBs) at both ends of the element, facilitating the physical excision of the transposon from its donor site and its subsequent integration into a new target locus (Hickman & Dyda, 2016; Wells & Feschotte, 2020).

Class I TEs possess the potential to play a crucial role in regulating the chromosomal architecture and expression of structural genes (Arvas et al., 2023). In addition, retrotransposons are subdivided into two major categories depending on their structure and transposition cycle: Long terminal repeat (LTR) retrotransposons and non-LTR retrotransposons (Cordaux & Batzer, 2009). LTR retrotransposons, also known as endogenous retroviruses (ERVs), characterized by the presence of LTRs, exhibit both structural and phylogenetic similarities with retroviruses (Ramakrishnan et al., 2023; Luqman-Fatah et al., 2024). Nonetheless, unlike retroviruses, LTR retrotransposons typically lack the *envelope* (*env*) gene required for infecting animal or insect cells, with a few exceptions (Ty3/Gypsy superfamily) (Ramakrishnan et al., 2023). Structurally, a functional LTR element consists of three regions: U3 (unique, 3′ end), R (repeat), and U5 (unique, 5' end) (Pluta et al., 2020; Horvath et al., 2024). The U3 is situated upstream of the transcription start site (TSS), while the U5 is positioned downstream of the TTS (Zhang et al., 2014). The U3 region encompasses the basal promoter, a core enhancer and regulatory motifs which participate in transcriptional regulation (Münch et al., 2005; Zhang et al., 2014). Moreover, U5 region may include additional regulatory elements (Horvath et al., 2024). The R region, positioned between the U3 and U5 regions, comprises both the start and termination sites for transcription (Uren et al., 2005; Pluta et al., 2020). The fundamental structure of an LTR-RT comprises two identical LTRs flanked by target site duplications (TSDs), a primer binding site (PBS) that acts as minus priming site for reverse transcription, and a polypurine tract (PPT) that serves as plus priming site for reverse transcription (Yin et al., 2013; Kalendar et al., 2019). The internal region located between the two LTRs constitutes the coding sequence of the element, encompassing the gag and pol domains which are related with transposition and integration mechanisms (Vangelisti et al., 2020). In particular, gag is responsible for the encoding a major structural proteins including the capsid (CA), nucleocapsid (NC), and the synthesis of reverse transcription while pol encodes several essential enzymes crucial for the processing of RE transcripts, including reverse transcriptase (RT), ribonuclease H (RNH), integrase (INT) as well as protease (PR) (Bennetzen, 2000; Ustyantsev et al., 2015; Dodonova et al., 2019; Kalendar et al., 2021). LTR retrotransposons are classified into five superfamilies: Ty1/Copia, Ty3/Gypsy, Bel-Pao, retrovirales, as well as ERV-like elements based on the phylogenetic relationships of their RT sequences, proliferating devices, gag-pol domain architecture and structural characteristics (Nouroz et al., 2015). Each group of transposons is associated with non-autonomous forms, which are missing one or more sequences required for transposition (Hassan et al., 2024). In addition, LTR retrotransposons comprise two distinct non-autonomous forms: terminal-repeat retrotransposons in miniature (TRIM) and large retrotransposon derivatives (LARD) (Kalendar et al., 2021).

Retrotransposons represent the most abundant transposable elements within plant genomes (Huang et al., 2017) and LTR retrotransposons constitute the major proportion among TEs (Nouroz et al., 2015). In this context, the activation or silencing of LTR retrotransposons in plants has the potential to induce epigenetic modifications, promising a candidate for the development of genetic engineering tools that provide many advantages for genome regulation and stability (Ramakrishnan et al., 2023). Additionality, LTR elements are termed human endogenous retroviruses (HERVs) in humans, which constitute approximately 8% of the human genome (Giménez-Orenga & Oltra, 2021). It is worth noting that HERVs have emerged as promising therapeutic targets owing to their variable expression levels across a wide range of malignancies (Serafino et al., 2009; Cherkasova et al., 2011; Balestrieri et al., 2018) and their established involvement in various oncogenic pathways (Stricker et al., 2023).

Non-LTR retrotransposons, also referred to as poly (A) retroelements or target-primed (TP), are characterized by the absence of LTRs and transpose via mechanisms which are different from LTR retrotransposons (Han, 2010). In addition, non-LTR retrotransposons consist of Long Interspersed Nuclear Elements (LINEs), Short Interspersed Nuclear Elements (SINEs), and SINE-variable number of tandem repeat (VNTR)- *Alu* (SVA) elements (Luqman-Fatah et al., 2024). LINEs encompass several superfamilies, including I, R2, Jockey, L1, and RTE while SINEs are classified into the tRNA, 5S and 7SL superfamilies (Hassan et al., 2024). LINE-1 or L1, an autonomous non-LTR retrotransposon in mammals, encodes two essential polypeptides open reading frame 1 (ORF1) and ORF2 which are required for its mobilization. On the other hand, SINEs are non-autonomous forms and their mobilization depend on L1 proteins (Dewannieux & Heidmann, 2005; Grandi & An, 2013). Additionally, Dictyostelium discoideum TE (DIRS), categorized within Class I TEs, is further subdivided into the superfamilies Ngaro and VIPER (Hassan et al., 2024).

Retrotransposons constitute approximately 42% of the human genome and LINEs representing the most substantial proportion of human genome at 20.4%, followed by SINEs at 13.1%, LTRs at 9.1%, as well as SVA elements which is a non-autonomous non-LTR retrotransposon at 0.1% (Ostertag et al., 2003; Tang et al., 2018; Ali et al., 2021; Luqman-Fatah et al., 2024).

Class II TEs are non-viral molecules that have been extensively utilized for genome manipulation or restructuring in both cell lines and living organisms, not only enabling the identification of genes and molecular pathways involved in disease mechanisms and pathogen pathogenesis but also offering a promising alternative tools to viral systems in gene therapy research due to their various advantageous properties (Muñoz-López & García-Pérez, 2010; Albieri et al., 2010). Additionality, DNA transposons in eukaryotes are categorized into subclasses, including "cut and paste" transposons, rolling circle (RC) transposons (Helitrons), tyrosine recombinase transposons (Cryptons) as well as self-replicating transposons (Mavericks) (Bao et al., 2010). Autonomous DNA transposons are characterized by the presence of at least one ORF encoding a transposase enzyme responsible for catalyzing the transposition process, and are typically flanked by two terminal inverted repeats (TIRs) (Bao et al., 2010). The transposase recognizes TIRs to catalyze the excision of the transposon DNA segment, which is integrated into a distinct genomic position (Ma et al., 2023). In addition, the insertion process leads to the duplication of the target site DNA, resulting in TSDs that act as distinctive signatures characteristic of each DNA transposon; notably, the length of the TSD constitutes a crucial feature in the classification of Class II TEs (Roffler & Wicker, 2015). For instance, Polintons also known as Mavericks are very large transposons characterized by long TIRs and possess the coding capacity for multiple proteins (Haapa-Paananen et al., 2014). In contrast, RC transposons or Helitrons, lack TIRs and do not encode any proteins analogous to known transposases (thought to transpose via a replicative RC mechanism which is similar to bacterial IS91 elements) (Kapitonov & Jurka, 2001; Garcillán-Barcia & de la Cruz, 2002; Castanera et al., 2014). DNA transposons are classified into distinct families based on their sequence, TSDs and/or TIRs, and have been grouped into 23 superfamilies to date (Bao et al., 2009; Ma et al., 2023). In addition, Miniature inverted-repeat transposable elements (MITEs), a group of non-autonomous Class II TEs, are widespread in eukaryotic genomes and contribute to genome architecture and evolutionary dynamics (Klai et al., 2022). Structurally, MITEs are characterized by a relatively small size (approximately 50 to 800 base pairs), the presence of short TIRs, TSDs at both ends with a high adenine/thymine (A/T) content, and high copy numbers (Crescente et al., 2018; Li et al., 2024). Despite lacking coding capacity, MITEs are mobilized by the transposase enzymes encoded by their autonomous counterparts (Yaakov et al., 2012). Most MITEs are classified into two main superfamilies based on the similarity of their TIRs and TSD sequence signatures: the *Tourist*-like sub-group, characterized by 3-bp TAA TSDs and the *Stowaway*-like sub-group, characterized by 2-bp TA TSDs ([a]Bureau & Wessler, 1994; [b]Bureau & Wessler, 1994). Additionality, most MITEs originated from autonomous DNA transposons, such as *PIF/Harbinger-like*, *Mutator-like*, *hAT-like*, and *Tc1/Mariner-like* elements. For instance, *Tourist-like* MITEs originated from *PIF/Harbinger-like* elements, while *Stowaway-like* MITEs derived from the *Tc1/mariner-like* elements (Stelmach et al., 2017; Macko-Podgórni et al., 2021).

2. Functional Roles of TEs in Genome and Cellular Dynamics

TEs constitute a prominent part of the human genome and possess the capacity to introduce novel enhancers or promoters that modulate cellular gene expression (Fueyo et al., 2022; Mosaddeghi et al., 2023). In addition, TEs exert significant regulatory effects on mammalian gene expression at the transcriptional level through both *cis*- and *trans*-acting mechanisms (Fueyo et al., 2022). They also influence regulatory networks, contribute to genomic rearrangements and drive genetic diversity (Feschotte, 2008; Serrato-Capuchina & Matute, 2018). The Encyclopedia of DNA Elements (ENCODE) project aims to construct a comprehensive map of all functional elements encoded in the human and mouse genomes by employing a variety of high-throughput approaches (Davis et al., 2018). Similarly, Functional Annotation of Mouse/Mammalian Genome (FANTOM) project is an international consortium and provides comprehensive expression profiles (Lizio et al., 2019). These large-scale genomic analyses have indicated that TEs can exhibit pronounced activity in a cell type-specific manner (Karttunen et al., 2023), and are capable of regulating not only their own cell-specific transcription but also the transcription of neighboring genes (Lykoskoufis et al., 2024).

TEs contribute to a large percentage of non-coding RNAs' (ncRNAs) transcription and can serve as functional domains of long non-coding RNAs (lncRNAs) (Tsagakis et al., 2020; Park et al., 2022). Importantly, a significant number of lncRNA sequence elements are derived from TEs and are involved in a wide-range of regulatory functions (Hadjiargyrou & Delihas, 2013). As an example, lncRNA embedded-TEs can play a fundamental role in regulating lncRNA expression, subcellular localization, and tissue-specific activity (Fort et al., 2021). Moreover, miRNAs derived from TEs (MDTEs) possess the capacity regulate gene expression at post-transcriptional level and have been categorized into three types (Qin et al., 2015; Kim et al., 2023). As is well documented, TEs are classified into

SINE, LINE, LTR, and DNA transposon classes in the human genome (Du et al., 2024) and each of these TE classes have different contributions for three types of MDTEs (Qin et al., 2015). Furthermore, emerging evidence stated that MDTEs promote carcinogenesis by directly or indirectly interacting with cancer-associated genes (Kim et al., 2023). For instance, hsa-miR-4454, a HERV-derived miRNA, has been exhibited oncogenic potential by targeting the suppressor genes *DNAJB4* and *SASH1* in non-muscle-invasive bladder cancer (Park et al., 2023).

Accumulating evidence has indicated that dysregulation of TE is implicated in various pathophysiological processes, including cancer, autoimmune disorders as well as inflammatory diseases (Burns, 2017; Marasca et al., 2020). Additionally, it is well established that TEs can contribute to genomic and epigenomic instability via both transposition-dependent and -independent mechanisms which potentially leading to various physiological derangements, such as cellular dysfunction and cell death (Hsu et al., 2021; Bhat et al., 2022). For instance, prior investigation has stated that TEs' abnormal activation and/or mobilization has the potential for contributing to genomic instability in neurodegenerative disease (Guo et al., 2018). Importantly, a potential link has been proposed between altered TE expression and associated genomic instability, both of which are implicated in Tau mediated neurodegenerative mechanisms (Guo et al., 2018). Recent studies have highlighted that SINE are implicated in various human diseases, including a wide range of age-related conditions and have suggested that therapies targeting SINE RNAs may offer promising prospects for the treatment of age-associated disorders (Shah et al., 2024). In addition, the derepression of LTRs has been implicated as a critical factor in the pathogenesis of human lymphomas, potentially offering diagnostic, prognostic, and therapeutic significance (Lamprecht et al., 2010). For instance, literature indicated that hypomethylation of LTR promoters has the potential to promote carcinogenesis in B cell-derived Hodgkin's lymphoma by dysregulating the expression of the colony-stimulating factor 1 receptor (CSF1R), a known proto-oncogene (Lamprecht et al., 2010). Additionality, retrotransposons, particularly LINE-1 elements, are frequently found to be hypomethylated in various types of cancer, including chronic lymphocytic leukemia (Barrow et al., 2021), hepatocellular carcinoma (Ramzy et al., 2011), non-small cell lung cancer (Daskalos et al., 2009), breast cancer (Zeggar et al., 2020), gastric cancer (Hong et al., 2018), epithelial ovarian cancer (Pattamadilok et al., 2008), prostate cancer (Fiano et al., 2017) as well as colorectal cancer (Antelo et al., 2012).

The insertion of TEs into coding regions of the genome has the potential to induce missense, nonsense, or frameshift mutations leading to alterations in the genomic sequence (Bhat et al., 2022). In addition, TE insertions have been associated with human diseases; for instance, a *de novo* insertion of a LINE-1 element into exon 14 of the factor VIII gene has been identified as the cause of hemophilia A (Kazazian et al., 1988). Moreover, Alu insertions have been related with risks for various human diseases, including Lynch-like syndrome (Solassol et al., 2019), hereditary breast and ovarian cancer (Bouras et al., 2021), leukemia (Ade et al., 2013), Alport syndrome (Knebelmann et al., 1995), and hyper-IgM with immunodeficiency syndrome (Apoil et al., 2007). On the other hand, a recent study reported that 10 polymorphic TE insertions are potentially linked to the pathogenesis of neurological and psychiatric disorders as candidates for causative roles (Ahn et al., 2023). Additionally, insertion of a LINE-1 element into the dystrophin gene resulted in exon 44 skipping during splicing of the dystrophin mRNA precursor, leading to Duchenne muscular dystrophy (Narita et al., 1993).

TE-mediated genomic alterations, such as deletions and chromosomal rearrangements, have been implicated in a wide spectrum of human diseases, including Von Hippel Lindau disease (Franke et al., 2009), breast and ovarian cancer (Armaou et al., 2007), Sandhoff disease (Neote et al., 1990), hereditary diffuse gastric cancer (Oliveira et al., 2009), and hematolymphoid neoplasms (Rodić et al., 2013). In addition, several types of transposable elements can facilitate the formation of intragenic polyadenylation signals, giving rise to novel cleavage sites and thereby contributing to the enrichment of the human transcriptome (Lavi & Carmel, 2018). Moreover, a growing body of evidence indicates that TE-mediated insertions, particularly involving retroelements such as Alu and LINE-1, can give rise to novel polyadenylation sites (PAS), which have been implicated in the development of a variety of human diseases, including haemophilia (LINE 1 insertion) (Mukherjee et al., 2004), autoimmune lymphoproliferative syndrome (Alu insertion) (Tighe et al., 2002) as well as X-linked dilated cardiomyopathy (LINE 1 insertion) (Yoshida et al., 1998). Similary, TE-mediated exonization (i.e., creation of new exons), which contributes to the expansion of human proteome diversity and TE-mediated alternative splicing, such as intron retention have been involved in several diseases, including tumorigenesis for a number of different cancers (Smart et al., 2018; Attig et al., 2019; Clayton et al., 2020).

TE enhancers play a significant role in early embryonic development, germ cell differentiation, and the determination of cell fate (Hsu et al., 2021). In human pluripotent stem cells, TEs serve as key targets for RNA-binding proteins (Ma et al., 2022) and are integral to driving cellular transitions and phenotypic plasticity (Eskier et al., 2025). Furthermore, the pivotal connection between TEs and stem cells resides in genetic engineering, a transformative approach that plays a crucial role in unraveling disease mechanisms and developing cutting-edge gene- and cell-based therapies (Schumann et al., 2019).

There is a plethora of evidence that TEs hold promise as potential biomarkers for both diagnosis and prognosis (Zhu et al., 2021; Xu et al., 2025). For instance, TE expression has been implicated as an significant factor for patient prognosis in colorectal cancer (Zhu et al., 2021). In addition, the clinical significance and diagnostic value of HERV elements have been assessed in gastric cancer (Xu et al., 2025). It has been revealed that higher HERV expression is associated with larger tumor size, increased lymphatic metastasis, and higher histological grade, suggesting that HERVs may indicate gastric cancer progression and serve as promising diagnostic biomarkers (Xu et al., 2025). Moreover, hypomethylation of LINE-1 elements has been proposed as a predictive biomarker for therapeutic response in human hepatocellular carcinoma (HCC) and has also been associated with worse overall survival in HCC patients (Anwar et al., 2019). In this context, TE-based strategies can represent a promising therapeutic approach in cancer treatment (Lee et al., 2024; Wang et al., 2024).

Numerous native and reconstructed transposons have been identified to date, several of which have been employed as tools in genomics research including, Sleeping Beauty (SB) (Kebriaei et al., 2017), Tol1 (Koga et al., 2007), Himar1 (Keravala et al., 2006), PiggyBac (PB) (Feschotte, 2006), Passport (Clark et al., 2009), Hermes (Gangadharan et al., 2010), Transposable element of Oryzias latipes, number 2 (Tol2) (Kawakami, 2007), Tn5 (Li et al., 2020), Frog Prince (FP) (Miskey et al., 2003) as well as Minos (Pavlopoulos et al., 2007). In particular, SB, PB, and Tol2 are the most widely studied transposon-based gene delivery systems in basic research and preclinical applications (Sandoval-Villegas et al., 2021).

3. TEs as Tools for Genome Engineering in Human

TEs have gained significant attention as versatile tools at the forefront of life science research, with applications ranging from basic research to therapeutic innovation (Han et al., 2023). These elements serve essential functions as genetic and molecular biology tools, particularly in fields such as genetic engineering and human gene therapy (Bourque et al., 2018; Schmitz & Querques, 2024).

In research, various types of transposons have been evaluted for human gene therapy applications (VandenDriessche et al., 2009; Di Matteo et al., 2012; Bhat et al., 2022). Nevertheless, SB, PB, and Tol2 transposons have emerged as the preferred tools for cell engineering, owing to their advantageous characteristics, including ease of manipulation in experimental setups, efficient gene transfer in human cell types as well as a comprehensive understanding of the transposition mechanism (Schumann et al., 2019).

The **SB transposon**, a member of the Tc1/mariner superfamily, was synthetically reconstructed from salmonid fish genomes using moleculer pylogenetic approaches (Ivics et al., 2004; Voigt et al., 2016). The SB transposon system represents an efficient non-viral gene delivery platform and demonstrates markedly higher activity in vertebrates compared to the other tested transposon systems (Fischer et al., 2001; Izsvák & Ivics, 2004).

In its natural configuration, the SB transposon is approximately 1.6 kilobases (kb) in length and comprises two main components: the transposase, referred to as SBase, and the integration cassette, referred to as the transposon (Di Matteo et al., 2012; [b]Tipanee et al., 2017). Moreover, the SB transposon contains 210–250 base pair (bp) inverted repeats (IRs) at its termini, with directly repeated DNA sequence motifs positioned at the ends of each (Ivics et al., 1997). Additionally, SB transposase is characterized as a 360-amino-acid DNA-binding protein that encompasses distinct functional domains responsible for transposon binding, catalysis, and nuclear localization (Di Matteo et al., 2012). Moreover, the formation of a nucleoprotein complex stated as the synaptic complex constitutes a crucial step in the life cycle of SB transposition (Ochmann & Ivics, 2021). In addition, the pT2 is commonly employed as the parental plasmid in SB transposition applications (Cui et al., 2002; Turunen et al., 2016).

Functionally, the SB transposase comprises several conserved domains that are critical for its activity (Dupuy, 2010). Initially, the transposase contains a bipartite DNA-binding domain (PAI and RED), which confer sequence-specific binding to IRs are situated at the N-terminal region (Colloms et al., 1994; Izsvák et al., 2002). In particularly, the N-terminal PAI subdomain has been demonstrated to play a predominant role in mediating interactions with the transposase-binding sites and AT-hook motif has been identified as a functional subdomain that contributes to sequence-specific DNA binding (Izsvák et al., 2002; Battista et al., 2024). Moreover, the catalytic domain of the transposase located at the C-terminal region and is characterized by the DDE motif (Yuan & Wessler, 2011). This evolutionarily conserved catalytic triad is common to recombinase, transposase, and viral integrases and is critically involved in mediating the DNA breakage and integration reactions (Hickman & Dyda, 2015; Wang et al., 2017). Importantly, this domain catalyzes the "cut and paste" transposition reaction in vertebrate cells, thereby underpinning the mobility of transposable elements (Ivics et al., 1997). Notably, SB transposon systems generate characteristically distinct footprints at excision sites across different cell types, proposing that alternative repair machineries function in coordination with transposition (Liu et al., 2004). In addition, mutations occurring in the terminal nucleotides affect excision activity, but do not affect transposase binding in SB-based transposition (Liu et al., 2004).

The transposition efficiency of the SB system decreases at approximately a logarithmic rate with increasing insert size (Izsvák et al., 2000). Previous studies have demonstrated that the SB system is capable of transposing transgenes up to approximately 10 kb in length; nevertheless, its transposition efficiency declines markedly when the length of the transposable element gets longer than 4 kb (Zayed et al., 2004). In addition, the regulation of SB transposition is orchestrated not only by transposon- but also by host-encoded factors (Ivics & Izsvák, 2015; Devaraj et al., 2023). Moreover, the participation of certain host factors in this process may lead to different transposition efficiency depending on species- or cell type-specific variations (Izsvák et al., 2009). Additionally, the transposition efficiency is influenced by the ratio between SB transposase to transposon (Geurts et al., 2003).

The SB transposon stands as a landmark in the application of transposition-mediated gene delivery systems in vertebrates (Izsvák et al., 2000). In more detail, the SB system is recognized as a powerful tool due to its numerous advantageous features (Amberger & Ivics, 2020): i) SB transposon system is considered a relatively safe vector for transposition, as it exhibits a close-to-random integration profile within the human genome, which potentially contributes to the enhanced safety (Swierczek et al., 2012; Kebriaei et al., 2017) ii) this transposon system also demonstrates target site specificity by integrating into TA-dinucleotide sequences, offering a safer alternative to viral vectors (Liu et al., 2005) iii) the enhanced stability of synaptic complex may represent one possible factor contributing to the efficient transposition of SB in vertebrate cells (Izsvák et al., 2002) iv) SB-mediated system can provide not only high-level stable gene transfer but also long-term gene expression (Podetz-Pedersen et al., 2016; Hudecek et al., 2017) v) the relatively low immunogenicity of the SB system represents a key advantage over viral vectors in gene delivery applications (Sowińska et al., 2019) vi) the SB transposon system also reduces the risk of rearrangements related to the expression cassette which is part of a transposing unit of DNA (Izsvák & Ivics, 2004; Ivics & Izsvák, 2006).

The SB transposon is a well-characterized DNA transposable element that offers simplicity, cost-effectiveness, and favorable safety features for potential human applications (Holstein et al., 2018). However, the integration and continued expression of the transposase may pose potential risks, as it may give rise to unintended re-integration and re-mobilization, leading to increased the risk of insertional mutagenesis (Wilber et al., 2006). In this context, further optimization of the SB system is required, including strategies to avoid the risk of insertional inactivation and to improve its efficacy as a molecular tool (Harmening et al., 2023). Another limitation of SB transposon system is overproduction inhibition which leads to reduced transpositional activity at higher transposase concentrations (Wilson et al., 2005). Nevertheless, the engineering of transposase/DNA-binding domain chimeras, exemplified by zinc finger/SB transposase chimera, has been shown to attenuate overproduction inhibition, potentially offering certain advantages over the native enzyme (Wilson et al., 2005).

Additionally, several hyperactive versions of the SB transposon system such as SB10, SB11 and SB100X have been developed to enhance transpositional activity by manipulating either the SBase coding sequence or the IR regions of the transposon (Zayed et al., 2004; Baus et al., 2005). Among these, SB11 exhibits approximately three-fold higher activity compared to the first-generation SB transposase (Hudecek et al., 2017). Moreover, the combination of SB12 (a hyperactive SB variant) with the pT3 transposon (a hyperactive SB transposon) enhances SB transposition by two to four times relative to the native SB system (Zayed et al., 2004; Wilson et al., 2005). Furthermore, SB100X exhibits approximately a 100-fold enhancement in efficiency compared to the first generation transposase and demonstrates the highest efficiency (24%) compared with SB11 (1.23%) (Mátés et al., 2009; Xue et al., 2009). Additionally, the transposition efficiency of hySB100X is enhanced by approximately 30% relative to that of SB100X (Moretti et al., 2022).

The SB system, a plasmid-based transposon platform, offer a safer profile compared to integrative viral vectors (Swierczek et al., 2012). Alongside this, clustered regularly interspaced short palindromic repeats

(CRISPR)/CRISPR-associated protein 9 (Cas9) technology represents a powerful gene editing tool and lentiviral vectors serve as one of the primary platforms for delivering the CRISPR/Cas9 system to achieve high transduction efficiency (Ortinski et al., 2017). However, potential biosafety risks associated with lentiviral vectors may impact their progress into clinical applications (Ma et al., 2021). In this context, the combination of SB transposons with CRISPR/Cas9 enables high-efficiency gene transfection with a reliable biosafety profile for gene delivery applications (Ma et al., 2021). Furthermore, recent advancements have paved the way for the development of SB-based viral hybrid platforms that combine the integrative features of the SB system with the high-efficiency nucleic acid delivery capabilities of non-integrating viral vectors (Kebriaei et al., 2017).

The **PB transposon**, formerly named IFP2, was originally isolated from a mutant baculovirus cultured in *Trichoplusia ni* (TN-368) cells in the 1980s (Fraser et al., 1983). The PB transposon has been widely utilized in research on insect transgenesis including the red flour beetle *Tribolium castaneum* (Wang et al., 2008). However, subsequent studies have revealed that taxonomic distribution for PB transposon has significantly broadened to encompass various eukaryotic organisms (Sarkar et al., 2003; Guo et al., 2023) and several piggyBac-like elements (PLEs) have been identified in other baculoviruses or species (Xu et al., 2006; Carpes et al., 2009; Pagan et al., 2010; Guo et al., 2023).

The PB, a short inverted-repeat-type DNA transposable element, is approximately 2,472 bp in length and is characterized by specific 13 bp TIRs and additional 19 bp internal inverted repeats (Cary et al., 1989; Elick et al., 1997). In addition, a well-defined PB comprises a single ORF encoding a 594-amino acid transposase (PBase) with a predicted molecular mass of 68 kDa that is required for transposition and likely excision (Elick et al., 1996; Lee et al., 2011). Structurally, PBase consists of three distinct regions: an acidic N-terminal domain of approximately 100 amino acids (aa), a central domain of about 400 aa including the DDD/E motif, and a cysteine-rich domain of roughly 90 aa (Helou et al., 2021). Functionally, a catalytic domain with a characteristic DDE/D triad interacts with divalent metal ions during the transposition process, whereas the C-terminal domain of PBase contains a Zn^{2+}-binding plant homeodomain finger and may promote binding to transposon DNA in a chromatin context (Junop & Haniford, 1997; Yusa, 2015). Additionally, PB has exhibited substantially higher transposition activity compared to early-generation SBase and Tol2 transposases; however, its efficiency remains lower than that of the hyperactive SB100X transposase system (Wu et al., 2006; Hou et al., 2015).

Furthermore, engineered hyperactive PBase (hyPBase) exhibits enhanced transposition activity compared to previous PBase with a distinct insertion pattern (Meir et al., 2013).

The PB-based gene delivery system is a powerful tool owing to its several advantageous features (Inada et al., 2015): i) exhibits a higher cargo capacity relative to commonly utilized viral vectors employed in gene transfer applications (Li et al., 2013), ii) Unlike SB transposons, it displays precise excision from the genome and does not leave a footprint mutation at the original transposition site (Moretti et al., 2022) iii) transposition is host-factor independent and is functional in wide variety of organisms (Ding et al., 2005; Ye et al., 2015) iv) demonstrates low toxicity and long-term expression (Saridey et al., 2009; Di Matteo et al., 2012) v) displays stable integration (Wen et al., 2020) vi) possesses high transposition efficiency and a lack of overproduction inhibition (to some extent) which is a considerable limitation associated with the SB system (Wilson et al., 2007; Grabundzija et al., 2010). However, several challenges related to the efficiency and safety of the PB system need to be addressed and optimized for clinical applications (Meir et al., 2013).

The PB system also exhibits a typical "cut-and-paste" (a non-replicative) transposition reaction (Zheng et al., 2019). In contrast to SB transposon, the PB preferentially integrates into target sites including TTAA sequences (Cary et al., 1989). In addition, the PB transposon system is a useful genetic engineering tool for genome research, including human gene therapy and genetic manipulation, particularly transgenesis and insertional mutagenesis (Feschotte, 2006; Rad et al., 2010; Woodard & Wilson, 2015). Conventionally, the PB-based genetic manipulation platform utilizes two separate plasmids (*trans*): the PB transposase expression cassette is carried by a helper plasmid, while the gene of interest flanked by two TRDs is carried by a donor plasmid (Meir et al., 2013). On the other hand, it is possible to deliver both the transposase and the transposon cargo on the same plasmid (*cis*) (Urschitz et al., 2010). Additionally, pXL-BacII is commonly utilized as the parental plasmid in PB transposition systems (O'Brochta et al., 2011; Cao et al., 2013). Moreover, animal transgenesis research constitutes a pivotal approach to investigating disease pathophysiology and generating preclinical models of human disorders (Woodard & Wilson, 2015), while insertional mutagenesis mediated by the PB transposon holds significant potential as a strategy for identifying cancer-related genes (Rad et al., 2010). Furthermore, the PB transposon mediated system represents a versatile technology for the genetic modification of therapeutically significant cell types, such as induced pluripotent stem cells (iPSCs) (Yusa, 2011) and human T lymphocytes (Nakazawa et al., 2009).

The combination of PB transposons and the CRISPR/Cas9 system represents a promising advancement in genome engineering, with the potential to serve as a robust tool and offer valuable opportunities for both *in vitro* and *in vivo* applications (Cheng et al., 2016; Li et al., 2017). For instance, recent studies have reported that PB-engineered GPC3-specific CAR-T cell therapy demonstrates potent cytotoxic activity against hepatocellular carcinoma cells, highlighting its potential as a promising therapeutic strategy for patients in clinical settings (Wang et al., 2020). Furthermore, the PB transposon-based CRISPR/Cas9 system enables stable expression of CRISPR components in human pluripotent stem cells (hPSCs) and this platform allows the knockout of both protein coding genes and lncRNAs in hPSCs, with efficiencies reaching up to 99% (Jiang et al., 2022).

The **Tol2,** a DNA-based transposable element, was discovered in the medaka fish (*Oryzias latipes*), which is a small freshwater teleost (Urasaki et al., 2006). It represents a naturally occurring active transposon identified in vertebrate genomes (Kawakami & Noda, 2004) and functions in a wide range of species, including zebrafish, chicken, Xenopus, mouse as well as human (Kawakami, 2007).

Tol2 is approximately 4.7 kb in length and comprises three introns and four exons that encode 117, 352, 102, and 118 aa, constituting an ORF which encodes a functional transposase (Koga et al., 1999; Koga & Hori, 2001). In this context, various isoforms of transposases have been identified, of which the 649 aa isoform represents the most active variant both *in vivo* and *in vitro* (Ni et al., 2016). Additionally, Tol2 not only exhibits DNA sequence similarity to transposases of the *hAT* family transposons (Kawakami & Shima, 1999), but also shares a wide range of features with the other *hAT* members such as short TIRs at each end of the element (Hickman, 2005).

Structurally, the Tol2 transposition system comprises a transposon-donor plasmid harboring the Tol2 construct and an expression plasmid capable of providing transposase activity (Kawakami et al., 2016). Importantly, Tol2 vectors containing 200 bp 5′ end as well as 150 bp 3′ end are capable of transposition indicating that these sequences encompassing TIRs and subterminal regions are both essential and sufficient for transposition (Urasaki et al., 2006). In addition, a novel Tol2 donor plasmid (referred to as pTol2mini-cassette) was developed by replacing the long terminal repeats of the Tol2ends-cassette with minimal repeat sequences, without reducing transpositional efficiency. Moreover, this minimal Tol2 construct exhibited approximately a three-fold increase in transposition activity compared to the full-length Tol2 system (Meir et al., 2011). Furthermore, a recent study demonstrated that codon optimization of the Tol2 transposase enhances both its enzymatic activity and the frequency of transposition events *in vitro* and *in vivo* (Keng et al., 2009). As an example, the codon-optimized Tol2 transposase (named as iTol2) exhibited ~ two-fold increase in activity compared to the endogenous Tol2 transposase derived from medaka fish in functional assays using cultured HeLa cells (Keng et al., 2009). Additionally, the epitope-tagged Tol2 transposase protein (His-Tol2) has the potential to serve as a novel source of transposase in genetic engineering applications (Ni et al., 2016). Furthermore, a previous report suggests that the application of His-Tol2, purified from *E. coli* may offer advantages to generate low mosaic transgenic animals with a high germline transmission rate (Ni et al., 2016). Moreover, active recombinant Tol2 protein represents an important novel tool for a range of applications, encompassing the biochemical analysis of the transposition process, gene discovery, and molecular-based therapeutic research (Ni et al., 2016).

Tol2 functions via a "cut-and-paste" mechanism and does not cause alterations such as rearrangements or modifications at the target site, except for the generation of 8-bp TSDs at the integration sites (Kawakami, 2007; Urasaki et al., 2008). In addition, the Tol2 transposon system generates footprints of varying lengths (Parinov et al., 2004). The Tol2 transposon system exhibits a high cargo capacity and is capable of delivering genetic material up to approximately 10–11 kb without a significant reduction in transposition efficiency (Balciunas et al., 2006; Kawakami, 2007). In contrast to SB and PB transposons, Tol2 does not exhibit a preference for specific target sequences, such as TA or TTAA sequences and is instead associated with a weak consensus sequence (Kawakami, 2007; Kondrychyn et al., 2009). Like SB and PB, Tol2 systems enable long-term transgene expression accompanied by minimal signs of silencing in human cells (Grabundzija et al., 2010). Emerging evidence indicates that Tol2 transposase does not exhibit significant overproduction inhibition within the tested range of transposase concentrations (Balciunas et al., 2006). Nonetheless, it remains unclear whether the Tol2 system is entirely free from this inhibition due to limited experimental conditions, as the transposase levels may have remained below the threshold necessary for detecting inhibition (Kawakami, 2007). On the other hand, Tol2 transposases have been reported in a recent study to be less affected by this mechanism compared to SB (Grabundzija et al., 2010). Additionally, Tol2 has the ability to transpose across a broad range of temperatures, including 25°C to 26°C in zebrafish and 37°C to 38°C in chicken (Kawakami, 2007). Emerging research has highlighted that Tol2 demonstrates high efficiency in numerous cell lines compared to the SB system (Wu et al., 2006). However, SB and PB exhibit higher transposition efficiency than Tol2 in the context of non-restrictive conditions (Grabundzija et al., 2010).

Tol2 transposon based system represents a promising platform for gene therapy applications, owing to its efficacy in generation of insertional mutagenesis (Kawakami et al., 1998) and transgenic animal models such as mouse (Yang, 2016), frog ([a]Kawakami et al., 2004), chicken (Sato et al., 2007), and zebrafish (Suster et al., 2009). Moreover, Tol2 transposon system can be utilized in the development of gene trap approach which enables the identification of novel genes and contribute to analysis of their biological importance or enhancer trap method (Cecconi & Meyer, 2000; [b]Kawakami et al., 2004). Furthermore, a previous study proposed that the Tol2 transposon system could serve as a genetic tool for the development of novel gene transfer, mutagenesis, and transgenesis in mammals, but biological aspects should be carefully considered (Kawakami & Noda, 2004). In addition, Tol2-based vectors have been employed for transfection in various mammalian cell types, including embryonic stem cells (ESCs) (Kawakami & Noda, 2004), iPSCs (Imamura et al., 2016) as well as human lymphocytes (Tsukahara et al., 2015). Additionally, the Tol2 transposon mediated vector system serves as a useful tool for generating stably transfected primary cultured cells and is appropriate for studying the circadian clock, an essential biological mechanism in mammals that regulates numerous physiological functions (Yagita et al., 2010). Moreover, the Tol2 transposon system has been employed in the manufacturing of CAR-T cells due to its ability to ensure stable expression of CAR (Tsukahara et al., 2015). For instance, it could be applied for the stable transfer of CD19-CAR to primary human T cells, offering a potential therapeutic strategy for the treatment of refractory B-cell malignancies (Tsukahara et al., 2015).

4. Transposon-Based Gene Therapy: Therapeutic Strategies in Fundamental and Preclinical Studies

TEs have exhibited significant prognostic and predictive potential across a broad spectrum of diseases (Harris et al., 2010; Barry et al., 2015; Panda et al., 2018; Zhang et al., 2019; Ohtani et al., 2020). However, SB, PB, and

Tol2 transposon systems have emerged as the most widely utilized and promising transposon platforms for gene therapy in the context of basic and preclinical research (Di Matteo et al., 2012).

In the realm of regenerative medicine research, stem and progenitor cells have been identified as key players with remarkable therapeutic potential, serving as relevant targets for gene- and cell-based therapies (Ferrari et al., 2021; Hussen et al., 2024). Notably, PB or SB mediated gene transfer enabled stable gene integration in mesenchymal stem cells (MSCs) (Belay et al., 2010; Wen et al., 2014). Moreover, MSCs genetically engineered via hyperactive SB or PB based transposon systems preserved their ability to differentiate into osteogenic, myogenic and adipogenic lineages (Belay et al., 2010). Furthermore, the hyperactive SB100X system achieved stable gene transfer into human hematopoietic stem cells (Xue et al., 2009). Additionally, SB100X-mediated gene transfer has been applied to myoblasts and satellite cells to develop an *ex vivo* gene therapy strategy for muscular dystrophy ([a]Tipanee et al., 2017). Similarly, the PB-based transposon system has been utilized to deliver therapeutic genes into myoblasts, paving the way for a novel gene therapy approach targeting Duchenne muscular dystrophy (Loperfido et al., 2016). In addition, SB100X has been demonstrated to mediate stable transposition in iPSCs, which represent promising adult stem cells for the treatment of genetic or degenerative diseases (VandenDriessche et al., 2009; [a]Tipanee et al., 2017).

A broad spectrum of other clinically relevant cell types has been effectively targeted by SB- and PB-based gene therapy in various diseases, as summarized in Table 1 (for SB-mediated transposon systems) and Table 2 (for PB-mediated transposon systems). However, the Tol2 transposon remains relatively limited in the context of gene therapy, particularly in comparison to SB and PB transposons. To date, it has been indicated that the Tol2 transposon system can be involved in CD19-CAR-based T-cell therapy, offering a potential therapeutic approach for refractory B-cell malignancies (Tsukahara et al., 2015).

Table 1. Representative Research Illustrating Basic and Preclinical Applications of SB-Based Transposon Systems in Disease Models

Diseases	Description	Transposon/transposase	References
Hereditary tyrosinemia type I	Hepatocytes transfected with the SB-based transposon are capable of supporting liver repopulation, resulting in long-lasting correction of the phenotype associated with fumarylacetoacetate hydrolase deficiency.	SB11	(Montini et al., 2002; Wilber et al., 2007)
Huntington disease	The SB-mediated approach with RNA interference was able to mediate the downregulation of huntingtin gene expression.	SB10	(Chen et al., 2005)
Pulmonary fibrosis	SB-based therapy with human indoleamine-2,3-dioxygenase constituted a promising therapeutic strategy for the management of chronic complications following lung transplantation.	hSB17	(Liu et al., 2006)
Glioblastoma	SB-mediated strategy could enhance the efficacy of immunogene therapy in glioma-bearing mice.	SB13	(Wu et al., 2007)

Mucopolysaccharidosis type I (MPS I)	SB-based technology contributed to the improvement of several clinical manifestations of MPS I disease in an immunodeficient mouse model, as evidenced by pathology and radiographic assessments.	SB11	(Aronovich et al., 2009)
Pulmonary fibrosis	SB-based miR-29b therapy demonstrated the potential to prevent and treat bleomycin-induced pulmonary fibrosis in mice.	SB11	(Xiao et al., 2012)
Alzheimer's disease (AD)	A novel clinical-grade cell line, NGC0211, was generated using an optimized transposase system, resulting in a greater than 10-fold increase in nerve growth factor (NGF) expression, which represents a promising therapeutic candidate for AD.	SB100X	(Fjord-Larsen et al., 2012)
Lymphoma	Anti-CD19 CAR T cells generated using the advanced SB technology resulted in the eradication of lymphoma cells in a xenograft model.	SB100X- minicircle vector (MC)	(Monjezi et al., 2017)

Pancreatic cancer	Engineering of functional NK-92MI mesothelin-CAR T cells with a SB-based technology triggered proinflammatory signals, including granzyme B and IFN-γ and enhanced cytotoxicity against pancreatic cancer cells.	SB11- MC	(Batchu et al., 2019)
Age-related macular degeneration	SB-engineered cells including rat retinal pigment epithelial cells and rat iris pigment epithelial cells overexpressed pigment epithelium-derived factor (PEDF) and appeared to reduce choroidal neovascularization and restore the physiological vascular endothelial growth factor/PEDF balance.	SB100X-pFAR4	(Hernandez et al., 2019)
Acute myeloid leukemia (AML)	Generation of CD33 CAR cytokine-induced killer (CIK) cells by utilizing the hyperactive transposase-pT4 vector exhibited *in vivo* activity against chemotherapy resistant or residual AML cells which are key drivers of AML relapse.	SB100X	(Rotiroti et al., 2020)

Table 2. Representative Research Illustrating Basic and Preclinical Applications of PB-Based Transposon Systems in Disease Models

Diseases	Description	Transposon/transposase	References
Ovarian cancer	PB-mediated strategy combined with polyethylenimine enabled sustained transgene expression and significant tumor-growth inhibition, as confirmed by histological analyses demonstrating extensive lymphocyte infiltration and necrosis in a ovarian-cancer model.	recombinant plasmid PB (Act-RFP, HSV-tk)	(Kang et al., 2009)
α1-antitrypsin deficiency (A1ATD)	Combinatorial approach involving zinc finger nucleases (ZFNs) and the PB platform in human iPSCs could enable biallelic correction of the Glu342Lys point mutation in the SERPINA1 gene, which plays a crucial role in the pathogenesis of A1ATD.	pCMV-hyPBase	(Yusa et al., 2011)
β-thalassemia	PB-CRISPR/Cas9 technology demonstrated significant potential for the seamless correction of hemoglobin beta gene mutations in patient-specific iPSCs.	hyperactive PBase (hyPBase)	(Xie et al., 2014)
Melanoma	PhiC31 (φC31) recombinase/PB-based system mediated long term and high-level of transgene expression in adipose-derived mesenchymal stem cells (ADSCs). IFNγ-	the vector pmhyGENIE-3 (including EGFP gene, a hyperactive self	(Bahrambeigi et al., 2014)

	expressing ADSCs prevented tumor growth and angiogenesis, upregulated PD-L1 expression, inhibited the systemic increase of $CD4^{+}CD25^{+}Foxp3^{+}$ regulatory T cells, and extended the survival of mice.	inactivating PB sequence and PB transposon)	
von Willebrand disease (vWD)	Engineered PB transposon system held promise for enabling long-term gene transfer for the treatment of vWD.	iPB7	(Johnson et al., 2016)
Duchenne muscular dystrophy	PB-mediated technology provided full-length dystrophin expression and contributed to functional improvement in dystrophic muscles.	PB	(Iyer et al., 2018)
Kidney-related disease	PB-based transposon system mediated the reprogramming of HK2 cells (adult human kidney epithelial cells) to a nephron progenitor-like state with functional nephrogenic potential.	a hyperactive PB transposase plasmid (p-EF-1α-HA-m7pB)	(Vanslambrouck et al., 2019)
Recessive dystrophic epidermolysis bullosa (RDEB)	PB-based technology provided the gene mutation correction with footprint-free during the gene editing process in iPSC-RDEB26 cells in conjunction with a combination of the CRISPR/Cas9 system.	pCMV-PBase-Bsd	(Itoh et al., 2020)

Neuroblastoma (NB)	Combinatorial strategy with PB-GD2-CAR-T cells and a MEK inhibitor (i.e., trametinib) demonstrated potential synergistic benefits for the clinical management of NB by enhancing antitumor efficacy in a xenograft model, irrespective of the MAPK pathway mutation status in tumor cells.	pCMV-PB transposase plasmid	(Tomida et al., 2021)
HER2 positive solid tumor	PB-based HER2-specific CAR-T cells exhibited not only significant antitumor efficacy *in vitro* but also shrank HER2-positive tumors *in vivo*.	pCMV-PB transposase plasmid	(Nakamura et al., 2021)

5. Transposon-Based Gene Therapy: Advances in Clinical Applications

TE-based therapeutic strategies have demonstrated considerable promise in clinical investigations. For instance, a single-arm Phase II trial of Lamivudine, a nucleoside reverse transcriptase inhibitor that targets LINE, Satellite, and ERV, in patients who have progressed on systemic therapy for metastatic colorectal cancer carrying TP53 mutations was completed (clinicaltrials.gov ID: NCT03144804) (Rajurkar et al., 2022). In addition, a Phase II clinical trial which evaluated the effect of neoadjuvant soy isoflavone administration on LINE-1 methylation in patients with head and neck squamous cell carcinoma was conducted (NCT02007200) (Rozek et al., 2019). Moreover, further clinical trials have been carried out to assess the therapeutic potential of TE–based approaches in various malignancies, including metastatic castration-resistant prostate cancer (Phase II; NCT00964002) (Houédé et al., 2014), ovarian cancer (Phase II; NCT0 1696032) (Oza et al., 2020) as well as advanced solid tumors (Phase I; NCT01537744) (Gaillard et al., 2019).

Additionally, the encouraging results emerged in preclinical studies have indicated that gene therapy strategies based on SB and PB transposon systems represent highly promising approaches for clinical investigations (Kebriaei et al., 2017; Sun et al., 2021). The first approved Phase I clinical trial application utilizing early-generation SB transposon technology involved the generation of CD19-specific CAR-T cells for the treatment of advanced non-Hodgkin lymphoma and acute lymphoblastic leukemia following hematopoietic stem cell transplantation in the autologous (NCT00968760) or allogeneic settings (NCT01497184) (Kebriaei et al., 2016). In addition, a number of clinical protocols have been conducted employing CD19-specific CAR-T cells, differing in aspects such as lymphodepletion therapy, CAR generations, T cell origin as well as administered cell doses (NCT01362452, NCT02529813, and NCT01653 717). Moreover, a Phase I/II clinical trial (NCT05194735) has been conducted, utilizing the administration of autologous T cells engineered via the SB transposon/transposase system to express neoantigen-specific T-cell receptors in patients with relapsed or refractory solid tumors (Levy & Gros, 2022).

As evidenced by completed/ongoing research, a gene therapy strategy involving the SB transposon system to genetically modify clinical-grade T cells to target CD19, marking a pivotal advancement in translational medicine (Singh et al., 2014). In a related context, natural killer (NK) cell-based therapies exhibit considerable potential in the field of bench-to-bedside research (Sakamoto et al., 2015; Park et al., 2024). Importantly, recent findings have introduced a game-changing approach for CAR-NK cell engineering utilizing a SB-based system and minimized DNA vectors (termed as minicircles) for the first time (Bexte et al., 2024). Notably, SB-generated CAR-NK cells exhibited high and stable CAR expression, which constitutes a critical determinant of CAR cell therapies (Bexte et al., 2024). In addition, employing of minicircle to express SB transposase and CARs significantly enhanced the viability of genetically modified T cells and gene transfer rate ([a]Tipanee et al., 2017). These advancements render minicircle-mediated SB CAR transposition a promising strategy for engineering clinical-grade CAR-T cells (Prommersberger et al., 2022). Moreover, a Phase I/II trial (NCT03389035) recently reported that donor-derived CD19 CAR-cytokine-induced killer cells engineered using the SB system demonstrated antileukemic activity without inducing severe toxicities in patients with B-cell acute lymphoblastic leukemia (Magnani et al., 2020).

The CARAMBA, which is funded by an EU Horizon 2020 grant (Grant Agreement ID: 754658), is the first clinical trial (Phase I/IIA; EudraCT: 2019-001264-30) based on virus-free CAR-T cells in Europe. It also represents the first clinical trial to utilize advanced SB transposon technology worldwide (Prommersberger et al., 2021). As a part of the project, the consortium selected the SLAMF7 which has been identified as a strategic therapeutic target in multiple myeloma (MM) (Chu et al., 2023). Moreover, the feasibility, anti-myeloma efficacy as well as safety of autologous SLAMF7 CAR-T cells were systematically assessed in the CARAMBA trial for treatment of the MM (Prommersberger et al., 2021).

Although the SB system, which was the first transposon ever used in patients, remains the most extensively utilized transposon in clinical trials, PB has recently entered the clinical stage as a promising alternative. Specifically, the first-in-human Phase I study (the Australian CARTELL trial, NHMRC identifier:1102172) which represented PB transposon system into clinic, aimed to evaluate the safety and efficacy of PB-engineered CD19-specific chimeric antigen receptor (CAR19)-T cells in patients with relapsed or refractory $CD19^+$ malignancies following human leukocyte antigen (HLA)-matched sibling donor hematopoietic stem cell transplantation (Bishop et al., 2019; Irving et al., 2021). Preliminary findings indicated that the safety and activity profiles were similar to those of CAR19 T cells generated using viral vectors (Bishop et al., 2019). Nevertheless, serious adverse events were reported, with two of the ten treated patients developing malignant CAR19-T cell tumors (Bishop et al.,

2021). In addition, a significant advance has been achieved with P-BCMA-101 autologous T stem cell memory (Tscm) CAR-T cells engineered via the PB platform for the treatment of patients with relapsed/refractory MM (NCT03288493). In this context, 90 patients have been treated with P-BCMA-101 and early outcomes demonstrated a 73% overall response rate in combination with Rituximab, accompanied by a favorable safety profile (Costello et al., 2021). Moreover, the efficacy of P-PSMA-101, an autologous CAR-T therapy utilizing the PB transposon system, was examined in a Phase I trial (NCT04249947) involving patients with metastatic castration-resistant prostate cancer (Slovin et al., 2022). Additionally, a Phase I clinical trial (NCT03182816) was conducted to evaluate the feasibility and safety of epidermal growth factor receptor (EGFR)- specifc CAR-T cells engineered using the PB system in patients with advanced relapsed/refractory non-small cell lung cancer (Zhang et al., 2021). Accordingly, nine patients received treatment, and none experienced grade 4 adverse events or severe cytokine release syndrome (Zhang et al., 2021). Although most patients experienced varying degrees of adverse events, all were manageable and did not result in severe or refractory adverse outcomes (Zhang et al., 2021).

6. Conclusions

TEs are repetitive DNA sequences with the capacity to mobilize within a genome and exert a broad range of functions in both physiological processes and pathological conditions, thereby contributing significantly to genome dynamics (Izsvák & Ivics, 2004; Kawakami et al., 2017). Moreover, transposons have gained attention as promising vectors for gene therapy, offering the potential to overcome several limitations associated with conventional viral vector systems ([b]Tipanee et al., 2017). Furthermore, considerable progress has been recorded in transposon-mediated technologies which demonstrate substantial potential for developing powerful genomic tools (Wang et al., 2024). As aforementioned, several transposable elements have been demonstrated to act as facilitators of efficient transposition in vertebrate model systems and have been utilized as tools in genomics research (Ivics & Izsvák, 2010). In particular, SB, PB, and Tol2, are the most widely studied transposon-based gene delivery systems, represent complementary tools in mammalian cells, offering significant advantages for gene transfer strategies in a wide range of research settings including gene/cell therapy and regenerative medicine. Despite the promising and encouraging outcomes obtained from extensive fundemantal studies, preclinical and clinical investigations, transposon-based therapies need further rigorous evaluation of their efficacy and safety through controlled pivotal trials.

References

Ade, C., Roy-Engel, A.M., & Deininger, P.L. (2013). Alu elements: an intrinsic source of human genome instability. *Current Opinion in Virology, 3*(6), 639–645. https://doi.org/10.1016/j.coviro.2013.09.002

Ahn, H.W., Worman, Z.F., Lechsinska, A., Payer, L.M., Wang, T., Malik, N., Li, W., Burns, K.H., Nath, A., & Levin, H.L. (2023). Retrotransposon insertions associated with risk of neurologic and psychiatric diseases. *EMBO Reports, 24*(1), e55197. https://doi.org/10.15252/embr.202255197

Albieri, I., Onorati, M., Calabrese, G., Moiana, A., Biasci, D., Badaloni, A., Camnasio, S., Spiliotopoulos, D., Ivics, Z., Cattaneo, E., & Consalez, G.G. (2010). A DNA transposon-based approach to functional screening in neural stem cells. *Journal of Biotechnology, 150*(1), 11–21. https://doi.org/10.1016/j.jbiotec.2010.07.027

Ali, A., Han, K., & Liang, P. (2021). Role of transposable elements in gene regulation in the human genome. *Life (Basel, Switzerland), 11*(2), 118. https://doi.org/10.3390/life11020118

Amberger, M., & Ivics, Z. (2020). Latest advances for the Sleeping Beauty transposon system: 23 years of insomnia but prettier than ever: refinement and recent innovations of the Sleeping Beauty transposon system enabling novel, nonviral genetic engineering applications. *BioEssays: News and Reviews in Molecular, Cellular and Developmental Biology, 42*(11), e2000136. https://doi.org/10.1002/bies.202000136

Antelo, M., Balaguer, F., Shia, J., Shen, Y., Hur, K., Moreira, L., Cuatrecasas, M., Bujanda, L., Giraldez, M.D., Takahashi, M., Cabanne, A., Barugel, M.E., Arnold, M., Roca, E.L., Andreu, M., Castellvi-Bel, S., Llor, X., Jover, R., Castells, A., Boland, C.R., …& Goel, A. (2012). A high degree of LINE-1 hypomethylation is a unique feature of early-onset colorectal cancer. *PloS One, 7*(9), e45357. https://doi.org/10.1371/journal.pone.0045357

Anwar, S.L., Hasemeier, B., Schipper, E., Vogel, A., Kreipe, H., & Lehmann, U. (2019). LINE-1 hypomethylation in human hepatocellular carcinomas correlates with shorter overall survival and CIMP phenotype. *PloS One, 14*(5), e0216374. https://doi.org/10.1371/journal.pone.0216374

Apoil, P.A., Kuhlein, E., Robert, A., Rubie, H., & Blancher, A. (2007). HIGM syndrome caused by insertion of an AluYb8 element in exon 1 of the CD40LG gene. *Immunogenetics, 59*(1), 17–23. https://doi.org/10.1007/ s00251-006-0175-5

Armaou, S., Konstantopoulou, I., Anagnostopoulos, T., Razis, E., Boukovinas, I., Xenidis, N., Fountzilas, G., & Yannoukakos, D. (2007). Novel genomic rearrangements in the BRCA1 gene detected in greek breast/ovarian cancer patients. *European Journal of Cancer (Oxford, England:1990), 43*(2), 443–453. https://doi.org/10.1016/j.ejca.2006.09.021

Aronovich, E.L., Bell, J.B., Khan, S.A., Belur, L.R., Gunther, R., Koniar, B., Schachern, P.A., Parker, J.B., Carlson, C.S., Whitley, C.B., McIvor, R.S., Gupta, P., & Hackett, P.B. (2009). Systemic correction of storage disease in MPS I NOD/SCID mice using the sleeping beauty transposon system. *Molecular Therapy: the Journal of the American Society of Gene Therapy, 17*(7), 1136–1144. https://doi.org/10.1038/mt.2009.87

Arvas, Y.E., Marakli, S., Kaya, Y., & Kalendar, R. (2023). The power of retrotransposons in high-throughput genotyping and sequencing. *Frontiers in Plant Science, 14*, 1174339. https://doi.org/10.3389/fpls.2023.1174339

Attig, J., Young, G.R., Hosie, L., Perkins, D., Encheva-Yokoya, V., Stoye, J.P., Snijders, A.P., Ternette, N., & Kassiotis, G. (2019). LTR retroelement expansion of the human cancer transcriptome and immunopeptidome revealed by de novo transcript assembly. *Genome Research, 29*(10), 1578–1590. https://doi.org/10.1101/gr.248922.119

Ayarpadikannan, S., & Kim, H.S. (2014). The impact of transposable elements in genome evolution and genetic instability and their implications in various diseases. *Genomics & Informatics, 12*(3), 98–104. https://doi.org/10.5808/GI.2014.12.3.98

Bahrambeigi, V., Ahmadi, N., Moisyadi, S., Urschitz, J., Salehi, R., & Haghjooy Javanmard, S. (2014). PhiC31/PiggyBac modified stromal stem cells: effect of interferon γ and/or tumor necrosis factor (TNF)-related apoptosis-inducing ligand (TRAIL) on murine melanoma. *Molecular Cancer, 13*, 255. https://doi.org/10.1186/1476-4598-13-255

Balciunas, D., Wangensteen, K.J., Wilber, A., Bell, J., Geurts, A., Sivasubbu, S., Wang, X., Hackett, P.B., Largaespada, D.A., McIvor, R.S., & Ekker, S.C. (2006). Harnessing a high cargo-capacity transposon for genetic applications in vertebrates. *PLoS Genetics, 2*(11), e169. https://doi.org/10.1371/journal.pgen.0020169

Balestrieri, E., Argaw-Denboba, A., Gambacurta, A., Cipriani, C., Bei, R., Serafino, A., Sinibaldi-Vallebona, P., & Matteucci, C. (2018). Human endogenous retrovirus K in the crosstalk between cancer cells microenvironment and plasticity: a new perspective for combination therapy. *Frontiers in Microbiology, 9*, 1448. https://doi.org/10.3389/fmicb.2018.01448

Bao, W., Jurka, M.G., Kapitonov, V.V., & Jurka, J. (2009). New superfamilies of eukaryotic DNA transposons and their internal divisions. *Molecular Biology and Evolution, 26*(5), 983–993. https://doi.org/10.1093/molbev/msp013

Bao, W., Kapitonov, V.V., & Jurka, J. (2010). Ginger DNA transposons in eukaryotes and their evolutionary relationships with long terminal repeat retrotransposons. *Mobile DNA, 1*(1), 3. https://doi.org/10.1186/1759-8753 1-3

Barrow, T.M., Wong Doo, N., Milne, R.L., Giles, G.G., Willmore, E., Strathdee, G., & Byun, H.M. (2021). Analysis of retrotransposon subfamily DNA methylation reveals novel early epigenetic changes in chronic lymphocytic leukemia. *Haematologica, 106*(1), 98–110. https://doi.org/10.3324/haematol.2019.228478

Barry, K.H., Moore, L.E., Liao, L.M., Huang, W.Y., Andreotti, G., Poulin, M., & Berndt, S.I. (2015). Prospective study of DNA methylation at LINE-1 and Alu in peripheral blood and the risk of prostate cancer. *The Prostate*, *75*(15), 1718–1725. https://doi.org/10.1002/pros.23053

Batchu, R.B., Gruzdyn, O.V., Tavva, P.S., Kolli, B.K., Dachepalli, R., Weaver, D.W., & Gruber, S.A. (2019). Engraftment of mesothelin chimeric antigen receptor using a hybrid Sleeping Beauty/minicircle vector into NK-92MI cells for treatment of pancreatic cancer. *Surgery, 166*(4), 503–508. https://doi.org/10.1016/j.surg.2019.05.047

Battista, S., Fedele, M., Secco, L., Ingo, A.M.D., Sgarra, R., & Manfioletti, G. (2024). Binding to the other side: the AT-hook DNA-binding domain allows nuclear factors to exploit the DNA minor groove. *International Journal of Molecular Sciences, 25*(16), 8863. https://doi.org/10.3390/ijms25168863

Baus, J., Liu, L., Heggestad, A.D., Sanz, S., & Fletcher, B.S. (2005). Hyperactive transposase mutants of the Sleeping Beauty transposon. *Molecular Therapy: the Journal of the American Society of Gene Therapy*, *12*(6), 1148–1156. https://doi.org/10.1016/j.ymthe.2005.06.484

Begum, A.A., Toth, I., Hussein, W.M., & Moyle, P.M. (2019). Advances in targeted gene delivery. *Current Drug Delivery, 16*(7), 588–608. https://doi.org/10.2174/1567201816666190529072914

Belay, E., Mátrai, J., Acosta-Sanchez, A., Ma, L., Quattrocelli, M., Mátés, L., Sancho-Bru, P., Geraerts, M., Yan, B., Vermeesch, J., Rincón, M.Y., Samara-Kuko, E., Ivics, Z., Verfaillie, C., Sampaolesi, M., Izsvák, Z., Vandendriessche, T., & Chuah, M.K. (2010). Novel hyperactive transposons for genetic modification of induced pluripotent and adult stem cells: a nonviral paradigm for coaxed differentiation. *Stem Cells (Dayton, Ohio), 28*(10), 1760–1771. https://doi.org/10.1002/stem.501

Bennetzen J.L. (2000). Transposable element contributions to plant gene and genome evolution. *Plant Molecular Biology, 42*(1), 251–269. http://doi.org/10.1023/A:1006344508454

Bexte, T., Botezatu, L., Miskey, C., Gierschek, F., Moter, A., Wendel, P., Reindl, L.M., Campe, J., Villena-Ossa, J.F., Gebel, V., Stein, K., Cathomen, T., Cremer, A., Wels, W.S., Hudecek, M., Ivics, Z., & Ullrich, E. (2024). Engineering of potent CAR NK cells using non-viral Sleeping Beauty transposition from minimalistic DNA vectors. *Molecular Therapy: the Journal of the American Society of Gene Therapy, 32*(7), 2357–2372. https://doi.org/10.1016/j.ymthe.2024.05.022

Bhagat, M., Kamal, R., Sharma, J., Kaur, K., Sharma, A., Singh, T.G., Bhatia, R., & Awasthi, A. (2024). Gene therapy: towards a new era of medicine. *AAPS PharmSciTech, 26*(1), 17. https://doi.org/10.1208/s12249-024-03010-6

Bhat, A., Ghatage, T., Bhan, S., Lahane, G.P., Dhar, A., Kumar, R., Pandita, R.K., Bhat, K.M., Ramos, K.S., & Pandita, T.K. (2022). Role of transposable elements in genome stability: implications for health and disease. *International Journal of Molecular Sciences, 23*(14), 7802. https://doi.org/10.3390/ijms23147802

Bishop, D.C., Clancy, L.E., Burgess, J., Mathew, G., Atkins, E., Advic, S., Maddock, K., Street, J., Moezzi, L., Simms, R., Stephen, K., O'Brien, T., Shaw, P.J., Gottlieb, D., Blyth, E., & Micklethwaite, K. (2019). Matched sibling donor-derived piggybac CAR19 T cells induce remission of relapsed/refractory CD19+ malignancy following haematopoietic stem cell transplant. *Cytotherapy, 21*, S9. https://doi.org/10.1016/j.jcyt.2019.03.562

Bishop, D.C., Clancy, L.E., Simms, R., Burgess, J., Mathew, G., Moezzi, L., Street, J.A., Sutrave, G., Atkins, E., McGuire, H.M., Gloss, B.S., Lee, K., Jiang, W., Maddock, K., McCaughan, G., Avdic, S., Antonenas, V., O'Brien, T.A., Shaw, P.J., Irving, D.O., …& Micklethwaite, K.P. (2021). Development of CAR T-cell lymphoma in 2 of 10 patients effectively treated with piggyBac-modified CD19 CAR T cells. *Blood, 138*(16), 1504–1509.

https://doi.org/10.1182/blood.2021010813

Bouras, A., Leone, M., Bonadona, V., Lebrun, M., Calender, A., & Boutry-Kryza, N. (2021). Identification and characterization of new *Alu* element insertion in the *BRCA1* exon 14 associated with hereditary breast and ovarian cancer. *Genes, 12*(11), 1736. https://doi.org/10.3390/genes12111736

Bourque, G., Burns, K.H., Gehring, M., Gorbunova, V., Seluanov, A., Hammell, M., Imbeault, M., Izsvák, Z., Levin, H.L., Macfarlan, T.S., Mager, D.L., & Feschotte, C. (2018). Ten things you should know about transposable elements. *Genome Biology, 19*(1), 199. https://doi.org/10.1186/s13059-018-1577-z

[a]Bureau, T.E., & Wessler, S.R. (1994). Mobile inverted-repeat elements of the tourist family are associated with the genes of many cereal grasses. *Proceedings of the National Academy of Sciences of the United States of America, 91*(4), 1411–1415. https://doi.org/10.1073/pnas.91.4.1411

[b]Bureau, T.E., & Wessler, S.R. (1994). Stowaway: a new family of inverted repeat elements associated with the genes of both monocotyledonous and dicotyledonous plants. *The Plant Cell, 6*(6), 907–916. https://doi.org/10.1105/tpc.6.6.907

Burns K.H. (2017). Transposable elements in cancer. *Nature Reviews. Cancer, 17*(7), 415–424. https://doi.org/10.1038/nrc.2017.35

Cao, Y., Rui, B., Wellems, D.L., Li, M., Chen, B., Zhang, D., & Pan, W. (2013). Identification of piggyBac-mediated insertions in Plasmodium berghei by next generation sequencing. *Malaria Journal, 12*, 287. https://doi.org/10.1186/1475-2875-12-287

Carpes, M.P., Nunes, J.F., Sampaio, T.L., Castro, M.E., Zanotto, P.M., & Ribeiro, B.M. (2009). Molecular analysis of a mutant Anticarsia gemmatalis multiple nucleopolyhedrovirus (AgMNPV) shows an interruption of an inhibitor of apoptosis gene (iap-3) by a new class-II piggyBac-related insect transposon. *Insect Molecular Biology, 18*(6), 747–757. https://doi.org/10.1111/j.1365-2583.2009.00917.x

Cary, L.C., Goebel, M., Corsaro, B.G., Wang, H.G., Rosen, E., & Fraser, M.J. (1989). Transposon mutagenesis of baculoviruses: analysis of Trichoplusia ni transposon IFP2 insertions within the FP-locus of nuclear polyhedrosis viruses. *Virology, 172*(1), 156–169. https://doi.org/10.1016/0042-6822(89)90117-7

Castanera, R., Pérez, G., López, L., Sancho, R., Santoyo, F., Alfaro, M., Gabaldón, T., Pisabarro, A.G., Oguiza, J.A., & Ramírez, L. (2014). Highly expressed captured genes and cross-kingdom domains present in Helitrons create novel diversity in Pleurotus ostreatus and other fungi.

BMC Genomics, 15(1), 1071. https://doi.org/10.1186/1471-2164-15-1071

Cecconi, F., & Meyer, B.I. (2000). Gene trap: a way to identify novel genes and unravel their biological function. *FEBS Letters, 480*(1), 63–71. https://doi.org/10.1016/s0014-5793(00)01779-8

Chen, Z.J., Kren, B.T., Wong, P.Y., Low, W.C., & Steer, C.J. (2005). Sleeping Beauty-mediated down-regulation of huntingtin expression by RNA interference. *Biochemical and Biophysical Research Communications, 329*(2), 646–652. https://doi.org/10.1016/j.bbrc.2005.02.024

Cheng, M., Jin, X., Mu, L., Wang, F., Li, W., Zhong, X., Liu, X., Shen, W., Liu, Y., & Zhou, Y. (2016). Combination of the clustered regularly interspaced short palindromic repeats (CRISPR)-associated 9 technique with the piggybac transposon system for mouse in utero electroporation to study cortical development. *Journal of Neuroscience Research, 94*(9), 814–824. https://doi.org/10.1002/jnr.23776

Cherkasova, E., Malinzak, E., Rao, S., Takahashi, Y., Senchenko, V.N., Kudryavtseva, A.V., Nickerson, M.L., Merino, M., Hong, J.A., Schrump, D.S., Srinivasan, R., Linehan, W.M., Tian, X., Lerman, M.I., & Childs, R.W. (2011). Inactivation of the von Hippel-Lindau tumor suppressor leads to selective expression of a human endogenous retrovirus in kidney cancer. *Oncogene, 30*(47), 4697–4706. https://doi.org/10.1038/onc.2011.179

Chu, E., Wu, J., Kang, S.S., & Kang, Y. (2023). SLAMF7 as a promising immunotherapeutic target in multiple myeloma treatments. *Current Oncology (Toronto, Ont.), 30*(9), 7891–7903. https://doi.org/10.3390/curroncol30090573

Clark, K.J., Carlson, D.F., Leaver, M.J., Foster, L.K., & Fahrenkrug, S.C. (2009). Passport, a native Tc1 transposon from flatfish, is functionally active in vertebrate cells. *Nucleic Acids Research, 37*(4), 1239–1247. https://doi.org/10.1093/nar/gkn1025

Clayton, E.A., Rishishwar, L., Huang, T.C., Gulati, S., Ban, D., McDonald, J.F., & Jordan, I.K. (2020). An atlas of transposable element-derived alternative splicing in cancer. *Philosophical Transactions of the Royal Society of London. Series B, Biological Sciences, 375*(1795), 20190342. https://doi.org/10.1098/rstb.2019.0342

Colloms, S.D., van Luenen, H.G., & Plasterk, R.H. (1994). DNA binding activities of the Caenorhabditis elegans Tc3 transposase. *Nucleic Acids Research, 22*(25), 5548–5554. https://doi.org/10.1093/nar/22.25.5548

Colonna Romano, N., & Fanti, L. (2022). Transposable elements: major players in shaping genomic and evolutionary patterns. *Cells, 11*(6), 1048. https://doi.org/10.3390/cells11061048

Cordaux, R., & Batzer, M.A. (2009). The impact of retrotransposons on human genome evolution. *Nature Reviews. Genetics, 10*(10), 691–703. https://doi.org/10.1038/nrg2640

Costello, C., Derman, B.A., Kocoglu, M.H., Deol, A., Ali, A.A., Gregory, T.,…. & Shah, N. (2021). Clinical trials of BCMA-targeted CAR-T cells utilizing a novel non-viral transposon system. *Blood, 138*, 3858. https://doi: 10.1182/blood-2021-151672

Crescente, J.M., Zavallo, D., Helguera, M., & Vanzetti, L.S. (2018). MITE Tracker: an accurate approach to identify miniature inverted-repeat transposable elements in large genomes. *BMC Bioinformatics, 19*(1), 348. https://doi.org/10.1186/s12859-018-2376-y

Cui, Z., Geurts, A.M., Liu, G., Kaufman, C.D., & Hackett, P.B. (2002). Structure-function analysis of the inverted terminal repeats of the sleeping beauty transposon. *Journal of Molecular Biology, 318*(5), 1221–1235. https://doi.org/10.1016/s0022-2836(02)00237-1

Daskalos, A., Nikolaidis, G., Xinarianos, G., Savvari, P., Cassidy, A., Zakopoulou, R., Kotsinas, A., Gorgoulis, V., Field, J.K., & Liloglou, T. (2009). Hypomethylation of retrotransposable elements correlates with genomic instability in non-small cell lung cancer. *International Journal of Cancer, 124*(1), 81–87. https://doi.org/10.1002/ijc.23849

Davis, C.A., Hitz, B.C., Sloan, C.A., Chan, E.T., Davidson, J.M., Gabdank, I., Hilton, J.A., Jain, K., Baymuradov, U.K., Narayanan, A.K., Onate, K.C., Graham, K., Miyasato, S.R., Dreszer, T.R., Strattan, J.S., Jolanki, O., Tanaka, F.Y., & Cherry, J.M. (2018). The encyclopedia of DNA elements (ENCODE): data portal update. *Nucleic Acids Research, 46*(D1), D794–D801. https://doi.org/10.1093/nar/gkx1081

Devaraj, A., Singh, M., Narayanavari, S.A., Yong, G., Chen, J., Wang, J., Becker, M., Walisko, O., Schorn, A., Cseresznyés, Z., Raskó, T., Radscheit, K., Selbach, M., Ivics, Z., & Izsvák, Z. (2023). HMGXB4 targets *Sleeping Beauty* transposition to germinal stem cells. *International Journal of Molecular Sciences, 24*(8), 7283. https://doi.org/10.3390/ijms24087283

Dewannieux, M., & Heidmann, T. (2005). LINEs, SINEs and processed pseudogenes: parasitic strategies for genome modeling. *Cytogenetic and Genome Research, 110*(1-4), 35–48. https://doi.org/10.1159/000084936

Di Matteo, M., Belay, E., Chuah, M.K., & Vandendriessche, T. (2012). Recent developments in transposon-mediated gene therapy. *Expert Opinion on Biological Therapy, 12*(7), 841–858.

https://doi.org/10.1517/14712598.2012.684875

Ding, S., Wu, X., Li, G., Han, M., Zhuang, Y., & Xu, T. (2005). Efficient transposition of the piggyBac (PB) transposon in mammalian cells and mice. *Cell, 122*(3), 473–483. https://doi.org/10.1016/j.cell.2005.07.013

Dodonova, S.O., Prinz, S., Bilanchone, V., Sandmeyer, S., & Briggs, J.A.G. (2019). Structure of the Ty3/Gypsy retrotransposon capsid and the evolution of retroviruses. *Proceedings of the National Academy of Sciences of the United States of America, 116*(20), 10048–10057. https://doi.org/10.1073/pnas.1900931116

Du, A.Y., Chobirko, J.D., Zhuo, X., Feschotte, C., & Wang, T. (2024). Regulatory transposable elements in the encyclopedia of DNA elements. *Nature Communications, 15*(1), 7594. https://doi.org/10.1038/s41467-024-51921-6

Dupuy A.J. (2010). Transposon-based screens for cancer gene discovery in mouse models. *Seminars in Cancer Biology, 20*(4), 261–268. https://doi.org/10.1016/j.semcancer.2010.05.003

Elick, T.A., Bauser, C.A., & Fraser, M.J. (1996). Excision of the piggyBac transposable element in vitro is a precise event that is enhanced by the expression of its encoded transposase. *Genetica, 98*(1), 33–41. https://doi.org/10.1007/BF00120216

Elick, T.A., Lobo, N., & Fraser, M.J., Jr (1997). Analysis of the cis-acting DNA elements required for piggyBac transposable element excision. *Molecular & General Genetics: MGG, 255*(6), 605–610. https://doi.org/10.1007/s004380050534

Eskier, D., Yetkin, S., Arslan, N., Karakülah, G., & Alotaibi, H. (2025). Exploring regulatory roles of transposable elements in EMT and MET through data-driven analysis: insights from regulaTER. *Journal of Molecular Biology, 437*(2), 168887. https://doi.org/10.1016/j.jmb.2024.168887

Ferrari, G., Thrasher, A.J., & Aiuti, A. (2021). Gene therapy using haematopoietic stem and progenitor cells. *Nature Reviews. Genetics, 22*(4), 216–234. https://doi.org/10.1038/s41576-020-00298-5

Feschotte C. (2006). The piggyBac transposon holds promise for human gene therapy. *Proceedings of the National Academy of Sciences of the United States of America, 103*(41), 14981–14982. https://doi.org/10.1073/pnas.0607282103

Feschotte C. (2008). Transposable elements and the evolution of regulatory networks. *Nature Reviews. Genetics, 9*(5), 397–405. https://doi.org/10.1038/nrg2337

Fiano, V., Zugna, D., Grasso, C., Trevisan, M., Delsedime, L., Molinaro, L., Gillio-Tos, A., Merletti, F., & Richiardi, L. (2017). LINE-1 methylation status in prostate cancer and non-neoplastic tissue adjacent to tumor in association with mortality. *Epigenetics, 12*(1), 11–18. https://doi.org/10.1080/15592294.2016.1261786

Fischer, S.E., Wienholds, E., & Plasterk, R.H. (2001). Regulated transposition of a fish transposon in the mouse germ line. *Proceedings of the National Academy of Sciences of the United States of America, 98*(12), 6759–6764. https://doi.org/10.1073/pnas.121569298

Fjord-Larsen, L., Kusk, P., Emerich, D.F., Thanos, C., Torp, M., Bintz, B., Tornøe, J., Johnsen, A.H., & Wahlberg, L.U. (2012). Increased encapsulated cell biodelivery of nerve growth factor in the brain by transposon-mediated gene transfer. *Gene Therapy, 19*(10), 1010–1017. https://doi.org/10.1038/gt.2011.178

Fort, V., Khelifi, G., & Hussein, S.M.I. (2021). Long non-coding RNAs and transposable elements: a functional relationship. *Biochimica et Biophysica Acta. Molecular Cell Research, 1868*(1), 118837. https://doi.org/10.1016/j.bbamcr.2020.118837

Franke, G., Bausch, B., Hoffmann, M.M., Cybulla, M., Wilhelm, C., Kohlhase, J., Scherer, G., & Neumann, H.P. (2009). Alu-Alu recombination underlies the vast majority of large VHL germline deletions: molecular characterization and genotype-phenotype correlations in VHL patients. *Human Mutation, 30*(5), 776–786. https://doi.org/10.1002/humu.20948

Fraser, M.J., Smith, G.E., & Summers, M.D. (1983). Acquisition of host cell DNA sequences by baculoviruses: relationship between host DNA insertions and FP mutants of Autographa californica and Galleria mellonella nuclear polyhedrosis viruses. *Journal of Virology, 47*(2), 287–300. https://doi.org/10.1128/JVI.47.2.287-300.1983

Fueyo, R., Judd, J., Feschotte, C., & Wysocka, J. (2022). Roles of transposable elements in the regulation of mammalian transcription. *Nature Reviews. Molecular Cell Biology*, *23*(7), 481–497. https://doi.org/10.1038/s41580-022-00457-y

Gaillard, S.L., Zahurak, M., Sharma, A., Durham, J.N., Reiss, K.A., Sartorius-Mergenthaler, S., Downs, M., Anders, N.M., Ahuja, N., Rudek, M. A., & Azad, N. (2019). A phase 1 trial of the oral DNA methyltransferase inhibitor CC-486 and the histone deacetylase inhibitor romidepsin in advanced solid tumors. *Cancer, 125*(16), 2837–2845. https://doi.org/10.1002/cncr.32138

Gangadharan, S., Mularoni, L., Fain-Thornton, J., Wheelan, S.J., & Craig, N.L. (2010). DNA transposon Hermes inserts into DNA in nucleosome-free regions in vivo. *Proceedings of the National Academy of Sciences of the United States of America, 107*(51), 21966–21972.

https://doi.org/10.1073/pnas.1016382107
Garcillán-Barcia, M.P., & de la Cruz, F. (2002). Distribution of IS91 family insertion sequences in bacterial genomes: evolutionary implications. *FEMS Microbiology Ecology, 42*(2), 303–313. https://doi.org/10.1111/j.1574-6941.2002.tb01020.x
Geurts, A.M., Yang, Y., Clark, K.J., Liu, G., Cui, Z., Dupuy, A.J., Bell, J.B., Largaespada, D.A., & Hackett, P.B. (2003). Gene transfer into genomes of human cells by the sleeping beauty transposon system. *Molecular Therapy: the Journal of the American Society of Gene Therapy, 8*(1), 108–117. https://doi.org/10.1016/s1525-0016(03)00099-6
Giménez-Orenga, K., & Oltra, E. (2021). Human endogenous retrovirus as therapeutic targets in neurologic disease. *Pharmaceuticals (Basel, Switzerland), 14*(6), 495. https://doi.org/10.3390/ph14060495
Ginn, S.L., Mandwie, M., Alexander, I.E., Edelstein, M., & Abedi, M.R. (2024). Gene therapy clinical trials worldwide to 2023-an update. *The Journal of Gene Medicine, 26*(8), e3721. https://doi.org/10.1002/jgm.3721
Grabundzija, I., Irgang, M., Mátés, L., Belay, E., Matrai, J., Gogol-Döring, A., Kawakami, K., Chen, W., Ruiz, P., Chuah, M.K., VandenDriessche, T., Izsvák, Z., & Ivics, Z. (2010). Comparative analysis of transposable element vector systems in human cells. *Molecular Therapy: the Journal of the American Society of Gene Therapy, 18*(6), 1200–1209. https://doi.org/10.1038/mt.2010.47
Grandi, F.C., & An, W. (2013). Non-LTR retrotransposons and microsatellites: partners in genomic variation. *Mobile Genetic Elements, 3*(4), e25674. https://doi.org/10.4161/mge.25674
Guo, C., Jeong, H.H., Hsieh, Y.C., Klein, H.U., Bennett, D.A., De Jager, P. L., Liu, Z., & Shulman, J.M. (2018). Tau activates transposable elements in Alzheimer's disease. *Cell Reports, 23*(10), 2874–2880. https://doi.org/10.1016/j.celrep.2018.05.004
Guo, M., Addy, G.A., Yang, N., Asare, E., Wu, H., Saleh, A.A., Shi, S., Gao, B., & Song, C. (2023). *PiggyBac* transposon mining in the small genomes of animals. *Biology, 13*(1), 24. https://doi.org/10.3390/biology13010024
Haapa-Paananen, S., Wahlberg, N., & Savilahti, H. (2014). Phylogenetic analysis of maverick/polinton giant transposons across organisms. *Molecular Phylogenetics and Evolution, 78*, 271–274. https://doi.org/10.1016/j.ympev.2014.05.024
Hadjiargyrou, M., & Delihas, N. (2013). The intertwining of transposable elements and non-coding RNAs. *International Journal of Molecular Sciences, 14*(7), 13307–13328. https://doi.org/10.3390/ijms140713307

Han J.S. (2010). Non-long terminal repeat (non-LTR) retrotransposons: mechanisms, recent developments, and unanswered questions. *Mobile DNA, 1*(1), 15. https://doi.org/10.1186/1759-8753-1-15

Han, M., Perkins, M.H., Novaes, L.S., Xu, T., & Chang, H. (2023). Advances in transposable elements: from mechanisms to applications in mammalian genomics. *Frontiers in Genetics, 14*, 1290146. https://doi.org/10.3389/fgene.2023.1290146

Harmening, N., Johnen, S., Izsvák, Z., Ivics, Z., Kropp, M., Bascuas, T., Walter, P., Kreis, A., Pajic, B., & Thumann, G. (2023). Enhanced biosafety of the Sleeping Beauty transposon system by using mRNA as source of transposase to efficiently and stably transfect retinal pigment epithelial cells. *Biomolecules, 13*(4), 658. https://doi.org/10.3390/biom13040658

Harris, C.R., Normart, R., Yang, Q., Stevenson, E., Haffty, B.G., Ganesan, S., Cordon-Cardo, C., Levine, A.J., & Tang, L.H. (2010). Association of nuclear localization of a long interspersed nuclear element-1 protein in breast tumors with poor prognostic outcomes. *Genes & Cancer*, *1*(2), 115–124. https://doi.org/10.1177/1947601909360812

Hassan, A.H., Mokhtar, M.M., & El Allali, A. (2024). Transposable elements: multifunctional players in the plant genome. *Frontiers in Plant Science*, *14*, 1330127. https://doi.org/10.3389/fpls.2023.1330127

Helou, L., Beauclair, L., Dardente, H., Arensburger, P., Buisine, N., Jaszczyszyn, Y., Guillou, F., Lecomte, T., Kentsis, A., & Bigot, Y. (2021). The C-terminal domain of piggyBac transposase is not required for DNA transposition. *Journal of Molecular Biology, 433*(7), 166805. https://doi.org/10.1016/j.jmb.2020.166805

Hernandez, M., Recalde, S., Garcia-Garcia, L., Bezunartea, J., Miskey, C., Johnen, S., Diarra, S., Sebe, A., Rodriguez-Madoz, J.R., Pouillot, S., Marie, C., Izsvák, Z., Scherman, D., Kropp, M., Prosper, F., Thumann, G., Ivics, Z., Garcia-Layana, A., & Fernandez-Robredo, P. (2019). Preclinical evaluation of a cell-based gene therapy using the Sleeping Beauty transposon system in choroidal neovascularization. *Molecular Therapy. Methods & Clinical Development, 15*, 403–417. https://doi.org/10.1016/j.omtm.2019.10.013

Hickman, A.B., & Dyda, F. (2015). Mechanisms of DNA transposition. *Microbiology Spectrum, 3*(2), MDNA3–2014. https://doi.org/10.1128/microbiolspec.MDNA3-0034-2014

Hickman, A. B., & Dyda, F. (2016). DNA transposition at work. *Chemical Reviews, 116*(20), 12758-12784. https://doi: 10.1021/acs.chemrev.6b00003.

Hickman, A.B., Perez, Z.N., Zhou, L., Musingarimi, P., Ghirlando, R., Hinshaw, J.E., Craig, N.L., & Dyda, F. (2005). Molecular architecture of a eukaryotic DNA transposase. *Nature Structural & Molecular Biology, 12*(8), 715–721. https://doi.org/10.1038/nsmb970

Holstein, M., Mesa-Nuñez, C., Miskey, C., Almarza, E., Poletti, V., Schmeer, M., Grueso, E., Ordóñez Flores, J.C., Kobelt, D., Walther, W., Aneja, M.K., Geiger, J., Bonig, H.B., Izsvák, Z., Schleef, M., Rudolph, C., Mavilio, F., Bueren, J.A., Guenechea, G., & Ivics, Z. (2018). Efficient non-viral gene delivery into human hematopoietic stem cells by minicircle Sleeping Beauty transposon vectors. *Molecular Therapy: the Journal of the American Society of Gene Therapy, 26*(4), 1137–1153. https://doi.org/10.1016/j.ymthe.2018.01.012

Hong, J.H., Jin, E.H., Kim, S., Song, K.S., & Sung, J.K. (2018). LINE-1 hypomethylation is inversely correlated with UHRF1 overexpression in gastric cancer. *Oncology Letters, 15*(5), 6666–6670. https://doi.org/10.3892/ol.2018.8121

Horvath, J., Jedlicka, P., Kratka, M., Kubat, Z., Kejnovsky, E., & Lexa, M. (2024). Detection and classification of long terminal repeat sequences in plant LTR-retrotransposons and their analysis using explainable machine learning. *BioData Mining, 17*(1), 57. https://doi.org/10.1186/s13040-024-00410-z

Hou, X., Du, Y., Deng, Y., Wu, J., & Cao, G. (2015). Sleeping Beauty transposon system for genetic etiological research and gene therapy of cancers. *Cancer Biology & Therapy, 16*(1), 8–16. https://doi.org/10.4161/15384047.2014.986944

Houédé, N., Pulido, M., Mourey, L., Joly, F., Ferrero, J.M., Bellera, C., Priou, F., Lalet, C., Laroche-Clary, A., Raffin, M.C., Ichas, F., Puech, A., & Piazza, P.V. (2014). A phase II trial evaluating the efficacy and safety of efavirenz in metastatic castration-resistant prostate cancer. *The Oncologist, 19*(12), 1227–1228. https://doi.org/10.1634/theoncologist.2014-0345

Hsu, P.S., Yu, S.H., Tsai, Y.T., Chang, J.Y., Tsai, L.K., Ye, C.H., Song, N. Y., Yau, L.C., & Lin, S.P. (2021). More than causing (epi)genomic instability: emerging physiological implications of transposable element modulation. *Journal of Biomedical Science, 28*(1), 58. https://doi.org/10.1186/s12929-021-00754-2

Huang, Y., Luo, L., Hu, X., Yu, F., Yang, Y., Deng, Z., Wu, J., Chen, R., & Zhang, M. (2017). Characterization, genomic organization, abundance, and chromosomal distribution of ty1-copia tetrotransposons in erianthus arundinaceus. *Frontiers in Plant Science, 8*, 924. https://doi.org/10.3389/fpls.2017.00924

Hudecek, M., Izsvák, Z., Johnen, S., Renner, M., Thumann, G., & Ivics, Z. (2017). Going non-viral: the Sleeping Beauty transposon system breaks on through to the clinical side. *Critical Reviews in Biochemistry and Molecular Biology*, *52*(4), 355–380. https://doi.org/10.1080/10409238.2017.1304354

Hussen, B.M., Taheri, M., Yashooa, R.K., Abdullah, G.H., Abdullah, S.R., Kheder, R.K., & Mustafa, S.A. (2024). Revolutionizing medicine: recent developments and future prospects in stem-cell therapy. *International Journal of Surgery (London, England), 110*(12), 8002–8024. https://doi.org/10.1097/JS9.0000000000002109

Imamura, K., Sahara, N., Kanaan, N.M., Tsukita, K., Kondo, T., Kutoku, Y., Ohsawa, Y., Sunada, Y., Kawakami, K., Hotta, A., Yawata, S., Watanabe, D., Hasegawa, M., Trojanowski, J.Q., Lee, V.M., Suhara, T., Higuchi, M., & Inoue, H. (2016). Calcium dysregulation contributes to neurodegeneration in FTLD patient iPSC-derived neurons. *Scientific Reports, 6*, 34904. https://doi.org/10.1038/srep34904

Inada, E., Saitoh, I., Watanabe, S., Aoki, R., Miura, H., Ohtsuka, M., Murakami, T., Sawami, T., Yamasaki, Y., & Sato, M. (2015). PiggyBac transposon-mediated gene delivery efficiently generates stable transfectants derived from cultured primary human deciduous tooth dental pulp cells (HDDPCs) and HDDPC-derived iPS cells. *International Journal of Oral Science, 7*(3), 144–154. https://doi.org/10.1038/ijos.2015.18

Irving, M., Lanitis, E., Migliorini, D., Ivics, Z., & Guedan, S. (2021). Choosing the right tool for genetic engineering: clinical lessons from chimeric antigen receptor-T cells. *Human Gene Therapy, 32*(19-20), 1044–1058. https://doi.org/10.1089/hum.2021.173

Itoh, M., Kawagoe, S., Tamai, K., Nakagawa, H., Asahina, A., & Okano, H.J. (2020). Footprint-free gene mutation correction in induced pluripotent stem cell (iPSC) derived from recessive dystrophic epidermolysis bullosa (RDEB) using the CRISPR/Cas9 and piggyBac transposon system. *Journal of Dermatological Science, 98*(3), 163–172. https://doi.org/10.1016/j.jdermsci.2020.04.004

Ivics, Z., Hackett, P.B., Plasterk, R.H., & Izsvák, Z. (1997). Molecular reconstruction of Sleeping Beauty, a Tc1-like transposon from fish, and its transposition in human cells. *Cell, 91*(4), 501–510. https://doi.org/10.1016/s0092-8674(00)80436-5

Ivics, Z., & Izsvák, Z. (2006). Transposons for gene therapy!. *Current Gene Therapy, 6*(5), 593–607. https://doi.org/10.2174/156652306778520647

Ivics, Z., & Izsvák, Z. (2010). The expanding universe of transposon technologies for gene and cell engineering. *Mobile DNA, 1*(1), 25. https://doi.org/10.1186/1759-8753-1-25

Ivics, Z., & Izsvák, Z. (2015). Sleeping Beauty transposition. *Microbiology Spectrum, 3*(2), MDNA3–2014. https://doi.org/10.1128/microbiolspec.MDNA3-0042-2014

Ivics, Z., Kaufman, C.D., Zayed, H., Miskey, C., Walisko, O., & Izsvák, Z. (2004). The Sleeping Beauty transposable element: evolution, regulation and genetic applications. *Current Issues in Molecular Biology, 6*(1), 43–56. https://doi.org/10.21775/cimb.006.043

Iyer, P.S., Mavoungou, L.O., Ronzoni, F., Zemla, J., Schmid-Siegert, E., Antonini, S., Neff, L.A., Dorchies, O.M., Jaconi, M., Lekka, M., Messina, G., & Mermod, N. (2018). Autologous cell therapy approach for Duchenne Muscular Dystrophy using PiggyBac transposons and mesoangioblasts. *Molecular Therapy: the Journal of the American Society of Gene Therapy, 26*(4), 1093–1108. https://doi.org/10.1016/j.ymthe.2018.01.021

Izsvák, Z., Chuah, M.K., Vandendriessche, T., & Ivics, Z. (2009). Efficient stable gene transfer into human cells by the Sleeping Beauty transposon vectors. *Methods (San Diego, Calif.), 49*(3), 287–297. https://doi.org/10.1016/j.ymeth.2009.07.001

Izsvák, Z., & Ivics, Z. (2004). Sleeping beauty transposition: biology and applications for molecular therapy. *Molecular Therapy: the Journal of the American Society of Gene Therapy, 9*(2), 147–156. https://doi.org/10.1016/j.ymthe.2003.11.009

Izsvák, Z., Ivics, Z., & Plasterk, R.H. (2000). Sleeping Beauty, a wide host-range transposon vector for genetic transformation in vertebrates. *Journal of Molecular Biology, 302*(1), 93–102. https://doi.org/10.1006/jmbi.2000.4047

Izsvák, Z., Khare, D., Behlke, J., Heinemann, U., Plasterk, R.H., & Ivics, Z. (2002). Involvement of a bifunctional, paired-like DNA-binding domain and a transpositional enhancer in Sleeping Beauty transposition. *The Journal of Biological Chemistry, 277*(37), 34581–34588. https://doi.org/10.1074/jbc.M204001200

Jiang, Y., Hoenisch, R.C., Chang, Y., Bao, X., Cameron, C.E., & Lian, X.L. (2022). Robust genome and RNA editing via CRISPR nucleases in PiggyBac systems. *Bioactive Materials, 14*, 313–320. https://doi.org/10.1016/j.bioactmat.2022.01.046

Johnson, B.A., Chauhan, A.K., & Staber, J.M. (2016). Long-term expression of von Willebrand factor via Piggybac-mediated gene transfer. *Blood, 128*(22): B3511-3511.

https://doi.org/10.1182/blood.V128.22.3511.3511
Junop, M.S., & Haniford, D.B. (1997). Factors responsible for target site selection in Tn10 transposition: a role for the DDE motif in target DNA capture. *The EMBO Journal, 16*(10), 2646–2655. https://doi.org/10.1093/emboj/16.10.2646

Kalendar, R., Amenov, A., & Daniyarov, A. (2019). Use of retrotransposon-derived genetic markers to analyse genomic variability in plants. *Functional Plant Biology: FPB*, *46*(1), 15–29. https://doi.org/10.1071/FP18098

Kalendar, R., Muterko, A., & Boronnikova, S. (2021). Retrotransposable elements: DNA fingerprinting and the assessment of genetic diversity. *Methods in Molecular Biology (Clifton, N.J.), 2222*, 263–286. https://doi.org/10.1007/978-1-0716-0997-2_15

Kang, Y., Zhang, X., Jiang, W., Wu, C., Chen, C., Zheng, Y., Gu, J., & Xu, C. (2009). Tumor-directed gene therapy in mice using a composite nonviral gene delivery system consisting of the piggyBac transposon and polyethylenimine. *BMC Cancer, 9*, 126. https://doi.org/10.1186/1471-2407-9-126

Kapitonov, V.V., & Jurka, J. (2001). Rolling-circle transposons in eukaryotes. *Proceedings of the National Academy of Sciences of the United States of America, 98*(15), 8714–8719. https://doi.org/10.1073/pnas.151269298

Karttunen, K., Patel, D., Xia, J., Fei, L., Palin, K., Aaltonen, L., & Sahu, B. (2023). Transposable elements as tissue-specific enhancers in cancers of endodermal lineage. *Nature Communications, 14*(1), 5313. https://doi.org/10.1038/s41467-023-41081-4

[a]Kawakami, K., Imanaka, K., Itoh, M., & Taira, M. (2004). Excision of the Tol2 transposable element of the medaka fish Oryzias latipes in Xenopus laevis and Xenopus tropicalis. *Gene, 338*(1), 93–98. https://doi.org/10.1016/j.gene.2004.05.013

[b]Kawakami, K., Takeda, H., Kawakami, N., Kobayashi, M., Matsuda, N., & Mishina, M. (2004). A transposon-mediated gene trap approach identifies developmentally regulated genes in zebrafish. *Developmental Cell, 7*(1), 133–144. https://doi.org/10.1016/j.devcel.2004.06.005

Kawakami K. (2007). Tol2: a versatile gene transfer vector in vertebrates. *Genome Biology, 8 Suppl 1*(Suppl 1), S7. https://doi.org/10.1186/gb-2007-8-s1-s7

Kawakami, K., Asakawa, K., Muto, A., & Wada, H. (2016). Tol2-mediated transgenesis, gene trapping, enhancer trapping, and Gal4-UAS system. *Methods in Cell Biology, 135*, 19–37. https://doi.org/10.1016/bs.mcb.2016.01.011

Kawakami, K., Koga, A., Hori, H., & Shima, A. (1998). Excision of the tol2 transposable element of the medaka fish, Oryzias latipes, in zebrafish, Danio rerio. *Gene, 225*(1-2), 17–22. https://doi.org/10.1016/s0378-1119(98)00537-x

Kawakami, K., Largaespada, D.A., & Ivics, Z. (2017). Transposons as tools for functional genomics in vertebrate models. *Trends Genet, 33*(11):784-801. https://doi:10.1016/j.tig.2017.07.006

Kawakami, K., & Noda, T. (2004). Transposition of the Tol2 element, an Ac-like element from the Japanese medaka fish Oryzias latipes, in mouse embryonic stem cells. *Genetics, 166*(2), 895–899. https://doi.org/10.1534/genetics.166.2.895

Kawakami, K., & Shima, A. (1999). Identification of the Tol2 transposase of the medaka fish Oryzias latipes that catalyzes excision of a nonautonomous Tol2 element in zebrafish Danio rerio. *Gene, 240*(1), 239–244. https://doi.org/10.1016/s0378-1119(99)00444-8

Kazazian, H.H., Jr, Wong, C., Youssoufian, H., Scott, A.F., Phillips, D.G., & Antonarakis, S.E. (1988). Haemophilia A resulting from de novo insertion of L1 sequences represents a novel mechanism for mutation in man. *Nature, 332*(6160), 164–166. https://doi.org/10.1038/332164a0

Kebriaei, P., Izsvák, Z., Narayanavari, S.A., Singh, H., & Ivics, Z. (2017). Gene therapy with the Sleeping Beauty transposon system. *Trends in Genetics: TIG, 33*(11), 852–870. https://doi.org/10.1016/j.tig.2017.08.008

Kebriaei, P., Singh, H., Huls, M.H., Figliola, M.J., Bassett, R., Olivares, S., Jena, B., Dawson, M.J., Kumaresan, P.R., Su, S., Maiti, S., Dai, J., Moriarity, B., Forget, M.A., Senyukov, V., Orozco, A., Liu, T., McCarty, J., Jackson, R.N., Moyes, J.S., …& Cooper, L.J. (2016). Phase I trials using Sleeping Beauty to generate CD19-specific CAR T cells. *The Journal of Clinical Investigation, 126*(9), 3363–3376. https://doi.org/10.1172/JCI86721

Keng, V.W., Ryan, B.J., Wangensteen, K.J., Balciunas, D., Schmedt, C., Ekker, S.C., & Largaespada, D.A. (2009). Efficient transposition of Tol2 in the mouse germline. *Genetics*, *183*(4), 1565–1573. https://doi.org/10.1534/genetics.109.100768

Keravala, A., Liu, D., Lechman, E.R., Wolfe, D., Nash, J.A., Lampe, D.J., & Robbins, P.D. (2006). Hyperactive Himar1 transposase mediates transposition in cell culture and enhances gene expression in vivo. *Human Gene Therapy, 17*(10), 1006–1018. https://doi.org/10.1089/hum.2006.17.1006

Kim, W.R., Park, E.G., Lee, D.H., Lee, Y.J., Bae, W.H., & Kim, H.S. (2023). The tumorigenic role of circular RNA-microRNA axis in cancer. *International Journal of Molecular Sciences, 24*(3), 3050. https://doi.org/10.3390/ijms24033050

Klai, K., Zidi, M., Chénais, B., Denis, F., Caruso, A., Casse, N., & Mezghani Khemakhem, M. (2022). Miniature inverted-repeat transposable elements (MITEs) in the two lepidopteran genomes of *Helicoverpa armigera* and *Helicoverpa zea*. *Insects, 13*(4), 313. https://doi.org/10.3390/insects13040313

Knebelmann, B., Forestier, L., Drouot, L., Quinones, S., Chuet, C., Benessy, F., Saus, J., & Antignac, C. (1995). Splice-mediated insertion of an Alu sequence in the COL4A3 mRNA causing autosomal recessive Alport syndrome. *Human Molecular Genetics, 4*(4), 675–679. https://doi.org/10.1093/hmg/4.4.675

Koga, A., & Hori, H. (2001). The Tol2 transposable element of the medaka fish: an active DNA-based element naturally occurring in a vertebrate genome. *Genes & Genetic Systems, 76*(1), 1–8. https://doi.org/10.1266/ggs.76.1

Koga, A., Shimada, A., Kuroki, T., Hori, H., Kusumi, J., Kyono-Hamaguchi, Y., & Hamaguchi, S. (2007). The Tol1 transposable element of the medaka fish moves in human and mouse cells. *Journal of Human Genetics, 52*(7), 628–635. https://doi.org/10.1007/s10038-007-0161-2

Koga, A., Suzuki, M., Maruyama, Y., Tsutsumi, M., & Hori, H. (1999). Amino acid sequence of a putative transposase protein of the medaka fish transposable element Tol2 deduced from mRNA nucleotide sequences. *FEBS Letters, 461*(3), 295–298. https://doi.org/10.1016/s0014-5793(99)01479-9

Kondrychyn, I., Garcia-Lecea, M., Emelyanov, A., Parinov, S., & Korzh, V. (2009). Genome-wide analysis of Tol2 transposon reintegration in zebrafish. *BMC Genomics, 10*, 418. https://doi.org/10.1186/1471-2164-10-418

Lamprecht, B., Walter, K., Kreher, S., Kumar, R., Hummel, M., Lenze, D., Köchert, K., Bouhlel, M.A., Richter, J., Soler, E., Stadhouders, R., Jöhrens, K., Wurster, K.D., Callen, D.F., Harte, M.F., Giefing, M., Barlow, R., Stein, H., Anagnostopoulos, I., Janz, M., … & Mathas, S. (2010). Derepression of an endogenous long terminal repeat activates the CSF1R proto-oncogene in human lymphoma. *Nature Medicine, 16*(5), 571–579. https://doi.org/10.1038/nm.2129

Lavi, E., & Carmel, L. (2018). Alu exaptation enriches the human transcriptome by introducing new gene ends. *RNA Biology, 15*(6), 715–725. https://doi.org/10.1080/15476286.2018.1429880

Lee, C.Y., Li, J.F., Liou, J.S., Charng, Y.C., Huang, Y.W., & Lee, H.J. (2011). A gene delivery system for human cells mediated by both a cell-penetrating peptide and a piggyBac transposase. *Biomaterials, 32*(26), 6264–6276. https://doi.org/10.1016/j.biomaterials.2011.05.012

Lee, M., Jr, Ahmad, S.F., & Xu, J. (2024). Regulation and function of transposable elements in cancer genomes. *Cellular and Molecular Life Sciences: CMLS, 81*(1), 157. https://doi.org/10.1007/s00018-024-05195-2

Levy, P.L., & Gros, A. (2022). Fast track to personalized TCR T cell therapies. *Cancer Cell, 40*(5), 447–449. https://doi.org/10.1016/j.ccell.2022.04.013

Li, N., Jin, K., Bai, Y., Fu, H., Liu, L., & Liu, B. (2020). Tn5 transposase applied in genomics research. *International Journal of Molecular Sciences, 21*(21), 8329. https://doi.org/10.3390/ijms21218329

Li, R., Yao, J., Cai, S., Fu, Y., Lai, C., Zhu, X., Cui, L., & Li, Y. (2024). Genome-wide characterization and evolution analysis of miniature inverted-repeat transposable elements in Barley (*Hordeum vulgare*). *Frontiers in Plant Science, 15*, 1474846. https://doi.org/10.3389/fpls.2024.1474846

Li, R., Zhuang, Y., Han, M., Xu, T., & Wu, X. (2013). piggyBac as a high-capacity transgenesis and gene-therapy vector in human cells and mice. *Disease Models & Mechanisms, 6*(3), 828–833. https://doi.org/10.1242/dmm.010827

Li, S., Zhang, A., Xue, H., Li, D., & Liu, Y. (2017). One-step piggyBac transposon-based CRISPR/Cas9 activation of multiple genes. *Molecular Therapy. Nucleic Acids, 8*, 64–76. https://doi.org/10.1016/j.omtn.2017.06.007

Li, X., Le, Y., Zhang, Z., Nian, X., Liu, B., & Yang, X. (2023). Viral vector-based gene therapy. *International Journal of Molecular Sciences, 24*(9), 7736. https://doi.org/10.3390/ijms24097736

Liu, G., Aronovich, E.L., Cui, Z., Whitley, C.B., & Hackett, P.B. (2004). Excision of Sleeping Beauty transposons: parameters and applications to gene therapy. *The journal of Gene Medicine, 6*(5), 574–583. https://doi.org/10.1002/jgm.486

Liu, G., Geurts, A.M., Yae, K., Srinivasan, A.R., Fahrenkrug, S.C., Largaespada, D.A., Takeda, J., Horie, K., Olson, W.K., & Hackett, P.B. (2005). Target-site preferences of Sleeping Beauty transposons. *Journal of Molecular Biology, 346*(1), 161–173. https://doi.org/10.1016/j.jmb.2004.09.086

Liu, H., Liu, L., Fletcher, B.S., & Visner, G.A. (2006). Sleeping Beauty-based gene therapy with indoleamine 2,3-dioxygenase inhibits lung allograft fibrosis. *FASEB Journal: Official Publication of the Federation of American Societies for Experimental Biology, 20*(13), 2384–2386. https://doi.org/10.1096/fj.06-6228fje

Lizio, M., Abugessaisa, I., Noguchi, S., Kondo, A., Hasegawa, A., Hon, C.C., de Hoon, M., Severin, J., Oki, S., Hayashizaki, Y., Carninci, P., Kasukawa, T., & Kawaji, H. (2019). Update of the FANTOM web resource: expansion to provide additional transcriptome atlases. *Nucleic Acids Research, 47*(D1), D752–D758. https://doi.org/10.1093/nar/gky1099

Loperfido, M., Jarmin, S., Dastidar, S., Di Matteo, M., Perini, I., Moore, M., Nair, N., Samara-Kuko, E., Athanasopoulos, T., Tedesco, F.S., Dickson, G., Sampaolesi, M., VandenDriessche, T., & Chuah, M.K. (2016). piggyBac transposons expressing full-length human dystrophin enable genetic correction of dystrophic mesoangioblasts. *Nucleic Acids Research, 44*(2),744–760. https://doi.org/10.1093/nar/gkv1464

Lundstrom K. (2023). Viral vectors in gene therapy: where do we stand in 2023?. *Viruses, 15*(3), 698. https://doi.org/10.3390/v15030698

Luqman-Fatah, A., Nishimori, K., Amano, S., Fumoto, Y., & Miyoshi, T. (2024). Retrotransposon life cycle and its impacts on cellular responses. *RNA Biology, 21*(1), 11–27. https://doi.org/10.1080/15476286.2024.2409607

Lykoskoufis, N.M.R., Planet, E., Ongen, H., Trono, D., & Dermitzakis, E.T. (2024). Transposable elements mediate genetic effects altering the expression of nearby genes in colorectal cancer. *Nature Communications, 15*(1), 749. https://doi.org/10.1038/s41467-023-42405-0

Ma, G., Babarinde, I.A., Zhou, X., & Hutchins, A.P. (2022). Transposable elements in pluripotent stem cells and human disease. *Frontiers in Genetics, 13*, 902541. https://doi.org/10.3389/fgene.2022.902541

Ma, H., Wang, M., Zhang, Y.E., & Tan, S. (2023). The power of "controllers": transposon-mediated duplicated genes evolve towards neofunctionalization. *Journal of Genetics and Genomics = Yi chuan xue bao, 50*(7), 462–472. https://doi.org/10.1016/j.jgg.2023.04.003

Ma, K., Li, W., Zhu, G., Sun, S., Chi, H., Yin, Y., Diao, H., Xing, X.J., Guo, Z., Wang, L., Xu, W., Cui, C., & Xu, J. (2021). Functionalized PDA/DEX-PEI@HA nanoparticles combined with sleeping-beauty transposons for multistage targeted delivery of CRISPR/Cas9 gene. *Biomedicine & Pharmacotherapy = Biomedecine & Pharmacotherapie, 142*, 112061. https://doi.org/10.1016/j.biopha.2021.112061

Macko-Podgórni, A., Machaj, G., & Grzebelus, D. (2021). A Global landscape of miniature inverted-repeat transposable elements in the carrot genome. *Genes, 12*(6), 859. https://doi.org/10.3390/genes12060859

Magnani, C.F., Gaipa, G., Lussana, F., Belotti, D., Gritti, G., Napolitano, S., Matera, G., Cabiati, B., Buracchi, C., Borleri, G., Fazio, G., Zaninelli, S., Tettamanti, S., Cesana, S., Colombo, V., Quaroni, M., Cazzaniga, G., Rovelli, A., Biagi, E., Galimberti, S., … & Biondi, A. (2020). Sleeping Beauty-engineered CAR T cells achieve antileukemic activity without severe toxicities. *The Journal of Clinical Investigation, 130*(11), 6021–6033. https://doi.org/10.1172/JCI138473

Marasca, F., Gasparotto, E., Polimeni, B., Vadalà, R., Ranzani, V., & Bodega, B. (2020). The sophisticated transcriptional response governed by transposable elements in human health and disease. *International Journal of Molecular Sciences, 21*(9), 3201. https://doi.org/10.3390/ijms21093201

Mátés, L., Chuah, M.K., Belay, E., Jerchow, B., Manoj, N., Acosta-Sanchez, A., Grzela, D.P., Schmitt, A., Becker, K., Matrai, J., Ma, L., Samara-Kuko, E., Gysemans, C., Pryputniewicz, D., Miskey, C., Fletcher, B., VandenDriessche, T., Ivics, Z., & Izsvák, Z. (2009). Molecular evolution of a novel hyperactive Sleeping Beauty transposase enables robust stable gene transfer in vertebrates. *Nature Genetics, 41*(6), 753–761. https://doi.org/10.1038/ng.343

Meir, Y.J., Lin, A., Huang, M.F., Lin, J.R., Weirauch, M.T., Chou, H.C., Lin, S.J., & Wu, S.C. (2013). A versatile, highly efficient, and potentially safer piggyBac transposon system for mammalian genome manipulations. *FASEB Journal: Official Publication of the Federation of American Societies for Experimental Biology, 27*(11), 4429–4443. https://doi.org/10.1096/fj.12-223586

Meir, Y.J., Weirauch, M.T., Yang, H.S., Chung, P.C., Yu, R.K., & Wu, S.C. (2011). Genome-wide target profiling of piggyBac and Tol2 in HEK 293: pros and cons for gene discovery and gene therapy. *BMC Biotechnology, 11*, 28. https://doi.org/10.1186/1472-6750-11-28

Miskey, C., Izsvák, Z., Plasterk, R.H., & Ivics, Z. (2003). The Frog Prince: a reconstructed transposon from Rana pipiens with high transpositional activity in vertebrate cells. *Nucleic Acids Research, 31*(23), 6873–6881. https://doi.org/10.1093/nar/gkg910

Monjezi, R., Miskey, C., Gogishvili, T., Schleef, M., Schmeer, M., Einsele, H., Ivics, Z., & Hudecek, M. (2017). Enhanced CAR T-cell engineering using non-viral Sleeping Beauty transposition from minicircle vectors. *Leukemia, 31*(1), 186–194.

https://doi.org/10.1038/leu.2016.180

Montini, E., Held, P.K., Noll, M., Morcinek, N., Al-Dhalimy, M., Finegold, M., Yant, S.R., Kay, M.A., & Grompe, M. (2002). In vivo correction of murine tyrosinemia type I by DNA-mediated transposition. *Molecular Therapy: the Journal of the American Society of Gene Therapy, 6*(6), 759–769. https://doi.org/10.1006/mthe.2002.0812

Moretti, A., Ponzo, M., Nicolette, C.A., Tcherepanova, I.Y., Biondi, A., & Magnani, C.F. (2022). The past, present, and future of non-viral CAR T cells. *Frontiers in Immunology, 13*, 867013. https://doi.org/10.3389/fimmu.2022.867013

Mosaddeghi, P., Farahmandnejad, M., & Zarshenas, M.M. (2023). The role of transposable elements in aging and cancer. *Biogerontology, 24*(4), 479–491. https://doi.org/10.1007/s10522-023-10028-z

Mukherjee, S., Mukhopadhyay, A., Banerjee, D., Chandak, G.R., & Ray, K. (2004). Molecular pathology of haemophilia B: identification of five novel mutations including a LINE 1 insertion in Indian patients. *Haemophilia: The Official Journal of the World Federation of Hemophilia, 10*(3), 259–263. https://doi.org/10.1111/j.1365-2516.2004.00895.x

Muñoz-López, M., & García-Pérez, J.L. (2010). DNA transposons: nature and applications in genomics. *Current Genomics, 11*(2), 115–128. https://doi.org/10.2174/138920210790886871

Münch, J., Rajan, D., Rücker, E., Wildum, S., Adam, N., & Kirchhoff, F. (2005). The role of upstream U3 sequences in HIV-1 replication and CD4+ T cell depletion in human lymphoid tissue ex vivo. *Virology, 341*(2), 313–320. https://doi.org/10.1016/j.virol.2005.07.023

Nakamura, K., Yagyu, S., Hirota, S., Tomida, A., Kondo, M., Shigeura, T., Hasegawa, A., Tanaka, M., & Nakazawa, Y. (2021). Autologous antigen-presenting cells efficiently expand *piggyBac* transposon CAR-T cells with predominant memory phenotype. *Molecular Therapy. Methods & Clinical Development, 21*, 315–324. https://doi.org/10.1016/j.omtm.2021.03.011

Nakazawa, Y., Huye, L.E., Dotti, G., Foster, A.E., Vera, J.F., Manuri, P.R., June, C.H., Rooney, C.M., & Wilson, M.H. (2009). Optimization of the PiggyBac transposon system for the sustained genetic modification of human T lymphocytes. *Journal of Immunotherapy (Hagerstown, Md.: 1997), 32*(8), 826–836. https://doi.org/10.1097/CJI.0b013e3181ad762b

Narita, N., Nishio, H., Kitoh, Y., Ishikawa, Y., Ishikawa, Y., Minami, R., Nakamura, H., & Matsuo, M. (1993). Insertion of a 5' truncated L1 element into the 3' end of exon 44 of the dystrophin gene resulted in skipping of the exon during splicing in a case of Duchenne muscular dystrophy. *The Journal of Clinical Investigation, 91*(5), 1862–1867. https://doi.org/10.1172/JCI116402

Neote, K., McInnes, B., Mahuran, D.J., & Gravel, R.A. (1990). Structure and distribution of an Alu-type deletion mutation in sandhoff disease. *The Journal of Clinical Investigation, 86*(5), 1524–1531. https://doi.org/10.1172/JCI114871

Ni, J., Wangensteen, K.J., Nelsen, D., Balciunas, D., Skuster, K.J., Urban, M.D., & Ekker, S.C. (2016). Active recombinant Tol2 transposase for gene transfer and gene discovery applications. *Mobile DNA, 7*, 6. https://doi.org/10.1186/s13100-016-0062-z

Nouroz, F., Noreen, S., & Heslop-Harrison, J.S. (2015). Identification and evolutionary genomics of novel LTR retrotransposons in Brassica. *Turkish Journal of Biology, 39*(5), 740–757. https://doi.org/10.3906/biy-1501-77

O'Brochta, D.A., Alford, R.T., Pilitt, K.L., Aluvihare, C.U., & Harrell, R.A. 2nd (2011). piggyBac transposon remobilization and enhancer detection in Anopheles mosquitoes. *Proceedings of the National Academy of Sciences of the United States of America, 108*(39), 16339–16344. https://doi.org/10.1073/pnas.1110628108

Ochmann, M.T., & Ivics, Z. (2021). Jumping ahead with Sleeping Beauty: mechanistic insights into cut-and-paste transposition. *Viruses, 13*(1), 76. https://doi.org/10.3390/v13010076

Ohtani, H., Ørskov, A.D., Helbo, A.S., Gillberg, L., Liu, M., Zhou, W., Ungerstedt, J., Hellström-Lindberg, E., Sun, W., Liang, G., Jones, P.A., & Grønbæk, K. (2020). Activation of a subset of evolutionarily young transposable elements and innate immunity are linked to clinical responses to 5-Azacytidine. *Cancer Research, 80*(12), 2441–2450. https://doi.org/10.1158/0008-5472.CAN-19-1696

Oliveira, C., Senz, J., Kaurah, P., Pinheiro, H., Sanges, R., Haegert, A., Corso, G., Schouten, J., Fitzgerald, R., Vogelsang, H., Keller, G., Dwerryhouse, S., Grimmer, D., Chin, S.F., Yang, H.K., Jackson, C.E., Seruca, R., Roviello, F., Stupka, E., Caldas, C., … & Huntsman, D. (2009). Germline CDH1 deletions in hereditary diffuse gastric cancer families. *Human Molecular Genetics, 18*(9), 1545–1555. https://doi.org/10.1093/hmg/ddp046

O'Reilly, M., Shipp, A., Rosenthal, E., Jambou, R., Shih, T., Montgomery, M., Gargiulo, L., Patterson, A., & Corrigan-Curay, J. (2012). NIH oversight of human gene transfer research involving retroviral, lentiviral, and adeno-associated virus vectors and the role of the NIH recombinant DNA advisory committee. *Methods in Enzymology, 507*, 313–335. https://doi.org/10.1016/B978-0-12-386509-0.00016-8

Ortinski, P.I., O'Donovan, B., Dong, X., & Kantor, B. (2017). Integrase-deficient lentiviral vector as an all-in-one platform for highly efficient CRISPR/Cas9-mediated gene editing. *Molecular Therapy. Methods & Clinical Development, 5*, 153–164. https://doi.org/10.1016/j.omtm.2017.04.002

Ostertag, E.M., Goodier, J.L., Zhang, Y., & Kazazian, H.H. Jr (2003). SVA elements are nonautonomous retrotransposons that cause disease in humans. *American Journal of Human Genetics, 73*(6), 1444–1451. https://doi.org/10.1086/380207

Oza, A.M., Matulonis, U.A., Alvarez Secord, A., Nemunaitis, J., Roman, L. D., Blagden, S.P., Banerjee, S., McGuire, W.P., Ghamande, S., Birrer, M.J., Fleming, G.F., Markham, M.J., Hirte, H.W., Provencher, D.M., Basu, B., Kristeleit, R., Armstrong, D.K., Schwartz, B., Braly, P., Hall, G. D., … & Matei, D. (2020). A randomized phase II trial of epigenetic priming with guadecitabine and carboplatin in platinum-resistant, recurrent ovarian cancer. *Clinical Cancer Research: an Official Journal of the American Association for Cancer Research, 26*(5), 1009–1016. https://doi.org/10.1158/1078-0432.CCR-19-1638

Pagan, H.J., Smith, J.D., Hubley, R.M., & Ray, D.A. (2010). PiggyBac-ing on a primate genome: novel elements, recent activity and horizontal transfer. *Genome Biology and Evolution, 2*, 293–303. https://doi.org/10.1093/gbe/evq021

Panda, A., de Cubas, A.A., Stein, M., Riedlinger, G., Kra, J., Mayer, T., Smith, C.C., Vincent, B.G., Serody, J.S., Beckermann, K.E., Ganesan, S., Bhanot, G., & Rathmell, W.K. (2018). Endogenous retrovirus expression is associated with response to immune checkpoint blockade in clear cell renal cell carcinoma. *JCI Insight, 3*(16), e121522. https://doi.org/10.1172/jci.insight.121522

Parinov, S., Kondrichin, I., Korzh, V., & Emelyanov, A. (2004). Tol2 transposon-mediated enhancer trap to identify developmentally regulated zebrafish genes in vivo. *Developmental Dynamics: an Official Publication of the American Association of Anatomists, 231*(2), 449–459. https://doi.org/10.1002/dvdy.20157

Park, E.G., Ha, H., Lee, D.H., Kim, W.R., Lee, Y.J., Bae, W.H., & Kim, H.S. (2022). Genomic analyses of non-coding RNAs overlapping transposable elements and its implication to human diseases. *International Journal of Molecular Sciences, 23*(16), 8950. https://doi.org/10.3390/ijms23168950

Park, E.G., Lee, Y.J., Huh, J.W., Park, S.J., Imai, H., Kim, W.R., Lee, D.H., Kim, J.M., Shin, H.J., & Kim, H.S. (2023). Identification of microRNAs derived from transposable elements in the *Macaca mulatta* (Rhesus Monkey) genome. *Genes, 14*(11), 1984. https://doi.org/10.3390/genes14111984

Park, H., Kim, G., Kim, N., Ha, S., & Yim, H. (2024). Efficacy and safety of natural killer cell therapy in patients with solid tumors: a systematic review and meta-analysis. *Frontiers in Immunology, 15*, 1454427. https://doi.org/10.3389/fimmu.2024.1454427

Pattamadilok, J., Huapai, N., Rattanatanyong, P., Vasurattana, A., Triratanachat, S., Tresukosol, D., & Mutirangura, A. (2008). LINE-1 hypomethylation level as a potential prognostic factor for epithelial ovarian cancer. *International Journal of Gynecological Cancer: Official Journal of the International Gynecological Cancer Society, 18*(4), 711–717. https://doi.org/10.1111/j.1525-1438.2007.01117.x

Pavlopoulos, A., Oehler, S., Kapetanaki, M.G., & Savakis, C. (2007). The DNA transposon Minos as a tool for transgenesis and functional genomic analysis in vertebrates and invertebrates. *Genome Biology, 8 Suppl 1*(Suppl 1), S2. https://doi.org/10.1186/gb-2007-8-s1-s2

Pluta, A., Jaworski, J.P., & Cortés-Rubio, C.N. (2020). Balance between retroviral latency and transcription: based on HIV Model. *Pathogens (Basel, Switzerland), 10*(1), 16. https://doi.org/10.3390/pathogens10010016

Podetz-Pedersen, K.M., Olson, E.R., Somia, N.V., Russell, S.J., & McIvor, R.S. (2016). A broad range of dose optima achieve high-level, long-term gene expression after hydrodynamic delivery of Sleeping Beauty transposons using hyperactive SB100x transposase. *Molecular Therapy. Nucleic Acids, 5*(1), e279. https://doi.org/10.1038/mtna.2015.54

Prommersberger, S., Monjezi, R., Shankar, R., Schmeer, M., Hudecek, M., Ivics, Z., & Schleef, M. (2022). Minicircles for CAR T cell production by Sleeping Beauty transposition: a technological overview. *Methods in Molecular Biology (Clifton, N.J.), 2521*, 25–39. https://doi.org/10.1007/978-1-0716-2441-8_2

Prommersberger, S., Reiser, M., Beckmann, J., Danhof, S., Amberger, M., Quade-Lyssy, P., Einsele, H., Hudecek, M., Bonig, H., & Ivics, Z. (2021). CARAMBA: a first-in-human clinical trial with SLAMF7 CAR-T cells prepared by virus-free Sleeping Beauty gene transfer to treat multiple myeloma. *Gene Therapy, 28*(9), 560–571. https://doi.org/10.1038/s41434-021-00254-w

Qin, S., Jin, P., Zhou, X., Chen, L., & Ma, F. (2015). The role of transposable elements in the origin and evolution of microRNAs in human. *PloS One, 10*(6), e0131365. https://doi.org/10.1371/journal.pone.0131365

Rad, R., Rad, L., Wang, W., Cadinanos, J., Vassiliou, G., Rice, S., Campos, L.S., Yusa, K., Banerjee, R., Li, M.A., de la Rosa, J., Strong, A., Lu, D., Ellis, P., Conte, N., Yang, F.T., Liu, P., & Bradley, A. (2010). PiggyBac transposon mutagenesis: a tool for cancer gene discovery in mice. *Science (New York, N.Y.), 330*(6007), 1104–1107. https://doi.org/10.1126/science.1193004

Rajurkar, M., Parikh, A.R., Solovyov, A., You, E., Kulkarni, A.S., Chu, C., Xu, K.H., Jaicks, C., Taylor, M.S., Wu, C., Alexander, K.A., Good, C.R., Szabolcs, A., Gerstberger, S., Tran, A.V., Xu, N., Ebright, R.Y., Van Seventer, E.E., Vo, K.D., Tai, E.C., … & Ting, D.T. (2022). Reverse transcriptase inhibition disrupts repeat element life cycle in colorectal cancer. *Cancer Discovery, 12*(6), 1462–1481. https://doi.org/10.1158/2159-8290.CD-21-1117

Ramakrishnan, M., Papolu, P.K., Mullasseri, S., Zhou, M., Sharma, A., Ahmad, Z., Satheesh, V., Kalendar, R., & Wei, Q. (2023). The role of LTR retrotransposons in plant genetic engineering: how to control their transposition in the genome. *Plant Cell Reports, 42*(1), 3–15. https://doi.org/10.1007/s00299-022-02945-z

Ramzy, I.I., Omran, D.A., Hamad, O., Shaker, O., & Abboud, A. (2011). Evaluation of serum LINE-1 hypomethylation as a prognostic marker for hepatocellular carcinoma. *Arab Journal of Gastroenterology: the Official Publication of the Pan-Arab Association of Gastroenterology, 12*(3), 139–142. https://doi.org/10.1016/j.ajg.2011.07.002

Rodić, N., Zampella, J.G., Cornish, T.C., Wheelan, S.J., & Burns, K.H. (2013). Translocation junctions in TCF3-PBX1 acute lymphoblastic leukemia/lymphoma cluster near transposable elements. *Mobile DNA, 4*(1), 22. https://doi.org/10.1186/1759-8753-4-22

Roffler, S., & Wicker, T. (2015). Genome-wide comparison of asian and african rice reveals high recent activity of DNA transposons. *Mobile DNA, 6*, 8. https://doi.org/10.1186/s13100-015-0040-x

Rotiroti, M.C., Buracchi, C., Arcangeli, S., Galimberti, S., Valsecchi, M.G., Perriello, V.M., Rasko, T., Alberti, G., Magnani, C.F., Cappuzzello, C., Lundberg, F., Pande, A., Dastoli, G., Introna, M., Serafini, M., Biagi, E., Izsvák, Z., Biondi, A., & Tettamanti, S. (2020). Targeting CD33 in chemoresistant AML patient-derived xenografts by CAR-CIK cells modified with an improved SB transposon system. *Molecular Therapy: the Journal of the American Society of Gene Therapy, 28*(9), 1974–1986. https://doi.org/10.1016/j.ymthe.2020.05.021

Rozek, L.S., Virani, S., Bellile, E.L., Taylor, J.M.G., Sartor, M.A., Zarins, K.R., Virani, A., Cote, C., Worden, F.P., Mark, M.E.P., McLean, S.A.,

Duffy, S.A., Yoo, G.H., Saba, N.F., Shin, D.M., Kucuk, O., & Wolf, G.T. (2019). Soy isoflavone supplementation increases long interspersed nucleotide element-1 (LINE-1) methylation in head and neck squamous cell carcinoma. *Nutrition and Cancer, 71*(5), 772–780. https://doi.org/10.1080/01635581.2019.1577981

Sakamoto, N., Ishikawa, T., Kokura, S., Okayama, T., Oka, K., Ideno, M., Sakai, F., Kato, A., Tanabe, M., Enoki, T., Mineno, J., Naito, Y., Itoh, Y., & Yoshikawa, T. (2015). Phase I clinical trial of autologous NK cell therapy using novel expansion method in patients with advanced digestive cancer. *Journal of Translational Medicine, 13*, 277. https://doi.org/10.1186/s12967-015-0632-8

Sandoval-Villegas, N., Nurieva, W., Amberger, M., & Ivics, Z. (2021). Contemporary transposon tools: a review and guide through mechanisms and applications of Sleeping Beauty, piggyBac and Tol2 for genome engineering. *International Journal of Molecular Sciences, 22*(10), 5084. https://doi.org/10.3390/ijms22105084

Saridey, S.K., Liu, L., Doherty, J.E., Kaja, A., Galvan, D.L., Fletcher, B.S., & Wilson, M.H. (2009). PiggyBac transposon-based inducible gene expression in vivo after somatic cell gene transfer. *Molecular Therapy: the Journal of the American Society of Gene Therapy, 17*(12), 2115–2120. https://doi.org/10.1038/mt.2009.234

Sarkar, A., Sim, C., Hong, Y.S., Hogan, J.R., Fraser, M.J., Robertson, H.M., & Collins, F.H. (2003). Molecular evolutionary analysis of the widespread piggyBac transposon family and related "domesticated" sequences. *Molecular Genetics and Genomics: MGG, 270*(2), 173–180. https://doi.org/10.1007/s00438-003-0909-0

Sato, Y., Kasai, T., Nakagawa, S., Tanabe, K., Watanabe, T., Kawakami, K., & Takahashi, Y. (2007). Stable integration and conditional expression of electroporated transgenes in chicken embryos. *Developmental Biology, 305*(2), 616–624. https://doi.org/10.1016/j.ydbio.2007.01.043

Sayed, N., Allawadhi, P., Khurana, A., Singh, V., Navik, U., Pasumarthi, S.K., Khurana, I., Banothu, A.K., Weiskirchen, R., & Bharani, K.K. (2022). Gene therapy: comprehensive overview and therapeutic applications. *Life Sciences, 294*, 120375. https://doi.org/10.1016/j.lfs.2022.120375

Schmitz, M., & Querques, I. (2024). DNA on the move: mechanisms, functions and applications of transposable elements. *FEBS Open Bio, 14*(1), 13–22. https://doi.org/10.1002/2211-5463.13743

Schumann, G.G., Fuchs, N.V., Tristán-Ramos, P., Sebe, A., Ivics, Z., & Heras, S.R. (2019). The impact of transposable element activity on therapeutically relevant human stem cells. *Mobile DNA, 10*, 9. https://doi.org/10.1186/s13100-019-0151-x

Serafino, A., Balestrieri, E., Pierimarchi, P., Matteucci, C., Moroni, G., Oricchio, E., Rasi, G., Mastino, A., Spadafora, C., Garaci, E., & Vallebona, P.S. (2009). The activation of human endogenous retrovirus K (HERV-K) is implicated in melanoma cell malignant transformation. *Experimental Cell Research, 315*(5), 849–862. https://doi.org/10.1016/j.yexcr.2008.12.023

Serrato-Capuchina, A., & Matute, D.R. (2018). The role of transposable elements in speciation. *Genes, 9*(5), 254. https://doi.org/10.3390/genes9050254

Shah, S., Yu, S., Zhang, C., Ali, I., Wang, X., Qian, Y., & Xiao, T. (2024). Retrotransposon SINEs in age-related diseases: mechanisms and therapeutic implications. *Ageing Research Reviews, 101*, 102539. https://doi.org/10.1016/j.arr.2024.102539

Singh, H., Huls, H., Kebriaei, P., & Cooper, L.J. (2014). A new approach to gene therapy using Sleeping Beauty to genetically modify clinical-grade T cells to target CD19. *Immunological Reviews, 257*(1), 181–190. https://doi.org/10.1111/imr.12137

Slovin, S.F., Dorff, T.B., Falchook, G.S., Wei, X.X., Gao, X., McKay, R.R., Oh, D.Y., Wibmer, A.G., Spear, M.A., McCaigue, J., Shedlock, D.J., Dhar, M., Coronella, J., Martin, C.E., Ghodussi, M., Murphy, A., & Ostertag, E.M. (2022). Phase 1 study of P-PSMA-101 CAR-T cells in patients with metastatic castration-resistant prostate cancer (mCRPC). *Journal of Clinical Oncology, 40*, 98–98. https://doi.org/10.1200/JCO.2022.40.6_suppl.098

Smart, A.C., Margolis, C.A., Pimentel, H., He, M.X., Miao, D., Adeegbe, D., Fugmann, T., Wong, K.K., & Van Allen, E.M. (2018). Intron retention is a source of neoepitopes in cancer. *Nature Biotechnology, 36*(11), 1056–1058. https://doi.org/10.1038/nbt.4239

Solassol, J., Larrieux, M., Leclerc, J., Ducros, V., Corsini, C., Chiésa, J., Pujol, P., & Rey, J.M. (2019). Alu element insertion in the MLH1 exon 6 coding sequence as a mutation predisposing to Lynch syndrome. *Human Mutation, 40*(6), 716–720. https://doi.org/10.1002/humu.23725

Sowińska, W., Wawro, M., Solecka, A., & Kasza, A. (2019). Potential limitations of the Sleeping Beauty transposon use in gene expression studies. *Acta Biochimica Polonica, 66*(3), 263–268. https://doi.org/10.18388/abp.2019_2839

Stelmach, K., Macko-Podgórni, A., Machaj, G., & Grzebelus, D. (2017). Miniature inverted repeat transposable element insertions provide a source of intron length polymorphism markers in the carrot (*Daucus carota* L.). *Frontiers in Plant Science, 8*, 725. https://doi.org/10.3389/fpls.2017.00725

Stricker, E., Peckham-Gregory, E.C., & Scheurer, M.E. (2023). CancerHERVdb: human endogenous retrovirus (HERV) expression database for human cancer accelerates studies of the retrovirome and predictions for HERV-based therapies. *Journal of Virology, 97*(6), e0005923. https://doi.org/10.1128/jvi.00059-23

Sun, Y., Liu, G., & Huang, Y. (2021). Applications of *piggyBac* transposons for genome manipulation in stem cells. *Stem Cells International, 2021*, 3829286. https://doi.org/10.1155/2021/3829286

Suster, M.L., Sumiyama, K., & Kawakami, K. (2009). Transposon-mediated BAC transgenesis in zebrafish and mice. *BMC Genomics, 10*, 477. https://doi.org/10.1186/1471-2164-10-477

Swierczek, M., Izsvák, Z., & Ivics, Z. (2012). The Sleeping Beauty transposon system for clinical applications. *Expert Opinion on Biological Therapy, 12*(2), 139–153. https://doi.org/10.1517/14712598.2012.642358

Tamura, R., & Toda, M. (2020). Historic overview of genetic engineering technologies for human gene therapy. *Neurologia Medico-Chirurgica, 60*(10), 483–491. https://doi.org/10.2176/nmc.ra.2020-0049

Tang, R., & Xu, Z. (2020). Gene therapy: a double-edged sword with great powers. *Molecular and Cellular Biochemistry, 474*(1-2), 73–81. https://doi.org/10.1007/s11010-020-03834-3

Tang, W., & Liang, P. (2024). The identification of retro-DNAs in primate genomes as DNA transposons mobilizing via retrotransposition. *F1000Research, 12*, 255. https://doi.org/10.12688/f1000research.130043.3

Tang, W., Mun, S., Joshi, A., Han, K., & Liang, P. (2018). Mobile elements contribute to the uniqueness of human genome with 15,000 human-specific insertions and 14 Mbp sequence increase. *DNA Research: an International Journal for Rapid Publication of Reports on Genes and Genomes, 25*(5), 521–533. https://doi.org/10.1093/dnares/dsy022

Tighe, P.J., Stevens, S.E., Dempsey, S., Le Deist, F., Rieux-Laucat, F., & Edgar, J.D. (2002). Inactivation of the Fas gene by Alu insertion: retrotransposition in an intron causing splicing variation and autoimmune lymphoproliferative syndrome. *Genes and Immunity, 3*, S66–S70. https://doi.org/10.1038/sj.gene.6363864

[a]Tipanee, J., Chai, Y.C., VandenDriessche, T., & Chuah, M.K., 2017. Preclinical and clinical advances in transposon-based gene therapy. *Bioscience Reports, 37*(6), BSR20160614. https://doi.org/10.1042/BSR20160614

[b]Tipanee, J., VandenDriessche, T., & Chuah, M.K., 2017. Transposons: moving forward from preclinical studies to clinical trials. *Human Gene Therapy, 28*(11), 1087–1104. https://doi.org/10.1089/hum.2017.128

Tomida, A., Yagyu, S., Nakamura, K., Kubo, H., Yamashima, K., Nakazawa, Y., Hosoi, H., & Lehara, T. (2021). Inhibition of MEK pathway enhances the antitumor efficacy of chimeric antigen receptor T cells against neuroblastoma. *Cancer Science, 112*(10), 4026–4036. https://doi.org/10.1111/cas.15074

Tsagakis, I., Douka, K., Birds, I., & Aspden, J.L. (2020). Long non-coding RNAs in development and disease: conservation to mechanisms. *The Journal of Pathology, 250*(5), 480–495. https://doi.org/10.1002/path.5405

Tsukahara, T., Iwase, N., Kawakami, K., Iwasaki, M., Yamamoto, C., Ohmine, K., Uchibori, R., Teruya, T., Ido, H., Saga, Y., Urabe, M., Mizukami, H., Kume, A., Nakamura, M., Brentjens, R., & Ozawa, K. (2015). The Tol2 transposon system mediates the genetic engineering of T-cells with CD19-specific chimeric antigen receptors for B-cell malignancies. *Gene Therapy, 22*(2), 209–215. https://doi.org/10.1038/gt.2014.104

Turunen, T.A., Kurkipuro, J., Heikura, T., Vuorio, T., Hytönen, E., Izsvák, Z., & Ylä-Herttuala, S. (2016). Sleeping Beauty transposon vectors in liver-directed gene delivery of LDLR and VLDLR for gene therapy of familial hypercholesterolemia. *Molecular Therapy: the Journal of the American Society of Gene Therapy, 24*(3), 620–635. https://doi.org/10.1038/mt.2015.221

Urasaki, A., Asakawa, K., & Kawakami, K. (2008). Efficient transposition of the Tol2 transposable element from a single-copy donor in zebrafish. *Proceedings of the National Academy of Sciences of the United States of America, 105*(50), 19827–19832. https://doi.org/10.1073/pnas.0810380105

Urasaki, A., Morvan, G., & Kawakami, K. (2006). Functional dissection of the Tol2 transposable element identified the minimal cis-sequence and a highly repetitive sequence in the subterminal region essential for transposition. *Genetics, 174*(2), 639–649. https://doi.org/10.1534/genetics.106.060244

Uren, A.G., Kool, J., Berns, A., & van Lohuizen, M. (2005). Retroviral insertional mutagenesis: past, present and future. *Oncogene, 24*(52), 7656–7672. https://doi.org/10.1038/sj.onc.1209043

Urschitz, J., Kawasumi, M., Owens, J., Morozumi, K., Yamashiro, H., Stoytchev, I., Marh, J., Dee, J.A., Kawamoto, K., Coates, C.J., Kaminski, J.M., Pelczar, P., Yanagimachi, R., & Moisyadi, S. (2010). Helper-independent piggyBac plasmids for gene delivery approaches: strategies for avoiding potential genotoxic effects. *Proceedings of the National Academy of Sciences of the United States of America, 107*(18), 8117–8122. https://doi.org/10.1073/pnas.1003674107

Ustyantsev, K., Novikova, O., Blinov, A., & Smyshlyaev, G. (2015). Convergent evolution of ribonuclease h in LTR retrotransposons and retroviruses. *Molecular Biology and Evolution, 32*(5), 1197–1207. https://doi.org/10.1093/molbev/msv008

VandenDriessche, T., Ivics, Z., Izsvák, Z., & Chuah, M.K. (2009). Emerging potential of transposons for gene therapy and generation of induced pluripotent stem cells. *Blood, 114*(8), 1461–1468. https://doi.org/10.1182/blood-2009-04-210427

Vangelisti, A., Mascagni, F., Usai, G., Natali, L., Giordani, T., & Cavallini, A. (2020). Low long terminal repeat (LTR)-retrotransposon expression in leaves of the marine phanerogam Posidonia Oceanica L. *Life (Basel, Switzerland), 10*(3), 30. https://doi.org/10.3390/life10030030

Vanslambrouck, J.M., Woodard, L.E., Suhaimi, N., Williams, F.M., Howden, S.E., Wilson, S.B., Lonsdale, A., Er, P.X., Li, J., Maksimovic, J., Oshlack, A., Wilson, M.H., & Little, M.H. (2019). Direct reprogramming to human nephron progenitor-like cells using inducible piggyBac transposon expression of SNAI2-EYA1-SIX1. *Kidney International, 95*(5), 1153–1166. https://doi.org/10.1016/j.kint.2018.11.041

Voigt, F., Wiedemann, L., Zuliani, C., Querques, I., Sebe, A., Mátés, L., Izsvák, Z., Ivics, Z., & Barabas, O. (2016). Sleeping Beauty transposase structure allows rational design of hyperactive variants for genetic engineering. *Nature Communications, 7*, 11126. https://doi.org/10.1038/ncomms11126

Wang, J., Du, Y., Wang, S., Brown, S.J., & Park, Y. (2008). Large diversity of the piggyBac-like elements in the genome of Tribolium castaneum. *Insect Biochemistry and Molecular Biology, 38*(4), 490–498. https://doi.org/10.1016/j.ibmb.2007.04.012

Wang, P., Qin, W., Liu, T., Jiang, D., Cui, L., Liu, X., Fang, Y., Tang, X., Jin, H., & Qian, Q. (2020). PiggyBac-engineered T cells expressing a glypican-3-specific chimeric antigen receptor show potent activities against hepatocellular carcinoma. *Immunobiology, 225*(1), 151850. https://doi.org/10.1016/j.imbio.2019.09.009

Wang, Y., Pryputniewicz-Dobrinska, D., Nagy, E.É., Kaufman, C.D., Singh, M., Yant, S., Wang, J., Dalda, A., Kay, M.A., Ivics, Z., & Izsvák, Z. (2017). Regulated complex assembly safeguards the fidelity of Sleeping Beauty transposition. *Nucleic Acids Research, 45*(1), 311–326. https://doi.org/10.1093/nar/gkw1164

Wang, Z.Y., Ge, L.P., Ouyang, Y., Jin, X., & Jiang, Y.Z. (2024). Targeting transposable elements in cancer: developments and opportunities. *Biochimica et Biophysica Acta. Reviews on Cancer, 1879*(5), 189143. https://doi.org/10.1016/j.bbcan.2024.189143

Wells, J.N., & Feschotte, C. (2020). A field guide to eukaryotic transposable elements. *Annual Review of Genetics, 54,* 539–561. https://doi.org/10.1146/annurev-genet-040620-022145

Wen, S., Zhang, H., Li, Y., Wang, N., Zhang, W., Yang, K., Wu, N., Chen, X., Deng, F., Liao, Z., Zhang, J., Zhang, Q., Yan, Z., Liu, W., Zhang, Z., Ye, J., Deng, Y., Zhou, G., Luu, H.H., Haydon, R.C., … & Wei, G. (2014). Characterization of constitutive promoters for piggyBac transposon-mediated stable transgene expression in mesenchymal stem cells (MSCs). *PloS One, 9*(4), e94397. https://doi.org/10.1371/journal.pone.0094397

Wen, W., Song, S., Han, Y., Chen, H., Liu, X., & Qian, Q. (2020). An efficient screening system in yeast to select a hyperactive piggyBac transposase for mammalian applications. *International Journal of Molecular Sciences, 21*(9), 3064. https://doi.org/10.3390/ijms21093064

Wilber, A., Frandsen, J.L., Geurts, J.L., Largaespada, D.A., Hackett, P.B., & McIvor, R.S. (2006). RNA as a source of transposase for Sleeping Beauty-mediated gene insertion and expression in somatic cells and tissues. *Molecular Therapy: the Journal of the American Society of Gene Therapy, 13*(3), 625–630. https://doi.org/10.1016/j.ymthe.2005.10.014

Wilber, A., Wangensteen, K.J., Chen, Y., Zhuo, L., Frandsen, J.L., Bell, J.B., Chen, Z.J., Ekker, S.C., McIvor, R.S., & Wang, X. (2007). Messenger RNA as a source of transposase for sleeping beauty transposon-mediated correction of hereditary tyrosinemia type I. *Molecular Therapy: the Journal of the American Society of Gene Therapy, 15*(7), 1280–1287. https://doi.org/10.1038/sj.mt.6300160

Wilson, M.H., Coates, C.J., & George, A.L., Jr (2007). PiggyBac transposon-mediated gene transfer in human cells. *Molecular Therapy:*

the Journal of the American Society of Gene Therapy, 15(1), 139–145. https://doi.org/10.1038/sj.mt.6300028

Wilson, M.H., Kaminski, J.M., & George, A.L., Jr (2005). Functional zinc finger/sleeping beauty transposase chimeras exhibit attenuated overproduction inhibition. *FEBS Letters, 579*(27), 6205–6209. https://doi.org/10.1016/j.febslet.2005.10.004

Woodard, L.E., & Wilson, M.H. (2015). piggyBac-ing models and new therapeutic strategies. *Trends in Biotechnology, 33*(9), 525–533. https://doi.org/10.1016/j.tibtech.2015.06.009

Wu, A., Oh, S., Ericson, K., Demorest, Z.L., Vengco, I., Gharagozlou, S., Chen, W., Low, W. C., & Ohlfest, J.R. (2007). Transposon-based interferon gamma gene transfer overcomes limitations of episomal plasmid for immunogene therapy of glioblastoma. *Cancer Gene Therapy, 14*(6), 550–560. https://doi.org/10.1038/sj.cgt.7701045

Wu, S.C., Meir, Y.J., Coates, C.J., Handler, A.M., Pelczar, P., Moisyadi, S., & Kaminski, J.M. (2006). piggyBac is a flexible and highly active transposon as compared to sleeping beauty, Tol2, and Mos1 in mammalian cells. *Proceedings of the National Academy of Sciences of the United States of America, 103*(41), 15008–15013. https://doi.org/10.1073/pnas.0606979103

Xiao, J., Meng, X.M., Huang, X.R., Chung, A.C., Feng, Y.L., Hui, D.S., Yu, C.M., Sung, J.J., & Lan, H.Y. (2012). miR-29 inhibits bleomycin-induced pulmonary fibrosis in mice. *Molecular Therapy: the Journal of the American Society of Gene Therapy, 20*(6), 1251–1260. https://doi.org/10.1038/mt.2012.36

Xie, F., Ye, L., Chang, J.C., Beyer, A.I., Wang, J., Muench, M.O., & Kan, Y.W. (2014). Seamless gene correction of β-thalassemia mutations in patient-specific iPSCs using CRISPR/Cas9 and piggyBac. *Genome Research, 24*(9), 1526–1533. https://doi.org/10.1101/gr.173427.114

Xu, H.F., Xia, Q.Y., Liu, C., Cheng, T.C., Zhao, P., Duan, J., Zha, X.F., & Liu, S.P. (2006). Identification and characterization of piggyBac-like elements in the genome of domesticated silkworm, Bombyx mori. *Molecular Genetics and Genomics: MGG, 276*(1), 31–40. https://doi.org/10.1007/s00438-006-0124-x

Xu, J., Liu, J., Wang, Y., Peng, L., Li, W., Ji, L., Yang, Y., You, B., Huang, Y., Fang, S., Ni, P., Zhang, W., & Zhou, C. (2025). Transcriptomics of HERVs reveals clinico-biological characterization of LTR5_Hs and HERVS71 loci in gastric cancer. *Translational Oncology, 56*, 102369. https://doi.org/10.1016/j.tranon.2025.102369

Xue, X., Huang, X., Nodland, S.E., Mátés, L., Ma, L., Izsvák, Z., Ivics, Z., LeBien, T.W., McIvor, R.S., Wagner, J.E., & Zhou, X. (2009). Stable gene transfer and expression in cord blood-derived CD34+ hematopoietic stem and progenitor cells by a hyperactive Sleeping Beauty transposon system. *Blood, 114*(7), 1319–1330. https://doi.org/10.1182/blood-2009-03-210005

Yaakov, B., Ceylan, E., Domb, K., & Kashkush, K. (2012). Marker utility of miniature inverted-repeat transposable elements for wheat biodiversity and evolution. *TAG. Theoretical and Applied Genetics. Theoretische und angewandte Genetik, 124*(7), 1365–1373. https://doi.org/10.1007/s00122-012-1793-y

Yagita, K., Yamanaka, I., Emoto, N., Kawakami, K., & Shimada, S. (2010). Real-time monitoring of circadian clock oscillations in primary cultures of mammalian cells using Tol2 transposon-mediated gene transfer strategy. *BMC Biotechnology, 10*, 3. https://doi.org/10.1186/1472-6750-10-3

Yang, Y., Wang, W., Huang, T., Ruan, W., & Cao, G. (2016). Transgenesis of Tol2-mediated seamlessly constructed BAC mammary gland expression vectors in Mus musculus. *Journal of Biotechnology, 218*, 66–72. https://doi.org/10.1016/j.jbiotec.2015.11.024

Ye, L., You, Z., Qian, Q., Zhang, Y., Che, J., Song, J., & Zhong, B. (2015). TAL effectors mediate high-efficiency transposition of the piggyBac transposon in silkworm Bombyx mori L. *Scientific Reports, 5*, 17172. https://doi.org/10.1038/srep17172

Yin, H., Kanasty, R.L., Eltoukhy, A.A., Vegas, A.J., Dorkin, J.R., & Anderson, D.G. (2014). Non-viral vectors for gene-based therapy. *Nature Reviews. Genetics, 15*(8), 541–555. https://doi.org/10.1038/nrg3763

Yin, H., Liu, J., Xu, Y., Liu, X., Zhang, S., Ma, J., & Du, J. (2013). TARE1, a mutated Copia-like LTR retrotransposon followed by recent massive amplification in tomato. *PloS One, 8*(7), e68587. https://doi.org/10.1371/journal.pone.0068587

Yoshida, K., Nakamura, A., Yazaki, M., Ikeda, S., & Takeda, S. (1998). Insertional mutation by transposable element, L1, in the DMD gene results in X-linked dilated cardiomyopathy. *Human Molecular Genetics, 7*(7), 1129–1132. https://doi.org/10.1093/hmg/7.7.1129

Yuan, Y.W., & Wessler, S.R. (2011). The catalytic domain of all eukaryotic cut-and-paste transposase superfamilies. *Proceedings of the National Academy of Sciences of the United States of America, 108*(19), 7884–7889. https://doi.org/10.1073/pnas.1104208108

Yudaeva, A., Kostyusheva, A., Kachanov, A., Brezgin, S., Ponomareva, N., Parodi, A., Pokrovsky, V.S., Lukashev, A., Chulanov, V., & Kostyushev,

D. (2024). Clinical and translational landscape of viral gene therapies. *Cells, 13*(22), 1916. https://doi.org/10.3390/cells13221916

Yusa, K. (2015). piggyBac Transposon. *Microbiology Spectrum, 3*(2), MDNA3–2014.https://doi.org/10.1128/microbiolspec.MDNA3-0028-2014

Yusa, K., Rashid, S.T., Strick-Marchand, H., Varela, I., Liu, P.Q., Paschon, D.E., Miranda, E., Ordóñez, A., Hannan, N.R., Rouhani, F.J., Darche, S., Alexander, G., Marciniak, S.J., Fusaki, N., Hasegawa, M., Holmes, M.C., Di Santo, J.P., Lomas, D.A., Bradley, A., & Vallier, L. (2011). Targeted gene correction of α1-antitrypsin deficiency in induced pluripotent stem cells. *Nature, 478*(7369), 391–394. https://doi.org/10.1038/nature10424

Zayed, H., Izsvák, Z., Walisko, O., & Ivics, Z. (2004). Development of hyperactive sleeping beauty transposon vectors by mutational analysis. *Molecular Therapy: the Journal of the American Society of Gene Therapy, 9*(2), 292–304. https://doi.org/10.1016/j.ymthe.2003.11.024

Zeggar, H.R., How-Kit, A., Daunay, A., Bettaieb, I., Sahbatou, M., Rahal, K., Adouni, O., Gammoudi, A., Douik, H., Deleuze, J.F., & Kharrat, M. (2020). Tumor DNA hypomethylation of LINE-1 is associated with low tumor grade of breast cancer in Tunisian patients. *Oncology Letters, 20*(2), 1999–2006. https://doi.org/10.3892/ol.2020.11745

Zhang, L., Yan, L., Jiang, J., Wang, Y., Jiang, Y., Yan, T., & Cao, Y. (2014). The structure and retrotransposition mechanism of LTR-retrotransposons in the asexual yeast Candida albicans. *Virulence, 5*(6), 655–664. https://doi.org/10.4161/viru.32180

Zhang, R., Zhang, F., Sun, Z., Liu, P., Zhang, X., Ye, Y., Cai, B., Walsh, M.J., Ren, X., Hao, X., Zhang, W., & Yu, J. (2019). LINE-1 retrotransposition promotes the development and progression of lung squamous cell carcinoma by disrupting the tumor-suppressor gene FGGY. *Cancer Research, 79*(17), 4453–4465. https://doi.org/10.1158/0008-5472.CAN-19-0076

Zhang, Y., Zhang, Z., Ding, Y., Fang, Y., Wang, P., Chu, W., Jin, Z., Yang, X., Wang, J., Lou, J., & Qian, Q. (2021). Phase I clinical trial of EGFR-specific CAR-T cells generated by the piggyBac transposon system in advanced relapsed/refractory non-small cell lung cancer patients. *Journal of Cancer Research and Clinical Oncology, 147*(12), 3725–3734. https://doi.org/10.1007/s00432-021-03613-7

Zheng, Y., Li, Z.R., Yue, R., Fu, Y.L., Liu, Z.Y., Feng, H.Y., Li, J.G., & Han, S.Y. (2019). PiggyBac transposon system with polymeric gene carrier transfected into human T cells. *American Journal of Translational Research, 11*(11), 7126–7136.

Zhu, X., Fang, H., Gladysz, K., Barbour, J.A., & Wong, J.W.H. (2021). Overexpression of transposable elements is associated with immune evasion and poor outcome in colorectal cancer. *European Journal of Cancer (Oxford, England: 1990), 157*, 94–107. https://doi.org/10.1016/j.ejca.2021.08.003

Zu, H., & Gao, D. (2021). Non-viral vectors in gene therapy: recent development, challenges, and prospects. *The AAPS Journal, 23*(4), 78. https://doi.org/10.1208/s12248-021-00608-7

Author Biography

Dr. Yasemin Kartal is a faculty member at Kırklareli University, Faculty of Medicine, Department of Physiology. She obtained her PhD degrees both from Hacettepe University, Faculty of Medicine, Department of Physiology, and Ankara University, Institute of Health Sciences, specializing in Interdisciplinary Forensic Sciences-Forensic Chemistry and Forensic Toxicology. Her research integrates diverse disciplines within the medical sciences, including physiology, molecular biology, biotechnology, genetics, bioinformatics, and toxicology.

Dr. Kartal is dedicated to advancing scientific knowledge through rigorous research and academic studies, with the belief that *science is the only true guide in life*. Her work is particularly focused on elucidating the underlying physiological and molecular mechanisms of cancer and rare diseases. Additionality, she seeks to contribute to the development of innovative diagnostic and therapeutic strategies through interdisciplinary approaches.

PART III:

PHYSICAL METHODS FOR GENE DELIVERY

CHAPTER 15

SONOPORATION

SIMGE UNAY,[1] MEHMET DINCER BILGIN,[2] MEHMET BILGEN[3]

[1]Usak University, Faculty of Medicine, Department of Biophysics, Usak, Türkiye
[2]Aydin Adnan Menderes University, Faculty of Medicine, Department of Biophysics, Aydin, Türkiye
[3]Aydin Adnan Menderes University, Faculty of Medicine, Department of Biophysics, Aydin, Türkiye

Abstract

Sonoporation is an emerging and innovative non-viral gene delivery technique that uses ultrasound waves to enhance cell membrane permeability, facilitating the efficient entry of genetic material into cells. The process involves the use of microbubbles that are typically composed of lipid, protein, or polymer shells filled with gas. When subjected to ultrasound energy, the microbubbles oscillate or expand and contract, which further leads to the formation of smaller bubbles that collapse rapidly, generating shear forces and microstreaming effects. These forces can momentarily disrupt the cell membrane, allowing the genetic material to enter the cell through transient membrane openings. This effect does not rely on viral vectors, reducing concerns about immune responses or insertional mutagenesis associated with viral-based gene delivery methods. One of the main advantages of sonoporation is its ability to deliver genetic material with high precision, targeting specific tissues or organs through localized ultrasound application. Additionally, by adjusting the ultrasound parameters (e.g., frequency, intensity, pulse duration), the efficiency of gene transfer can be fine-tuned, making sonoporation highly adaptable for a range of therapeutic applications. This makes it particularly suitable for gene therapies in areas like oncology, genetic disorders, and vaccines, where precise control over the delivery site and timing is crucial for success. Despite its potential, challenges remain in optimizing the technique for clinical use. Factors such as ultrasound frequency, microbubble size and composition, and treatment duration require careful optimization to enhance the efficiency and reproducibility of gene delivery. Furthermore, understanding the biological effects of sonoporation on different cell types and tissues is essential to minimize potential toxicity and maximize therapeutic outcomes. In conclusion, sonoporation presents a promising, non-invasive approach for gene delivery, offering a safer alternative to viral-based methods. Continued research and technological advancements will be key to unlocking its full potential in clinical gene therapy and precision medicine.

1. Introduction

Sonoporation, a technique that uses ultrasound waves in combination with microbubbles to transiently permeabilize cell membranes, has garnered significant attention as a promising non-viral gene delivery method (Baig et al., 2024). This approach exploits the physical properties of microbubbles, which, when exposed to low-frequency ultrasound, oscillate, producing localized mechanical forces and cavitation. These forces disrupt the lipid bilayer of cell membranes, allowing for the entry of genetic material into the cell (Fig.1.1). The process is highly controllable, allowing for the targeted delivery of materials to specific tissues or organs, making it a particularly appealing method for localized gene therapy applications (Delalande et al., 2015; van Rooij et al., 2016). This chapter is dedicated to explaining the principles of sonoporation technique and describing its applications in medicinal biotechnology.

2. Mechanisms of Sonoporation

Ultrasound is commonly used for imaging and examining organs and soft tissues (Bachu et al., 2021). Ultrasound's benefits of being non-invasive, non-radioactive, convenient, and economical make it a popular tool in clinical practice (Tang et al., 2018; Yang et al., 2019). Additionally, ultrasound has demonstrated good compatibility with several technologies for disease therapy during the past few decades, particularly ultrasound-mediated gene therapy. Delivering therapeutic molecules to the target region via plasma membranes and endothelial barriers to tissues or cells is the key to the drug delivery system (Bez et al., 2019). Effective aggregation at particular locations lessens adverse effects on healthy tissues (Y. Zhang et al., 2013). It is widely known that using ultrasound in conjunction with gas-filled microbubbles can improve intracellular gene or medication delivery in a non-invasive, virus-free manner (Jones et al., 2018; Luo et al., 2017).

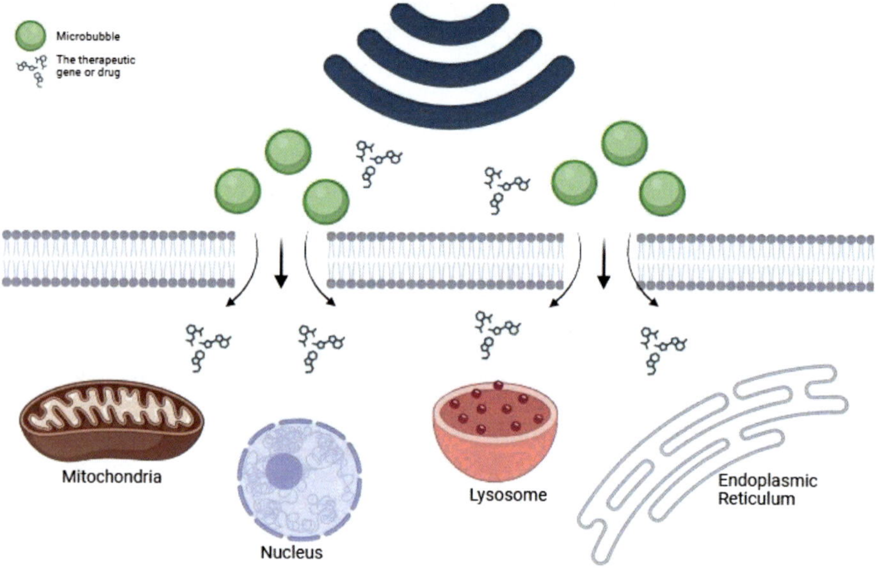

Figure 1.1. Mechanism of Sonoporation (Revised) (Krut et al., 2022). Created in BioRender. Unay, S. (2026) https://BioRender.com/8a7idan

The process of cavitation, or the creation, expansion, and disintegration of gas bubbles in a liquid upon exposure to ultrasonic waves, is closely related to the mechanism underlying sonoporation. The permeabilization of the cell membrane depends on several steps in the process. High-frequency sound waves, or ultrasound waves, move mechanically through a variety of materials, including water, tissues, and cells. Sonoporation usually uses frequencies between 20 kHz and several MHz, with lower frequencies (20-100 kHz) being more successful at creating cavitation (Lentacker et al., 2014; Tu & Yu, 2022).

One of the major advantages of sonoporation over other gene delivery techniques is its ability to offer high spatial and temporal control. By adjusting ultrasound parameters such as frequency, intensity, and duration of exposure, researchers can fine-tune the process for optimal gene transfer efficiency while minimizing potential cellular damage. Moreover, sonoporation can be performed non-invasively, without the need for invasive surgical procedures or viral vector-mediated delivery, which reduces the risk of complications and side effects. Despite its promising potential, sonoporation is still in the early stages of development, and there remain significant challenges to overcome before it can become a widely adopted clinical technique. Factors such as ultrasound frequency, microbubble characteristics, and treatment protocols need to be optimized for different tissue types and diseases. Additionally, understanding the biological effects of sonoporation on various cell types is crucial for minimizing toxicity and improving therapeutic outcomes (Lin et al., 2017).

Both continuous and pulsed types of ultrasound delivery are possible. Pulsed ultrasound is typically recommended because it can better manage the cavitation effect and lower the risk of heat damage to adjacent tissues. The ultrasonic waves' frequency and strength directly influence the size, development, and behavior of cavitation bubbles (Quarato et al., 2023).

2.1. Microbubbles

Ultrasound is usually combined with microbubbles, gas-filled spheres a few micrometers in diameter. These bubbles are frequently stabilized by a shell made of lipids, polymers, or other biocompatible substances to stop them from dissolving too quickly. Together with the therapeutic medicines to be administered, the microbubbles are added to the system (Al-Jawadi & Thakur, 2020). Microbubbles used for biomedical purposes typically range from 0.5 to 10 μm (Chowdhury et al., 2017). A significant portion of the total microbubble volume consists of a single, integral component known as the gas core. The shell serves as a barrier between the encapsulated gas and the surrounding aqueous environment. Various materials can be used as shell components, including lipids (approximately 3 nm thick), proteins (15–20 nm thick), and polymers (100–200 nm thick) (Zeng et al., 2022). Lipid molecules are held together by physical interactions such as hydrophobic forces and van der Waals interactions. Proteins are linked to each other through covalent disulfide bonds, while polymer chains are covalently cross-linked and/or entangled to form a bulk-like material (Sirsi & Borden, 2009).

Microbubbles have been used as ultrasound contrast agents in clinical applications for many years. These agents enhance sensitivity and image contrast for targeted regions during ultrasound imaging. Beyond their role as contrast agents, microbubbles are also utilized for the delivery of drugs and nucleic acids (such as mRNA and siRNA). Therapeutic agents encapsulated within microbubbles can be released at the desired site upon ultrasound-induced microbubble rupture. This approach enables targeted drug delivery while also minimizing potential side effects (e.g., those associated with chemotherapy drugs). The combination of microbubbles and ultrasound has been demonstrated as a novel and promising strategy for delivering therapeutic agents to tumors (Chowdhury et al., 2017).

The shells of microbubbles are essential to prevent their dissolution in the physiological environment and to inhibit gas diffusion. Based on their shell properties, microbubbles can be classified as soft-shelled or hard-shelled microbubbles (Shakya et al., 2024). The shell of soft-shelled microbubbles is typically composed of phospholipids and is only a few nanometers thick. The flexible phospholipid structure allows microbubbles to readily respond to the compression and rarefaction phases of ultrasound waves. In contrast, hard-shelled microbubbles have thicker and more rigid polymer or protein coatings, making them more stable but less responsive to oscillation (Escoffre & Bouakaz, 2019). The phospholipid-based shell forms an adhesive monolayer through the use of long and saturated fatty acid chains, ensuring stability while allowing oscillations induced by ultrasound to remain coherent. Additionally, phospholipids can be easily functionalized, enabling the production of targeted and drug-loaded microbubbles. To prolong the circulation time of microbubbles in the bloodstream, polyethylene glycol (PEG) chains are often incorporated into the microbubble shell. These PEG chains provide steric hindrance, preventing microbubble aggregation and protecting them from interactions with blood components that trigger clearance by the reticuloendothelial system (RES) (Abou-Saleh et al., 2019).

The microbubbles expand and contract as a result of pressure changes brought on by the ultrasonic waves as they travel through the medium (H. Li et al., 2022; Sun et al., 2020). The cavitation process revolves around this oscillating characteristic (Türkkol, 2022; Turkkol et al., 2025). There are two types of cavitation, inertical and stable cavitation of microbubbles. Microbubble oscillation amplitude increases with each cycle under high-intensity ultrasound exposure, ultimately resulting in microbubble collapse. Inertial cavitation is created when the microbubble breaks up into multiple smaller microbubbles upon collapse. The shock waves and strong shear strains applied by collapsing microbubbles produce surface disruption and pore development. Liquid jets are created when microbubbles collide asymmetrically with cell membranes. Shock waves and liquid jets have enough energy to enter blood arteries in addition to piercing nearby cell membranes. The size of the generated holes is determined by ultrasound parameters like pressure, exposure duration, and pulse repetition frequency. These parameters affect the distribution of bigger medicines or drug carriers. Cell membrane pore development caused by ultrasound-targeted microbubble destruction (UTMD) permits cytosolic distribution, which is essential for gene therapy since it can promote DNA endocytic uptake (Wischhusen & Padilla, 2019). Inertial cavitation causes severe mechanical and chemical attacks that result in membrane perforation and enhanced vascular permeability, in addition to the biophysical effects mentioned for stable cavitation. Microbubbles improve medication delivery even when they do not come into direct contact with cell surfaces because inertial cavitation has effects across longer distances. Inertial cavitation creates bigger membrane pores, ranging from hundreds of nanometers to several micrometers, in contrast to stable cavitation (He et al., 2022; Zhao et al., 2023).

2.2. Cell Membrane Disruption

During sonoporation, the mechanical forces produced by cavitation cause the cell membrane to rupture. Microbubbles develop and contract close to the cell membrane as a result of ultrasound-induced cavitation, creating significant shear stresses that distort the lipid bilayer (Escoffre & Bouakaz, 2019). These forces cause the membrane to temporarily open up, allowing larger molecules—like medications, nucleic acids, or imaging agents—to get past the normally selective barrier. Shear tension, hydrodynamic effects, and mechanical stress brought on by cavitation all contribute to the breakdown of cell membranes during sonoporation (Kim et al., 2021; Zevnik & Dular, 2022). When microbubbles collapse, the membrane experiences strong shear pressures that may cause temporary pores to emerge. The size, ultrasonic intensity, and proximity of the microbubbles to the membrane all affect the shear stress's magnitude (Csuka et al., 2016; Lipatova et al., 2019). Hydrodynamic Effects are high-velocity jets generated by collapsing bubbles that directly hit the cell membrane, creating localized forces that facilitate membrane disruption (Polgár et al., 2022). These fluid shear forces contribute to the formation of nanoscale pores. Cavitation-triggered mechanical stress is the result of microbubbles expanding and contracting quickly, which puts pressure on the membrane and eventually causes pore formation by generating compressive and tensile stresses in the surrounding fluid. The intensity of the ultrasonic waves, the kind of microbubbles employed, and the length of exposure are some variables that can affect the size, quantity, and stability of these pores. Crucially, the cell membrane usually reseals after the ultrasonic exposure stops, reducing the likelihood of irreversible cell damage (She et al., 2024).

2.3. Reversibility of Membrane Permeabilization

One of its main benefits is that membrane disruption during sonoporation is reversible. Cell membrane integrity usually returns after the ultrasonic exposure is over. The temporary cavitation-induced holes reseal within seconds to minutes, allowing the cell to resume its typical state. Sonoporation differs from other methods, such as electroporation, in that it does not pose the risk of irreversible membrane damage (Qi & Liu, 2024). Therapeutic chemicals can enter cells under control thanks to sonoporation's reversible nature, which eliminates the requirement for the cell membrane to be permanently altered. When targeting healthy cells, this property is particularly crucial because it lowers the possibility of unintentional cellular injury or necrosis (Ambattu et al., 2025; Pereno et al., 2018).

2.4. Factors Affecting Sonoporation Efficiency

Sonoporation success is dependent on several critical parameters that control the cavitation process and the cell membrane's subsequent permeability. For effective drug or gene delivery and to minimize possible harm to nearby tissues, these variables need to be carefully adjusted (T.-Y. Wang et al., 2014).

2.4.1. Ultrasound Parameters

Ultrasound parameters include duty cycle, exposure time, pulse duration, frequency, and acoustic intensity, among others (L. Zhang et al., 2022). Higher ultrasound frequencies (e.g., 1–10 MHz) produce more localized effects with less cavitation intensity, whereas lower frequencies (e.g., 20–100 kHz) produce stronger cavitation and greater mechanical stress, which promotes membrane breakdown. There is a direct correlation between the strength of cavitation forces and the ultrasonic wave intensity. Although they may potentially raise the possibility of heat harm to nearby tissues, higher intensities can cause more substantial membrane disturbances. Reducing negative consequences while maintaining an adequate cavitation intensity is crucial. In sonoporation, pulsed ultrasound is frequently utilized to provide regulated cavitation and avoid excessive heat accumulation. To create effective cavitation while preventing heat damage, the duty cycle (the percentage of time the ultrasound is active within a certain period) and pulse duration (the amount of time the ultrasound is on) must be tuned (Boissenot et al., 2016).

2.4.2. Microbubble Characteristics

Microbubble size has an impact on cavitation behavior; larger microbubbles typically cause more intense inertial cavitation, whereas smaller microbubbles are better at producing stable cavitation (Böhmer et al., 2010; Song et al., 2015). Smaller microbubbles have lower stability due to their higher Laplace pressure. Additionally, microbubbles within this size range exhibit a resonance frequency within the 1–10 MHz range, which corresponds to the operating frequency of transducers used in medical ultrasound imaging. The resonance frequency refers to the frequency at which microbubble oscillations are maximized (Shakya et al., 2024). The intended effect and the particular target tissue determine the ideal size. The efficacy of sonoporation is also influenced by the microbubble concentration in the medium; higher concentrations often result in more cavitation events and greater membrane rupture. On the other hand, an overly high concentration may cause undue harm. Furthermore, the stability, behavior under ultrasonic exposure, and biocompatibility of microbubbles are all significantly influenced by the composition of their shell. Shells made of polymers or lipids are frequently utilized to improve the stability and functionality of microbubbles (Shapiro et al., 2016; L. Zhang et al., 2022).

At low acoustic pressures, microbubbles oscillate linearly, undergoing compression and expansion proportional to the pressure wave. At high acoustic pressures, microbubbles oscillate nonlinearly: they expand more rapidly than they compress and continue to grow until they collapse. microbubbles undergoing stable cavitation exert forces on adjacent endothelial cells; they can be pushed against the cell barrier by acoustic radiation force, microstreaming effects around microbubbles can impact cell membranes, and microbubble oscillations can push and pull cells. microbubbles undergoing inertial cavitation have even stronger effects on cells: shock waves disrupt cell junctions, and liquid jets perforate cells (Wischhusen & Padilla, 2019).

2.4.3. Cell or Tissue Type

The response of the targeted cell to sonoporation depends on its kind (e.g., liver cells, muscle cells, or cancer cells). Since the mechanical strength of various tissues varies, it might be necessary to modify the ultrasound parameters for every application. For example, tumor cells may respond better to sonoporation because of their more permeable nature and changed membrane properties (Aksel et al., 2026; Jia et al., 2015; Y. Li et al., 2016; M. Wang et al., 2018).

3. Role of Sonoporation in Gene Therapy

The concept of ' smart drug delivery' has grown significantly in the last few decades as a sophisticated method of delivering medications or genes to particular parts of the patient's body with controlled dosage release, improved distribution efficiency, improved biocompatibility, and easy accessibility. In this sense, one of the most promising methods for accomplishing spatiotemporally regulated medication delivery to specific locations is ultrasound-activated mechanical force (Tu & Yu, 2022).

In gene therapy, sonoporation is important because it improves the transfer of genetic material into cells (Amador et al., 2021; Belling et al., 2020; Lentacker et al., 2014; Sennoga et al., 2017). In order to facilitate the effective transfer of therapeutic genes, it briefly permeabilizes the cell membrane using ultrasound waves and microbubbles (Rinaldi et al., 2018). Ultrasound waves create cavitation and other mechanical forces that cause microbubbles to expand and oscillate. This expansion and contraction cause the cell membrane to develop tiny holes that let big molecules like DNA or RNA enter the cells (Du et al., 2021).

For gene therapy to be successful in treating cancer or genetic abnormalities, genes must be efficiently delivered to specific cells. On this point, sonoporation has several benefits (Lentacker et al., 2014; Sennoga et al., 2017). First of all, it offers a non-invasive way to distribute genes, negating the need for intricate surgical techniques. Second, by carefully adjusting the ultrasonic parameters, it is feasible to target particular organs or tissues while causing the least amount of harm to the healthy tissues around them. Third, sonoporation makes it possible to transport genes in a more controlled and temporary way, lowering the possibility of long-lasting genetic alterations that can cause unintended side effects. Furthermore, by providing a safer and more manageable alternative, sonoporation may be able to get around some of the drawbacks of conventional gene delivery techniques like viral vectors. This makes it a desirable choice for clinical gene therapy applications, particularly for illnesses requiring targeted and regulated gene delivery (Bai et al., 2015; Rinaldi et al., 2018; Shen et al., 2016; Tan et al., 2016; Yoon et al., 2017). Sonoporation has been effective in delivering plasmid DNA, siRNA, mRNA, and CRISPR-Cas9 components, among other types of genetic material, in preclinical experiments (Huang et al., 2022; Schwartz et al., 2021). Applications in cancer have been investigated, where localized delivery of immune-modulating sequences or tumor-suppressing genes can improve treatment results while lessening the side effects of radiation or chemotherapy (Bouakaz and Michel Escoffre, 2024; Mittal et al., 2024; Ricci et al., 2024).

Both in vitro and in vivo studies have demonstrated that sonoporation is an effective non-viral gene therapy approach across various organ systems (Belling et al., 2020; Rychak and Klibanov, 2014). However, its gene transfer efficiency has been reported to be lower than that of certain other non-viral techniques. Additionally, sonoporation may induce cell death due to disruption of the cell membrane. The application of ultrasonic energy to enhance gene therapy in specific cell types was first explored in the 1980s (Fechheimer et al., 1987). The ability of ultrasound waves to modulate the permeability of the plasma membrane facilitates gene delivery. To enhance the efficiency of sonoporation-mediated gene transfer, the use of ultrasound contrast agents, such as microbubbles, has been investigated and has since become widely adopted (Krut et al., 2022).

4. Conclusion

Sonoporation offers several benefits, such as minimum cytotoxicity, non-invasiveness, and the capacity to control gene delivery in both space and time, thus providing a precise, safe, and efficient substitute for traditional gene delivery techniques. It can be customized by varying ultrasonic parameters such as frequency, intensity, and pulse duration, which increases its versatility for a range of therapeutic uses. However, a number of obstacles need to be overcome before this method may be widely used in clinical settings. These include standardizing microbubble formulations, maximizing ultrasonic settings, and guaranteeing uniform therapeutic results across various cell types and tissues.

References

Abou-Saleh, R. H., McLaughlan, J. R., Bushby, R. J., Johnson, B. R., Freear, S., Evans, S. D., & Thomson, N. H. (2019). Molecular Effects of Glycerol on Lipid Monolayers at the Gas-Liquid Interface: Impact on Microbubble Physical and Mechanical Properties. *Langmuir*, *35*(31), 10097–10105.

https://doi.org/10.1021/ACS.LANGMUIR.8B04130/ASSET/IMAGES/LARGE/LA-2018-041307_0007.JPEG

Aksel, M., Bozkurt Girit, O., Ozmen, A., & Bilgin, M. D. (2026). The Comparison of Anticancer Efficiency of Methylene Blue- and Aluminum Phthalocyanine-Mediated Sonophotodynamic Therapy on Prostate Cancer Cells In Vitro. *Photobiomodulation, Photomedicine, and Laser Surgery*, *44*(5), 313–323. https://doi.org/10.1177/25785478261433604

Al-Jawadi, S., & Thakur, S. S. (2020). Ultrasound-responsive lipid microbubbles for drug delivery: A review of preparation techniques to optimise formulation size, stability and drug loading. *International Journal of Pharmaceutics*, *585*, 119559. https://doi.org/10.1016/J.IJPHARM.2020.119559

Amador, C., Shah, R., Ghiam, S., Kramerov, A. A., & Ljubimov, A. V. (2021). Gene Therapy in the Anterior Eye Segment. *Current Gene Therapy*, *22*, 104–131. https://doi.org/10.2174/1566523221666210423084233

Ambattu, L. A., Del Rosal, B., Conn, C. E., & Yeo, L. Y. (2025). High-frequency MHz-order vibration enables cell membrane remodeling and lipid microdomain manipulation. *Biophysical Journal*, *124*, 25–39. https://doi.org/10.1016/j.bpj.2024.10.007

Bachu, V. S., Kedda, J., Suk, I., Green, J. J., & Tyler, B. (2021). High-Intensity Focused Ultrasound: A Review of Mechanisms and Clinical Applications. *Annals of Biomedical Engineering*, *49*(9), 1975–1991. https://doi.org/10.1007/S10439-021-02833-9/TABLES/3

Bai, M., Shen, M., Teng, Y., Sun, Y., Li, F., Zhang, X., Xu, Y., Duan, Y., & Du, L. (2015). Enhanced therapeutic effect of Adriamycin on multidrug resistant breast cancer by the ABCG2-siRNA loaded polymeric nanoparticles assisted with Ultrasound. *Oncotarget*, *6*, 43779–43790. https://doi.org/10.18632/oncotarget.6085

Baig, M. A., Du, Y., Zan, Z., & Fan, Z. (2024). Influence of cell shape on sonoporation efficiency in microbubble-facilitated delivery using micropatterned cell arrays. *Scientific Reports*, *14*. https://doi.org/10.1038/s41598-024-81410-1

Belling, J. N., Heidenreich, L. K., Tian, Z., Mendoza, A. M., Chiou, T. T., Gong, Y., Chen, N. Y., Young, T. D., Wattanatorn, N., Park, J. H., Scarabelli, L., Chiang, N., Takahashi, J., Young, S. G., Stieg, A. Z., de Oliveira, S., Huang, T. J., Weiss, P. S., & Jonas, S. J. (2020). Acoustofluidic sonoporation for gene delivery to human hematopoietic stem and progenitor cells. *Proceedings of the National Academy of Sciences of the United States of America*, *117*, 10976–10982.

https://doi.org/10.1073/PNAS.1917125117

Bez, M., Foiret, J., Shapiro, G., Pelled, G., Ferrara, K. W., & Gazit, D. (2019). Nonviral ultrasound-mediated gene delivery in small and large animal models. *Nature Protocols*, *14*(4), 1015. https://doi.org/10.1038/S41596-019-0125-Y

Böhmer, M. R., Chlon, C. H. T., Raju, B. I., Chin, C. T., Shevchenko, T., & Klibanov, A. L. (2010). Focused ultrasound and microbubbles for enhanced extravasation. *Journal of Controlled Release*, *148*, 18–24. https://doi.org/10.1016/j.jconrel.2010.06.012

Boissenot, T., Bordat, A., Fattal, E., & Tsapis, N. (2016). Ultrasound-triggered drug delivery for cancer treatment using drug delivery systems: From theoretical considerations to practical applications. In *Journal of Controlled Release* (Vol. 241, pp. 144–163). Elsevier B.V. https://doi.org/10.1016/j.jconrel.2016.09.026

Bouakaz, A., & Michel Escoffre, J. (2024). From concept to early clinical trials: 30 years of microbubble-based ultrasound-mediated drug delivery research. *Advanced Drug Delivery Reviews*, *206*, 115199. https://doi.org/10.1016/J.ADDR.2024.115199

Chowdhury, S. M., Lee, T., & Willmann, J. K. (2017). Ultrasound-guided drug delivery in cancer. *Ultrasonography*, *36*(3), 171. https://doi.org/10.14366/USG.17021

Csuka, Z., Olšiak, R., & Fuszko, Z. (2016). Research of cavitation at high shear stress. *Strojnicky Casopis*, *66*, 7–16. https://doi.org/10.1515/scjme-2016-0006

Du, M., Li, Y., & Chen, Z. (2021). Sonoporation-Mediated Gene Transfection: A Novel Direction for Cell Reprogramming In Vivo. *Frontiers in Bioengineering and Biotechnology*, *9*, 803055. https://doi.org/10.3389/fbioe.2021.803055

Escoffre, J. M., & Bouakaz, A. (2019). Minireview: Biophysical Mechanisms of Cell Membrane Sonopermeabilization. Knowns and Unknowns. *Langmuir*, *35*(31). https://doi.org/10.1021/acs.langmuir.8b03538

Fechheimer, M., Boylan, J. F., Parker, S., Sisken, J. E., Patel, G. L., & Zimmer, S. G. (1987). Transfection of mammalian cells with plasmid DNA by scrape loading and sonication loading. *Proceedings of the National Academy of Sciences of the United States of America*, *84*, 8463–8467. https://doi.org/10.1073/pnas.84.23.8463

He, J., Liu, Z., Zhu, X., Xia, H., Gao, H., & Lu, J. (2022). Ultrasonic Microbubble Cavitation Enhanced Tissue Permeability and Drug Diffusion in Solid Tumor Therapy. *Pharmaceutics*, *14*. https://doi.org/10.3390/pharmaceutics14081642

Huang, J., Zhou, Y., Li, J., Lu, A., & Liang, C. (2022). CRISPR/Cas systems: Delivery and application in gene therapy. *Frontiers in Bioengineering and Biotechnology*, *10*, 942325. https://doi.org/10.3389/FBIOE.2022.942325

Jia, Y., Yuan, W., Zhang, K., Wang, J., Wang, P., Liu, Q., & Wang, X. (2015). Comparison of cell membrane damage induced by the therapeutic ultrasound on human breast cancer MCF-7 and MCF-7/ADR cells. *Ultrasonics Sonochemistry*, *26*, 128–135. https://doi.org/10.1016/j.ultsonch.2015.03.001

Jones, R. M., Deng, L., Leung, K., McMahon, D., O'Reilly, M. A., & Hynynen, K. (2018). Three-dimensional transcranial microbubble imaging for guiding volumetric ultrasound-mediated blood-brain barrier opening. *Theranostics*, *8*(11), 2909–2926. https://doi.org/10.7150/THNO.24911

Kim, C., Choi, W. J., Ng, Y., & Kang, W. (2021). Mechanically Induced Cavitation in Biological Systems. *Life (Basel, Switzerland)*, *11*. https://doi.org/10.3390/life11060546

Krut, Z., Gazit, D., Gazit, Z., & Pelled, G. (2022). Applications of Ultrasound-Mediated Gene Delivery in Regenerative Medicine. *Bioengineering 2022, Vol. 9, Page 190*, *9*(5), 190. https://doi.org/10.3390/BIOENGINEERING9050190

Lentacker, I., De Cock, I., Deckers, R., De Smedt, S. C., & Moonen, C. T. W. (2014). Understanding ultrasound induced sonoporation: Definitions and underlying mechanisms. In *Advanced Drug Delivery Reviews* (Vol. 72, pp. 49–64). Elsevier. https://doi.org/10.1016/j.addr.2013.11.008

Li, H., Zhang, Y., Shu, H., Lv, W., Su, C., & Nie, F. (2022). Highlights in ultrasound-targeted microbubble destruction-mediated gene/drug delivery strategy for treatment of malignancies. In *International Journal of Pharmaceutics* (Vol. 613). Elsevier B.V. https://doi.org/10.1016/j.ijpharm.2021.121412

Li, Y., Wang, P., Chen, X., Hu, J., Liu, Y., Wang, X., & Liu, Q. (2016). Activation of microbubbles by low-intensity pulsed ultrasound enhances the cytotoxicity of curcumin involving apoptosis induction and cell motility inhibition in human breast cancer MDA-MB-231 cells. *Ultrasonics Sonochemistry*, *33*, 26–36. https://doi.org/10.1016/j.ultsonch.2016.04.012

Lin, Y., Lin, L., Cheng, M., Jin, L., Du, L., Han, T., Xu, L., Yu, A. C. H., & Qin, P. (2017). Effect of acoustic parameters on the cavitation behavior of SonoVue microbubbles induced by pulsed ultrasound. *Ultrasonics Sonochemistry*, *35*(Pt A), 176–184.

https://doi.org/10.1016/J.ULTSONCH.2016.09.016

Lipatova, I. M., Losev, N. V., & Makarova, L. I. (2019). The influence of the combined impact of shear stress and cavitation on the structure and sorption properties of chitin. *Carbohydrate Polymers*, *209*, 320–327. https://doi.org/10.1016/j.carbpol.2019.01.038

Luo, W., Wen, G., Yang, L., Tang, J., Wang, J., Wang, J., Zhang, S., Zhang, L., Ma, F., Xiao, L., Wang, Y., & Li, Y. (2017). Dual-targeted and pH-sensitive doxorubicin prodrug-microbubble complex with ultrasound for tumor treatment. *Theranostics*, *7*(2), 452–465. https://doi.org/10.7150/thno.16677

Mittal, M., Kumari, A., Paul, B., Varshney, A., Bhavya, Saini, A., Verma, C., & Mani, I. (2024). Challenges and Opportunities of Gene Therapy in Cancer. *OBM Genetics 2024, Vol. 8, 219*, *8*(1), 1–501. https://doi.org/10.21926/OBM.GENET.2401219

Pereno, V., Aron, M., Vince, O., Mannaris, C., Seth, A., De Saint Victor, M., Lajoinie, G., Versluis, M., Coussios, C., Carugo, D., & Stride, E. (2018). Layered acoustofluidic resonators for the simultaneous optical and acoustic characterisation of cavitation dynamics, microstreaming, and biological effects. *Biomicrofluidics*, *12*. https://doi.org/10.1063/1.5023729

Polgár, M., Agarwal, C., Gogate, P., Németh, G., & Csóka, L. (2022). Using CFD simulations to investigate the shear stress in hydrodynamic cavitation reactors coupled with experimental validation using colony count measurements. *Scientific Reports*, *12*. https://doi.org/10.1038/s41598-022-20349-7

Qi, B., & Liu, S. (2024). Frequency-sensitive cell membrane dynamics under ultrasonic stimulation. In *Biophysical Journal*. Elsevier B.V. https://doi.org/10.1016/j.bpj.2024.11.3321

Quarato, C. M. I., Lacedonia, D., Salvemini, M., Tuccari, G., Mastrodonato, G., Villani, R., Fiore, L. A., Scioscia, G., Mirijello, A., Saponara, A., & Sperandeo, M. (2023). A Review on Biological Effects of Ultrasounds: Key Messages for Clinicians. *Diagnostics*, *13*(5), 855. https://doi.org/10.3390/DIAGNOSTICS13050855

Ricci, M., Barbi, E., Dimitri, M., Duranti, C., Arcangeli, A., & Corvi, A. (2024). Sonoporation, a Novel Frontier for Cancer Treatment: A Review of the Literature. *Applied Sciences 2024, Vol. 14, Page 515*, *14*(2), 515. https://doi.org/10.3390/APP14020515

Rinaldi, L., Folliero, V., Palomba, L., Zannella, C., Isticato, R., Di Francia, R., Berretta, M., de Sio, I., Adinolfi, L. E., Morelli, G., Lastoria, S., Altucci, L., Pedone, C., Galdiero, M., & Franci, G.

(2018). Sonoporation by microbubbles as gene therapy approach against liver cancer. *Oncotarget*, *9*, 32182–32190. https://doi.org/10.18632/oncotarget.25875

Rychak, J. J., & Klibanov, A. L. (2014). Nucleic acid delivery with microbubbles and ultrasound. In *Advanced Drug Delivery Reviews* (Vol. 72, pp. 82–93). Elsevier. https://doi.org/10.1016/j.addr.2014.01.009

Schwartz, M. R., Debski, A. C., & Price, R. J. (2021). Ultrasound-targeted nucleic acid delivery for solid tumor therapy. *Journal of Controlled Release*, *339*, 531–546. https://doi.org/10.1016/j.jconrel.2021.10.010

Sennoga, C. A., Kanbar, E., Auboire, L., Dujardin, P. A., Fouan, D., Escoffre, J. M., & Bouakaz, A. (2017). Microbubble-mediated ultrasound drug-delivery and therapeutic monitoring. In *Expert Opinion on Drug Delivery* (Vol. 14, pp. 1031–1043). Taylor and Francis Ltd. https://doi.org/10.1080/17425247.2017.1266328

Shakya, G., Cattaneo, M., Guerriero, G., Prasanna, A., Fiorini, S., & Supponen, O. (2024). Ultrasound-responsive microbubbles and nanodroplets: A pathway to targeted drug delivery. *Advanced Drug Delivery Reviews*, *206*, 115178. https://doi.org/10.1016/J.ADDR.2023.115178

Shapiro, G., Wong, A. W., Bez, M., Yang, F., Tam, S., Even, L., Sheyn, D., Ben-David, S., Tawackoli, W., Pelled, G., Ferrara, K. W., & Gazit, D. (2016). Multiparameter evaluation of in vivo gene delivery using ultrasound-guided, microbubble-enhanced sonoporation. *Journal of Controlled Release*, *223*, 157–164. https://doi.org/10.1016/j.jconrel.2015.12.001

She, Y., Ren, R., & Jiang, N. (2024). Mechanical stress can regulate temporomandibular joint cavitation via signalling pathways. In *Developmental Biology* (Vol. 507, pp. 1–8). Elsevier Inc. https://doi.org/10.1016/j.ydbio.2023.12.006

Shen, Z. Y., Xia, G. L., Wu, M. F., Ji, L. Y., & Li, Y. J. (2016). The effects of percutaneous ethanol injection followed by 20-kHz ultrasound and microbubbles on rabbit hepatic tumors. *Journal of Cancer Research and Clinical Oncology*, *142*, 373–378. https://doi.org/10.1007/s00432-015-2034-y

Sirsi, S. R., & Borden, M. A. (2009). Microbubble Compositions, Properties and Biomedical Applications. *Bubble Science Engineering and Technology*, *1*(1–2), 3. https://doi.org/10.1179/175889709X446507

Song, K. H., Fan, A. C., Brlansky, J. T., Trudeau, T., Gutierrez-Hartmann, A., Calvisi, M. L., & Borden, M. A. (2015). High efficiency molecular delivery with sequential low-energy sonoporation bursts. *Theranostics*, *5*, 1419–1427. https://doi.org/10.7150/thno.13033

Sun, S., Wang, P., Sun, S., & Liang, X. (2020). Applications of Micro/Nanotechnology in Ultrasound-based Drug Delivery and Therapy for Tumor. *Current Medicinal Chemistry*, *28*, 525–547. https://doi.org/10.2174/0929867327666200212100257

Tan, J. K. Y., Pham, B., Zong, Y., Perez, C., Maris, D. O., Hemphill, A., Miao, C. H., Matula, T. J., Mourad, P. D., Wei, H., Sellers, D. L., Horner, P. J., & Pun, S. H. (2016). Microbubbles and ultrasound increase intraventricular polyplex gene transfer to the brain. *Journal of Controlled Release*, *231*, 86–93. https://doi.org/10.1016/j.jconrel.2016.02.003

Tang, W., Yang, Z., Wang, S., Wang, Z., Song, J., Yu, G., Fan, W., Dai, Y., Wang, J., Shan, L., Niu, G., Fan, Q., & Chen, X. (2018). Organic Semiconducting Photoacoustic Nanodroplets for Laser-Activatable Ultrasound Imaging and Combinational Cancer Therapy. *ACS Nano*, *12*(3), 2610–2622. https://doi.org/10.1021/ACSNANO.7B08628

Tu, J., & Yu, A. C. H. (2022). Ultrasound-Mediated Drug Delivery: Sonoporation Mechanisms, Biophysics, and Critical Factors. In *BME Frontiers* (Vol. 2022). American Association for the Advancement of Science. https://doi.org/10.34133/2022/9807347

Türkkol, A. (2022). *Demonstration of the effect of ultrasonic cavitation on apoptosis induced by chlorine E6 mediated sonodynamic therapy for PC3 cell line* [Master Thesis]. Aydin Adnan Menderes University / Institute of Health Sciences .

Turkkol, A., Kolac, U. K., Donmez Yalcin, G., Bilgin, M. D., Yalcin, A., & Bilgen, M. (2025). Enhancing Sonodynamic Therapy in Prostate Cancer: Cavitation-Induced Cytotoxicity and Mitochondrial Unfolded Protein Response Disruption. *Cell Biochemistry and Biophysics*, *83*(3). https://doi.org/10.1007/S12013-025-01717-2,

van Rooij, T., Skachkov, I., Beekers, I., Lattwein, K. R., Voorneveld, J. D., Kokhuis, T. J. A., Bera, D., Luan, Y., van der Steen, A. F. W., de Jong, N., & Kooiman, K. (2016). Viability of endothelial cells after ultrasound-mediated sonoporation: Influence of targeting, oscillation, and displacement of microbubbles. *Journal of Controlled Release : Official Journal of the Controlled Release Society*, *238*, 197–211. https://doi.org/10.1016/J.JCONREL.2016.07.037

Wang, M., Zhang, Y., Cai, C., Tu, J., Guo, X., & Zhang, D. (2018). Sonoporation-induced cell membrane permeabilization and cytoskeleton disassembly at varied acoustic and microbubble-cell parameters. *Scientific Reports*, *8*. https://doi.org/10.1038/s41598-018-22056-8

Wang, T.-Y., Wilson, K. E., Machtaler, S., & Willmann, J. K. (2014). Ultrasound and Microbubble Guided Drug Delivery: Mechanistic Understanding and Clinical Implications. *Current Pharmaceutical Biotechnology*, *14*(8), 743. https://doi.org/10.2174/1389201014666131226114611

Wischhusen, J., & Padilla, F. (2019). Ultrasound Molecular Imaging with Targeted Microbubbles for Cancer Diagnostics: From Bench to Bedside. *IRBM*, *40*(1), 3–9. https://doi.org/10.1016/J.IRBM.2018.10.007

Yang, C., Li, Y., Du, M., & Chen, Z. (2019). Recent advances in ultrasound-triggered therapy. *Journal of Drug Targeting*, *27*(1), 33–50. https://doi.org/10.1080/1061186X.2018.1464012

Yoon, S., Wang, P., Peng, Q., Wang, Y., & Shung, K. K. (2017). Acoustic-transfection for genomic manipulation of single-cells using high frequency ultrasound. *Scientific Reports*, *7*. https://doi.org/10.1038/s41598-017-05722-1

Zeng, W., Yue, X., & Dai, Z. (2022). Ultrasound contrast agents from microbubbles to biogenic gas vesicles. *Medical Review*, *3*(1), 31. https://doi.org/10.1515/MR-2022-0020

Zevnik, J., & Dular, M. (2022). Cavitation bubble interaction with compliant structures on a microscale: A contribution to the understanding of bacterial cell lysis by cavitation treatment. *Ultrasonics Sonochemistry*, *87*. https://doi.org/10.1016/j.ultsonch.2022.106053

Zhang, L., Lin, Z., Zeng, L., Zhang, F., Sun, L., Sun, S., Wang, P., Xu, M., Zhang, J., Liang, X., & Ge, H. (2022). Ultrasound-induced biophysical effects in controlled drug delivery. In *Science China Life Sciences* (Vol. 65, pp. 896–908). Science Press (China). https://doi.org/10.1007/s11427-021-1971-x

Zhang, Y., Chan, H. F., & Leong, K. W. (2013). Advanced materials and processing for drug delivery: the past and the future. *Advanced Drug Delivery Reviews*, *65*(1), 104–120. https://doi.org/10.1016/J.ADDR.2012.10.003

Zhao, X., Wright, A., & Goertz, D. E. (2023). An optical and acoustic investigation of microbubble cavitation in small channels under therapeutic ultrasound conditions. *Ultrasonics Sonochemistry*, *93*. https://doi.org/10.1016/j.ultsonch.2023.106291

Author Biographies

Asst. Prof. Simge Unay graduated from Başkent University Department of Biomedical Engineering in 2015. She completed her master's degree in 2018 and her doctorate in 2022 under the supervision of Prof. Dr. Mehmet Dinçer BILGIN at Aydın Adnan Menderes University Institute of Health Sciences, Department of Biophysics. Between 2022-2024, she worked as a faculty member at Lokman Hekim University Faculty of Medicine, Department of Biophysics in Ankara. Since 2024, she has been working as a faculty member at Uşak University Faculty of Medicine, Department of Biophysics. Her research interests include cancer biophysics, neurobiophysics, photodynamic diagnosis, and low-level laser therapy. She also investigates the treatment mechanism of chemotherapy-induced peripheral neuropathy.

Prof. Dr. Mehmet Dinçer Bilgin is a medical doctor and biophysicist at Aydın Adnan Menderes University Medical Faculty in Aydın, Turkey, where he has served as the Head of the Biophysics Department since 2001. He graduated from Ankara University Medical Faculty in Ankara, Turkey, earned his PhD in Biophysics from the Illinois Institute of Technology in Chicago, USA, and completed postdoctoral research in Cellular Biophysics at Northwestern University in Chicago, USA.

Prof. Bilgin's research focuses on developing noninvasive methods for diagnosing and treating cancer, including photodynamic and sonodynamic therapies. He also investigates noninvasive approaches for conditions such as parasitic infestations, peripheral neural disorders, and diabetic neuropathy. His broader research interests include tissue optics, laser therapies, therapeutic ultrasound (such as low-intensity pulsed ultrasound), biomedical applications of electromagnetic waves, and nonlinear analysis of biological signals. Recently, his research group has been studying the sono-photodynamic effects of various sensitizers in the treatment of prostate, breast, and gastrointestinal cancers.

Prof. Dr. Mehmet Bilgen has been involved in educational and collaborative research activities in the areas of theoretical, experimental and medical physics, nondestructive testing, engineering, biomedicine, biotechnology, experiments with animal models and development of disease-oriented therapies.

CHAPTER 16

PHOTOPORATION FOR MEMBRANE TRANSFER IN CELLS

MEHRAN AKSEL, MEHMET DINÇER BILGIN, MEHMET BILGEN

Department of Biophysics, Faculty of Medicine, Adnan Menderes University, Aydin 09010, Türkiye

Abstract

Photoporation is an emerging light-based technique that enables transient and localized permeabilization of the cell membrane, thereby facilitating the delivery or transfer of biomolecules and organelles. This chapter provides a comprehensive overview of the fundamental mechanisms underlying photoporation, beginning with an introduction to its historical development and the principles of light–tissue interaction. The applications of photoporation in areas such as drug delivery, gene transfer, immunotherapy, and regenerative medicine are highlighted, demonstrating its versatility and translational potential. Challenges and limitations—including photothermal damage, variability in cellular response, and the need for precise control of irradiation parameters—are critically analyzed to inform future optimization strategies. The chapter also explores future directions, with particular emphasis on integrating photoporation with nanotechnology, real-time imaging, and machine learning for enhanced precision and safety. The discussion concludes with a summary of key insights and a perspective on the emerging trends that may shape photoporation as a next-generation platform for membrane transfer in both fundamental research and clinical applications.

Keywords: Photoporation, Tissue-Light interaction, Cell membrane permeabilization, Gene transfer, Optoporation.

1. Introduction

All living organisms and cells are surrounded by a membrane that serves as a selective physical barrier between their internal and external environments. This barrier is crucial for regulating the entry and exit of essential substances such as ions, nutrients, and waste materials, thereby maintaining cellular homeostasis. However, in various biomedical applications, including gene therapy, targeted drug delivery, and regenerative medicine, the transfer of genetic materials or other substances across the cell membrane into the cytoplasm is often required beyond the natural processes. To facilitate such transfers, several physical methods have been proposed to induce temporary (i.e., transient) membrane permeabilization. These methods are utilized to study, monitor, or modify the behavior of transfected cells (Rau & Rentmeister, 2017).

Pioneered in the 1980s, photoporation (or optoporation) has emerged as an innovative technique in bio-photonics, attracting significant attention in the context of membrane permeabilization (Ramon et al., 2021). The approach is particularly useful in biological research, as it enables manipulating cell functionalities. Unlike others, the method does not require physical or biological contact with the cells. It utilizes light (laser) to induce the passage of substances across the cell membrane (Fig. 1.).

The light exposure creates transient pores in the membrane and renders the membrane temporarily permeable that accompanies non-toxic uptake of new drugs, the delivery of macromolecules, or even the performance of cellular surgery(Xiong et al. 2016; Shinde et al. 2021; Xiong et al. 2023). The cell surface is illuminated by a light pulse, characterized by a sufficiently short duration and appropriate wavelength. As the energy of the incident light is absorbed by the cell membrane, its volume rapidly expands, resulting in the formation of transient pores. The size of the pores and their lifetime are significantly influenced by the localized energy distribution within the irradiated volume. The mechanism is complex and depends on various parameters, including laser pulse duration, intensity, wavelength, and the photothermal properties of the membrane. Currently, photoporation can be grouped into a few types, such as nanosecond pulsed, resting state, and femtosecond pulsed. Each type has its own advantages and applications.

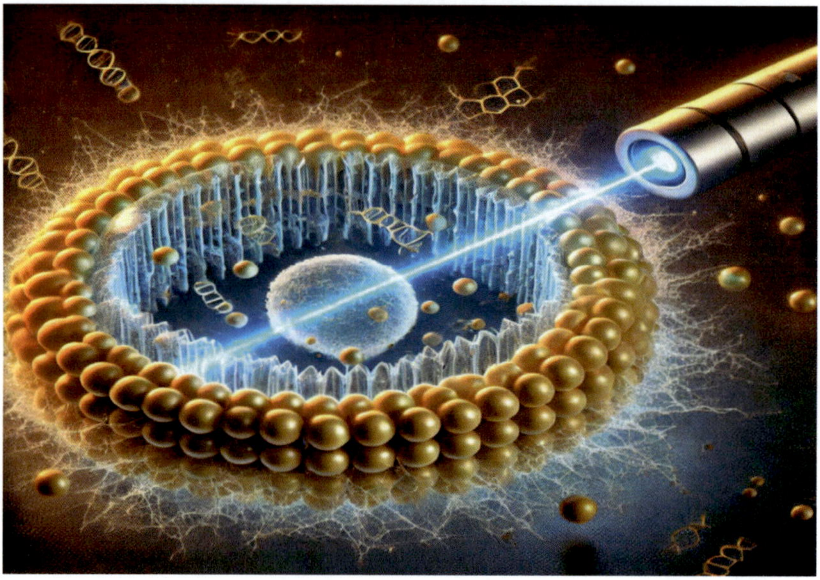

Fig.1. The mechanism of photoporation.

2. Light-Tissue Interaction

The biological and physical mechanisms of photoporation are multifaceted and depend on factors and interactions with the cellular microenvironment. The interaction of light with cellular components encompasses a series of biochemical and biophysical events triggered by physiological stimuli to maintain cellular homeostasis. This bio-photonic interaction is influenced by factors such as the broadness of the optical spectrum, the diversity of cell types, and the intrinsic properties of tissues (Krasnikov et al., 2019). Furthermore, the complexity of the mechanical, thermal, and optical behaviors of cells and the extracellular environment complicates the wide-reaching interplay between light and biological responses (Fuqiang et al., 2022). Although the complete and comprehensive modeling of a living cell from a bio-photonics perspective remains a significant challenge, the existing body of knowledge provides a substantial understanding of the fundamental principles underlying this phenomenon.

When laser energy is absorbed by the cell membrane, localized heat generation occurs. This heat induces phase transitions in the lipid bilayer, resulting in transient membrane defects that permit the entry of substances.

Excessive heat generation can lead to protein denaturation and permanent membrane damage. The efficiency of photoporation is influenced by laser parameters, including fluence, pulse duration, and exposure time (Fuqiang et al., 2022). For instance, membrane permeabilization can be achieved with a single ultrashort pulse lasting either 300 fs or 650 fs within a power range of 0.5 - 2.0 mW. Furthermore, when 20 - 40 laser pulses, each lasting 875 fs, are applied, it has been observed that the impact of pulse count on efficiency gradually decreases when the pulse duration exceeds 800 fs (Fraire et al., 2020).

The relationship between membrane penetration efficiency and laser pulse energy has been investigated in terms of its temporal evolution. The findings show that efficiency initially rises rapidly, peaking around 450 fs, and subsequently decreases sharply. Additionally, the relationship between pulse width and membrane penetration efficiency has been explored in greater detail. For pulse widths shorter than 1 ps, penetration efficiency increases significantly with pulse duration, rising from approximately 10% at 0.354 ps to about 45% at 765 fs, after which a slight decrease occurs. These findings highlight the complex interplay of parameters affecting photoporation efficiency and emphasize the importance of optimizing these factors for improved membrane permeabilization (Breunig et al., 2022; Pylaev et al., 2021).

Among the other mechanisms of photoporation, vapor nanobubble and opto-mechanical effects can also be observed. At higher laser fluences, the surrounding liquid reaches its boiling point, resulting in the formation of bubbles. These bubbles expand and collapse, generating shock waves that create pores in the cell membrane. The size and lifespan of the bubbles determine the extent of permeabilization. Another significant effect of photoporation is the opto-mechanical effect, wherein the rapid expansion and collapse of nanobubbles generate fluid shear forces that disrupt the membrane structure. In femtosecond laser-mediated photoporation, multiphoton ionization can generate reactive oxygen species (ROS), which induce oxidative stress(Aksel et al., 2020, 2021, 2024). This oxidative stress leads to membrane perforation through lipid peroxidation and protein modifications (Fraire et al., 2020; Ramon et al., 2021; Rudhall et al., 2012).

In summary, photoporation results from the cumulative effects of multiple interactions with the cell membrane. The biological effects on cells, particularly the ability to form pores, can be enhanced by increasing laser fluence, increasing the number of laser pulses, or reducing cell density.

3. Applications of Photoporation

Photoporation is a groundbreaking method that can effectively facilitate the entry of a broad range of exogenous biomolecules into the cell environment, thereby enhancing the possibilities for precise genetic manipulation. Genetic materials can be delivered through transient pores generated in the cell membrane by femtosecond lasers. It offers high transfection efficiency, low cytotoxicity, and broad compatibility with various biomolecules utilized in diverse cellular applications. These advantageous attributes position it as a particularly versatile option within the expansive and ever-evolving gene delivery arena, successfully delivering a multitude of therapeutic genes into an extraordinarily diverse array of cell types and demonstrating its remarkable adaptability in a plethora of experimental contexts and extensive applicability (Arun Kumar, 2021).

When photoporation is combined with pigment particles, as well as gold particles and gold-nanorods, it can produce promising results across an extensive variety of cell types, significantly enhancing its utility in gene therapies for targeted applications. Transfected genes can be successfully expressed in a variety of cellular contexts, and this impressive capability enables targeted treatments in the ongoing battle against genetic disorders, various types of cancers, and a growing list of infectious diseases that continually challenge healthcare professionals. For instance, a notably efficient delivery of the p53 gene, the TNF plasmid, and a nano-promoter into primary immune cells, MCF-7 cells, and mitotic cells can be achieved, resulting in the successful expression of several crucial therapeutic genes (Huang et al., 2022; Jahangiri-Manesh et al., 2022; Kanu et al., 2022; Ashish Kumar et al., 2024).

Beyond its significant implications for treating diseases in the medical field, the applications of photoporation continue to expand in multifaceted and innovative ways, tightly interwoven with remarkable advancements in biomedical research. Vaccination, which represents a critical initial step in the prevention of infectious diseases, is showing promising potential through the use of photoporation that can enhance immune responses significantly. In intriguing research studies, a replication-deficient influenza virus was ingeniously engineered to express the green fluorescent protein gene, thus paving the way for a novel and potentially transformational approach to vaccine development. This synthesized novel virus served as an experimental vaccine in mouse models, allowing for exhaustive studies on its efficacy and overall effectiveness in generating protective immunity (Bu et al., 2022; Jeong et al., 2021; Landreth et al., 2020).

Notably, the influenza virus vaccine group that was administered via the photoporation method exhibited an impressive increase in splenocyte responses to viral infections, accompanied by a remarkable rise in IgG levels that were found in mouse serum, indicating the robust immune activation prompted by this innovative delivery technique. This highlights the advantage of developing vaccines swiftly by encoding the spike proteins of infectious pathogens for which vaccines have not yet been established, thereby opening new avenues for exploration in the research of vaccines and their development. Furthermore, the utilization of a vaccine cocktail containing various viral components can facilitate concurrent administration by encoding different viral components into the genomes of immune cells selectively and strategically. Observations made in mouse models indicated a broad-spectrum viral response from this innovative and comprehensive vaccination approach, showcasing the potential efficacy of combinatorial strategies that could significantly enhance modern vaccine design (Kastenschmidt et al., 2023; O'Gorman et al., 2014).

Furthermore, the oncolytic adenovirus (OA) platform delivery system—which was effectively introduced into tumorous cells—has proven advantageous due to its remarkable ability to achieve high selectivity and efficient transfection of genes specifically into tumor cells, allowing for targeted therapeutic interventions that can significantly improve patient outcomes. Comprehensive examinations of the cytotoxicity and apoptotic outcomes of the delivered gene revealed some surprising findings that warrant further exploration and thorough scrutiny. It was determined that three specific genes, previously thought to be unrelated to apoptosis, actually led to significant cell death by increasing the concentration of the gene conjugated with the OA virus, complicating the understanding of gene interactions at a cellular level (Raes et al., 2020; Sung & Kim, 2019).

As the prominent dawn of synthetic biology unfolds on the research landscape, scientists have also begun to explore the delivery of guide RNA and dCas9 complexes or DNA into the cells of E. coli and K562, successfully resulting in the production of the α-GFP protein, showcasing the remarkable versatility of photoporation in diverse biological systems and its utility across different experimental frameworks. Furthermore, in sharp contrast to traditional gene delivery research, which typically focuses on curing specific diseases through singular gene expression in one particular cell type, the emerging strategy anticipates the creation of potentially new life forms that can be harnessed in the ever-evolving and dynamic field of genetic engineering (Alimi et al., 2021; Layachi et al., 2023; Taha et al., 2022).

These pioneering and forward-thinking approaches aim to enable the implementation of intelligent behavior in genetically modified organisms, representing a promising new beginning for innovative developments that could reshape our understanding of intricate biological systems and processes. However, it is important to note that despite the exhilarating possibilities that lie ahead, the applicability of these advanced methods in the medical realm remains largely unconfirmed as of now, requiring careful validation and extensive testing. Consequently, there remains a pressing need for further follow-up research that should encompass the scalability of large sample quantities, the expansion of application systems within the body, and the assurance of reproducibility in results across various experimental conditions, emphasizing the necessity of rigorous scientific inquiry (Haleem et al., 2022; S. Roy et al., 2022). Photoporation applications are summarized in Table-1.

4. Challenges and Limitations of Photoporation

Despite its wide adoption in biological research, especially in high-throughput drug screening and transfections, some conventional techniques may be tedious or unsuitable for specific applications. In contrast, photonic technologies—originally developed for bioimaging—have attracted growing attention as compelling alternatives. These methods offer rapid, contactless, and chemical-free membrane transfer capabilities, making them highly promising for advanced cellular manipulation (Luo et al., 2021; Xiong et al., 2023).

To date, the applications of photoporation have covered the fundamental biological research, cancer therapy and drug delivery, so much so, that it may eventually become an irreplaceable method in the life science. Nonetheless, there exist many challenges and limitations going along with this frontier technique. Foremost, and similar to other photonic techniques, the first challenge lies in the light absorption and diffusion into the biological tissues. As is widely known, the spectra of interest for photoporation lies in the UV or visible range, which have very limited penetration depth in the tissues. The need for high intensity, in term of MW/cm^2 or TW/cm^2, can also cross thresholds of stimulating unintended bio-effects in living organisms. In particular, current photoporation methods

Table 1. The summary of applications of photoporation

Researcher	Years	Cell Types	Agents	Light Dose	Pulse Duration	doi
McGraw et al.	2024	HN31, NOM9, peripheral blood mononuclear cells (PBMCs), CT1258, ZMTH3, DU145, CHO, Saccharomyces cerevisiae, HeLa, Jurkat cells.	Gold nanoparticles (AuNPs), carbon-based nanoparticles, graphene quantum dots (QDs), iron oxide nanoparticles.	532 nm (PL-2250 Nd:YAG laser), 1064 nm (Nd:YAG laser), 800 nm (Ti:sapphire laser), 561 nm (Opolette HE 355 LD laser).	70 ps , 5–9 ns, 35 fs, 100 fs.	(McGraw et al., 2024)
Du et al.	2023	HN31, NOM9, peripheral blood mononuclear cells (PBMCs)	Gold nanoparticles (AuNPs)	532 nm (PL-2250 Nd:YAG laser)	70 ps	(Du et al., 2024)
Goemaere et al.	2023	RAW264.7 murine macrophage-like cells.	Polydopamine nanoparticles (PDNPs) as photoporation sensitizers, FITC-dextran 500 kDa (FD500) as cargo molecules.	0.95 J/cm², 1.12 J/cm², 1.33 J/cm².	3 ns	(Goemaere et al., 2023)

Raes et al.	2021	H1299-EGFP (human non-small cell lung cancer cell line). Murine mesenchymal stem cells (mMSCs) expressing EGFP. Primary human T cells.	Gold nanoparticles (AuNPs) as photoporation sensitizers. Cas9 RNP (ribonucleoprotein) complexes for gene editing. Alexa Fluor 647 10 kDa dextran as a model macromolecule	0.84 J/cm^2 1.26 J/cm^2 1.60 J/cm^2	3 ns	(Raes et al., 2021)
Kumar et al.	2021	RAW264.7 murine macrophage-like cells	Carbon Black (CB) nanoparticles, Calcein, Propidium Iodide (PI)	25–88 mJ/cm^2	5–9 ns	(S. Kumar et al., 2021)
Du et al.	2021	HeLa (human cervical cancer) adherent cells.	Gold nanoparticles (AuNPs) as photoporation sensitizers, FITC-dextran (10 kDa) as a cargo molecule.	1.28 J/cm^2, 2.56 J/cm^2, 3.84 J/cm^2, 6.4 J/cm^2.	6 ns	(Du et al., 2021)
Hosokawa et al.	2011	Various vertebrate embryo cells (e.g., zebrafish, chick, shark, mouse)	Dextran, morpholino oligonucleotides (MOs), DNA plasmids, mRNA	400 nJ/pulse	120 fs	(Hosokawa et al., 2011)

Liu et al.	2018	HeLa cells	Graphene quantum dots (GQDs), fluorescently tagged phalloidin, nanobodies, SNAP-tags	0.47 J/cm² for AuNPs, 0.23 J/cm² for GQDs	7 ns	(Liu et al., 2018)
Liu et al.	2020	HeLa cells (adherent cells), Jurkat cells (suspension cells)	Graphene quantum dots (GQD), reduced graphene oxide (rGO), polyethylene glycol (PEG), polyethyleneimine (PEI)	0.89 J/cm²	2 ps	(Liu et al., 2020)
Duan et al.	2017	C2C12 myoblast cells	Hydrogen peroxide (H_2O_2)	55 mW	100 fs	(Duan et al., 2017)
Mitchell et al.	2013	Tobacco BY-2 cells (intact plant cells)	Propidium iodide (PI), Calcein, Flucrescein-conjugated dextrans (various sizes)	0.07 W to 1.8 W	140 fs	(Mitchell et al., 2013)
Mitchell et al.	2013	Tobacco BY-2 plant cells	Membrane-impermeant fluorescent dyes	800 nm	2 ps	(Raes et al., 2020)
Mohan et al.	2021	HeLa cells	Propidium iodide (PI) dye	7 mJ pulse energy at 650 nm wavelength	5 ns	(Mohan et al., 2021)

Maeno et al.	2018	Euglena gracilis (photosynthetic unicellular motile microalgae)	Fluorogenic peptide aptamers (FPBP), Mannitol	80 nJ pulse energy at 800 nm wavelength	100 fs	(Maeno et al., 2018)
Layachi et al.	2023	HeLa WT cancer cells	Gold nanoparticles (AuNP), FITC-Dextran 10 kDa	2.6 J/cm²	5 ns	(Layachi et al., 2023)
Xiong et al.	2018	Primary hippocampal neurons	Gold nanoparticles (AuNPs), Phalloidin (fluorescent actin-binding dye)	2 J/cm²	7 ns	(Xiong et al., 2018)
Antkowiak et al.	2010	Chinese hamster ovary (CHO-K1) cells	Propidium iodide (PI), Calcein AM	800 nm femtosecond laser	180 fs	
Maeno et al.	2018	Euglena gracilis (photosynthetic unicellular motile microalgae)	Fluorogenic peptide aptamers (FPBP), Mannitol	80 nJ pulse energy at 800 nm wavelength	100 fs	(Rukmana et al., 2019)

may suffer greatly from the optical shield posed by the plasma membrane of the living cell. Current photonic exposure schemes may give rise to the compromised cell viability in a substantial number of cell types. The reason behind such an inconsistent outcome is poorly understood and limits widely the applications of photoporation. However, the implementation of standardization protocols can be particularly complex, given the unique configuration and optical properties of each cell kind. As a forefront technique, the scope of the use of photoporation technology is still somehow limited by the gaps in the current technological arsenal as well as by the demands of the developmental efforts. Above aside, it is also important to notice the ethical dimension of the use of photoporation, the irreversible or long-term damaging to the tissues and living organisms in general(Sreedevi & Suresh, 2023).

5. Future Directions and Emerging Trends

Recent years have witnessed extensive endeavors in the innovation of new techniques and the development of novel solution strategies to improve and unravel the best photoporation applications. It has certainly emerged as a new and intriguing method of gene delivery, while its inherent flexibility undoubtedly offers fascinating prospects for future research and clinical application, it is essential to underscore that various unresolved issues and applications continue to require detailed attention and rigorous investigation. Only through sustained inquiry can the full potential of photoporation be realized to achieve great advancements in biotechnology and medical treatment. The top research challenges and the emerging trends remain in the theoretical, experimental and numerical work of the micro/nanoscale laser-induced techniques. The potential future directions and the broad disciplines of the ongoing and further research are visionary imagined, which is anticipated to inspire and lead to the scientific discoveries and innovative developments. Interdisciplinary convergence where laser photonics and biological studies neede to be integrated into the computational analysis, physical experimentations and mathematical examinations should foster the science breakthroughs and industrial innovations(Heinemann et al., 2022; M. Roy & Roy, 2021; Zhou et al., 2024). Future 3D manufacturing techniques which are ground on trial-and-error control by the illumination of photophysics are expected to largely reduce the energy quality, and time consumption in diverse fields such as agricultural applications and biotechnology. Possible collaborations of the artificial intelligence, machine learning, and optimal sensing for the integrated approach of the automatic predict and versatile control should also inspire further contributions in scientific investigation and practical use.

6. Conclusion and summary

As life sciences push the boundaries of biology, innovative experimental techniques like photoporation gain importance. This novel method enables precise internalization of molecules into cells using light-triggered permeation. Grasping the principles behind photoporation is crucial for its successful application, fostering ongoing innovation and enhancements in the field.

Photoporation has numerous in vitro and in vivo applications, from fundamental cellular research to clinical cancer therapy. The most significant advancements are seen in tissue applications, quickly adopted by labs, fostering vibrant research. With specific wavelengths, photoporation demonstrates impressive tissue selectivity and scalability via implantable devices. A deeper understanding of the processes involved and ongoing technological advancements will address challenges in micromirror control, transient phenomena, endoscopy-compatible light delivery, and high-power light sources. This progress may lead to novel medical interventions, potentially transforming biological sciences. The future of photoporation holds vast opportunities across life sciences, with many research avenues still to explore.

References

Aksel, M., Bozkurt-Girit, O., & Bilgin, M. D. (2020). Pheophorbide a-mediated sonodynamic, photodynamic and sonophotodynamic therapies against prostate cancer. *Photodiagnosis and Photodynamic Therapy*, *31*, 101909. 10.1016/j.pdpdt.2020.101909

Aksel, M., Erdoğan, Ö., & Bilgin, M. (2024). The Investigation of Efficiency of Pheophorbide-A Mediated Sonodynamic Therapy on Prostate Cancer 3D Cell Culture Model. *International Journal of Pure and Applied Sciences*, *10*(1), 47-56. 10.29132/ijpas.1393943

Aksel, M., Kesmez, Ö., Yavaş, A., & Bilgin, M. D. (2021). Titaniumdioxide mediated sonophotodynamic therapy against prostate cancer. *Journal of Photochemistry and Photobiology B: Biology*, *225*. 10.1016/j.jphotobiol.2021.112333

Alimi, L. O., Alyami, M. Z., Chand, S., Baslyman, W., & Khashab, N. M. (2021). Coordination-based self-assembled capsules (SACs) for protein,

CRISPR-Cas9, DNA and RNA delivery. *Chemical Science*. 10.1039/d0sc05975g

Breunig, H. G., König, A., & König, K. (2022). *Femtosecond-laser induced membrane optoporation for transfection and cell reprogramming*. 10.1117/12.2607258

Bu, L., Chen, B., Xing, L., Cai, X., Liang, S., Zhang, L., … Song, W. (2022). Generation of a pdmH1N1 2018 Influenza A Reporter Virus Carrying a mCherry Fluorescent Protein in the PA Segment. *Frontiers in Cellular and Infection Microbiology*, *11*. 10.3389/fcimb. 2021. 827790

Du, X., Wang, J., Chen, L., Zhang, Z., & Yao, C. (2021). Delivery of foreign materials into adherent cells by gold nanoparticle-mediated photoporation. *Membranes*, *11*(8). 10.3390/membranes11080550

Du, X., Zhao, M., Jiang, L., Pang, L., Wang, J., Lv, Y., … Wu, R. (2024). A mini-review on gene delivery technique using nanoparticles-mediated photoporation induced by nanosecond pulsed laser. *Drug Delivery*. 10.1080/10717544.2024.2306231

Duan, X., Wan, J. M. F., & Mak, A. F. T. (2017). Oxidative Stress Alters the Morphological Responses of Myoblasts to Single-Site Membrane Photoporation. *Cellular and Molecular Bioengineering*, *10*(4). 10.1007/s12195-017-0488-5

Fraire, J. C., Houthaeve, G., Liu, J., Raes, L., Vermeulen, L., Stremersch, S., … Braeckmans, K. (2020). Vapor nanobubble is the more reliable photothermal mechanism for inducing endosomal escape of siRNA without disturbing cell homeostasis. *Journal of Controlled Release*, *319*. 10.1016/j.jconrel.2019.12.050

Fuqiang, W., Xinping, Z., Yan, D., Hongliang, Y., Shi, X., Yang, L., & Ziming, C. (2022). Progress in radiative transfer in porous medium: A review from macro scale to pore scale with experimental test. *Applied Thermal Engineering*, *210*. 10.1016/j.applthermaleng.2022.118331

Goemaere, I., Punj, D., Harizaj, A., Woolston, J., Thys, S., Sterck, K., … Braeckmans, K. (2023). Response Surface Methodology to Efficiently Optimize Intracellular Delivery by Photoporation. *International Journal of Molecular Sciences*, *24*(4). 10.3390/ijms24043147

Haleem, A., Javaid, M., Pratap Singh, R., & Suman, R. (2022). Medical 4.0 technologies for healthcare: Features, capabilities, and applications. *Internet of Things and Cyber-Physical Systems*. 10.1016/j.iotcps. 2022.04.001

Heinemann, D., Zabic, M., Terakawa, M., & Boch, J. (2022). Laser-based molecular delivery and its applications in plant science. *Plant Methods*. 10.1186/s13007-022-00908-9

Hosokawa, Y., Ochi, H., Iino, T., Hiraoka, A., & Tanaka, M. (2011). Photoporation of biomolecules into single cells in living vertebrate embryos induced by a femtosecond laser amplifier. *PLoS ONE*, *6*(11). 10.1371/journal.pone.0027677

Huang, L., Zhou, M., Abbas, G., Li, C., Cui, M., Zhang, X. E., & Wang, D. B. (2022). A Cancer Cell Membrane-Derived Biomimetic Nanocarrier for Synergistic Photothermal/Gene Therapy by Efficient Delivery of CRISPR/Cas9 and Gold Nanorods. *Advanced Healthcare Materials*, *11*(16). 10.1002/adhm.202201038

Jahangiri-Manesh, A., Mousazadeh, M., Taji, S., Bahmani, A., Zarepour, A., Zarrabi, A., … Azimzadeh, M. (2022). Gold Nanorods for Drug and Gene Delivery: An Overview of Recent Advancements. *Pharmaceutics*. 10.3390/pharmaceutics14030664

Jeong, H., Lee, C. S., Lee, J., Lee, J., Hwang, H. S., Lee, M., & Na, K. (2021). Hemagglutinin Nanoparticulate Vaccine with Controlled Photochemical Immunomodulation for Pathogenic Influenza-Specific Immunity. *Advanced Science*, *8*(23). 10.1002/advs.202100118

Kanu, G. A., Parambath, J. B. M., Abu Odeh, R. O., & Mohamed, A. A. (2022). Gold Nanoparticle-Mediated Gene Therapy. *Cancers*. 10.3390/cancers14215366

Kastenschmidt, J. M., Sureshchandra, S., Jain, A., Hernandez-Davies, J. E., de Assis, R., Wagoner, Z. W., … Wagar, L. E. (2023). Influenza vaccine format mediates distinct cellular and antibody responses in human immune organoids. *Immunity*, *56*(8). 10.1016/j.immuni.2023.06.019

Krasnikov, I., Seteikin, A., & Roth, B. (2019). Advances in the simulation of light–tissue interactions in biomedical engineering. *Biomedical Engineering Letters*. 10.1007/s13534-019-00123-x

Kumar, Arun. (2021). Photoporation developed as an effective nonviral gene delivery system. *MRS Bulletin*, *46*(9). 10.1557/s43577-021-00177-2

Kumar, Ashish, Nahak, B. K., Gupta, P., Santra, T. S., & Tseng, F. G. (2024). Laser-Induced Intracellular Delivery: Exploiting Gold-Coated Spiky Polymeric Nanoparticles and Gold Nanorods under Near-Infrared Pulses for Single-Cell Nano-Photon-Poration. *Micromachines*, *15*(2). 10.3390/mi15020168

Kumar, S., Lazau, E., Kim, C., Thadhani, N. N., & Prausnitz, M. R. (2021). Serum protects cells and increases intracellular delivery of molecules by nanoparticle-mediated photoporation. *International Journal of Nanomedicine*, *16*. 10.2147/IJN.S307027

Landreth, S., Lu, Y., Pandey, K., & Zhou, Y. (2020). A replication-defective influenza virus vaccine confers complete protection against H7N9 viral infection in mice. *Vaccines*, *8*(2). 10.3390/vaccines 8020207

Layachi, M., Treizebré, A., Hay, L., Gilbert, D., Pesez, J., D'Acremont, Q., … Courtade, E. (2023). Novel opto-fluidic drug delivery system for efficient cellular transfection. *Journal of Nanobiotechnology*, *21*(1). 10.1186/s12951-023-01797-3

Liu, J., Li, C., Brans, T., Harizaj, A., Van de Steene, S., De Beer, T., … Braeckmans, K. (2020). Surface functionalization with polyethylene glycol and polyethyleneimine improves the performance of graphene-based materials for safe and efficient intracellular delivery by laser-induced photoporation. *International Journal of Molecular Sciences*, *21*(4). 10.3390/ijms21041540

Liu, J., Xiong, R., Brans, T., Lippens, S., Parthoens, E., Zanacchi, F. C., … Braeckmans, K. (2018). Repeated photoporation with graphene quantum dots enables homogeneous labeling of live cells with extrinsic markers for fluorescence microscopy. *Light: Science and Applications*, *7*(1). 10.1038/s41377-018-0048-3

Luo, T., Nie, Y., Lu, J., Bi, Q., Cai, Z., Song, X., … Jin, R. (2021). Iron doped carbon dots based nanohybrids as a tetramodal imaging agent for gene delivery promotion and photothermal-chemodynamic cancer synergistic theranostics. *Materials and Design*, *208*. 10.1016/j.matdes. 2021.109878

Maeno, T., Uzawa, T., Kono, I., Okano, K., Iino, T., Fukita, K., … Hosokawa, Y. (2018). Targeted delivery of fluorogenic peptide aptamers into live microalgae by femtosecond laser photoporation at single-cell resolution. *Scientific Reports*, *8*(1). 10.1038/s41598-018-26565-4

McGraw, E., Laurent, G. M., & Avila, L. A. (2024). Nanoparticle-Mediated Photoporation: Expanding Horizons in Drug Delivery. *Nanoscale Advances*, *6*(20), 5007-5019. 10.1039/D4NA00122B

Mitchell, C. A., Kalies, S., Cizmár, T., Heisterkamp, A., Torrance, L., Roberts, A. G., … Dholakia, K. (2013). Femtosecond optoinjection of intact tobacco BY-2 cells using a reconfigurable photoporation platform. *PLoS ONE*, *8*(11). 10.1371/journal.pone.0079235

Mohan, L., Kar, S., Mahapatra, P. S., Nagai, M., & Santra, T. S. (2021). Fabrication of TiO2microspikes for highly efficient intracellular delivery by pulse laser-assisted photoporation. *RSC Advances*, *11*(16). 10.1039/d0ra09785c

O'Gorman, W. E., Huang, H., Wei, Y. L., Davis, K. L., Leipold, M. D., Bendall, S. C., … Davis, M. M. (2014). The Split Virus Influenza

Vaccine rapidly activates immune cells through Fcγ receptors. *Vaccine*, *32*(45). 10.1016/j.vaccine.2014.07.115

Pylaev, T. E., Efremov, Y., Avdeeva, E. S., Antoshin, A. A., Shpichka, A. I., Khlebnikova, T. M., … Khlebtsov, N. G. (2021). Optoporation and Recovery of Living Cells under Au Nanoparticle Layer-Mediated NIR-Laser Irradiation. *ACS Applied Nano Materials*, *4*(12). 10.1021/acsanm.1c02734

Raes, L., Pille, M., Harizaj, A., Goetgeluk, G., Van Hoeck, J., Stremersch, S., … Braeckmans, K. (2021). Cas9 RNP transfection by vapor nanobubble photoporation for ex vivo cell engineering. *Molecular Therapy Nucleic Acids*, *25*. 10.1016/j.omtn.2021.08.014

Raes, L., Stremersch, S., Fraire, J. C., Brans, T., Goetgeluk, G., De Munter, S., … Braeckmans, K. (2020). Intracellular Delivery of mRNA in Adherent and Suspension Cells by Vapor Nanobubble Photoporation. *Nano-Micro Letters*, *12*(1). 10.1007/s40820-020-00523-0

Ramon, J., Xiong, R., De Smedt, S. C., Raemdonck, K., & Braeckmans, K. (2021). Vapor nanobubble-mediated photoporation constitutes a versatile intracellular delivery technology. *Current Opinion in Colloid and Interface Science*. 10.1016/j.cocis.2021.101453

Rau, K., & Rentmeister, A. (2017). Making the Message Clear: Concepts for mRNA Imaging. *ACS Central Science*, *3*(7). 10.1021/acscentsci.7b00251

Roy, M., & Roy, A. (2021). The Rise of Interdisciplinarity in Engineering Education in the Era of Industry 4.0: Implications for Management Practice. *IEEE Engineering Management Review*, *49*(3). 10.1109/EMR.2021.3095426

Roy, S., Meena, T., & Lim, S. J. (2022). Demystifying Supervised Learning in Healthcare 4.0: A New Reality of Transforming Diagnostic Medicine. *Diagnostics*. 10.3390/diagnostics12102549

Rudhall, A. P., Antkowiak, M., Tsampoula, X., Mazilu, M., Metzger, N. K., Gunn-Moore, F., & Dholakia, K. (2012). Exploring the ultrashort pulse laser parameter space for membrane permeabilisation in mammalian cells. *Scientific Reports*, *2*. 10.1038/srep00858

Rukmana, T. I., Moran, G., Méallet-Renault, R., Ohtani, M., Demura, T., Yasukuni, R., & Hosokawa, Y. (2019). Enzyme-Assisted Photoinjection of Megadalton Molecules into Intact Plant Cells Using Femtosecond Laser Amplifier. *Scientific Reports*, *9*(1). 10.1038/s41598-019-54124-y

Shinde, A., Kar, S., Nagai, M., Tseng, F. G., & Santra, T. S. (2021). Light-Induced Cellular Delivery and Analysis. Dans *Handbook of Single-Cell Technologies*. 10.1007/978-981-10-8953-4_4

Sreedevi, P. R., & Suresh, K. (2023). Cold atmospheric plasma mediated cell membrane permeation and gene delivery-empirical interventions and pertinence. *Advances in Colloid and Interface Science*. 10.1016/j.cis.2023.102989

Sung, Y. K., & Kim, S. W. (2019). Recent advances in the development of gene delivery systems. *Biomaterials Research*. 10.1186/s40824-019-0156-z

Taha, E. A., Lee, J., & Hotta, A. (2022). Delivery of CRISPR-Cas tools for in vivo genome editing therapy: Trends and challenges. *Journal of Controlled Release*. 10.1016/j.jconrel.2022.01.013

Xiong, R., Sauvage, F., Fraire, J. C., Huang, C., De Smedt, S. C., & Braeckmans, K. (2023). Photothermal Nanomaterial-Mediated Photoporation. *Accounts of Chemical Research*, *56*(6). 10.1021/acs.accounts.2c00770

Xiong, R., Verstraelen, P., Demeester, J., Skirtach, A. G., Timmermans, J. P., De Smedt, S. C., … Braeckmans, K. (2018). Selective labeling of individual neurons in dense cultured networks with nanoparticle-enhanced photoporation. *Frontiers in Cellular Neuroscience*, *12*. 10.3389/fncel.2018.00080

Zhou, Q., Liu, Q., Wang, Y., Chen, J., Schmid, O., Rehberg, M., & Yang, L. (2024). Bridging Smart Nanosystems with Clinically Relevant Models and Advanced Imaging for Precision Drug Delivery. *Advanced Science*. 10.1002/advs.202308659

Author Biographies

Assistant Prof. Dr. Mehran Aksel graduated from Eskişehir Osmangazi University and pursed Master of Science from Osmangazi University of Eskisehir, Turkey in year 2011. He is earned Ph.D. in Department of Biophysics, Adnan Menderes University of Aydin, Turkey in 2019. He serves in the Department of Biophysics at Aydın Adnan Menderes University Faculty of Medicine. His academic studies focus on the intersection of biophysics with medicine and biomedical technology. He particularly concentrates on innovative approaches in cancer treatment, including sonophotodynamic therapy, nanomaterial applications, and mechanisms of cell death. He develops projects that integrate molecular biology, biochemistry, and biophysics by employing both experimental animal models and cell culture studies. As an educator, he teaches not only biophysics but also courses that span different disciplines such as sports biomechanics, biomedical technologies, and the biophysics of the nervous system, providing students with an interdisciplinary perspective.

Prof. Dr. Mehmet Dinçer Bilgin graduated from Ankara University Faculty of Medicine and earned his Ph.D. in Biophysics at the Illinois Institute of Technology (Chicago, USA) between 1994 and 1999. During his doctorate, he worked on photodynamic therapy at Ravenswood Hospital's Wenske Laser Center and later conducted postdoctoral research in cellular biophysics at Northwestern University Feinberg School of Medicine. Since 2000, he has been the Chair of the Department of Biophysics at Aydın Adnan Menderes University Faculty of Medicine. He became Associate Professor in 2006 and Professor in 2011, becoming the second medical doctor in Turkey to achieve this in Biophysics. He has supervised 9 master's and 12 Ph.D. theses and contributed to 15 projects funded by TÜBİTAK or TÜSEB. His research interests include cancer therapies such as photodynamic and sonodynamic treatments, laser–tissue interactions, the medical use of non-ionizing radiation, ultrasound, and neuroscience. **ORCID:** 0000-0003-0754-0854

Prof. Dr. Mehmet Bilgen has been involved in educational and collaborative research activities in the areas of theoretical, experimental and medical physics, nondestructive testing, engineering, biomedicine, biotechnology, experiments with animal models and development of disease-oriented therapies.

CHAPTER 17

ELECTROPORATION PRINCIPLES AND APPLICATIONS

ELÇIN ÖZGÜR BÜYÜKATALAY[1], HANDAN KAYHAN[2,3]

[1] Gazi University Faculty of Medicine, Department of Biophysics, Ankara, Türkiye
[2] Gazi University Faculty of Medicine, Department of Adult Hematology, Ankara, Türkiye
[3] Exo Life Biotechnology Ltd. Co., Ankara, Türkiye

Abstract

Electroporation has emerged as a pivotal physical method for delivering genetic materials and therapeutic molecules into cells through transient membrane permeabilization. This chapter provides a comprehensive examination of electroporation technology, from fundamental biophysical principles to cutting-edge technological innovations.

We begin by elucidating the molecular mechanisms of membrane permeabilization, including the pore formation cascade (hydrophobic to hydrophilic transitions), water wire formation and lipid reorganization revealed through molecular dynamics simulations, and biphasic membrane resealing kinetics. Critical operational parameters are systematically analyzed, encompassing electrical variables (field strength, pulse duration, pulse number), biological factors (cell geometry, membrane composition), and environmental conditions (buffer composition, temperature). DNA uptake mechanisms are examined in detail, revealing the synergistic roles of electrophoresis, diffusion, and endocytosis-like processes.

The chapter then explores technological innovations transforming electroporation into precision delivery platforms. Microfluidic systems enable high-throughput processing with real-time monitoring and minimal sample volumes, demonstrated through semi-continuous flow devices and droplet-based platforms. Nanoscale approaches, including nanochannel electroporation and nanostraw systems, achieve unprecedented precision by focusing electric fields to subcellular membrane regions, delivering biomolecules at dramatically reduced voltages with maintaining high cell viability. Force-controlled nanofluidic delivery (FluidFM) extends spatial precision to individual subcellular structures. This comprehensive overview provides essential knowledge for optimizing electroporation protocols and advancing therapeutic applications in gene delivery and cellular engineering.

Keywords: Electroporation, Microfluidics, Membrane pore Dynamics, Nanoelectroporation, transfection

1. Introduction

The successful translation of gene therapy from bench to bedside hinges critically on the development of safe, efficient delivery systems capable of transporting therapeutic genetic material across cellular membranes. Among the diverse array of available delivery modalities, electroporation stands out as a physical method that circumvents many limitations inherent to viral vectors and chemical transfection agents (Neumann et al. 1982). First demonstrated in the early 1980s for DNA transfer into mouse lymphoma cells, electroporation has undergone remarkable evolution from a laboratory curiosity to a therapeutic platform in clinical use, with applications spanning oncology, immunotherapy, and infectious disease prevention (Neumann et al. 1982; Daud et al. 2008).

The fundamental premise of electroporation—also termed electropermeabilization—involves applying brief electrical pulses to cells or tissues, thereby creating transient aqueous pores in the plasma membrane through which normally impermeant molecules can traverse. This approach offers several distinct advantages. Unlike viral vectors, electroporation imposes no theoretical limit on cargo size, enabling delivery of large plasmids, linear DNA fragments, and even chromosomal segments (Potter, Weir, and Leder 1984). The direct cytoplasmic delivery bypasses endosomal entrapment and degradation, a common pitfall of chemical transfection methods (Golzio, Teissié, and Rols 2002). Moreover, the transient nature of membrane permeabilization minimizes long-term cellular perturbation while achieving high transfection efficiencies across diverse cell types, including traditionally difficult-to-transfect primary cells and stem cells.

Recent technological advances have expanded electroporation's clinical utility considerably. The development of standardized protocols for electrochemotherapy, which has received regulatory approval in several European countries, has made this modality an established treatment option for cutaneous metastases (Marty et al. 2006). Irreversible electroporation has carved a niche in ablative oncology for tumors adjacent to critical structures where thermal methods pose unacceptable risks (Martin et al. 2013). Perhaps most significantly, electroporation-mediated delivery of CRISPR-Cas9 components has enabled ex vivo genome editing of therapeutic cells, with early clinical trials in β-thalassemia and sickle cell disease demonstrating remarkable therapeutic responses (CRISPR Therapeutics 2021).

This chapter examines electroporation through multiple lenses: the biophysical mechanisms governing membrane permeabilization, the critical parameters determining treatment outcomes, technological innovations enhancing precision and efficiency. Understanding these facets provides essential context for integrating electroporation into comprehensive gene therapy strategies.

2. Fundamental Principles of Electroporation

2.1 Biophysical Mechanisms of Membrane Permeabilization

The cell membrane, comprising a lipid bilayer approximately 5 nm thick, serves as the primary barrier to molecular exchange between intracellular and extracellular compartments. Under resting conditions, mammalian cells maintain a transmembrane potential of approximately -70 to -40 mV, with the cytoplasm negative relative to the extracellular space (Kotnik et al. 2012). When cells are exposed to external electric fields, an induced transmembrane voltage (iTMV) develops across the membrane, adding vectorially to the resting potential. The magnitude of this induced voltage depends on cell geometry, field orientation, and field strength, with spherical cells experiencing maximal voltage induction at poles aligned with the field vector.

2.1.1 The Pore Formation Cascade

Electroporation proceeds through a well-characterized sequence of events. When the total transmembrane voltage (resting plus induced) exceeds a critical threshold—typically 200 mV for mammalian cells (Rols and Teissié 1990)—the lipid bilayer undergoes structural destabilization. This threshold corresponds to external field strengths of approximately 0.7 to 1.5 kV/cm and remains remarkably constant across cell types despite variations in membrane biochemical composition, suggesting a fundamental biophysical basis rather than specific molecular interactions (Rols and Teissié 1990).

Initial membrane defects manifest as small hydrophobic pores approximately 1 nm in diameter, formed when thermal fluctuations create local membrane thinning coincident with high transmembrane voltage. These transient structures are energetically unstable and either reseal rapidly or, if the electric field persists, transition to larger hydrophilic pores (Glaser et al. 1988). The hydrophilic configuration, characterized by pore walls lined with phospholipid headgroups oriented toward the aqueous channel, exhibits significantly greater stability. Pore diameters can expand to tens of nanometers under sustained field exposure, with experimental evidence suggesting individual pores may reach 10 nm under extreme conditions (Hibino et al. 1991).

The temporal dynamics of pore formation and evolution have been captured through sophisticated imaging approaches. Hibino and colleagues demonstrated that pores form within microseconds of pulse application and can persist for seconds to minutes following field removal, depending on pulse parameters and cellular context (Hibino et al. 1991). This extended lifetime enables molecular transport through the permeabilized membrane, though larger molecules require longer permeabilization periods for efficient uptake.

2.1.2 Membrane Resealing and Cell Recovery

Following electroporation, cells must reseal membrane defects to restore barrier function and maintain viability. This resealing process exhibits biphasic kinetics. Small pores (< 5 nm) reseal within milliseconds through lipid relaxation and thermal fluctuations, essentially reversing the formation process. Larger pores require extended resealing periods—from minutes to hours—with the process showing strong temperature and ionic strength dependence (Kinosita and Tsong 1977). Resealing typically completes within minutes to hours, though complete restoration of membrane properties may require longer periods.

Temperature profoundly influences resealing kinetics. At 4°C, membrane fluidity decreases, slowing both pore formation and resealing. While this prolongs the permeabilization window—potentially enhancing uptake of slowly diffusing macromolecules—it also extends cellular vulnerability to osmotic stress and ionic imbalance. Conversely, elevated temperatures accelerate lipid dynamics and membrane repair mechanisms, potentially improving cell survival at the cost of reduced uptake efficiency. Most protocols employ 4°C for the electroporation step itself, followed by transfer to 37°C for recovery, balancing these competing considerations.

2.1.3 Alternative Permeabilization Mechanisms

Beyond the classical pore hypothesis, several complementary mechanisms contribute to membrane permeabilization, as revealed through advanced molecular dynamics simulations and experimental validations. These alternative pathways provide a more nuanced understanding of electroporation at the molecular level, particularly relevant for optimizing biotechnological applications where precise control over membrane permeability is critical.

Molecular dynamics simulations have revealed that strong electric fields (0.5-1.0 V/nm) induce water defects—essentially water molecules penetrating into the hydrophobic core of the bilayer—which can coalesce into single-file water wires bridging the membrane (Tarek 2005). This process occurs remarkably rapidly, with initial water finger formation observed within 200 ps to 4 ns depending on field strength. These water-filled channels may facilitate ion flux even in the absence of stable lipid pores, representing a "prepore" state that precedes classical pore formation.

Significantly, water penetration appears to initiate from both sides of the bilayer simultaneously, independent of field direction, suggesting that local field gradients at the water-lipid interface drive this phenomenon rather than bulk field orientation alone. These water wires subsequently expand in diameter and recruit lipid headgroups from the membrane-water interface, transforming hydrophobic pathways into stable hydrophilic pores lined by reoriented phospholipid headgroups.

Following water wire formation, a critical transition occurs as polar lipid headgroups migrate from the membrane surface toward the bilayer interior (Tarek 2005). This lipid reorganization, occurring on a timescale of 1-4 ns depending on field strength, represents the rate-limiting step for stable pore formation. The resulting structures exhibit irregular, non-cylindrical morphologies with mixed hydrophilic-hydrophobic surfaces—dramatically different from idealized toroidal pore models often depicted in conceptual frameworks.

Importantly, these pores maintain significant contact between transported molecules and lipid acyl chains, suggesting that molecular transport involves more complex mechanisms than simple diffusion through purely aqueous channels. This observation has implications for predicting permeability to different molecular species and designing protocols for size-selective delivery.

Upon field removal, electroporated membranes undergo spontaneous resealing through a sequence of events that essentially reverses pore formation. Molecular dynamics simulations demonstrate complete membrane reconstitution within 2-4 ns for pores stabilized by lipid headgroups, with smaller hydrophobic water wires resealing even faster (250-500 ps) (Tarek 2005). This rapid intrinsic resealing capability contrasts with experimental observations of much longer pore lifetimes (milliseconds to seconds), suggesting that factors beyond lipid dynamics—such as ionic stabilization, membrane composition, and cellular repair mechanisms—govern practical resealing kinetics.

Electrocompressive forces, arising from the Maxwell stress tensor at interfaces between media of differing dielectric constants, can compress and thin the membrane, reducing the energy barrier for defect formation (Weaver 2000). Additionally, transmembrane proteins undergo conformational changes in response to altered membrane voltage, potentially creating permeabilization pathways through protein channels or at lipid-protein interfaces. The relative contributions of these mechanisms likely vary depending on specific experimental conditions and membrane composition.

2.2 Critical Parameters Governing Electroporation Outcomes

Successful electroporation requires optimization across multiple interdependent parameters. These factors collectively determine the balance between achieving sufficient membrane permeabilization for efficient molecular uptake and maintaining cell viability.

2.2.1 Electrical Parameters

Field Strength

The electric field strength (E), defined as the voltage (V) divided by the electrode gap distance (d), represents the primary determinant of membrane permeabilization. For *in vitro* applications, optimal field strengths typically range from 100 to 1000 V/cm, with exact values depending on cell type, pulse duration, and desired outcomes (Miklavčič et al. 2014). Smaller cells generally require higher field strengths to achieve threshold transmembrane voltage, while larger cells permeabilize at lower field strengths. *In vivo* applications typically employ lower field strengths (100-400 V/cm) due to tissue heterogeneity and the need to minimize muscle contractions and tissue damage.

Pulse Duration and Waveform

Pulse duration critically influences both permeabilization efficiency and cell viability. Microsecond pulses (10-100 μs) represent the conventional choice for gene delivery, providing sufficient duration for pore formation and molecular uptake while limiting thermal effects and cell damage. The most commonly pulse frequency is eight of 100-μs-long pulses (Miklavčič et al. 2014). The pulse shape also matters: square wave pulses, which maintain constant voltage throughout the pulse duration, offer superior control and reproducibility compared to exponentially decaying pulses generated by capacitor discharge systems (Kotnik and Miklavčič 2006). Initially, capacitor discharge pulse generators were used, but square wave generators became more prominent due to their better reproducibility of pulses and control over electroporation (Miklavčič et al. 2014).

Recent investigations into nanosecond pulsed electric fields (nsPEF) have revealed distinct biological effects. Pulses shorter than 10 ns can penetrate intracellular membranes, permeabilizing organelles including mitochondria, endoplasmic reticulum, and nuclear envelope while leaving the plasma membrane relatively intact. For example, when 3-5 pulses of 60 ns duration were applied to human eosinophils, their intracellular granules were modified without causing permanent disruption of the plasma membrane (Schoenbach, Beebe, and Buescher 2001). This enables novel applications including intracellular calcium mobilization and selective organelle targeting, though gene delivery applications primarily employ longer microsecond pulses for plasma membrane permeabilization.

Pulse Number and Repetition Rate

Multiple pulses generally increase permeabilization efficiency and molecular uptake compared to single pulses, up to a point. Each successive pulse enlarges existing pores and creates additional defects, expanding the permeabilized membrane area. However, excessive pulse numbers increase cell mortality through cumulative membrane damage, ionic imbalance, and metabolic stress (Mir et al. 1999). Most protocols employ 1 to 8 pulses, with intervals ranging from milliseconds to seconds. The optimal pulse number represents a balance between uptake efficiency and cell viability, varying with cell type and application. For example, a highly efficient method for plasmid DNA transfer into muscle fibers has been developed, utilizing square-wave electric pulses. These pulses are characterized by low field strength (under 300 V/cm) and long duration (over 1 ms) (Mir et al. 1999).

2.2.2 Biological and Environmental Parameters

Cell Characteristics

Cell size and shapes directly influences electroporation outcomes through its effect on induced transmembrane voltage. The shape of a cell significantly influences how its Induced Transmembrane Voltage (ITV) is calculated, with different approaches used for regular versus irregular geometries. For cells with sufficiently regular shapes, such as spheres, spheroids, or cylinders, and that are far apart in dilute suspensions, the time dependence and spatial distribution of the ITV can be derived using analytical methods. This involves solving partial differential equations, which simplify to the Laplace equation in a steady state, and applying realistic boundary conditions to determine the electric potential across the membrane (Kotnik et al. 2012).

For a single spherical cell with a nonconductive plasma membrane, the steady-state Schwan equation is used:

$$\nabla\Psi_{\mathrm{m}} = \tfrac{3}{2}\, E\, R \cos\theta,$$

E is the electric field, *R* is the cell radius, and θ is the angle measured from the center of the cell with respect to the direction of the field. (Kotnik et al. 2012).

Generally, in electroporation, larger cells or tissues can be permeabilized with lower external field strengths compared to smaller cells because the potential drop across the membrane is proportional to the cell radius, meaning a larger cell experiences a greater transmembrane potential for the same external field. Cell membrane composition also matters: cholesterol content, lipid saturation, and membrane protein abundance all modulate permeabilization susceptibility and resealing kinetics. This means membranes with higher cholesterol content are less susceptible to permeabilization. (Tarek 2005).

Buffer Composition

The electroporation medium significantly impacts outcomes. Low-conductivity buffers reduce joule heating and enable higher field strengths or longer pulse durations before thermal damage occurs. However, cells require minimal ionic strength to maintain viability, necessitating balanced formulations. Most protocols employ buffers with conductivities between 0.1 and 2.0 mS/cm, incorporating low sodium chloride concentrations with osmotic balance provided by non-ionic compounds such as sucrose or mannitol (Pucihar et al. 2001).

Pucihar et al. investigated the influence of extracellular medium conductivity on the electropermeabilization and survival of cells across a broad range of conductivities (approximately 0.001 to 1.5 S/m). Cells were exposed to trains of eight rectangular electric pulses (100 μs duration, 1 Hz repetition frequency) with amplitudes ranging from 0 to 400 V. They found that the percentage of surviving cells increased as the medium conductivity decreased. Cells with highest conductivity showed the lowest 50% survival threshold (267 V), with other media showing higher thresholds in descending order of conductivity. In addition, the percentage of electropermeabilized cells remained unaffected by changes in medium conductivity (Pucihar et al. 2001).

Temperature

As noted previously, temperature influences membrane fluidity, pore dynamics, and cellular metabolism. Standard protocols perform electroporation at 4°C to reduce thermal effects and metabolic stress, then transfer cells to 37°C for recovery and DNA uptake. Some protocols maintain 4°C throughout to maximize pore lifetime for large cargo delivery, accepting reduced recovery rates.

2.3 DNA Uptake Mechanisms

The mechanisms by which DNA enters electroporated cells involve multiple processes acting in concert. It is a complex process where DNA's electrophoretic movement plays a crucial role, influencing membrane permeability and actively participating in the expansion and modification of electropores to facilitate its entry into the cell. Electrophoresis—the migration of charged molecules in electric fields—drives DNA toward the membrane and into pores, with the DNA backbone's negative charge ensuring movement toward the positive electrode (Sukharev et al. 1992).

The electrophoretic contribution is particularly significant during the pulse, when both field strength and pore size are maximal.

Following pulse termination, diffusion through enlarged pores continues to transport DNA, though at reduced efficiency. The presence of DNA in the cell suspension significantly increases membrane permeability to molecules like dextrans (Sukharev et al. 1992). Sukharev et al reported a two-pulse method was employed to distinguish between membrane electroporation and DNA electrophoresis. A short, high-intensity first pulse (6 kV/cm, 10 μs) creates pores efficiently but results in low transfection efficiency (TE). A subsequent longer, lower-amplitude second pulse (0.2 kV/cm, 10 ms), which alone does not cause poration or transfection, significantly enhances TE by about an order of magnitude when applied after the first pulse. While electropores are estimated to be 1-10 nm, and DNA molecules can be much larger (up to 2,000 nm for 150 kb), DNA's flexibility allows for orientation and deformation in an electric field, enabling its entry dextrans (Sukharev et al. 1992).

Recent evidence also implicates endocytosis-like processes for DNA uptake following electroporation. Unlike small molecules, which primarily enter through simple diffusion after an electric pulse, the entry of macromolecules such as DNA occurs through a multistep mechanism. For larger molecules (those with a molecular weight above 4 kDa), direct transfer to the cytoplasm is observed only if these macromolecules (e.g., proteins, DNA) are present during the application of the electric pulse. This suggests that the mechanism for macromolecule uptake differs significantly from that of small molecules. Membrane disruption triggers compensatory endocytosis to remove damaged membrane patches, potentially internalizing membrane-associated DNA in the process (Escoffre et al. 2009).

3. Technological Advancements in Electroporation Systems

3.1 Miniaturization: Micro- and Nanoelectroporation

Traditional bulk electroporation systems, employing cuvettes with millimeter-scale electrode gaps, have served effectively for decades. However, miniaturization to micro- and nanoscale dimensions has unlocked new capabilities while addressing persistent challenges.

3.1.1 Microfluidic Electroporation Platforms

Microfluidic electroporation platforms are microfluidic devices that combine fluidic channels at the micrometer scale with integrated electric fields to transiently permeabilize cell membranes for the delivery of nucleic acids and other cargos, enabling controlled, high-throughput transfection within a fluidic workflow. The core concept is the use of microfluidic channels where cells (with or without cargo) travel through regions with applied electric fields, permitting continuous flow or semi-continuous flow electroporation processes "Semi-continuous Flow Electroporation Chip for High Throughput Transfection on Mammalian Cells" (Wang et al. 2009). Wang et al, reported this device on K562 cells which were porated with unipolar square wave electric pulses (150V, 10-25 ms). As a result, transfection efficiency was 100% improved (from ~5% to ~10% for 25 ms pulse).

Zhan and colleagues developed a microfluidic device for cell electroporation within aqueous droplets formed in an oil phase. In the device, cell-containing droplets undergo electroporation as they flow past a pair of surface microelectrodes (~20 μm apart) with constant voltage applied. The duration and intensity of electroporation are controlled by droplet velocity (1.38-8.86 m/min), droplet dimensions (60-386 μm), electrode distance, and applied voltage (5-9 V), with transit times ranging from 0.37 to 21.6 ms. The system has been successfully used for transferring a plasmid vector encoding enhanced green fluorescent protein into cells. Critical factors in optimizing electroporation efficiency include the applied voltage (higher voltage increases transfection efficiency but reduces viability from ~68% at 4.7 V to ~14% at 7.1 V), droplet flow rate and dimensions, electrode distance, and the location of cells within the droplets. The study demonstrated that achieving optimal results requires a delicate balance between providing sufficient electrical shock for gene delivery and maintaining cell viability, with transfection efficiency being influenced by the combination of electrical parameters, droplet dimensions, and cell localization within the droplets (Zhan et al. 2009).

Microfluidic devices enable real-time monitoring of electroporation progress. Transparent channel materials (PDMS, glass) permit optical observation of cell behavior during and after pulse application. Integrated sensors can measure impedance changes or fluorescence signals reporting intracellular events, providing data for parameter characterization and assessment of electroporation effectiveness (Khine et al. 2005).

Despite these advantages, microfluidic electroporation faces several technical and practical challenges. Device fabrication using PDMS micromolding and surface micromachining for silicon molds requires specialized expertise and equipment (Khine et al. 2005). Operational challenges include maintaining system stability and preventing disruptions to flow patterns. Narrow channel geometries—such as the 4 μm × 3.1 μm cross-sectional trapping channels used by Khine et al. or the ~20 μm electrode gaps in Zhan et al.'s droplet system—demand precise fluidic control. Cell trapping requires careful pressure management; Khine et al. applied approximately -22 psi negative pressure via syringe to hydrodynamically trap individual HeLa cells, with the resulting viscoelastic deformation during trapping representing an additional process variable. In droplet-based systems, maintaining stable droplet generation and consistent dimensions is critical—Zhan et al. reported that droplet size (60-386 μm) directly influences electric field exposure duration and peak current, with transit times ranging from 0.37 to 21.6 ms depending on droplet velocity (1.38-8.86 m/min) and dimensions. Throughput limitations represent significant constraints for applications requiring large cell numbers. Single-cell devices like Khine's chip process cells sequentially with approximately 6.5 ms pulse duration per cell, and although parallel trapping capability was demonstrated, substantial device parallelization would be required for higher-throughput applications. Zhan's continuous-flow droplet approach offers higher throughput potential, but faces the challenge that increased voltage significantly reduces cell viability—from approximately 68% at 4.7 V to about 14% at 7.1 V—necessitating careful parameter balancing between transfection efficiency and cell survival.

Voltage optimization and monitoring present device-specific challenges. Khine et al. achieved electroporation at remarkably low applied voltages (0.76 ± 0.095 V, with average transmembrane potential of 0.51 ± 0.13 V) by focusing the electric field through geometric confinement, generating approximately 750 kV/cm field strength at the trapped membrane. This design exploits an approximately 80-fold resistance difference between the trapped and free membrane portions, arising from the difference in membrane surface areas inside versus outside the trapping channel. In contrast, Zhan et al.'s system required higher applied voltages (5-9 V) across the ~20 μm electrode gap, with electroporation parameters determined by the combination of voltage, droplet velocity, droplet dimensions, and cell location within droplets. Real-time monitoring adds complexity but enables detailed process characterization. Khine et al. used Ag/AgCl electrodes with patch clamp amplifiers to measure characteristic current "jumps" corresponding to drops in cell resistance during membrane poration (observed in 15 of 17

HeLa cells tested), and video microscopy at 30 fps for fluorescence analysis of Calcein AM escape and Trypan blue entrance. Their observations demonstrated membrane resealing within 60 seconds, evidenced by recovery of high resistance in second pulse sequences. Zhan et al. successfully delivered plasmid DNA encoding enhanced green fluorescent protein within isolated droplets, though they noted that transfection efficiency was affected by the combination of electrical parameters, droplet dimensions, and cell localization within droplets, indicating optimization remains empirical. Nevertheless, for applications requiring high-precision control, real-time monitoring, and minimal sample volumes—such as exploratory research with valuable or limited cell populations—microfluidic systems offer compelling benefits. The ability to electroporate at sub-volt levels with localized field focusing (Khine et al. 2005) or within isolated picoliter droplets (Zhan et al. 2009) represents capabilities extending beyond traditional bulk electroporation approaches.

3.1.2 Nanotechnology-Enhanced Electroporation

At the nanoscale, electroporation achieves unprecedented precision through nanochannel-based delivery systems. Nanochannel electroporation (NEP) employs a unique microchannel-nanochannel-microchannel architecture, where nanofabricated channels (~90 nm diameter) connect two microchannels (Boukany et al. 2011).

The System Design and Operation can be done by precisely positioning individual cells at the nanochannel tip using optical tweezers, while the transfection agent is loaded in the opposing microchannel. Upon application of voltage pulses (150-350 V), the nanochannel generates extremely high local electric field strengths (up to 70 MV/m), creating focused poration in a very small membrane area (<1% of cell surface).

Xie et al. (2013) developed a nanostraw-electroporation system using hollow alumina nanowires (~250 nm diameter, 1.5 μm height) fabricated on track-etched membranes, achieving highly efficient parallel transfection with dramatically reduced voltages (5-20 V). The key innovation lies in cellular engulfment of nanostraws during adhesion, creating intimate membrane-nanostraw interfaces that localize electric fields to cell surface area and enable uniform transfection across large cell populations. The system demonstrates >95% PI dye delivery and 81% plasmid transfection efficiency in CHO cells with >98% viability, operating as a temporal "valve" that opens transiently during pulsing and reseals within 10 minutes. Unlike diffusion-dominated conventional methods, biomolecule transport occurs primarily through electrophoresis during poration, as evidenced by dramatically reduced efficiency upon polarity reversal. The platform uniquely enables dose control (via plasmid concentration and pulse number modulation), high-yield co-transfection of multiple plasmids and sequential transfection with independent delivery events—capabilities difficult to achieve with stochastic bulk methods. Control experiments confirm that neither nanostraws alone nor electroporation through flat porous membranes achieve comparable efficiency, demonstrating the synergistic requirement of nanostraw geometry and localized field concentration for optimal performance (Xie et al. 2013).

3.1.3 Force-Controlled Nanofluidic Delivery (FluidFM)

FluidFM (fluid force microscopy) technology enables precise molecular delivery to single cells and even subcellular structures by combining atomic force microscopy principles with nanofluidic systems (Meister et al. 2009). The system is based on hollow silicon dioxide cantilevers containing a microfluidic channel, with solution dispensed through a submicrometer aperture opened by focused ion beam milling at the cantilever tip. The sensitive force feedback of AFM enables two distinct operational modes: (1) controlled perforation of the cell membrane at high force setpoints (≥3 nN) for intracellular injection (~10 fL volumes), and (2) gentle contact with the membrane at low force setpoints (<1 nN) for diffusion-mediated delivery of membrane-permeant dyes. Solution flow driven by hydrostatic pressure (typically 10 mbars) enables precise molecular delivery to targets beyond the resolution of optical microscopy, such as varicosity-like subcellular structures. Although the technique has inherently low throughput, its unique spatial precision offers new opportunities for tissue engineering and fundamental cell biology research.

4. Conclusions

Electroporation has matured from a basic laboratory technique into a sophisticated therapeutic platform with proven clinical utility. The fundamental biophysical principle—using electrical pulses to transiently permeabilize cell membranes—remains unchanged, but technological advances have dramatically expanded capabilities and applications.

Researchs elucidating membrane permeabilization mechanisms, systematic optimization of electrical and biological parameters, and technological innovations including microfluidics, advanced pulse generation, and image-guided electrode placement. Standardized protocols, validated through multi-center trials, have facilitated clinical adoption and regulatory approval.

Challenges remain. *In vivo* applications face limitations in tissue accessibility, field uniformity, and delivery efficiency. Immunogenicity concerns may restrict repeated treatments or specific patient populations. Broader clinical adoption requires additional training, equipment investment, and integration into clinical pathways.

Yet the trajectory is clear. Ongoing research into spatially selective electroporation, combination modalities, and personalized treatment approaches promises continued advancement. Expansion into cardiovascular, neurodegenerative, and ophthalmologic applications will test electroporation's versatility. Integration with next-generation genome editing tools—base editors, prime editors, epigenome editors—will enable increasingly sophisticated cellular modifications.

References

Boukany, P. E., Morss, A., Liao, W. C., Henslee, B., Jung, H., Zhang, X., Yu, B., Wang, X., Wu, Y., Li, L., Gao, K., Hu, X., Zhao, X., Hemminger, O., Lu, W., Lafyatis, G. P., & Lee, L. J. (2011). Nanochannel electroporation delivers precise amounts of biomolecules into living cells. *Nature Nanotechnology*, *6*(11), 747-754. https://doi.org/10.1038/nnano.2011.164

CRISPR Therapeutics. (2021, June 11). *CRISPR Therapeutics and Vertex announce positive safety and efficacy data from two phase 1/2 studies of investigational CRISPR/Cas9 gene-editing therapy CTX001® in severe hemoglobinopathies* [Press release]. https://crisprtx.gcs-web.com/

Daud, A. I., DeConti, R. C., Andrews, S., Urbas, P., Riker, A. I., Sondak, V. K., Munster, P. N., Sullivan, D. M., Ugen, K. E., Messina, J. L., & Heller, R. (2008). Phase I trial of interleukin-12 plasmid electroporation in patients with metastatic melanoma. *Journal of Clinical Oncology*, *26*(36), 5896-5903. https://doi.org/10.1200/JCO.2007.15.6794

Escoffre, J. M., Portet, T., Wasungu, L., Teissié, J., Dean, D., & Rols, M. P. (2009). What is (still) not known of the mechanism by which electroporation mediates gene transfer and expression in cells in vivo. *Molecular Biotechnology*, *41*(3), 286-295. ` https://doi.org/10.1007/s12033-008-9121-0

Glaser, R. W., Leikin, S. L., Chernomordik, L. V., Pastushenko, V. F., & Sokirko, A. I. (1988). Reversible electrical breakdown of lipid bilayers:

Formation and evolution of pores. *Biochimica et Biophysica Acta*, *940*(2), 275-287. https://doi.org/10.1016/0005-2736(88)90202-7

Golzio, M., Teissié, J., & Rols, M. P. (2002). Direct visualization at the single-cell level of electrically mediated gene delivery. *Proceedings of the National Academy of Sciences of the United States of America*, *99*(3), 1292-1297. https://doi.org/10.1073/pnas.022646499

Hibino, M., Shigemori, M., Itoh, H., Nagayama, K., & Kinosita, K., Jr. (1991). Membrane conductance of an electroporated cell analyzed by submicrosecond imaging of transmembrane potential. *Biophysical Journal*, *59*(1), 209-220. https://doi.org/10.1016/S0006-3495(91)82212-3

Khine, M., Lau, A., Ionescu-Zanetti, C., Seo, J., & Lee, L. P. (2005). A single cell electroporation chip. *Lab on a Chip*, *5*(1), 38-43. https://doi.org/10.1039/b408352k

Kinosita, K., Jr., & Tsong, T. Y. (1977). Formation and resealing of pores of controlled sizes in human erythrocyte membrane. *Nature*, *268*(5619), 438-441. https://doi.org/10.1038/268438a0

Kotnik, T., Kramar, P., Pucihar, G., Miklavčič, D., & Tarek, M. (2012). Cell membrane electroporation—Part 1: The phenomenon. *IEEE Electrical Insulation Magazine*, *28*(5), 14-23. https://doi.org/10.1109/MEI.2012.6268438

Kotnik, T., & Miklavčič, D. (2006). Theoretical evaluation of voltage inducement on internal membranes of biological cells exposed to electric fields. *Biophysical Journal*, *90*(2), 480-491. https://doi.org/10.1529/biophysj.105.070771

Martin, R. C., II, McFarland, K., Ellis, S., & Velanovich, V. (2013). Irreversible electroporation in locally advanced pancreatic cancer: Potential improved overall survival. *Annals of Surgical Oncology*, *20*(Suppl. 3), S443-S449. https://doi.org/10.1245/s10434-012-2736-1

Marty, M., Serša, G., Garbay, J. R., Gehl, J., Collins, C. G., Snoj, M., Billard, V., Geertsen, P. F., Larkin, J. O., Miklavčič, D., Pavlović, I., Paulin-Košir, S. M., Čemažar, M., Morsli, N., Rudolf, Z., Robert, C., O'Sullivan, G. C., & Mir, L. M. (2006). Electrochemotherapy—An easy, highly effective and safe treatment of cutaneous and subcutaneous metastases: Results of ESOPE (European Standard Operating Procedures of Electrochemotherapy) study. *European Journal of Cancer Supplements*, *4*(11), 3-13. https://doi.org/10.1016/j.ejcsup.2006.08.002

Meister, A., Gabi, M., Behr, P., Studer, P., Vörös, J., Niedermann, P., Bitterli, J., Polesel-Maris, J., Liley, M., Heinzelmann, H., & Zambelli, T. (2009). FluidFM: Combining atomic force microscopy and nanofluidics in a universal liquid delivery system for single cell applications. *Nano Letters*, *9*(6), 2501-2507. https://doi.org/10.1021/nl901384x

Miklavčič, D., Mali, B., Kos, B., Heller, R., & Serša, G. (2014). Electrochemotherapy: From the drawing board into medical practice. *Biomedical Engineering Online*, *13*, 29. https://doi.org/10.1186/1475-925X-13-29

Mir, L. M., Bureau, M. F., Gehl, J., Rangara, R., Rouy, D., Caillaud, J. M., Delaere, P., Branellec, D., Schwartz, B., & Scherman, D. (1999). High-efficiency gene transfer into skeletal muscle mediated by electric pulses. *Proceedings of the National Academy of Sciences of the United States of America*, *96*(8), 4262-4267. https://doi.org/10.1073/pnas.96.8.4262

Neumann, E., Schaefer-Ridder, M., Wang, Y., & Hofschneider, P. H. (1982). Gene transfer into mouse lyoma cells by electroporation in high electric fields. *EMBO Journal*, *1*(7), 841-845. https://doi.org/10.1002/j.1460-2075.1982.tb01257.x

Potter, H., Weir, L., & Leder, P. (1984). Enhancer-dependent expression of human kappa immunoglobulin genes introduced into mouse pre-B lymphocytes by electroporation. *Proceedings of the National Academy of Sciences of the United States of America*, *81*(22), 7161-7165. https://doi.org/10.1073/pnas.81.22.7161

Pucihar, G., Kotnik, T., Kandušer, M., & Miklavčič, D. (2001). The influence of medium conductivity on electropermeabilization and survival of cells in vitro. *Bioelectrochemistry*, *54*(2), 107-115. https://doi.org/10.1016/S1567-5394(01)00117-7

Rols, M. P., & Teissié, J. (1990). Electropermeabilization of mammalian cells. Quantitative analysis of the phenomenon. *Biophysical Journal*, *58*(6), 1089-1098. https://doi.org/10.1016/S0006-3495(90)82451-6

Schoenbach, K. H., Beebe, S. J., & Buescher, E. S. (2001). Intracellular effect of ultrashort electrical pulses. *Bioelectromagnetics*, *22*(6), 440-448. https://doi.org/10.1002/bem.71

Sukharev, S. I., Klenchin, V. A., Serov, S. M., Chernomordik, L. V., & Chizmadzhev, Y. A. (1992). Electroporation and electrophoretic DNA transfer into cells. The effect of DNA interaction with electropores. *Biophysical Journal*, *63*(5), 1320-1327. https://doi.org/10.1016/S0006-3495(92)81709-5

Tarek, M. (2005). Membrane electroporation: A molecular dynamics simulation. *Biophysical Journal*, *88*(6), 4045-4053. https://doi.org/10.1529/biophysj.104.050617

Wang, S., Zhang, X., Wang, W., & Lee, L. J. (2009). Semi-continuous flow electroporation chip for high-throughput transfection on mammalian cells. *Analytical Chemistry*, *81*(11), 4414-4421. https://doi.org/10.1021/ac9002672

Weaver, J. C. (2000). Electroporation of cells and tissues. *IEEE Transactions on Plasma Science*, *28*(1), 24-33. https://doi.org/10.1109/27.842820

Xie, X., Xu, A. M., Leal-Ortiz, S., Cao, Y., Garner, C. C., & Melosh, N. A. (2013). Nanostraw-electroporation system for highly efficient intracellular delivery and transfection. *ACS Nano*, *7*(5), 4351-4358. https://doi.org/10.1021/nn400874a

Zhan, Y., Wang, J., Bao, N., & Lu, C. (2009). Electroporation of cells in microfluidic droplets. *Analytical Chemistry*, *81*(5), 2027-2031. https://doi.org/10.1021/ac9001172

Author Biography

Prof. Dr. Elçin Özgür Büyükatalay is a professor at the Department of Biophysics, Faculty of Medicine, Gazi University, Ankara, Türkiye, and the Director of the Project Coordination Application and Research Center of Gazi University. Her research interests include electromagnetic field interactions with biological systems, hyperthermia, blood–brain barrier modulation, and applications in cancer and neuroscience. She has coordinated and contributed to several national and international research projects supported by TÜBİTAK, TÜSEB, COST Actions, and Horizon Europe programs. Prof. Büyükatalay has authored numerous articles in SCI-indexed journals and supervised graduate research in radiation biophysics and bioelectromagnetics. She also serves as a reviewer for international scientific journals and national funding programs.

Assoc. Prof. Handan Kayhan is a member of Gazi University Faculty of Medicine, Department of Hematology, and the founder and CEO of Exo Life Biotechnology Ltd. She specializes in Medical Biology and Genetics. Her research focuses on extracellular vesicles, cancer biology, regenerative medicine, and gene transfer systems. She has developed numerous magnetic nanoparticle-based techniques, including the exosome isolation method DrExo. She is the author of numerous publications and patents, and has 18 years of experience in laboratory quality management as an ISO 15189 and ISO 17025 auditor. She has expertise in RNAi/shRNA strategies, flow cytometry, cell culture, and a wide range of molecular techniques.

CHAPTER 18

MICROINJECTION PRECISION DELIVERY AT THE CELLULAR LEVEL

MUHAMMED ALI NALBANT[1]

[1]Bandirma Onyedi Eylül Unıversıty, Faculty of Medıcıne, Department of Medical Biology, Balıkesir, Türkiye.

Abstract

Microinjection represents one of the most precise and direct physical methods for gene delivery, enabling the introduction of nucleic acids, proteins, and other biologically active molecules into individual cells with micrometer-level control. This chapter provides a comprehensive overview of microinjection as a cornerstone technology in molecular biology, developmental genetics, and assisted reproductive technologies. The discussion begins with the historical evolution of microinjection, from its pioneering use in generating the first transgenic animals to its continuing importance in modern genetic engineering. The chapter outlines the essential components of a microinjection system—including microscopes, micromanipulators, microinjectors, and micropipettes—detailing their roles in ensuring precise targeting and reproducibility. Various procedural approaches, such as cytoplasmic and pronuclear injection, are described in the context of their biological objectives, emphasizing the technique's ability to bypass cellular barriers and deliver material directly to specific intracellular compartments. Applications range from transgenesis, gene therapy research, and CRISPR/Cas9-mediated genome editing to manipulation of embryos, oocytes, and stem cells, as well as clinical procedures like intracytoplasmic sperm injection (ICSI). The chapter also critically evaluates microinjection's advantages—including high single-cell efficiency, versatility, and temporal control—against its limitations, notably low throughput, labor intensity, and technical demands. A comparative analysis with alternative delivery systems (viral, chemical, and other physical methods) highlights microinjection's unique niche where precision is prioritized over scalability. Finally, recent innovations such as robotic automation, miniaturized nanoinjection systems, and integration with gene-editing platforms are discussed, suggesting that while microinjection is unlikely to become a large-scale therapeutic modality, it will remain indispensable for research and highly specialized clinical applications.

Keywords: Microinjection, Transgenesis, Intracellular Targeting, Reproductive Technologies, Nanoinjection

1. Introduction to Microinjection

Gene therapy holds immense promise for treating a vast array of human diseases by correcting genetic defects at their source. A cornerstone of this field is the development of effective delivery systems capable of transporting therapeutic genetic material into target cells. Among the diverse strategies employed, physical methods offer alternatives to viral and chemical vectors, often leveraging mechanical forces or fields to breach cellular barriers. Microinjection stands out within this category as a highly sophisticated technique characterized by its direct, mechanical approach to intracellular delivery.

Microinjection is a physical method of gene delivery involving the direct injection of genetic material into individual cells using a fine needle or micropipette. This technique has a long history in molecular biology and has played a pivotal role in gene transfer experiments since the early days of genetic engineering. In gene therapy, microinjection offers a highly precise (albeit labor-intensive) way to introduce therapeutic genes or gene-editing tools into target cells. This chapter provides a comprehensive overview of microinjection as a gene therapy delivery system, including its historical development, the technical procedure and equipment, advantages and disadvantages relative to other delivery methods, applications in treating or modeling disease, and recent advances, challenges, and future directions for its use in both experimental and clinical settings.

1.1 Defining Microinjection: A Mechanical Gateway into the Cell

Microinjection is a physical gene transfer method involving the direct introduction of exogenous materials -such as DNA, RNA, proteins, peptides, or even entire organelles—into a single living cell (Biology Notes Online, 2025) . This is achieved using an exceptionally fine glass needle, known as a micropipette, typically with a tip diameter in the micrometer or sub-micrometer range (Das et al., 2015). The process is meticulously controlled and observed under high-resolution microscopy (Biology Notes Online, 2025).

Fundamentally, microinjection operates as a mechanical tool. Unlike other physical methods such as electroporation or sonoporation, which utilize external fields (electric or acoustic, respectively) to induce transient permeability in cell membranes, microinjection relies on the physical force exerted by the micropipette to penetrate the cell membrane and/or nuclear envelope (Zhang & Yu, 2008). This direct mechanical breach is a defining characteristic, distinguishing microinjection from field-based permeabilization techniques. While field-based methods leverage inherent membrane properties to allow cargo entry, they often contend with variable efficiencies and the potential for widespread, albeit temporary, membrane disruption across a cell population (Das et al., 2015). Microinjection, conversely, bypasses natural cellular uptake mechanisms and membrane transport challenges entirely by creating a direct conduit into the cell's interior, albeit at the cost of localized physical trauma.

The primary advantage stemming from this direct mechanical approach is the unparalleled precision it offers. Microinjection allows for the delivery of precisely controlled volumes of substances to specific subcellular compartments, such as the cytoplasm or the nucleus (Biology Notes Online 2025). This capability ensures that the cargo reaches its intended site of action with minimal ambiguity, a feature highly valued in research and certain therapeutic applications (Zhang & Yu, 2008). This precision has rendered microinjection an invaluable tool across numerous domains, including molecular biology, genetics, developmental biology, assisted reproduction, and gene therapy research.

1.2 Historical Context and Evolution

The concept of microinjection dates back several decades, with early reports emerging around the 1970s. Initially, the technique was employed to introduce relatively large macromolecules into cells. Its potential was quickly recognized, and the method was adapted for the delivery of a wider array of biologically significant molecules, including DNA, RNA, enzymes, proteins, metabolites, ions, and even cellular organelles like mitochondria (Das et al., 2015). Early developmental work extensively utilized large cells like *Xenopus* eggs and animal embryos due to their size, which facilitated manipulation (News-Medical, 2025). A landmark application came with the generation of the first transgenic animals, where microinjection was instrumental in introducing foreign DNA into embryos, establishing its critical role in genetic engineering and biomedical research (Volobueva et al., 2019).

A landmark achievement in this period was the creation of the first transgenic animals using pronuclear microinjection. In 1980, Jon Gordon and Frank Ruddle demonstrated that injecting purified DNA into the nucleus of a fertilized mouse egg could result in the integration of that DNA into the mouse genome. In their experiments, a single-celled mouse embryo at the pronucleus stage was held in place and DNA was microinjected into one of its pronuclei; the embryo was then implanted into a foster mother and carried to term. This **pronuclear microinjection** technique led to live transgenic mice carrying the foreign gene in all their cells, proving that heritable gene transfer was possible. Notably, this DNA injection method was the first and remains a common technique for generating transgenic animals. Subsequent studies soon showed that the introduced genes could be expressed and even produce observable traits. For example, early transgenic mouse studies introduced a thymidine kinase (TK) gene (as done by Gordon and Ruddle) which integrated without a dramatic phenotype, followed shortly by experiments that injected growth hormone genes, resulting in mice that grew significantly larger than normal. These successes in the early 1980s set the stage for using microinjection to modify genomes and model diseases (Jones, 2011).

Around the same time, microinjection was also being applied to cultured cells. In 1980, Capecchi and colleagues reported that directly microinjecting DNA into the nucleus of cultured mammalian cells yielded substantially higher gene expression than more conventional means of adding DNA to cells (Katz et al., 2013). This showed that physical delivery into the nucleus could overcome many of the barriers that free DNA faces, albeit on a single-cell scale. Thus, by the early 1980s, microinjection had established itself as a viable gene delivery tool in research – from single cells in culture to one-cell embryos – allowing investigators to introduce and study genes in ways not previously possible.

However, as gene therapy moved toward clinical applications in the late 1980s and 1990s, microinjection faced competition from more scalable delivery systems. The first approved human gene therapy in 1990 used a viral vector (a retrovirus to deliver the ADA gene in immune cells), highlighting the practicality of vectors for treating large cell populations (Tamura & Toda, 2020). Viral methods offered the ability to transduce millions of cells, whereas microinjection remained limited in throughput.

Nonetheless, the historical contributions of microinjection were critical: it provided the first proof-of-concept for direct gene insertion into genomes and enabled the creation of innumerable transgenic and gene-modified animals that informed biomedical research and gene therapy strategies.

1.3 Fundamental Principles of Operation

The operational principle of microinjection is conceptually straightforward: physically penetrate the cell boundary with a micropipette and deposit the desired cargo directly inside. This is typically accomplished through a coordinated system involving three key elements: visualization, manipulation, and injection (Biology Notes Online, 2025).

1. **Visualization:** The entire procedure is carried out under a high-resolution microscope (often an inverted microscope equipped with phase contrast or Differential Interference Contrast (DIC) optics) allowing clear visualization of the target cell, the micropipette, and critical intracellular structures like the nucleus or pronuclei.
2. **Manipulation:** Micromanipulators are essential for controlling the position of the micropipette and often a second "holding" pipette with extreme precision, typically enabling movements in three dimensions with sub-micrometer accuracy. These devices counteract hand tremors and allow for the delicate maneuvers required to approach, penetrate, and withdraw from the cell without causing excessive damage.
3. **Injection:** A microinjector system is used to expel the substance contained within the micropipette into the cell. This is commonly achieved by applying controlled positive pressure (e.g., hydrostatic or gas pressure) to the back of the micropipette, forcing the liquid cargo out through the fine tip. Precise control over the applied pressure and duration allows for the delivery of specific volumes, often in the picoliter range (Smith, 2004).

The distinction between microinjection's direct mechanical insertion and the field-induced permeability of methods like electroporation dictates their respective strengths and weaknesses. Microinjection offers certainty of delivery to the targeted compartment for successfully injected cells but is inherently invasive and limited in throughput. Field-based methods can treat large populations simultaneously but face challenges related to variable uptake efficiency, cell viability, and ensuring cargo reaches the correct intracellular location (e.g., the nucleus for DNA) (Elaswad et al., 2018). This fundamental difference underscores why microinjection remains a critical tool for applications demanding single-cell precision, despite the development of higher-throughput alternatives.

2. The Microinjection Toolkit: Methodology and Equipment

Performing microinjection successfully requires specialized instrumentation and meticulous technique. The process involves preparing the cells, crafting the delivery tool (the micropipette), and executing the injection using a sophisticated setup that allows for precise control and visualization.

2.1 Core Components: Microscopes, Micromanipulators, Microinjectors

A functional microinjection workstation integrates several key pieces of equipment:

- **Microscope:** An inverted microscope is standard, allowing access to the sample from above while viewing through objectives positioned below the stage. High magnification (e.g., 20x, 40x objectives) and contrast-enhancing optics (Phase Contrast or DIC) are necessary for visualizing cellular details, particularly the nucleus or pronuclei in zygotes (Liu et al., 2013). The condenser must have a long working distance to accommodate the micromanipulation apparatus positioned above the stage.
- **Micromanipulators:** These are robotic arms that translate coarse hand movements into ultra-fine, stable movements of the micropipettes. Typically, two manipulators are used: one for the injection needle and one for a holding pipette. They provide precise control in X, Y, and Z axes, often with sub-micron resolution, and can be driven mechanically, hydraulically, or electronically (e.g., using piezoelectric actuators). Stability and smooth operation are paramount.
- **Microinjector:** This device delivers the injection pressure needed to expel the liquid cargo from the micropipette tip. Systems like the Eppendorf Transjector allow precise control over injection pressure (Pi), which forces the liquid out, and constant pressure (Po), a slight positive pressure maintained when not injecting to prevent capillary action from drawing medium into the needle or leakage of the injection solution. Injection is often triggered by a foot pedal. Gas-pressure regulated systems are used for delivering very small

volumes (News-Medical, 2025).

- **Holding Pipette System:** To stabilize the target cell or embryo during injection, a holding pipette with a smooth, fire-polished opening is used. This pipette is connected to a separate control system (e.g., Eppendorf CellTram Vario, often oil-filled) that allows gentle suction to be applied, holding the cell stationary against the pipette tip.
- **Vibration Isolation Table:** Due to the microscopic scale and precision required, microinjection setups are extremely sensitive to vibrations. An anti-vibration table (e.g., air table) is often essential to dampen ambient vibrations and ensure stability.
- **Optional Components:** Digital cameras connected to the microscope allow for recording, documentation, and demonstration purposes. Computer control systems can enhance automation and reproducibility (Evans, 2006).

2.2 The Micropipette: Crafting the Delivery Needle

The micropipette is the critical interface between the injection system and the cell. Its quality significantly impacts the success and viability of the procedure.

- **Fabrication:** Micropipettes are typically fabricated from borosilicate glass capillaries. A specialized instrument called a micropipette puller heats the capillary and pulls it under controlled tension to draw it out into two fine-tipped needles. The pulling parameters (heat, force, velocity) determine the taper and tip diameter.
- **Tip Characteristics:** The ideal tip is extremely fine yet robust enough to penetrate the cell membrane without excessive tearing. Tip diameters vary depending on the application: sub-micrometer (<0.5 μm) for precise nuclear injection, 0.5-5 μm is a commonly cited range, while tips for applications like ICSI might be larger (Butt et al., 2022). Achieving consistent, high-quality tips requires experience (News-Medical, 2025). The initial capillary often contains an internal filament, which aids in loading the injection solution into the needle tip via capillary action.
- **Opening the Tip:** Freshly pulled needles often have sealed tips. Just prior to injection, the tip must be opened. This is commonly done by gently tapping the injection needle against the holding pipette under microscopic view or sometimes by touching it against debris on the culture dish surface (Evans, 2006). The size of the opening affects

the flow rate and required injection pressure, necessitating pressure adjustments for each new needle (Liu et al., 2013).

2.3 Procedural Workflow: From Cell Preparation to Injection

While specific protocols vary depending on the cell type and application, the general workflow for microinjection shares common steps, exemplified by pronuclear injection (PNI) in mouse zygotes or injection into *C. elegans* gonads or catfish embryos:

1. **Cell/Embryo Preparation:** Target cells or embryos are collected and prepared. For PNI, this involves harvesting fertilized zygotes, often following superovulation protocols for donors. For *C. elegans*, young gravid adults are selected. Catfish require artificial fertilization (Elaswad et al., 2018). Cells are typically placed in a suitable medium (e.g., M2 medium for mouse zygotes outside CO_2 incubator, Holtfreter's solution for catfish) within an injection chamber, often a drop of medium under mineral oil to prevent evaporation and pH changes.
2. **Injection Solution Preparation:** The material to be injected (e.g., DNA solution for transgenesis, CRISPR components) is prepared. DNA solutions are often centrifuged to pellet any particulate matter that could clog the fine needle tip. Concentration is carefully adjusted (Thermo Fisher Scientific, 2025a). A tracking dye (e.g., phenol red, fluorescent markers) may be included to visualize the injection and identify injected cells later (Evans, 2006).
3. **Needle Loading:** Using a microloader tip or a drawn-out capillary, the injection solution is carefully loaded into the back of the micropipette, allowing capillary action along the internal filament to draw the liquid to the tip.
4. **Setup and Positioning:** The injection chamber is placed on the microscope stage. The loaded injection needle and the holding pipette are mounted onto their respective micromanipulators and carefully lowered into the medium drop. The needle tip is opened if necessary.
5. **Cell Immobilization:** A target cell or embryo is selected and gently immobilized using the holding pipette, applying minimal suction to hold it steady. For *C. elegans*, worms are immobilized by adherence to a dry agarose pad (Evans, 2006).
6. **Targeting and Penetration:** The microscope is focused on the target site (e.g., pronucleus, cytoplasm, gonad syncytium). The injection needle is brought into the same focal plane and precisely

positioned adjacent to the target. Penetration is achieved with a quick, smooth, controlled forward movement of the needle using the micromanipulator. Sometimes the needle must pass completely through the nucleus to breach the membrane.

7. **Injection:** Once the needle tip is confirmed to be inside the target compartment, the microinjector is activated (e.g., foot pedal pressed) to deliver a controlled volume of the solution. Successful injection is often confirmed by visual cues, such as the swelling of the pronucleus or visible flow within the *C. elegans* gonad (Evans, 2006). Injection pressure (Pi) and duration determine the volume delivered; constant pressure (Po) prevents backflow.
8. **Withdrawal:** After injection, the needle is carefully and smoothly withdrawn from the cell to minimize damage (Microbe Notes, 2025). The injected cell/embryo is released from the holding pipette and often moved to a separate area of the dish.
9. **Post-Injection Culture:** Injected cells/embryos are collected, washed, and transferred to appropriate culture conditions (e.g., M16 medium in CO_2 incubator for mouse embryos) to recover and continue development (Liu et al., 2013).

2.4 Variations: Cytoplasmic vs. Pronuclear Injection

The specific intracellular target dictates the type of microinjection performed:

- **Cytoplasmic Microinjection:** The cargo is delivered directly into the cytoplasm. This is the method of choice for substances intended to act within the cytoplasm, such as mRNA for translation, functional proteins or peptides, or RNA interference molecules. It is also the basis for ICSI, where a sperm cell is injected into the egg's cytoplasm. Delivering CRISPR/Cas9 ribonucleoprotein (RNP) complexes directly into the cytoplasm is also common (Synthego, 2025). While DNA can be injected into the cytoplasm, its subsequent journey to the nucleus for transcription or integration faces significant hurdles (Elaswad et al., 2018).
- **Pronuclear Microinjection (PNI):** The cargo, almost exclusively DNA for transgenesis or gene editing constructs, is injected directly into one of the pronuclei of a fertilized zygote. This strategy bypasses the cytoplasm and its degrading enzymes (nucleases) and delivers the DNA directly to the nuclear compartment, greatly increasing the likelihood of transient expression or stable integration into the host

genome (Elaswad et al., 2018). PNI has historically been the gold standard for creating transgenic founder animals (Volobueva et al., 2019).

The existence and specific protocols for these distinct injection types are not merely technical variations; they directly reflect the need to overcome fundamental biological barriers. Delivering DNA into the cytoplasm necessitates subsequent transport across the nuclear envelope, a process that is often inefficient and exposes the DNA to degradation (Elaswad et al., 2018). PNI circumvents these issues by placing the DNA payload directly within the nuclear boundary (Jinturkar et al., 2011). Conversely, cytoplasmic delivery is logical and efficient for RNA or proteins that function there. The requirement for sophisticated equipment and considerable operator skill further underscores that microinjection is a highly controlled method designed to precisely navigate and overcome these specific cellular compartments and defense mechanisms, rather than a simple brute-force entry (Zhang & Yu, 2008). The choice between cytoplasmic and nuclear injection is therefore critically linked to the nature of the cargo and the desired biological outcome, highlighting both the precision and the complexity of the technique.

3. Applications of Microinjection in Biological Research and Therapy

Microinjection's unique ability to deliver materials directly into individual cells with high precision has secured its place as a vital technique in various fields, from fundamental research to clinical applications like assisted reproduction. Its versatility allows for the manipulation of embryos, oocytes, stem cells, and various cultured cells for diverse purposes.

3.1 Pioneering Transgenesis: Creating Genetically Modified Organisms

Perhaps the most historically significant application of microinjection is in the creation of transgenic organisms. Pronuclear microinjection (PNI), the injection of foreign DNA directly into the pronucleus of a fertilized egg (zygote), remains a cornerstone method for generating genetically modified animals (Volobueva et al., 2019). This technique has been successfully applied across a wide range of species, including mice, rats, rabbits, pigs, sheep, cattle, fish (*e.g.*, zebrafish, catfish), invertebrates (*e.g.*, *C. elegans*, arthropods), and even in plant protoplasts.

The primary goal of transgenesis via PNI is typically to introduce a specific gene (transgene) into the organism's germline, allowing the modification to be passed down to subsequent generations (Shakweer et al., 2023). This enables researchers to:

- **Study gene function:** By overexpressing a gene or expressing a modified version.
- **Model human diseases:** By introducing genes associated with human genetic disorders into animals (e.g., ApoE3-Leiden mice for dysbetalipoproteinemia, various models for cardiovascular diseases, neurodegenerative diseases, metabolic disorders) (Wei et al., 2022).
- **Improve livestock traits:** By introducing genes for enhanced growth, milk production, or disease resistance (Kumar & Ratwan, 2016).

Despite its widespread use, PNI-based transgenesis has notable limitations. Efficiency, defined as the percentage of injected embryos that develop into transgenic offspring, is often low, particularly in larger animals like pigs, sheep, and cattle (often below 5%, sometimes less than 1%) (Hryhorowicz et al. 2020, 2). Efficiency in mice is generally higher but still variable (e.g., up to 20-30%) (Kumar & Ratwan, 2016). Furthermore, the integration of the transgene into the host genome is typically random (Wei et al., 2022). This random integration can lead to unpredictable levels of gene expression due to positional effects, mosaicism (where the transgene is present in only some cells of the founder animal), and potential disruption of endogenous genes at the insertion site (insertional mutagenesis) (Smith, 2004).

Even with these drawbacks, PNI microinjection persists as a primary tool, particularly for generating founder transgenic animals. This persistence highlights a key aspect of its utility: the high *value* placed on achieving germline transmission outweighs the low *volume* or efficiency of production. Creating even a few founder animals that can establish a transgenic line is often sufficient justification for the significant effort and resources required. This contrasts sharply with therapeutic applications where modifying large numbers of cells efficiently is paramount. The random integration issue, however, remains a significant concern, driving efforts to combine microinjection's delivery capability with targeted integration technologies like CRISPR/Cas9 or to explore alternative methods like somatic cell nuclear transfer (SCNT) using pre-modified cells (Volobueva et al., 2019).

3.2 Role in Assisted Reproductive Technologies (ART)

Microinjection plays an indispensable role in modern ART, primarily through Intracytoplasmic Sperm Injection (ICSI). Developed to overcome severe male infertility factors (e.g., low sperm count, poor motility, abnormal morphology), ICSI involves selecting a single sperm and injecting it directly into the cytoplasm of a mature oocyte using a specialized micropipette. This bypasses natural fertilization barriers and has enabled countless couples to conceive. The success of ICSI underscores the power of microinjection in scenarios where single-cell precision is the only viable path to a desired biological outcome.

There are two main types of injection in the ICSI procedure. One procedure is **cytoplasmic vs. nuclear injection.** DNA is often delivered into the nucleus to maximize gene expression, but in some cases cytoplasmic injection is used (for instance, injecting mRNA or protein that will later find its way to the nucleus, or when targeting organelles like injecting into an egg's cytoplasm). Another procedure is the use of a **piezo-electric drill or actuator** on the micropipette to facilitate penetration, commonly used in injecting mouse embryos or performing intracytoplasmic sperm injection (ICSI) in IVF; the rapid vibration reduces membrane resistance and trauma. The volumes injected are extremely small (femtoliters to picoliters), but the local concentration can be high. Because the DNA (or other material) is delivered directly inside the cell, microinjection bypasses the usual barriers of the plasma membrane and endosomal uptake – the genetic material is placed exactly where it needs to act, which is often the nucleus for gene expression.

Beyond ICSI, micromanipulation techniques closely related to microinjection are used in other ART procedures, such as:

- **Zona Pellucida Manipulation:** Techniques like zona dissection or laser-assisted hatching create openings in the zona pellucida (the outer layer of the egg) to facilitate embryo hatching or allow for preimplantation genetic diagnosis (PGD) by removing blastomeres for testing.
- **Somatic Cell Nuclear Transfer (SCNT):** While primarily a research tool for cloning, SCNT involves micromanipulation to remove the nucleus from an oocyte (enucleation) and microinjection to transfer a nucleus from a somatic cell into the enucleated oocyte (News-Medical, 2025).

3.3 A Tool for Gene Therapy Research: Delivery of Nucleic Acids and Gene Editing Tools

In the context of gene therapy research, microinjection serves as a valuable tool for delivering therapeutic nucleic acids directly into target cells. By physically bypassing cellular membranes and uptake pathways, it can efficiently deliver naked DNA plasmids or other genetic constructs into the cytoplasm or nucleus, avoiding issues like extracellular degradation or endosomal trapping that plague other non-viral methods. While its low throughput prevents direct clinical application for treating large cell populations, it is useful for proof-of-concept studies, validating gene function, and investigating cellular responses to gene delivery in vitro or in specific cells in vivo (e.g., muscle, skin, neural tissue) (Butt et al., 2022).

More recently, microinjection has become a preferred method for delivering components of genome editing systems, particularly CRISPR/Cas9, into cells and embryos (Zhang & Yu, 2008). The cargo can be delivered in various forms:

- **Plasmid DNA:** Encoding Cas9 and the guide RNA (gRNA).
- **mRNA:** Encoding Cas9, co-injected with gRNA.
- **Ribonucleoprotein (RNP) complexes:** Pre-assembled Cas9 protein and gRNA.

Injecting these components directly into zygotes (PNI or cytoplasmic injection) or early embryos allows for highly efficient gene editing to create knockout or knock-in animal models with specific genetic modifications. This combination leverages microinjection's precision delivery with CRISPR's targeted editing, overcoming the random integration limitations of traditional PNI transgenesis. Examples include generating gene-edited catfish, mice and zebrafish, and rabbits. Its utility in delivering gene editing tools also extends to human germline gene modification research, although this application remains ethically charged and technologically immature for clinical use (Smith, 2004).

3.4 Manipulating Stem Cells and Oocytes

Microinjection is frequently used to manipulate stem cells and oocytes for research purposes:

- **Embryonic Stem (ES) Cells:** Foreign DNA or other molecules can be microinjected into pluripotent ES cells in culture. These genetically modified ES cells can then be selected and subsequently injected (again, often using microinjection or aggregation techniques) into blastocysts to generate chimeric animals, where the modified cells contribute to various tissues, including the germline (News-Medical, 2025).

- **Induced Pluripotent Stem Cells (iPSCs):** Microinjection is also applicable for delivering gene editing tools or other constructs into iPSCs for research or potential therapeutic applications.
- **Oocytes:** Ooplasmic microinjection involves injecting substances directly into the cytoplasm of oocytes (immature eggs) for various research aims, such as studying oocyte maturation, fertilization processes, or early development.

3.5 Broader Applications: Delivering Proteins, Peptides, and Other Molecules

The utility of microinjection extends beyond nucleic acid delivery. Its mechanical nature makes it suitable for introducing a wide variety of molecules that might otherwise struggle to cross the cell membrane. This includes:

- Functional proteins and enzymes.
- Peptides and antibodies.
- Small molecule drugs, metabolites, and ions.
- Imaging agents or dyes for cell tracking.

This versatility makes it valuable in fields like cell biology for studying signal transduction pathways or protein function, and neuroscience, where delivering substances directly into primary neurons (which are often difficult to transfect by other means) is crucial.

4. Evaluating Microinjection as a Gene Delivery System

Microinjection presents a unique profile of strengths and weaknesses as a gene delivery method. Its evaluation hinges on balancing its exceptional precision and directness against significant limitations in throughput and ease of use.

4.1 Key Advantages

- **Precision and Targeting:** The most significant advantage is the ability to deliver a precisely controlled volume of cargo to a specific subcellular location, typically the cytoplasm or the nucleus. Nuclear targeting is particularly advantageous for DNA delivery, bypassing cytoplasmic degradation and facilitating access to the transcriptional machinery or integration sites.
- **High Single-Cell Efficiency:** For a cell that is successfully injected without lethal damage, the delivery of the cargo is essentially guaranteed (Das et al., 2015). This contrasts with population-based methods where only a fraction of cells may receive the cargo.
- **Cargo Versatility:** Microinjection is remarkably versatile regarding the type and size of cargo it can deliver. It is not limited by the biochemical properties that govern membrane transport or vector packaging. DNA, RNA (including siRNA), proteins, peptides, antibodies, drugs, and even organelles can be injected. It is particularly useful for delivering large DNA molecules (Butt et al., 2022).
- **Direct Access/Barrier Bypass:** The technique physically bypasses the cell membrane and associated biological barriers like the endosomal/lysosomal pathway, which can trap or degrade cargo delivered by other methods (especially chemical vectors). Nuclear injection further bypasses the nuclear envelope barrier for DNA (Elaswad et al., 2018).
- **Independence from Selection Markers:** Because delivery to the target cell is direct and often visually confirmed (potentially using co-injected dyes), there is typically no need for co-transfection with selectable marker genes (e.g., antibiotic resistance) to identify successfully modified cells, simplifying downstream workflows (Evans, 2006).
- **Relatively Low Cell Stress (Potentially):** When performed skillfully, the physical insult to the cell can be minimized. Compared to the potential immunogenicity of viral vectors or the widespread membrane disruption and potential toxicity of electroporation or chemical transfection, microinjection can be less stressful for the successfully injected individual cell, potentially leading to higher viability among those cells. It also requires smaller amounts of starting material (e.g., purified protein) compared to bulk methods.
- **Temporal Control:** Delivery can be precisely timed relative to specific stages of the cell cycle or developmental events.

4.2 Significant Limitations

- **Low Throughput/Scalability:** This is arguably the most significant drawback. Microinjection is inherently a single-cell technique. Manually injecting even a few hundred cells is extremely time-consuming. This makes it completely impractical for applications requiring the modification of large cell populations, such as systemic gene therapy or large-scale cell production for therapeutic use.
- **Labor Intensity and Time Consumption:** The manual process is tedious, demanding intense focus and dexterity from the operator over extended periods.
- **Technical Skill Requirement:** Achieving proficiency and reproducible results requires significant training and expertise (Das et al., 2015). Success rates can vary considerably based on operator skill.
- **High Cost of Equipment:** The necessary equipment, including a high-quality inverted microscope, precise micromanipulators, a microinjector, and potentially a vibration isolation table, represents a significant capital investment (Evans, 2006).
- **Potential for Cell Damage and Death:** Despite the potential for lower stress compared to some methods, the physical act of piercing the cell membrane with a needle is inherently invasive and can cause significant damage or cell death if not performed optimally. Injecting too large a volume can also disrupt cellular homeostasis. Careful optimization and appropriate controls are essential (Microbe Notes, 2025).
- **Cell Type Restrictions:** The technique is most easily applied to relatively large, robust cells, such as oocytes, zygotes, and early embryos (Butt et al., 2022). Adherent cultured cells are also commonly used. Injecting suspension cells is more challenging as they must be immobilized (e.g., by a holding pipette or specialized devices). Cells with small cytoplasmic volumes or nuclei can also be difficult to inject successfully (Das et al., 2015).
- **Random Integration (PNI Transgenesis):** As discussed previously, when used for traditional transgenesis via PNI, DNA integration into the host genome is typically random, leading to unpredictable expression patterns and the risk of insertional mutagenesis (Smith, 2004)

The evaluation of microinjection reveals a fundamental trade-off: it maximizes precision and control at the single-cell level but inherently sacrifices scalability and throughput. This precision-scalability dichotomy is not merely one limitation among others; it is the core characteristic that defines microinjection's unique application space. While methods like viral vectors or electroporation prioritize treating large populations, accepting compromises in individual cell control or introducing different safety concerns, microinjection excels where meticulous manipulation of individual cells is the primary goal. Consequently, it remains indispensable for research applications focused on single-cell analysis, the creation of founder organisms, or clinical procedures like ICSI, but it is poorly suited for therapies requiring the modification of millions or billions of cells. Ongoing advancements in automation aim to mitigate the throughput limitation, but the technique remains fundamentally a single-cell approach.

Table 4-1: Summary of Advantages and Disadvantages of Microinjection for Gene Delivery

Advantages	Disadvantages
High Precision & Targeting	Extremely Low Throughput/Scalability
High Single-Cell Efficiency	Highly Labor-Intensive & Time-Consuming
Broad Cargo Versatility (Size/Type)	Requires Significant Technical Skill & Training
Direct Intracellular Access	High Equipment Cost
Bypasses Uptake Barriers/Degradation	Potential for Cell Damage/Death
No Selection Markers Needed	Cell Type Limitations (Size, Adherence)
Relatively Low Stress (cf. some methods)	Random Integration (PNI Transgenesis)
Precise Temporal Control	Difficult for Large-Scale Analysis (e.g., Westerns)

5. Microinjection in Context: Comparison with Other Delivery Systems

Understanding the specific strengths and weaknesses of microinjection requires comparing it to other major gene delivery platforms, including alternative physical methods, viral vectors, and non-viral chemical approaches. Each strategy presents a distinct set of capabilities and challenges, positioning microinjection within a broader landscape of available tools.

5.1 Physical Delivery Methods

Physical methods employ forces or mechanical actions to overcome the cell membrane barrier.

- **Electroporation:** This technique uses high-voltage electric pulses to create transient pores in the cell membrane, allowing nucleic acids or other molecules in the surrounding medium to enter.
    - *Comparison:* Electroporation offers much higher throughput, capable of transfecting large populations of cells simultaneously, whereas microinjection is limited to single cells (Evans, 2006). Electroporation is generally faster and less technically demanding per cell population, though optimization is required. However, microinjection provides superior precision in delivery volume and subcellular targeting. Electroporation can cause significant cell death (viability often around 50%) and does not guarantee nuclear entry for DNA, while microinjection's viability depends heavily on skill but ensures delivery to the target site. Electroporation is widely used for cultured cells, bacteria, yeast, and plant protoplasts, while microinjection excels for embryos, oocytes, and specific research applications requiring single-cell manipulation. Equipment costs differ, with electroporators being distinct from the complex microscope/manipulator setup of microinjection. Identifying successfully electroporated cells can be difficult, whereas microinjected cells are often easily identifiable. Nucleofection is a specialized form of electroporation optimized for direct nuclear delivery (Synthego, 2025).
- **Gene Gun (Biolistics / Particle Bombardment):** This method uses high pressure (e.g., helium gas) to accelerate microscopic heavy-metal particles (e.g., gold, tungsten) coated with DNA or RNA directly into cells or tissues.

    - *Comparison:* The gene gun can transfect cells within intact tissues and is particularly useful for plant transformation and cells that are difficult to transfect by other means. It is less dependent on target cell characteristics than some methods. While invasive, it avoids the direct needle puncture of microinjection. However, it causes physical damage due to particle impact, can have high cell mortality rates, requires specialized equipment (the gene gun device), and offers less control over dosage and subcellular targeting compared to microinjection. Microinjection provides more precise control over delivery into individual, often isolated, cells or embryos.
- **Sonoporation:** Utilizes ultrasonic frequencies, often in conjunction with microbubbles (contrast agents), to induce cavitation, which temporarily disrupts cell membranes and enhances permeability.
    - *Comparison:* Sonoporation offers the potential for non-invasive delivery and can target cells deeper within tissues compared to methods requiring direct access. However, its efficiency is often relatively low, and controlling the process to avoid excessive cell damage can be challenging. Microinjection, while invasive, offers much higher efficiency and precision at the single-cell level.
- **Other Physical Methods:** Techniques like laser-mediated transfection (photoporation), magnetofection (using magnetic nanoparticles), hydrodynamic delivery (rapid injection of large volumes, primarily for liver targeting in vivo), and nanoinjection represent alternative physical strategies. Each operates on distinct principles and presents unique advantages (e.g., laser precision, magnetofection targeting potential, hydrodynamic in vivo efficiency for certain organs) and limitations compared to the direct mechanical approach of microinjection.

5.2 Viral Vector Systems

Viruses have evolved highly efficient mechanisms for entering cells and delivering their genetic material. Gene therapy often harnesses these capabilities using engineered viral vectors (e.g., retroviruses, lentiviruses, adenoviruses, adeno-associated viruses (AAVs)) stripped of their pathogenic components.

- *Comparison:* Viral vectors generally achieve much higher transduction efficiencies across large cell populations compared to the single-cell focus of microinjection. Many viral vectors (e.g., lentiviruses) can integrate into the host genome, potentially leading to stable, long-term gene expression, whereas microinjection typically results in transient expression unless combined with integrating elements or gene editing tools. However, viral vectors carry significant risks, including immunogenicity (triggering immune responses against the vector or transduced cells) and potential insertional mutagenesis if integration occurs randomly in detrimental locations. Microinjection avoids these specific biological risks, with its primary safety concern being physical cell damage. Viral vectors have limitations on the size of the genetic cargo they can package, whereas microinjection can potentially deliver very large DNA constructs (Butt et al., 2022). Manufacturing clinical-grade viral vectors is complex and expensive, while microinjection, though requiring expensive equipment and skill, is conceptually simpler in terms of cargo preparation (Smith, 2004).

5.3 Non-Viral Chemical Methods

These methods utilize synthetic or natural compounds (e.g., cationic lipids, polymers) to complex with nucleic acids, neutralize their charge, and facilitate entry into cells, often via endocytosis.

- *Comparison:* Chemical methods, like lipofection, are generally easier to perform for bulk transfection of cultured cells compared to the technically demanding nature of microinjection. They are often less expensive in terms of reagents per experiment for large populations. However, their efficiency can be highly variable depending on the cell type and reagent, and they often suffer from lower overall efficiency compared to viral vectors or the guaranteed single-cell delivery of microinjection. A major hurdle for chemical methods is overcoming the endosomal barrier; cargo can become trapped in endosomes and degraded in lysosomes before reaching the cytoplasm or nucleus. Microinjection completely bypasses this pathway (Elaswad et al., 2018). Chemical reagents can also exhibit cytotoxicity. While chemical vectors offer some protection to the cargo during delivery, microinjection offers unparalleled protection once the cargo is delivered directly into the target compartment (especially the nucleus).

Table 5-1: Comparative Analysis of Microinjection vs. Key Alternative Gene Delivery Methods

Feature	**Microinjection**	**Electroporation**	**Gene Gun (Biolistics)**	**Viral Vectors (General)**	**Lipofection (Chemical)**
Principle	Mechanical needle penetration	Electric pulse-induced pores	DNA-coated particle acceleration	Virus-mediated cell entry	Lipid-mediated fusion/endocytosis
Typical Efficiency	High per injected cell (~100%)	Moderate to High (variable)	Variable, good for some tissues	High population efficiency	Low to Moderate (variable)
Throughput/ Scalability	Very Low	High	Moderate	High	High
Precision (Targeting)	Very High (subcellular)	Low (population level)	Low to Moderate	Moderate (tropism/engineering)	Low (population level)
Major Advantages	Precision, Versatility, Direct Access	High throughput, Simple concept	Targets tissues, Plants	High efficiency, Stable expression possible	Ease of use (bulk), Low immunogenicity

Major Limitations	Low throughput, Skill/Cost, Damage	Cell death, Low precision	Cell damage, Superficial targets	Immunogenicity, Mutagenesis, Cost	Low efficiency, Endosomal escape, Toxicity
Typical Applications	Transgenesis, ICSI, Research	Cultured cells, Bacteria, Plants	Plants, Skin, Difficult cells	Gene therapy (in/ex vivo)	In vitro transfection
Cost Indication	High (Equipment)	Moderate	High (Device)	Very High (Clinical Grade)	Low to Moderate (Reagents)

This comparative analysis reveals that no single gene delivery method is universally superior. Each approach occupies a specific niche defined by its unique balance of efficiency, precision, safety, scalability, and cargo capacity. Microinjection's enduring value stems from its ability to provide unparalleled precision and direct intracellular access for individual cells, a capability unmatched by higher-throughput methods. It persists because it effectively addresses specific applications where the limitations of other methods (e.g., immunogenicity of viruses, inefficiency of endosomal escape for chemical vectors, lack of precision in electroporation) are prohibitive, and where its own major limitation (low throughput) is an acceptable trade-off for the required outcome. It fills a critical, albeit specialized, role within the diverse toolkit of gene delivery technologies.

6. Advancements and Future Directions

Despite being a mature technique, microinjection continues to evolve, driven by technological advancements aimed at overcoming its inherent limitations, primarily low throughput and reliance on operator skill, and by synergy with emerging biological tools like gene editing.

6.1 Overcoming Throughput Limitations: Automation and Robotics

The most significant efforts to improve microinjection focus on automation. Manual microinjection is slow, laborious, and suffers from variability due to operator fatigue and skill differences, often resulting in low overall success and survival rates. Robotic systems are being developed to address these issues by automating key steps of the process.

These automated systems typically integrate several advanced technologies:

- **Machine Vision:** Computer vision algorithms are used for automated cell detection, identification, and targeting, replacing manual searching under the microscope. Techniques include image segmentation and pattern recognition to locate cells or specific structures like the pronucleus.
- **Automated Cell Handling/Holding:** Systems are being developed to automatically orient and immobilize cells for injection, moving beyond the single-cell holding pipette. Methods include microfluidic channels that position cells, arrays of micro-wells or V-grooves, dielectrophoresis, or optical tweezers.

- **Robotic Manipulation:** High-precision robotic arms, often driven by piezoelectric actuators, provide rapid, repeatable, and accurate control of the injection needle's movement, including penetration and withdrawal.
- **Sensor Integration:** Force sensors integrated into the needle holder can detect membrane penetration, providing feedback to control injection depth and minimize damage. Vision sensors provide real-time monitoring of the process.
- **Optimized Injection Strategies:** Automation allows for the implementation of refined puncture strategies (e.g., using vibration assistance) and precise control over injection volume and pressure (Chi et al., 2020).

The goals of automation are to dramatically increase injection speed (throughput), improve consistency, enhance cell survival rates, and reduce the need for highly specialized manual labor. Significant progress has been made, particularly in systems designed for specific model organisms like zebrafish embryos. However, challenges remain, including robust autofocusing, reliable handling of diverse cell types (especially suspension cells), achieving nanoliter-picoliter volume control consistently, and developing universally applicable systems (Zhao et al., 2018).

6.2 Miniaturization: Towards Nanoinjection

Another avenue of development involves shrinking the injection tool itself. Traditional micropipettes, despite their fineness, still cause considerable physical disruption to the cell. Nanoinjection utilizes significantly smaller probes or "lances," potentially fabricated using Micro-Electro-Mechanical Systems (MEMS) technology, with dimensions on the nanometer scale (e.g., 100th the diameter of a human hair).

The primary anticipated advantage of nanoinjection is a drastic reduction in cell damage and invasiveness due to the much smaller penetration site, potentially leading to higher cell viability. Some nanoinjection concepts may also employ different delivery mechanisms, such as using localized electroporation at the nano-lance tip to facilitate DNA entry without fluid flow, potentially offering better control over delivery. While still largely developmental, nanoinjection represents a promising approach to refining the mechanical delivery process at an even smaller scale.

6.3 Synergy with Gene Editing Technologies

The rise of precise gene editing tools, especially CRISPR/Cas9, has created a powerful synergy with microinjection. Microinjection provides an efficient and direct route to deliver the necessary CRISPR components (Cas9 protein/mRNA and guide RNA, or RNP complexes) into the nucleus or cytoplasm of target cells, particularly zygotes and embryos (Thermo Fisher Scientific, 2025b). This combination allows researchers to leverage microinjection's delivery precision to achieve highly specific, targeted modifications of the genome, effectively overcoming the random integration problem associated with traditional PNI-based transgenesis. This synergy has accelerated the generation of precisely engineered animal models and cell lines for research.

6.4 Niche Roles in Future Therapeutic Strategies

Given its inherent limitations in scalability, microinjection is unlikely to become a mainstream method for direct in vivo gene therapy in large patient populations. However, it may find niche roles in specific therapeutic contexts:

- **Ex Vivo Cell Modification:** For therapies involving the genetic modification of cells outside the body (ex vivo), microinjection could potentially be used if only a small number of critical cells need modification and high precision is required. This might include certain types of stem cell therapy or specialized applications in ART (Jinturkar et al., 2011). The feasibility of such applications would likely depend heavily on advancements in automation to make the process more efficient and cost-effective.
- **Preclinical Research:** Microinjection will undoubtedly remain a crucial tool in preclinical research for generating transgenic and gene-edited animal models needed to study disease mechanisms and test therapeutic strategies (Volobueva et al., 2019).

These advancements automation, miniaturization, and synergy with gene editing represent concerted efforts to overcome the biological and physical constraints inherent in the microinjection technique. Automation targets the limitations of human operators; nanoinjection addresses the physical trauma of needle insertion; combining with CRISPR leverages delivery precision for genetic specificity. The trajectory suggests microinjection will evolve not into a mass-delivery platform but into a more refined, reliable, and accessible tool for specialized, high-value applications where its unique advantages are paramount, solidifying its niche in research and specific clinical areas like ART.

7. Conclusion

7.1 Microinjection's Enduring Value and Specific Niche

Microinjection stands as a testament to the power of direct physical intervention at the cellular level. It is a technique defined by its exceptional precision, allowing researchers and clinicians to deliver a wide array of molecules directly into the cytoplasm or nucleus of individual cells, bypassing complex biological barriers. This precision, however, comes at the cost of significant limitations in throughput, labor intensity, and technical demands.

Despite these challenges, microinjection holds an enduring and indispensable position in several key areas. It remains a foundational technique for generating transgenic founder animals, providing a direct route to germline modification essential for creating invaluable research models (Volobueva et al., 2019). In assisted reproductive technologies, particularly through ICSI, it offers a critical solution for infertility, demonstrating its clinical impact where single-cell manipulation is paramount. Furthermore, its relevance has been reinvigorated by the advent of gene editing technologies like CRISPR/Cas9, where microinjection serves as a highly effective method for delivering editing components into embryos and cells with the necessary precision (Zhang & Yu, 2008). In these domains, the value derived from successfully manipulating a single cell often outweighs the inherent inefficiency of the process.

7.2 Balancing Precision and Scalability in Gene Delivery

Microinjection occupies a unique niche within the diverse landscape of gene delivery systems. The field constantly grapples with balancing the competing demands of delivery efficiency, targeting precision, cargo capacity, safety, and scalability. No single method excels across all criteria. Viral vectors offer high efficiency but raise safety concerns; chemical methods are simpler for bulk use but face biological hurdles; other physical methods offer different trade-offs between invasiveness, efficiency, and throughput.

Microinjection distinguishes itself by prioritizing absolute precision and direct access over scalability. While unlikely to become a platform for widespread gene therapy due to its low throughput, it serves as a crucial tool for applications where modifying individual, high-value cells is the objective. The principles it embodies direct, controlled intracellular delivery continue to inspire innovation. Ongoing advancements in automation and miniaturization promise to mitigate some of its limitations, potentially expanding its utility within its specialized niche and ensuring its continued role as a powerful technique in the armamentarium of biological manipulation and gene delivery.

References

1. Biology Notes Online. (2025, May 2). *Microinjection - definition, types, principle, steps, applications.* https://biologynotesonline.com/microinjection/
2. Zhang, Y., & Yu, L. C. (2008). Microinjection as a tool of mechanical delivery. *Current Opinion in Biotechnology, 19*(5), 506–510. https://doi.org/10.1016/j.copbio.2008.07.005
3. Das, A. K., Gupta, P., & Chakraborty, D. (2015). Physical methods of gene transfer: Kinetics of gene delivery into cells: A review. *Agricultural Reviews, 36*(1), 61–67. https://doi.org/10.5958/0976-0741.2015.00007.0
4. Butt, M. H., Zaman, M., Ahmad, A., Khan, R., Mallhi, T. H., Hasan, M. M., Khan, Y. H., Hafeez, S., Massoud, E. E. S., Rahman, M. H., & Cavalu, S. (2022). Appraisal for the potential of viral and nonviral vectors in gene therapy: A review. *Genes, 13*(8), 1370. https://doi.org/10.3390/genes13081370
5. Liu, C., Xie, W., Gui, C., & Du, Y. (2013). Pronuclear microinjection and oviduct transfer procedures for transgenic mouse production. In *Methods in Molecular Biology* (Vol. 1027, pp. 217–232). https://doi.org/10.1007/978-1-60327-369-5_10
6. Meacham, J. M., Durvasula, K., Degertekin, F. L., & Fedorov, A. G. (2014). Physical methods for intracellular delivery: Practical aspects from laboratory use to industrial-scale processing. *Journal of Laboratory Automation, 19*(1), 1–18. https://doi.org/10.1177/2211068213494388
7. BYJU'S. (2025, May 2). *Difference between electroporation and microinjection.* https://byjus.com/biology/difference-between-electroporation-and-microinjection/

8. Khan, N. T. (2017). Non-viral mediated physical approach for gene delivery. *Drug Designing: Open Access, 6*(2). https://doi.org/10.4172/2169-0138.1000151
9. Du, X., Wang, J., Zhou, Q., Zhang, L., Wang, S., Zhang, Z., & Yao, C. (2018). Advanced physical techniques for gene delivery based on membrane perforation. *Drug Delivery, 25*(1), 1516–1525. https://doi.org/10.1080/10717544.2018.1480674
10. Creative Biolabs. (2025, May 2). *Overview of microinjection-based gene delivery.* https://www.creative-biolabs.com/gene-therapy/overview-of-microinjection-based-gene-delivery.htm
11. News-Medical. (2025, May 2). *Micromanipulation and microinjection techniques.* https://www.news-medical.net/life-sciences/Micromanipulation-and-Microinjection-Techniques.aspx
12. Volobueva, A. S., Orekhov, A. N., & Deykin, A. V. (2019). An update on the tools for creating transgenic animal models of human diseases – Focus on atherosclerosis. *Brazilian Journal of Medical and Biological Research, 52*(5), e8108. https://doi.org/10.1590/1414-431x20198108
13. Kumar, M., & Ratwan, P. (2016). Transgenic or genetically modified farm animals and their applications: A review. *Research & Reviews: Journal of Veterinary Science and Technology, 5*(3), 25–34.
14. Microbe Notes. (2025, May 2). *Microinjection: Definition, principle, steps, uses.* https://microbenotes.com/microinjection/
15. Smith, K. R. (2004). Gene therapy: The potential applicability of gene transfer technology to the human germline. *International Journal of Medical Sciences, 1*(2), 76–91. https://doi.org/10.7150/ijms.1.76
16. Thermo Fisher Scientific (a). (2025, May 2). *Demonstrated protocol: Embryo microinjection with CRISPR-Cas9 in mice and zebrafish.* https://www.thermofisher.com/us/en/home/life-science/genome-editing/genome-editing-learning-center/genome-editing-resource-library/genome-editing-application-notes/protocol-embryo-microinjection-crispr-cas9-mice-zebrafish.html
17. Elaswad, A., Khalil, K., Cline, D., Page-McCaw, P., Chen, W., Michel, M., Cone, R., & Dunham, R. (2018). Microinjection of CRISPR/Cas9 protein into channel catfish, *Ictalurus punctatus,* embryos for gene editing. *Journal of Visualized Experiments, (131),* 56275. https://doi.org/10.3791/56275

18. Chi, Z., Xu, Q., & Zhu, L. (2020). A review of recent advances in robotic cell microinjection. *IEEE Access, 8,* 8520–8532. https://doi.org/10.1109/ACCESS.2020.2964305
19. Evans, T. C. (2006). Transformation and microinjection. In *WormBook: The Online Review of C. elegans Biology* (pp. 1–15). https://www.ncbi.nlm.nih.gov/books/NBK19648/
20. Synthego. (2025, May 2). *CRISPR transfection protocols guide: How to select the best.* https://www.synthego.com/guide/how-to-use-crispr/transfection-protocols
21. Wei, J., Zhang, W., Li, J., Jin, Y., & Qiu, Z. (2022). Application of the transgenic pig model in biomedical research: A review. *Frontiers in Cell and Developmental Biology, 10,* 1031812. https://doi.org/10.3389/fcell.2022.1031812
22. Hryhorowicz, M., Lipiński, D., Hryhorowicz, S., Nowak-Terpiłowska, A., Ryczek, N., & Zeyland, J. (2020). Application of genetically engineered pigs in biomedical research. *Genes, 11*(6), 670. https://doi.org/10.3390/genes11060670
23. Shakweer, W. M. E., Krivoruchko, A. Y., Dessouki, S. M., & Khattab, A. A. (2023). A review of transgenic animal techniques and their applications. *Journal of Genetic Engineering and Biotechnology, 21*(1), 55. https://doi.org/10.1186/s43141-023-00502-z
24. Thermo Fisher Scientific (b). (2025, May 2). *Other physical methods of transfection.* https://www.thermofisher.com/us/en/home/references/gibco-cell-culture-basics/transfection-basics/methods/other-physical-transfection-methods.html
25. Cyagen. (2025, May 2). *Pronuclear injection (PNI) transgenic mice generation.* https://www.cyagen.com/us/en/community/technical-bulletin/transgenic-mice-generation.html
26. Park, F. (2007). Lentiviral vectors: Are they the future of animal transgenesis? *Physiological Genomics, 31*(2), 159–173. https://doi.org/10.1152/physiolgenomics.00069.2007
27. Okamura, E., Mizuno, S., Matsumoto, S., Murata, K., Tanimoto, Y., Tra, D. T. H., Suzuki, H., et al. (2023). Highly efficient transgenic mouse production using piggyBac and its application to rapid phenotyping at the founder generation. *Bioengineering.* https://doi.org/10.1101/2023.12.10.570953

28. Jinturkar, K. A., Rathi, M. N., & Misra, A. (2011). Gene delivery using physical methods. In *Challenges in delivery of therapeutic genomics and proteomics* (pp. 83–126). Elsevier. https://doi.org/10.1016/B978-0-12-384964-9.00003-7
29. Zhao, Y., Sun, H., Sha, X., Gu, L., Zhan, Z., & Li, W. (2018). A review of automated microinjection of zebrafish embryos. *Micromachines, 10*(1), 7. https://doi.org/10.3390/mi10010007
30. Jones, D. (2011). Genetic engineering of a mouse: Dr. Frank Ruddle and somatic cell genetics. *The Yale Journal of Biology and Medicine, 84*(2), 117–124.
31. Katz, M. G., Fargnoli, A. S., Williams, R. D., & Bridges, C. R. (2013). Gene therapy delivery systems for enhancing viral and nonviral vectors for cardiac diseases: Current concepts and future applications. *Human Gene Therapy, 24*(11), 914–927. https://doi.org/10.1089/hum.2013.2517
32. Tamura, R., & Toda, M. (2020). Historic overview of genetic engineering technologies for human gene therapy. *Neurologia Medico-Chirurgica, 60*(10), 483–491. https://doi.org/10.2176/nmc.ra.2020-0049

Author Biography

This chapter was written by Asst. Prof. Muhammed Ali NALBANT, a faculty member of Bandırma Onyedi Eylül University, Faculty of Medicine. Asst. Prof. Muhammed Ali NALBANT conducts studies in the fields of infertility genetics, cancer genetics and sports genetics. He conducts studies to increase the success rates of advanced laboratory technologies and microinjection in clinical IVF applications. He is also interested in antioxidant metabolism to prevent sperm and oocyte DNA damage in both male and female infertility.